NEURORADIOLOGY
KEY DIFFERENTIAL DIAGNOSES AND CLINICAL QUESTIONS

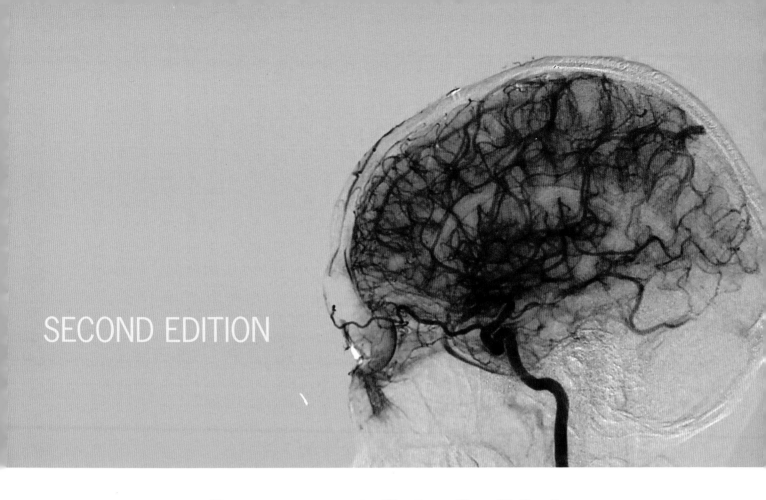

SECOND EDITION

NEURORADIOLOGY
KEY DIFFERENTIAL DIAGNOSES AND CLINICAL QUESTIONS

Juan E. Small, MD, MSc
Associate Professor of Radiology
Neuroradiology
Lahey Hospital and Medical Center
Burlington, Massachusetts

Pamela W. Schaefer, MD
Associate Director of Neuroradiology
Clinical Director of MRI
Department of Radiology
Massachusetts General Hospital
Boston, Massachusetts

Asha Sarma, MD
Assistant Professor
Radiology and Radiological Sciences
Vanderbilt University Medical Center
Nashville, Tennessee

Paul M. Bunch, MD
Associate Professor
Department of Radiology
Wake Forest University School of Medicine
Winston-Salem, North Carolina

ELSEVIER

Elsevier
1600 John F. Kennedy Blvd.
Ste 1800
Philadelphia, PA 19103-2899

NEURORADIOLOGY: KEY DIFFERENTIAL DIAGNOSES
AND CLINICAL QUESTIONS, SECOND EDITION   ISBN: 978-0-323-84761-2

Copyright © 2024 by Elsevier Inc. All rights reserved.

Notice

Previous edition copyrighted 2013.

Senior Content Strategist: Melanie Tucker
Senior Content Development Specialist: Shilpa Kumar
Publishing Services Manager: Shereen Jameel
Senior Project Manager: Manikandan Chandrasekaran
Design Direction: Brian Salisbury

Printed in India

Last digit is the print number: 9   8   7   6   5   4   3   2   1

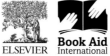

Working together
to grow libraries in
developing countries

www.elsevier.com • www.bookaid.org

Section Editors

Juan E. Small, MD, MSc
Associate Professor of Radiology
Neuroradiology
Lahey Hospital and Medical Center
Burlington, Massachusetts

Pamela W. Schaefer, MD
Associate Director of Neuroradiology
Clinical Director of MRI
Department of Radiology
Massachusetts General Hospital
Boston, Massachusetts

Asha Sarma, MD
Assistant Professor
Radiology and Radiological Sciences
Vanderbilt University Medical Center
Nashville, Tennessee

Paul M. Bunch, MD
Associate Professor
Department of Radiology
Wake Forest University School of Medicine
Winston-Salem, North Carolina

Stuart Pomerantz, MD
Associate Director of Neuro-CT
Neuroradiologist
Massachusetts General Hospital
Harvard Medical School
Boston, Massachusetts

Hillary R. Kelly, MD
Radiologist
Massachusetts Eye and Ear;
Neuroradiologist
Massachusetts General Hospital;
Assistant Professor
Department of Radiology
Harvard Medical School
Boston, Massachusetts

Tina Young Poussaint, MD, FACR
Lionel W. Young Chair in Radiology
Boston Children's Hospital
Professor of Radiology
Harvard Medical School
Boston, Massachusetts

Contributors

Jalil Afnan, MD, MRCS
Assistant Professor of Radiology
Vice-Chair
Department of Radiology
Lahey Hospital and Medical Center
Burlington, Massachusetts

Kenneth S. Allison, MD
Neuroradiologist
Radiology Imaging Associates
Englewood, Colorado

Ahmad Amer, MD
PGY1 Resident Physician
Transitional Year
Broward Health North
Deerfield Beach, Florida

Swetha Aribindi, BA, MD
Resident Physician
Department of Radiology
Wake Forest University School of Medicine
Winston-Salem, North Carolina

Nino Boals, MD
Staff Radiologist
Department of Radiology
Memphis VA Medical Center
Memphis, Tennessee

Fargol Booya, MD
Department of Radiology
Columbus Radiology
Laguna Niguel, California

Maria Braileanu, MD
Neuroradiology
Massachusetts General Hospital
Boston, Massachusetts

Riley Brazil, MD, MPH
Resident Physician
Washington State University
Pullman, Washington

Bhavana Budigi, MBBS, MD
Neuroradiology Fellow
Wake Forest University School of Medicine
Winston-Salem, North Carolina

Paul M. Bunch, MD
Associate Professor
Department of Radiology
Wake Forest University School of Medicine
Winston-Salem, North Carolina

Yuh-Shin Chang, MD, PhD
Diagnostic Neuroradiology
Massachusetts General Hospital
Boston, Massachusetts

Hui J. Jenny Chen, MD
Bay Imaging Consultants
Walnut Creek, California

Robert Chun Chen, MD
Senior Consultant
Department of Diagnostic Radiology
Singapore General Hospital
Singapore

Daniel B. Chonde, MD, PhD
Clinical Fellow
Department of Radiology
Massachusetts General Hospital
Boston, Massachusetts

Nathan M. Coleman, MD
Neuroradiology Clinical Fellow
Neuroradiology
Massachusetts General Hospital
Boston, Massachusetts

Mary E. Cunnane, MD
Chief, Department of Radiology
Massachusetts Eye and Ear
Assistant Professor of Radiology
Harvard Medical School
Boston, Massachusetts

Katharina Eikermann-Haerter, MD
Associate Professor
Department of Radiology
New York University
New York City, New York

Sara Emami, MD, CMD
Internist and Geriatrician
Massachusetts General Hospital
Harvard Medical School
Boston, Massachusetts

John M. Fagnou, MD
Clinical Assistant Professor
Diagnostic Imaging
University of Calgary
Calgary, Alberta
Canada

Chad William Farris, MD, PhD
Assistant Professor
Department of Radiology
Boston University Chobanian & Avedisian School of Medicine
Boston Medical Center
Boston, Massachusetts

Reza Forghani, MD, PhD
Professor of Radiology and Artificial Intelligence (AI) and
    Vice Chair of AI
Department of Radiology
University of Florida College of Medicine;
Norman Fixel Institute for Neurological Diseases
Gainesville, Florida

Alexandra M. Foust, DO
Pediatric Neuroradiology Fellow
Boston Children's Hospital
Boston, Massachusetts;
Assistant Professor
Department of Radiology
Vanderbilt University Medical Center
Nashville, Tennessee

Daniel Thomas Ginat, MD
Associate Professor
Department of Radiology
University of Chicago
Chicago, Illinois

Farahnaz Golriz, MD
Neuroradiology
Massachusetts General Hospital
Boston, Massachusetts

Emily Haas, MD
Resident Physician
Department of Radiology
Vanderbilt University Medical Center
Nashville, Tennessee

Kevin D. Hiatt, MD
Assistant Professor
Department of Radiology
Wake Forest University School of Medicine
Winston-Salem, North Carolina

Daniel Hill, MD
Neuroradiology Fellow
Department of Radiology
Massachusetts General Hospital
Boston, Massachusetts

Mai-Lan Ho, MD
Professor of Radiology
Vice Chair for Operations and Innovation
Medical Director of Radiology
Physician Director of Radiology Informatics
Division Director of Neuroradiology
University of Missouri
Columbia, Missouri

Jennifer Huang, MD, MEd
Resident Physician
Department of Radiology
Vanderbilt University Medical Center
Nashville, Tennessee

Scott Edward Hunter, MD, MBA
Radiologist
Neuroradiology
Midwest Radiology
Saint Paul, Minnesota

Jason M. Johnson, MD, MBA
Associate Professor
Neuroradiology
The University of Texas MD Anderson Cancer Center
Houston, Texas

Bashar Kako, MD
Diagnostic Radiology Fellow
Department of Radiology
Massachusetts General Hospital
Boston, Massachusetts

Shervin Kamalian, MD, MSc
Neuroradiologist
Beth Israel Deaconess Medical Center
Harvard Medical School
Boston, Massachusetts

Swapnil Khose, MD, MPH
Resident Physician
Department of Neurology
University of Texas Health Science Center
Houston, Texas

Hillary R. Kelly, MD
Radiologist
Massachusetts Eye and Ear;
Neuroradiologist
Massachusetts General Hospital;
Assistant Professor
Department of Radiology
Harvard Medical School
Boston, Massachusetts

Andrew R. King, MD
Neuroradiology Fellow
Department of Radiology
Wake Forest University School of Medicine
Winston-Salem, North Carolina

Girish Kori, MD
Section Chief
Neuroradiology
MAPMG, Kaiser Permanente
Rockville, Maryland

Jason Lauer, MD
Clinical Fellow
Department of Radiology, Division of Neuroradiology
Massachusetts General Hospital
Harvard Medical School
Boston, Massachusetts

Melissa Shuhui Lee, MBBS, FRCR
Consultant
Department of Diagnostic Radiology
Singapore General Hospital
Singapore

Mary D. Maher, MD
Assistant Professor of Radiology
Department of Radiology
University of Pennsylvania
Philadelphia, Pennsylvania

Simone Montoya, MD
Clinical Fellow
Division of Neuroradiology
Department of Radiology
Massachusetts General Hospital
Boston, Massachusetts

Gul Moonis, MD
Professor
Department of Radiology
NYU Langone Health
New York, New York

Josephine Mwikali Ndolo, MBChB, MMed
Radiologist
Pediatric, Neuroradiology and Nuclear Medicine
Radiology of Huntsville
Huntsville, Alabama

Daniel L. Noujaim, MD
Neuroradiologist
Department of Radiology
Henry Ford Hospital
Detroit, Michigan

Parth Y. Patel, MD
Resident Physician
Department of Radiology
Henry Ford Hospital
Detroit, Michigan

Halyna Pokhylevych, MD
PGY1 Resident Physician
Department of Radiology
University of Arkansas for Medical Sciences
Little Rock, Arkansas

Michael T. Preece, MD
Radiology Imaging Associates
Englewood, Colorado

Hamid Rajebi, MD
Emergency Radiologist
San Diego Imaging
San Diego, California

Jeffrey R. Sachs, MD
Associate Professor
Department of Radiology
Wake Forest University School of Medicine
Winston-Salem, North Carolina

Asha Sarma, MD
Assistant Professor
Radiology and Radiological Sciences
Vanderbilt University Medical Center
Nashville, Tennessee

Pamela W. Schaefer, MD
Associate Director of Neuroradiology
Clinical Director of MRI
Department of Radiology
Massachusetts General Hospital
Boston, Massachusetts

Juan E. Small, MD, MSc
Associate Professor of Radiology
Neuroradiology
Lahey Hospital and Medical Center
Burlington, Massachusetts

Henry Su, MD, PhD
South Shore Radiological Associates
South Weymouth, Massachusetts

Adam Sweeney, MD
Assistant Professor
Department of Radiology
Wake Forest University School of Medicine
Winston-Salem, North Carolina

Katharine Tansavatdi, MD
Neuroradiologist
Radsource, LLC
Brentwood, Tennessee

Nicholas A. Telischak, MD, MS
Assistant Professor
Radiology, Neurosurgery (courtesy)
Stanford, California

Kai Wang, MD
Diagnostic Radiology Resident
Department of Radiology
Vanderbilt University Medical Center
Nashville, Tennessee

David Wei Wen, MBBS, FRCR
Consultant
Department of Diagnostic Radiology
Singapore General Hospital
Singapore

Thomas G. West, MD
Associate Professor
Department of Radiology
Wake Forest University School of Medicinea
Winston-Salem, North Carolina

Brian Zipser, MD
Neuroradiologist
Transparent Imaging
Santa Monica, California

Preface

This book is based on the premise that carefully reviewing unknown cases is one of the most powerful techniques for mastering accurate imaging interpretation. Rather than presenting individual unknown cases, this book intentionally groups several unknown cases centered around a common theme in each chapter. These themes are often based on imaging findings (e.g., T1 hyperintense lesions, lucent temporal bone lesions) rather than diagnosis groups, which is purposely designed to simulate real-world radiology practice. Our collective experience as neuroradiology educators and clinicians has taught us that side-by-side comparing and contrasting of similar-appearing lesions is essential to building a database in the mind's eye that can be accessed during imaging interpretation. Thus, the format of this book was tailored to increase the reader's diagnostic accuracy and confidence. With these principles in mind, we encourage you to actively and carefully evaluate each chapter's grouping of cases and thoughtfully consider the most likely diagnoses before proceeding to the answers and associated discussion.

Juan E. Small, MD, MSc
Pamela W. Schaefer, MD
Asha Sarma, MD
Paul M. Bunch, MD

Acknowledgments

We would like to gratefully acknowledge Shilpa Kumar, Manikandan Chandrasekaran, Melanie Tucker, Joslyn Chaiprasert-Paguio, Lora Sickora, Pamela Hetherington, Sabina Borza, Rebecca Gaertner, Colleen McGonigal, Carrie Stetz, and all the support staff and illustrators at Elsevier for their help throughout this endeavor. We would also like to acknowledge our many mentors as well as the fellows, and residents at Massachusetts General Hospital, Brigham and Women's Hospital, Lahey Hospital and Medical Center, Vanderbilt University Medical Center, and Wake Forest University School of Medicine for their persistent hard work and dedication to neuroradiology.

How to Use This Book

Although this book does not have to be read in sequence from cover to cover, it is essential that the cases be approached as unknowns. Attempting to interpret several unknown cases at once can be overwhelming. To gain the most from this text, the cases within a series should first be interpreted individually. The main challenge is to formulate a specific differential diagnosis for each individual unknown case. We encourage readers to then compare and contrast cases within that series. The goal is to find the often subtle, key imaging characteristics that enable distinction among superficially similar disease entities. Each series of cases includes individual diagnoses, a description of findings, and a brief discussion of the various diagnostic considerations. This supportive text should be read only after going through the process of interpreting each case individually and comparing and contrasting the cases within each series. Additional cases illustrate other manifestations and considerations important for imaging interpretation. Major teaching points are highlighted at the end of each chapter. We sincerely hope that you benefit as much from reading this book as we have benefited from writing and editing it.

Contents

1

Computed Tomography Hyperdense Lesions

HENRY SU, MD, PHD

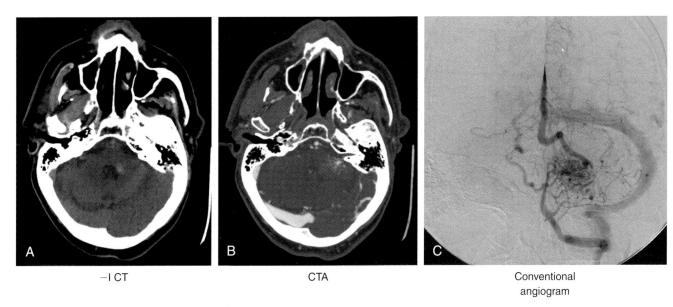

−I CT   CTA   Conventional
angiogram

CASE A: A 66-year-old presenting with sudden-onset left-sided weakness. *CT,* Computed tomography; *CTA,* CT angiogram.

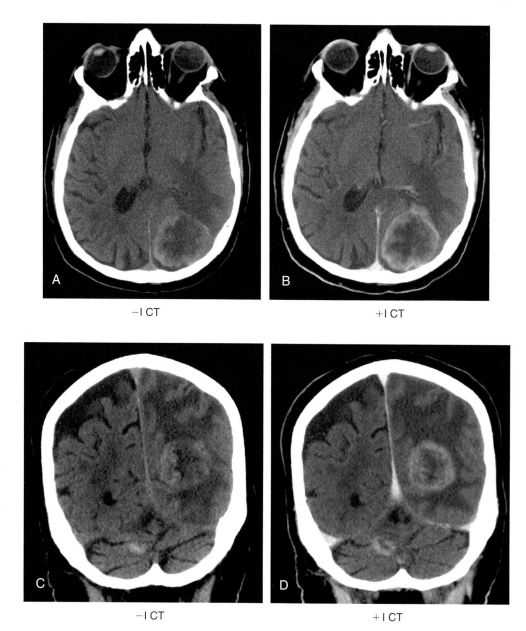

−I CT   +I CT

−I CT   +I CT

CASE B: A 77-year-old with a history of lung cancer. *CT,* Computed tomography.

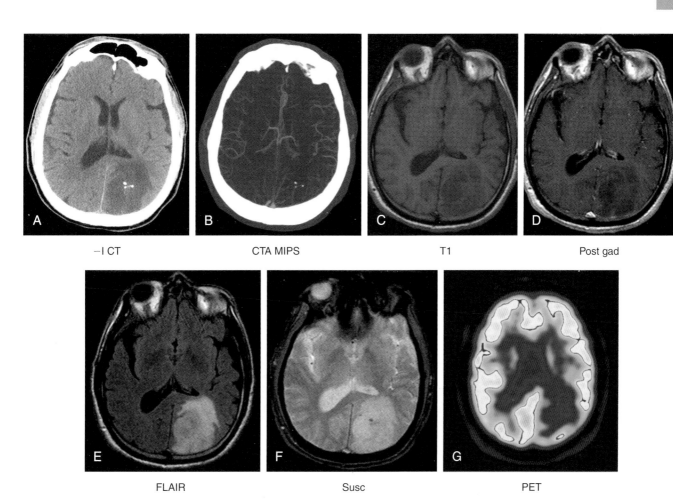

CASE C: A 73-year-old with depression, falls, and difficulty completing sentences. *CT,* Computed tomography; *CTA,* CT angiogram; *FLAIR,* fluid attenuated inversion recovery; *gad,* gadolinium; *MIPS,* maximum intensity projections; *PET,* positron emission tomography; *Susc,* susceptibility.

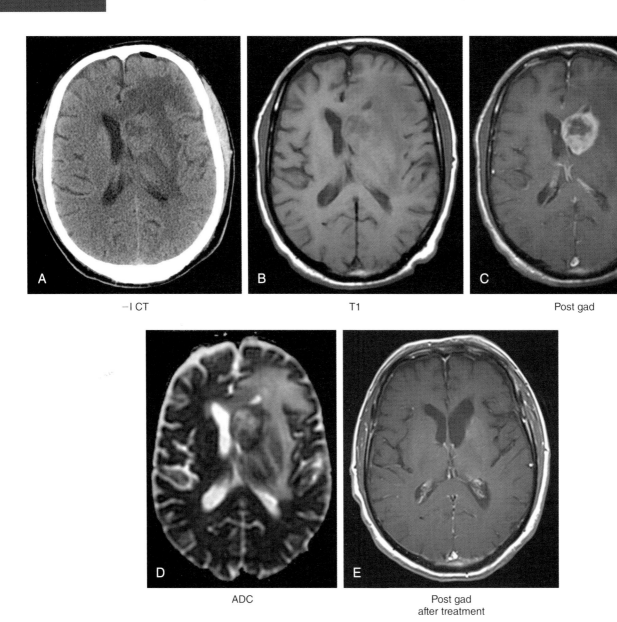

−I CT

T1

Post gad

ADC

Post gad
after treatment

CASE D: A 56-year-old with generalized tonic-clonic seizures. *ADC,* Apparent diffusion coefficient; *CT,* computed tomography; *gad,* gadolinium.

DESCRIPTION OF FINDINGS

- Case A: A small focus of hyperdensity is present in the left middle cerebellar peduncle. The CT angiogram demonstrates a tangle of vessels just lateral to this focus of hemorrhage. A conventional catheter angiogram confirms the presence of an arteriovenous malformation with arterial supply from the left anterior inferior cerebellar artery and pontine perforators and early filling of the straight, transverse, and sigmoid sinuses. The lesion was subsequently treated with liquid embolic material (not shown).
- Case B: A left occipital lesion demonstrates peripheral hyperdensity. There is surrounding edema with local mass effect and effacement of the left occipital horn. After administration of contrast, superimposed enhancement is seen along the peripheral portions of the mass. On the coronal reformats, an additional smaller hyperdense right cerebellar lesion with ring enhancement is noted. Given the patient's history of lung cancer, these findings are consistent with lung metastases.
- Case C: Small, discrete hyperdensities measuring 150 to 200 Hounsfield units (HU) are consistent with calcifications in the left occipital lobe. Surrounding parietal occipital hypodensity and effacement of the left ventricular atrium are noted. CT angiogram maximum intensity projection image does not demonstrate abnormal associated vessels. Gadolinium-enhanced, T1-weighted MRI shows no associated enhancement. Marked T2/FLAIR hyperintense signal is noted, correlating with the CT hypodensity. Gradient echo imaging shows calcific foci appearing as punctate foci of susceptibility. PET imaging demonstrates a predominantly hypometabolic lesion. Pathologic evaluation after surgical resection revealed an oligodendroglioma.
- Case D: A CT scan of the brain demonstrates a mass lesion centered in the left anterior basal ganglia. There is an irregular hyperdense rim with a hypodense center. On MRI, the rim enhances and has restricted diffusion characterized by hypointensity on the ADC images. The findings are suggestive of a hypercellular lesion with internal necrotic or cystic components. The patient was given a diagnosis of lymphoma, and marked improvement of the enhancing lesion occurred after IV methotrexate was administered.

Diagnosis

Case A: Intraparenchymal cerebellar hemorrhage resulting from an arteriovenous malformation

Case B: Metastatic lung cancer

Case C: Oligodendroglioma grade 2 (proven by pathology)

Case D: Lymphoma

Summary

The differential diagnosis of CT hyperdense lesions usually revolves around hemorrhagic products, calcifications, or hypercellular lesions. CT attenuation value of hyperdense lesions in the brain can be helpful in determining the etiology. Attenuation of hyperdense hemorrhage in the brain ranges from 60 to 100 HU. Calcifications typically have Hounsfield units in the hundreds. Care must be taken when measuring small hyperdensities because volume averaging can underestimate the Hounsfield units. MRI susceptibility-weighted images can also be helpful for differentiating these entities. Intraparenchymal hemorrhage demonstrates susceptibility (low signal) with marked enlargement or "blooming" of the hemorrhage compared with its actual size. Calcification typically shows low signal with little to no blooming. Dense cellular packing does not show susceptibility.

Determining the etiology of an intraparenchymal hemorrhage is important because it will affect prognosis, treatment, and management. CT angiography is highly sensitive and specific for identifying an underlying vascular lesion. Approximately 15% of intraparenchymal hemorrhages result from vascular lesions such as arteriovenous malformations and fistulae, aneurysms, dural venous sinus thrombosis, moyamoya disease, and vasculitis. If an underlying vascular lesion is not identified, common causes of intraparenchymal hemorrhage in elderly patients should be considered. Hemorrhages due to anticoagulation are usually large, lobar hemorrhages, and hypertensive hemorrhages typically are located in the deep gray nuclei, brainstem, and cerebellum.

If anticoagulation and hypertension are not considerations, a gadolinium-enhanced MRI with gradient echo sequences is obtained to evaluate for other causes, such as amyloid angiopathy, underlying neoplasms, and cavernous malformations. Amyloid angiopathy is characterized by a lobar hemorrhage with associated gray/white matter junction microhemorrhages and/or leptomeningeal hemosiderosis on susceptibility-weighted sequences. Neoplasms that produce intraparenchymal hemorrhage include high-grade gliomas and metastatic tumors, such as melanoma and renal cell carcinoma. Frequently, an underlying enhancing mass is identified after administration of IV gadolinium. However, an underlying mass can be obscured by the hemorrhage, and follow-up MRI is recommended if no clear cause for the parenchymal hemorrhage is identified and neoplasm remains in the differential diagnosis. Cavernous malformations may be the cause of acute intraparenchymal hemorrhage in children and young adults. They typically have a heterogenous "popcorn" appearance with a complete hemosiderin rim on T2-weighted images and no surrounding edema. After acute hemorrhage, there is edema and the hemosiderin rim may be obscured. Clues to the etiology are age and associated classic cavernous malformations in other brain locations (particularly in the familial form).

Calcifications can be either benign or associated with pathology. Intraparenchymal calcifications are nonspecific and can be seen in a variety of etiologies, including normal deposition in the basal ganglia, prior cerebral insult (e.g., infection, inflammation, or ischemia), vascular abnormalities (e.g., cavernous malformations, arteriovenous malformations, and fistulae), or neoplasms. Primary intraaxial central nervous system neoplasms that show calcifications include astrocytomas, oligodendrogliomas, or, rarely, glioblastomas. Case C is a grade 2 oligodendroglioma. Low-grade oligodendrogliomas are slowly growing neoplasms typically located in a cortical/subcortical location, most commonly in the frontal lobe. They may cause scalloping of the adjacent calvarium. The majority demonstrate calcification and about 50% show variable enhancement. Differentiation from other neoplasms is not definitively possible with imaging alone.

On CT, increased attenuation due to dense cellular packing usually is seen with lymphoma and other small, round, blue-cell tumors, such as peripheral neuroectodermal tumors and medulloblastomas, but increased density also can be seen in glioblastomas. Lymphoma is characteristically located in the deep white matter and deep gray nuclei. On MRI, the high cellularity is reflected by isointensity to brain parenchyma on T2-weighted images, and restricted diffusion with hyperintensity on diffusion-weighted images, and hypointensity on ADC maps. Lymphoma typically demonstrates avid homogenous enhancement in immunocompetent patients. In immunocompromised patients, lymphomas may demonstrate rim enhancement with nonenhancing regions of central necrosis. In contrast with acute hemorrhage, lymphomas do not have susceptibility. Lymphomas usually rapidly respond to treatment with IV methotrexate, radiation therapy, or steroids.

Differential Diagnosis

Acute hemorrhage
Calcification
Highly cellular neoplasms
Previous contrast

Pearls

- Underlying etiologies for acute intraparenchymal hemorrhage should be further assessed by CT angiogram.
- When patients with intraparenchymal hemorrhage have negative CT angiogram findings and no history of hypertension or anticoagulation, a gadolinium-enhanced MRI with gradient echo sequences should be performed to assess for underlying malignancy and amyloid angiopathy, respectively.
- Increased attenuation on CT examination due to dense cellular packing usually is seen with lymphoma and other small, round, blue-cell tumors. These lesions usually show dense, homogeneous enhancement and restricted diffusion and do not have susceptibility.
- Attenuation of hyperdense hemorrhage in the brain typically ranges from 60 to 100 HU, whereas calcifications typically have Hounsfield units in the hundreds. Calcifications have little to no blooming on susceptibility-weighted images, in contrast to hemorrhage, which has marked blooming.

Suggested Readings

Dainer HM, Smirniotopoulos JG: Neuroimaging of hemorrhage and vascular malformations, *Semin Neurol* 28(4):533–547, 2008.

Delgado Almondoz JE, Schaefer PW, Forero NP, et al: Diagnostic accuracy and yield of multidetector CT angiography in the evaluation of spontaneous intraparenchymal cerebral hemorrhage, *AJNR Am J Neuroradiol* 30(6):1213–1221, 2009.

Koeller KK, Rushing EJ: From the archives of the AFIP: oligodendroglioma and its variants: radiologic-pathologic correlation, *Radiographics* 25(6):1669–1688, 2005.

Koeller KK, Smirniotopoulos JG, Jones RV: Primary central nervous system lymphoma: radiologic-pathologic correlation, *Radiographics* 17(6):1497–1526, 1997.

Lee YY, Van Tassel P: Intracranial oligodendrogliomas: imaging findings in 35 untreated cases, *AJR Am J Roentgenol* 152(2):361–369, 1989.

Morris PG, Abrey LE: Therapeutic challenges in primary CNS lymphoma, Lancet Neurol 8(6):581–592, 2009.

Osborn AG: *Diagnostic neuroradiology*, St Louis, 1994, Mosby.

Stadnik TW, Chaskis C, Michotte A, et al: Diffusion-weighted MR imaging of intracerebral masses: comparison with conventional MR imaging and histologic findings, *AJNR Am J Neuroradiol* 22(5): 969–976, 2001.

2

T1 Hyperintense Lesions

HENRY SU, MD, PHD AND JUAN E. SMALL, MD, MSC

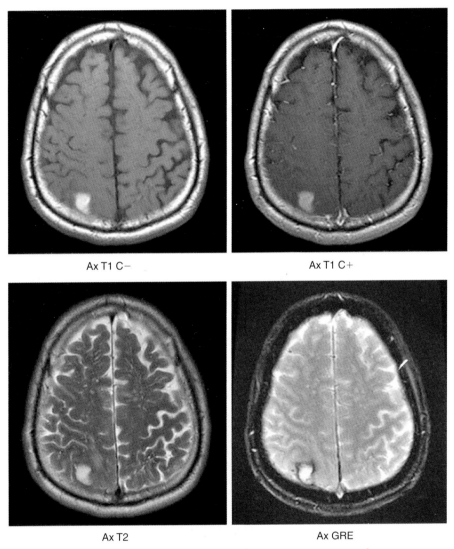

Ax T1 C−

Ax T1 C+

Ax T2

Ax GRE

CASE A: A 64-year-old with a history of amyloid angiopathy–related hemorrhages. *Ax*, Axial; *GRE*, Gradient refocused echo.

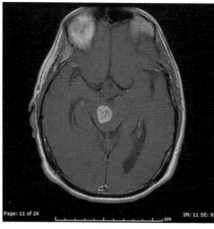
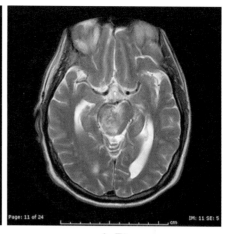

Ax T1 C−   Ax T1 C+   Ax T2

CASE B: A 64-year-old with a history of renal cell carcinoma, difficulty walking, and diplopia. *Ax*, Axial.

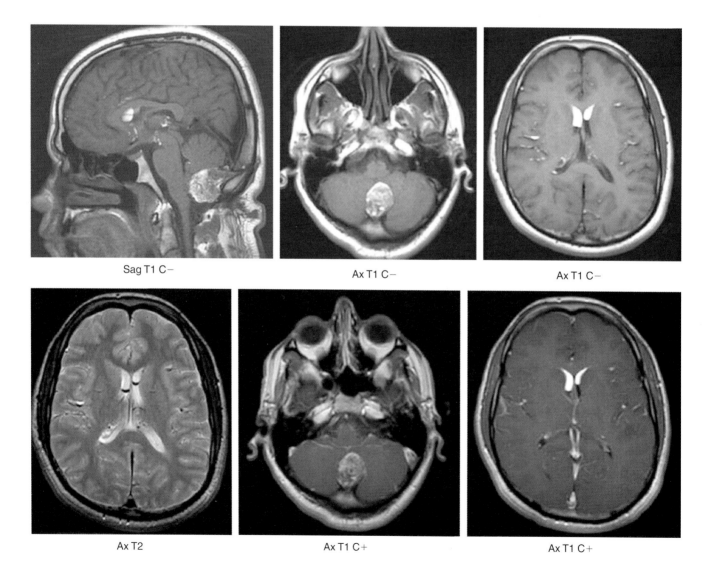

Sag T1 C−   Ax T1 C−   Ax T1 C−

Ax T2   Ax T1 C+   Ax T1 C+

CASE C: A 25-year-old presenting after sustaining trauma. *Ax*, Axial; *Sag*, sagittal.

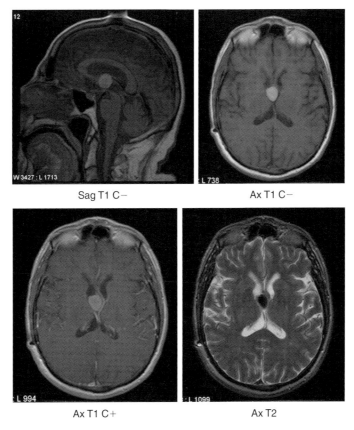

Sag T1 C−   Ax T1 C−

Ax T1 C+   Ax T2

CASE D: A 50-year-old presenting with a history of headaches. *Ax*, Axial; *Sag*, sagittal.

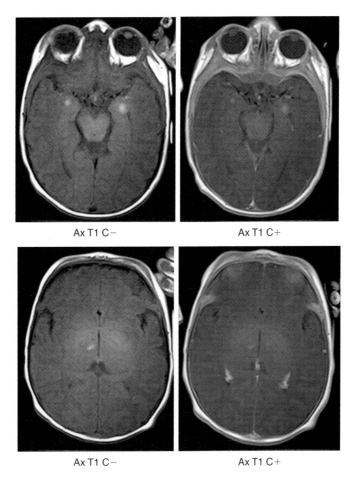

Ax T1 C−   Ax T1 C+

Ax T1 C−   Ax T1 C+

CASE E: A 2-month-old infant presenting with a giant congenital melanocytic nevus. *Ax*, Axial.

DESCRIPTION OF FINDINGS

- Case A: An oval, nonenhancing, T1 hyperintense right parietal abnormality is evident. Associated T2 hyperintensity and peripheral susceptibility are seen. There also is surrounding edema. The findings are consistent with a late subacute hemorrhage in a patient with a known history of amyloid angiopathy.
- Case B: A mass centered within the right cerebral peduncle demonstrates T1 hyperintense foci and heterogeneous T2 hyperintense signal with surrounding edema. The postcontrast T1-weighted image demonstrates an avidly enhancing mass consistent with a pathologically proven hemorrhagic renal cell carcinoma metastasis.
- Case C: A large heterogeneous mass with regions of T1 hyperintensity and an associated sinus tract is centered within the midline inferior posterior fossa. No enhancement is identified. There are fat-fluid levels in the frontal horns of the lateral ventricles with chemical shift artifact on the T2-weighted images as well as multiple small T1 hyperintense foci consistent with fat within the bilateral sylvian fissures. These findings are consistent with a ruptured dermoid cyst.
- Case D: A large, oval, well-circumscribed, T1 hyperintense, T2 hypointense, nonenhancing intraventricular mass is noted in the region of the foramen of Monro. The location and imaging characteristics of this lesion are consistent with a proteinaceous colloid cyst.
- Case E: There are bilateral medial temporal and right thalamic intraparenchymal as well as scattered leptomeningeal T1 hyperintense lesions. No associated enhancement is identified. These findings are consistent with melanocytic deposits in a patient with neurocutaneous melanosis.

Diagnosis

Case A: Late subacute hematoma in a patient with amyloid angiopathy

Case B: Hemorrhagic metastasis (renal cell carcinoma)

Case C: Ruptured dermoid cyst

Case D: Colloid cyst (with proteinaceous contents)

Case E: Neurocutaneous melanosis

Summary

Intrinsic T1 hyperintensity (T1 shortening) on MRI can be due to the presence of blood products, fat, melanin, proteinaceous material, or calcification.

Hemoglobin has different signal characteristics on MRI depending in its oxidative state. Subacute phase methemoglobin (both intracellular and extracellular) has intrinsic T1 hyperintense signal. Intracellular methemoglobin also demonstrates blooming in susceptibility-weighted sequences. A history of recent trauma or anticoagulation makes the diagnosis of T1 hyperintense intracranial hemorrhage straightforward. Patients with a history of hypertension may have deep gray nuclei and brainstem or cerebellar T1 hyperintense subacute hemorrhages. Lobar T1 hyperintense lesions with associated gray/white matter junction foci of susceptibility suggest amyloid angiopathy in older patients. Furthermore, in the appropriate clinical setting, intraparenchymal T1 hyperintense lesions should raise concern for metastatic disease. Intrinsic T1 signal can be seen in hemorrhagic metastases (e.g., renal cell, lung, thyroid). Intrinsic T1 hyperintensity associated with metastatic melanoma may be due to either hemorrhagic components or intrinsic T1 shortening from melanin. In many cases, an underlying mass can be identified on contrast-enhanced sequences. If an underlying mass is not identified, it is important to obtain follow-up imaging to rule out an underlying enhancing lesion initially obscured by the hemorrhage. In younger patients, T1 hyperintense hemorrhages may result from underlying vascular lesions such as cavernous malformations (a "popcorn" appearance with complete hemosiderin rim on gradient echo and T2-weighted sequences) or arteriovenous malformations.

Melanin-containing lesions, such as neurocutaneous melanosis, also should be considered in the differential diagnosis of T1 shortening when the clinical setting is appropriate. Neurocutaneous melanosis is a rare congenital phakomatosis associated with multiple cutaneous melanocytic nevi and benign or malignant central nervous system melanotic lesions. Its intracranial imaging characteristics are due to the proliferation of melanocytes in the leptomeninges or parenchyma. As such, multiple T1 hyperintense lesions generally are evident. Because symptoms usually manifest by 2 to 3 years of age, a pediatric patient with cutaneous lesions and these imaging characteristics should suggest this diagnosis despite its rarity. Hydrocephalus is seen in two-thirds of symptomatic patients due to obstruction of cerebrospinal fluid (CSF) flow.

Fat-containing lesions, such as lipomas or dermoid cysts, also should be considered in the differential diagnosis of T1 shortening. Dermoid cysts often are midline in sellar/parasellar, frontal, and posterior fossa locations and are believed to be due to early inclusion of surface ectoderm during embryogenesis. Twenty percent are associated with sinus tracts. When uncomplicated, these lesions are not associated with enhancement. Confirming the presence of fat is helpful with CT or fat-saturated sequences on MRI. T2 signal is variable. Dermoid cyst rupture can present with disseminated foci of intracranial T1 hyperintensity due to spillage of lipid contents into the subarachnoid space or intraventricular compartment. Because of density differences, lipid droplets or fat fluid levels are antidependent. Dermoid rupture can cause chemical meningitis due to meningeal irritation from the internal contents, which can result in leptomeningeal enhancement. Hydrocephalus may develop from blockage of arachnoid granulations.

Protein-containing lesions also should be considered in the differential diagnosis of T1 hyperintense lesions. The location of a protein-containing lesion is the most important clue to diagnosis. For instance, colloid cysts, which arise from the inferior aspect of the septum pellucidum, typically are present in the region of the foramen of Monro. These lesions are well-circumscribed, nonenhancing cystic lesions that are hyperintense on T1-weighted images when the protein/mucin content is relatively high. When a well-circumscribed, homogeneous, T1 hyperintense lesion is centered in the region of the pituitary gland, a craniopharyngioma or Rathke's cleft cyst should be considered.

Spectrum of Disease

See Fig. 2.1.

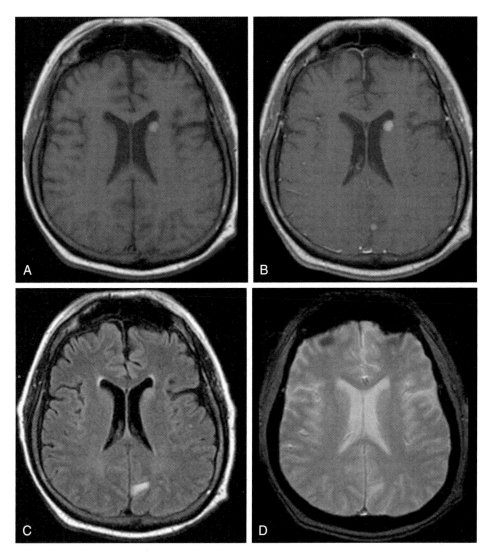

• **Fig. 2.1** A 56-year-old with history of metastatic melanotic melanoma. (A) Axial T1 precontrast image demonstrates a T1 hyperintense lesion centered in the left caudate nucleus. (B) Postcontrast T1 image also demonstrates a smaller enhancing lesion along the medial aspect of the left parietal lobe, with surrounding edema evident on (C) FLAIR. It is difficult to determine whether the caudate lesion enhances. Susceptibility blooming is not associated with the intrinsically T1 hyperintense lesion (D); the signal characteristics could be secondary to extracellular methemoglobin or melanin. The imaging characteristics of metastatic melanoma may vary from patient to patient depending on whether the lesions represent melanotic melanoma metastasis, amelanotic melanoma metastasis, or hemorrhagic metastasis.

Differential Diagnosis

Hemorrhagic lesions: Hematomas, hemorrhagic infarcts, hemorrhagic infections (e.g., herpes simplex encephalitis), hemorrhagic neoplasms, vascular malformations, and thrombosed aneurysms

Fatty lesions: Lipomas, dermoids, and teratomas

Melanin-containing lesions: Melanoma metastases and intraparenchymal and leptomeningeal melanosis

Protein-containing lesions: Colloid cysts, Rathke cleft cysts, craniopharyngioma, and atypical epidermoid

Calcified/ossified lesions or lesions with mineral accumulation: Endocrine/metabolic disorders, calcified neoplasms, and calcifying infections

Pearls

- An imaging interpretation error is to mistake intrinsic T1 hyperintensity for enhancement. The imaging interpreter should closely compare T1 precontrast and T1 postcontrast sequences to avoid this pitfall.
- Side-by-side scrutiny of precontrast and postcontrast sequences is invaluable for the identification of areas of subtle enhancement, a finding that markedly tailors the differential diagnosis.
- Follow-up imaging in the setting of a parenchymal hemorrhage is required to rule out an underlying enhancing vascular or neoplastic abnormality obscured by mass effect exerted by the hematoma.

Signs and Complications

- Dermoid cyst rupture with spilling of lipid components results in a chemical meningitis when the contents of the ruptured cyst involve the subarachnoid spaces. If spilled lipid obstructs arachnoid granulations, hydrocephalus may develop.
- Hydrocephalus is seen in two-thirds of symptomatic patients with neurocutaneous melanosis due to obstruction of CSF flow.

Suggested Readings

Atlas SW, Grossman J, Gomori JM, et al: MR imaging of intracranial metastatic melanoma, *J Comput Assist Tomogr* 11(4):577–582, 1987.

Cakirer S, Karaarslan E, Arslan A: Spontaneously T1-hyperintense lesions of the brain on MRI: a pictorial review, *Curr Probl Diagn Radiol* 32(5):194–217, 2003.

Huisman TA: Intracranial hemorrhage: ultrasound, CT and MRI findings, *Eur Radiol* 15(3):434–440, 2005.

Osborn AG, Preece MT: Intracranial cysts: radiologic-pathologic correlation and imaging approach, *Radiology* 239(3):650–664, 2006.

Stendel R, Pietilä TA, Lehmann K, et al: Ruptured intracranial dermoid cysts, *Surg Neurol* 57(6):391–398, 2002.

Zaheer A, Ozsunar Y, Schaefer PW: Magnetic resonance imaging of cerebral hemorrhagic stroke, *Top Magn Reson Imaging* 11(5):288–299, 2000.

3

Multiple Susceptibility Artifact Lesions

JUAN E. SMALL, MD, MSC

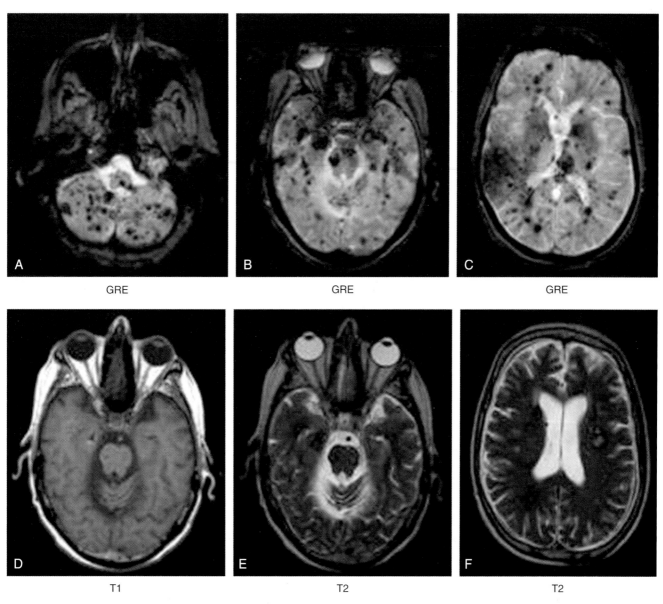

CASE A: A 48-year-old with a strong family history of cerebral microhemorrhage. *GRE,* Gradient refocused echo.

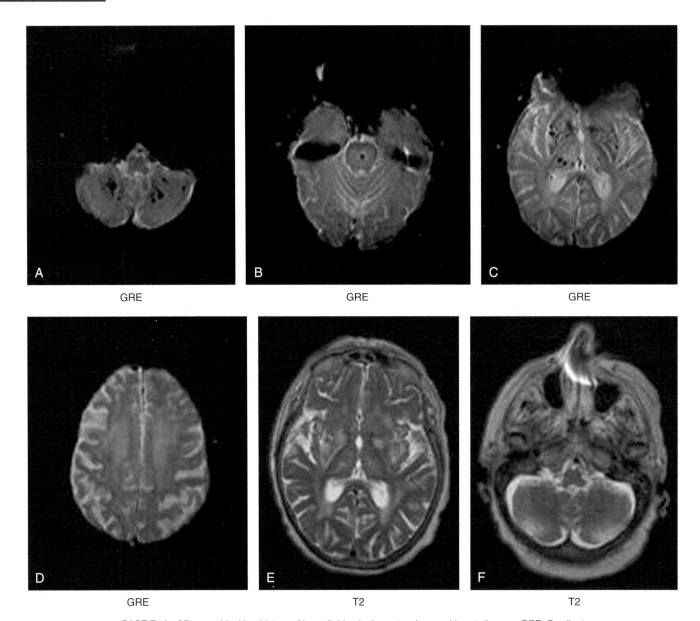

CASE B: An 87-year-old with a history of hyperlipidemia, hypertension, and heart disease. *GRE,* Gradient refocused echo.

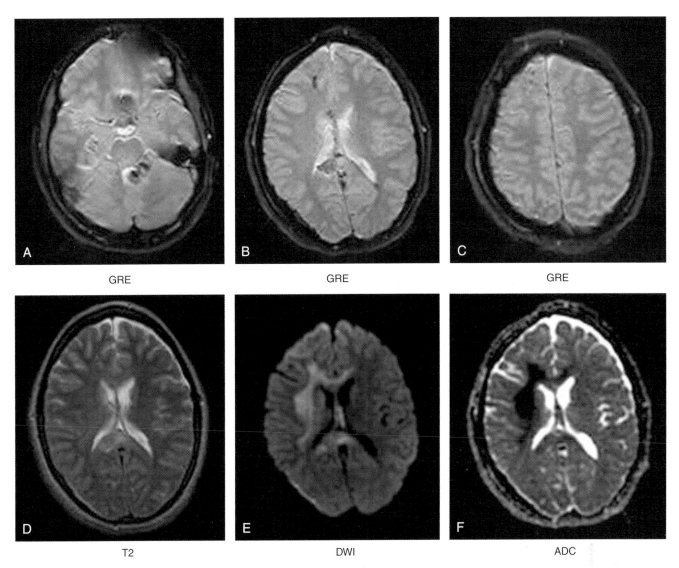

CASE C: An 18-year-old unrestrained driver after a motor vehicle accident. *ADC,* Apparent diffusion coefficient; *DWI,* diffusion-weighted imaging; *GRE,* gradient refocused echo.

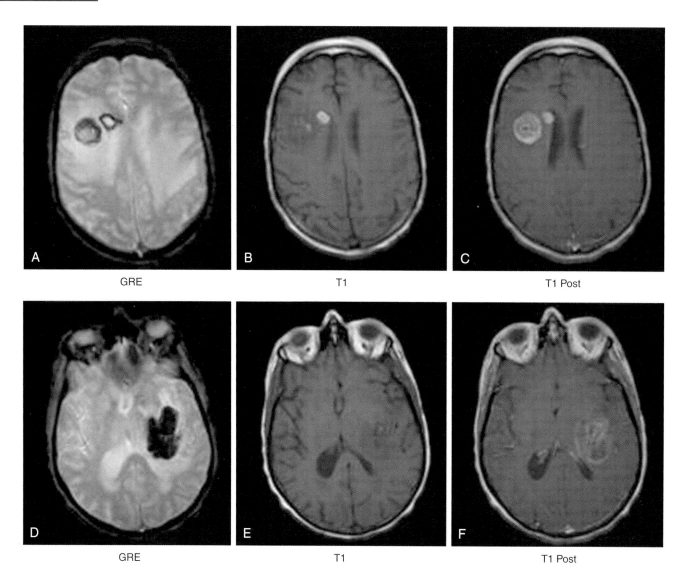

GRE

T1

T1 Post

GRE

T1

T1 Post

CASE D: A 65-year-old with a history of breast cancer presenting with difficulty walking. *GRE*, Gradient refocused echo.

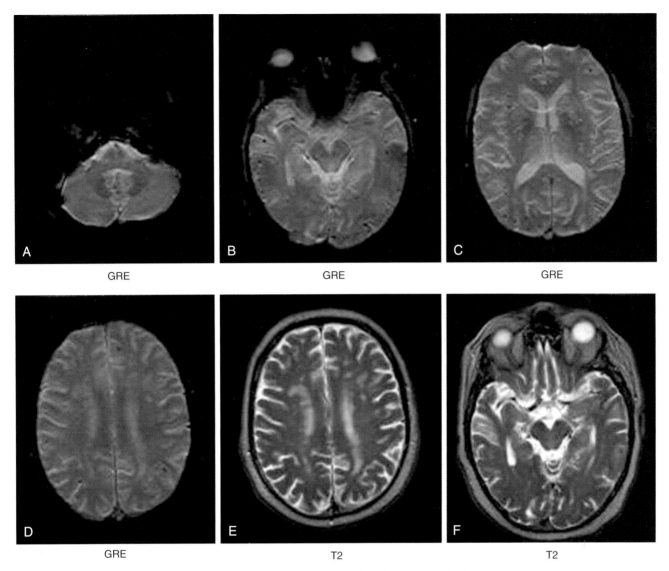

CASE E: A 64-year-old presenting with mild cognitive impairment. *GRE*, Gradient refocused echo.

DESCRIPTION OF FINDINGS

- Case A: Familial cavernous malformations: A patient with a familial history presents with multiple foci of susceptibility, the largest of which (pons, left corona radiata) demonstrate a typical "popcorn" appearance with central heterogeneity and circumferential complete rings of hypointense signal on T2-weighted images, without mass effect or edema.
- Case B: Hypertension: Multiple cerebral microhemorrhages involving the deep gray nuclei, brainstem, and cerebellum in a patient with a history of hypertension. There also are periventricular T2 hyperintense foci and bilateral deep gray nuclei lacunes.
- Case C: Diffuse axonal injury: A patient with a history of trauma with microhemorrhages involving the cerebral gray/white matter junctions, corpus callosum, and the left middle cerebellar peduncle. There is restricted diffusion in the genu and splenium of the corpus callosum as well as the right corona radiata.
- Case D: Hemorrhagic metastases (breast cancer): A patient with a history of malignancy with prominent foci of susceptibility, T1 hyperintensity, associated enhancement, and surrounding vasogenic edema.
- Case E: Amyloid angiopathy: A patient older than 60 years with multiple cerebral microhemorrhages in a peripheral pattern (cortical/subcortical distribution) sparing the deep white matter, basal ganglia, brainstem, and cerebellum. There is also moderate periventricular white matter T2 hyperintensity.

Diagnosis

Case A: Familial cavernous malformations
Case B: Hypertension
Case C: Diffuse axonal injury
Case D: Hemorrhagic metastases (breast cancer)
Case E: Amyloid angiopathy

Summary

Cerebral microhemorrhages appear as scattered punctate foci of susceptibility on gradient refocused echo (GRE)/susceptibility images. Typically, chronic microbleeds are associated with hypertension, amyloid angiopathy, and other causes of small vessel vasculopathy.

Microhemorrhages resulting from chronic hypertension typically are located in the deep gray nuclei, deep white matter, brainstem, and cerebellum. Approximately 56% of patients with an acute hypertensive hemorrhage have associated microbleeds. Patients with chronic hypertension usually have periventricular white matter T2/FLAIR hyperintensity.

Microhemorrhages resulting from amyloid angiopathy typically occur in patients older than 60 years, in a cortical/subcortical distribution with sparing of the deep white matter, basal ganglia, brainstem, and cerebellum. Approximately 75% of patients with a lobar hemorrhage resulting from amyloid angiopathy have associated microbleeds at gray/white matter junctions. Patients with amyloid angiopathy usually have periventricular white matter FLAIR/T2 hyperintensity and can also have leptomeningeal hemosiderosis. Patients with the rarer inflammatory form of amyloid angiopathy have associated vasogenic edema and leptomeningeal enhancement.

The diagnosis of hemorrhagic metastases should be considered when enhancing lesions with susceptibility and surrounding edema is seen. A study in the literature noted that 7% of melanoma metastases were identified best on GRE images. The most common hemorrhagic cerebral metastases are melanoma and renal cell carcinoma. Breast carcinoma and lung carcinoma hemorrhage less frequently but are the most common cerebral metastases and should be considered. Thyroid carcinoma and choriocarcinoma also produce hemorrhagic lesions, but they rarely metastasize to the brain.

Lobar or deep acute hemorrhage in young patients with additional foci of susceptibility can suggest the diagnosis of multiple cavernous malformations, especially if there is a classic heterogeneous lesion with a complete hemosiderin ring and no surrounding edema. In patients with a family history of this condition, an autosomal dominant inheritance pattern is seen. It is noteworthy that these familial lesions are not associated with developmental venous malformations.

In the setting of trauma, diffuse axonal injury should be considered. Microhemorrhage associated with diffuse axonal injury is most often seen at gray/white matter junctions and in the corpus callosum, subcortical and deep white matter, and dorsolateral brainstem. In addition to punctate foci of susceptibility, diffusion restriction may be seen at sites of diffuse axonal injury.

Lastly, any cause of vasculitis, whether infectious or inflammatory, should be considered. In particular, septic emboli, fungal infections, and radiation and chemotherapy changes should be considered in the appropriate clinical setting. In addition, causes of small vessel vasculopathy, such as sickle cell disease or cerebral autosomal dominant arteriopathy with subcortical infarcts and leukoencephalopathy, should be considered.

Spectrum of Disease

The spectrum of disease is detailed in the preceding section.

Differential Diagnosis

The differential diagnosis is provided in Table 3.1.

Pearls

Findings suggestive of hypertension include:
- "Central" predominant microhemorrhages involving the deep gray nuclei, deep white matter, brainstem, and cerebellum

TABLE 3.1 **Young vs. Older Patient**

Younger Patient	Older Patient
Infection	Supratentorial and peripheral: amyloid angiopathy
Diffuse axonal injury	Central predominant and cerebellum: hypertension
Multiple cavernous malformations	Other: metastases, infection

Findings suggestive of amyloid angiopathy include:
- Patients generally are older than 60 years
- A "peripheral" pattern with a cortical/subcortical distribution
- The deep white matter, basal ganglia, brainstem, and cerebellum generally are spared
- Leptomeningeal hemosiderosis

Findings suggestive of hemorrhagic metastases include:
- History of malignancy
- Enhancement associated with scattered foci of susceptibility with surrounding edema

Findings suggestive of multiple cavernous malformations include:
- History: young age and family history
- Lesions with typical popcorn appearance and complete hemosiderin ring

Signs and Complications

Signs and complications generally are related to acute hemorrhage and local mass effect. Patients with amyloid angiopathy and numerous microhemorrhages may present with dementia.

Suggested Readings

Blitstein MK, Tung GA: MRI of cerebral microhemorrhages, *AJR Am J Roentgenol* 189(3):720–725, 2007.

Chao CP, Kotsenas AL, Broderick DF: Cerebral amyloid angiopathy: CT and MR imaging findings, *Radiographics* 26(5):1517–1531, 2006.

Fazekas F, Kleinert R, Roob G, et al: Histopathologic analysis of foci of signal loss on gradient-echo T2*-weighted MR images in patients with spontaneous intracerebral hemorrhage: evidence of microangiopathy-related microbleeds, *AJNR Am J Neuroradiol* 20:637–642, 1999.

Gaviani P, Mullins ME, Braga TA, et al: Improved detection of metastatic melanoma by T2*-weighted imaging, *AJNR Am J Neuroradiol* 27(3):605–608, 2006.

Greenberg SM, Finklestein SP, Schaefer PW: Petechial hemorrhages accompanying lobar hemorrhage: detection by gradient-echo MRI, *Neurology* 46(6):1751–1754, 1996.

Kwa VI, Franke CL, Verbeeten B, et al: Silent intracerebral microhemorrhages in patients with ischemic stroke, Amsterdam Vascular Medicine Group, *Ann Neurol* 44:372–377, 1998.

Lee SH, Bae HJ, Ko SB, et al: Comparative analysis of the spatial distribution and severity of cerebral microbleeds and old lacunes, *J Neurol Neurosurg Psychiatry* 75(3):423–427, 2004.

Roob G, Schmidt R, Kapeller P, et al: MRI evidence of past cerebral microbleeds in a healthy elderly population, *Neurology* 52:991–994, 999.

4

Lobar Hemorrhage

SHERVIN KAMALIAN, MD, MSC AND SARA EMAMI, MD, CMD

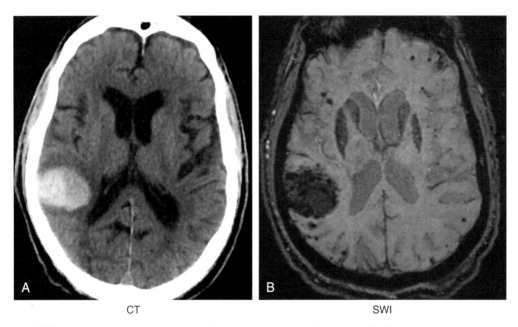

CASE A: An 83-year-old man who was found confused and disoriented. *CT,* Computed tomography; *SWI,* susceptibilityweighted imaging.

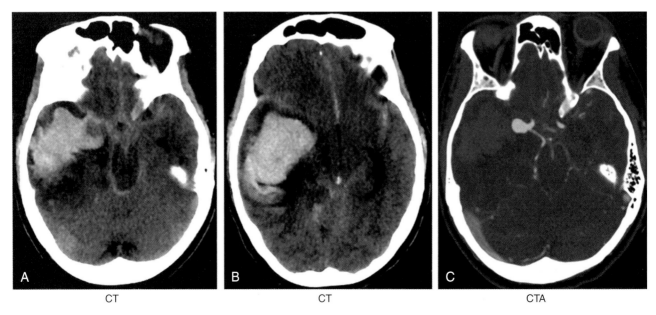

CASE B: A 62-year-old woman who collapsed. *CT,* Computed tomography; *CTA,* CT angiogram.

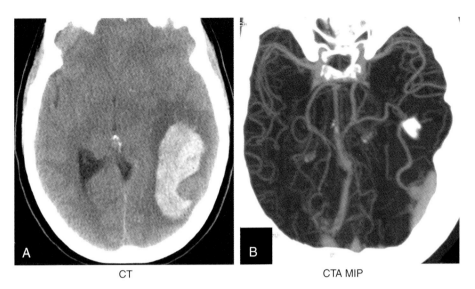

CT   CTA MIP

CASE C: A 43-year-old woman who woke up with a severe headache, confusion, and aphasia. *CT*, Computed tomography; *CTA*, CT angiogram; *MIP*, maximum intensity projection.

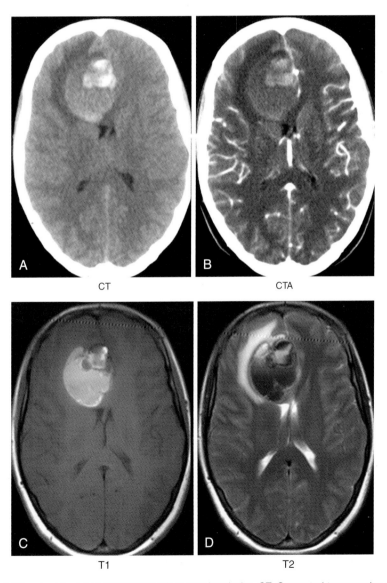

CT   CTA

T1   T2

CASE D: A 23-year-old woman presenting with severe headache. *CT*, Computed tomography; *CTA*, CT angiogram.

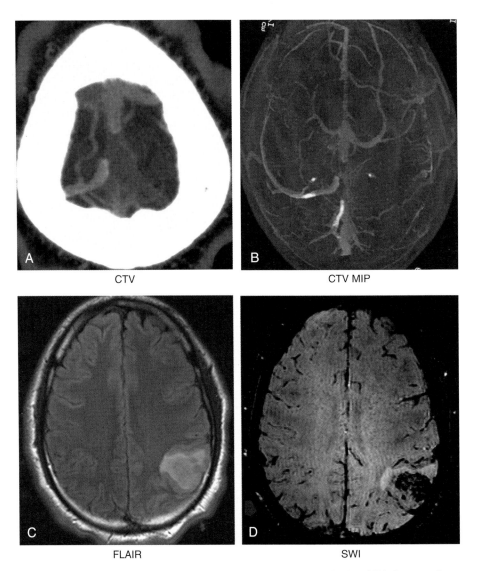

CTV | CTV MIP

FLAIR | SWI

CASE E: A 21-year-old man presenting with new onset, pulsatile headache. *CTV*, Computed tomography venography; *FLAIR*, fluid attenuated inversion recovery; *MIP*, maximum intensity projection; *SWI*, susceptibility-weighted imaging.

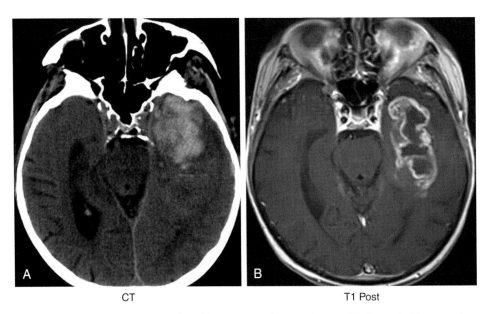

CT | T1 Post

CASE F: An 80-year-old man presenting with acute mental status change. *CT*, Computed tomography.

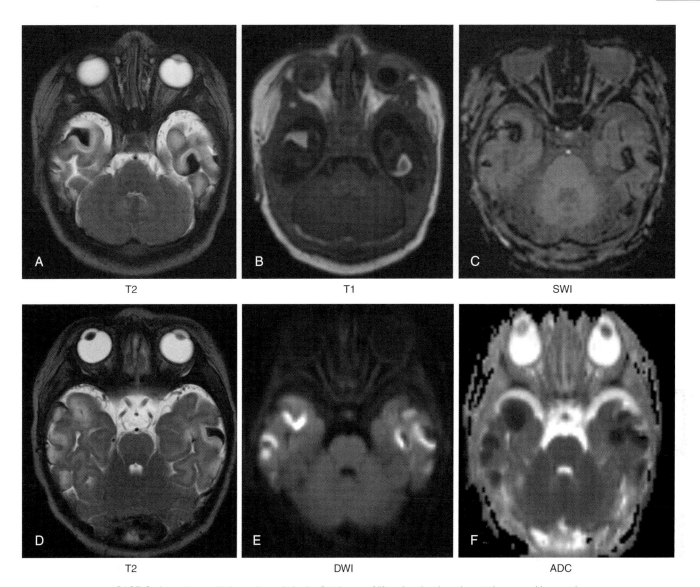

T2

T1

SWI

T2

DWI

ADC

CASE G: A newborn with hypoglycemia in the first hours of life, who developed central apnea with associated bradycardia on day 2 of life. *ADC*, Apparent diffusion coefficient; *DWI*, diffusion-weighted imaging; *SWI*, susceptibility-weighted imaging.

DESCRIPTION OF FINDINGS

- Case A: Acute intraparenchymal hemorrhage in the right posterior temporal lobe. Multiple scattered areas of peripheral cerebral microbleeds are suggestive of cerebral amyloid angiopathy.
- Case B: A large acute intraparenchymal hemorrhage in the right temporal lobe with surrounding vasogenic edema. There is a ruptured lobulated saccular aneurysm arising from the origin of the right posterior communicating artery. There are also scattered foci of subarachnoid hemorrhage.
- Case C: A large acute intraparenchymal hemorrhage in the left temporo-occipital region with surrounding vasogenic edema, due to a ruptured left temporo-occipital arteriovenous malformation (AVM). An enlarged left temporal artery arising from the left posterior cerebral artery supplies the AVM. There is a single draining vein into the left transverse/sigmoid sinus.
- Case D: Acute intraparenchymal hemorrhage in the right frontal lobe with surrounding vasogenic edema and no abnormal enhancement. Within the anterior hematoma is a lesion with a "popcorn" appearance on MRI with T2 hypointense rim and mixed signal intensity blood products on T1- and T2-weighted images. There is T1 hyperintense and T2 hypointense perilesional hemorrhage. The findings are suggestive of a giant cavernous malformation with recent hemorrhage. The lesion was resected and pathology confirmed the diagnosis.
- Case E: Left parietal lobe venous infarct with associated vasogenic edema and patchy hemorrhage in the territory of the left vein of Trolard. CTA confirmed thrombosis of the left vein of Trolard, extending into the mid-posterior segment of the superior sagittal sinus.
- Case F: Acute intraparenchymal hemorrhage in the left anterior temporal lobe, with surrounding vasogenic edema on CT and an associated mass with thick irregular rim enhancement on MRI, in the setting of pathology proven left temporal glioblastoma.
- Case G: T2 hypointense and T1 hyperintense crescentic hemorrhagic foci with associated susceptibility effect overlying the temporal cortices bilaterally which are separated from the adjacent cerebrospinal fluid (CSF) by smooth border, consistent with subpial hemorrhage. There is associated T2 hyperintensity and restricted diffusion, consistent with ischemia in the bilateral temporal cortex and subcortical white matter.

Diagnosis

Case A: Cerebral amyloid angiopathy
Case B: Ruptured saccular aneurysm
Case C: Arteriovenous malformation
Case D: Cavernous malformation
Case E: Cortical vein thrombosis
Case F: Glioblastoma
Case G: Subpial hemorrhage

Summary

Lobar hemorrhage is defined as a supratentorial intraparenchymal hemorrhage in the periphery of the cerebral lobes. By contrast, hypertensive hemorrhage is typically central, involving the basal ganglia, pons, and cerebellum.

In older patients, cerebral amyloid angiopathy and underlying neoplastic processes (metastatic or primary) are the most common causes of lobar hemorrhage, whereas in younger patients, vascular malformations and aneurysms are the most common causes. Occasionally, lobar hemorrhage can be seen in the spectrum of reversible cerebral vasoconstriction syndrome, including posterior reversible encephalopathy syndrome. Cortical vein and cerebral venous sinus thrombosis can occur in patients of all ages.

The subpial space is a potential space between the pia matter and the outermost layer of neural tissue called glia limitans. Subpial hemorrhage (SpH) typically occurs in neonates; however, it has also been reported in the adult population. The etiology of SpH is controversial, but it has been hypothesized as a primary insult to the end feet of the glia limitans, leading to a focal disruption of the basement membrane and subsequent rupture of small subpial vessels. This results in blood accumulation in the contained subpial space, causing increased pressure, similar to compartment syndrome in the skeletal muscles. Mass effect and disruption in the flow of the subpial veins result in focal cortical or subcortical infarction. On imaging, SpH appears as a crescentic hemorrhagic focus overlying the cerebral cortex separated from the adjacent CSF by a smooth border. In neonates, the most common presenting signs are apneic events and seizures with predominant involvement of the temporal lobes. In adults, the most common presenting signs and symptoms are seizures, headaches, and focal neurological symptoms.

After the detection of lobar hemorrhage on noncontrast CT, the next imaging step is head CT angiography, which is not only helpful to assess for an underlying vascular etiology (aneurysm, AVM, cortical or venous sinus thrombosis) but also helpful to identify active bleeding "spot sign" on the delayed image set for prognostication and management. The CTA spot sign is a focal contrast extravasation within the hematoma, indicative of active bleeding. This in turn predicts hematoma expansion and therefore poor outcome and may help guide more timely and aggressive medical or surgical management.

MRI is appropriate to evaluate for an underlying neoplastic process, amyloid angiopathy, or cavernous malformation. A cavernous malformation typically has a popcorn appearance with an internal signal heterogeneity and a complete T2 hypointense rim. Presence of T1 hyperintense and T2 hyperintense or hypointense perilesional signal is suggestive of cavernous malformation with recent hemorrhage, rather than a hemorrhagic mass. Of note, an underlying mass can be obscured by a lobar hemorrhage. If an underlying cause is not identified on the initial MRI and there is clinical concern for a primary or metastatic neoplastic process, a follow-up MRI is recommended after resolution of the hemorrhage. MRI of amyloid angiopathy demonstrates a lobar hemorrhage with associated microhemorrhages at gray white matter junctions and/or leptomeningeal hemosiderosis. Patients with inflammatory amyloid angiopathy have associated edema and leptomeningeal enhancement.

Spectrum of Disease

Cerebral amyloid angiopathy (CAA) has a wide spectrum of clinical manifestations. Symptoms may include intermittent headaches, episodes of confusion, and gradual cognitive impairment. If a lobar hemorrhage is large, patients present acutely with stroke-like symptoms, seizure, headache, vomiting, drowsiness, and coma. In general, clinical manifestations of lobar hemorrhage are related to the size and location of the hemorrhage.

Differential Diagnosis

Differential diagnosis is provided in Table 4.1.

Pearls

- CTA following identification of a lobar hemorrhage on CT should be obtained to search for an aneurysm, AVM, and arteriovenous fistula (AVF) or cerebral venous sinus thrombosis.
- CTA "spot sign" predicts hematoma expansion and therefore poor outcome. This may help guide a more timely and aggressive medical or surgical management.
- The diagnosis of CAA can be established using two major criteria:
  - Boston criteria incorporates clinical and MRI findings for definitive, probable, or possible diagnosis of CAA.
  - Edinburg criteria incorporates CT imaging features of lobar hemorrhage combined with APOE ε4 allele possession for high, intermediate, or low probability of CAA.
- Cavernous malformation typically has a "popcorn" appearance on MRI with a T2 hypointense rim. Presence of T1 hyperintense and T2 hyperintense or hypointense perilesional signal is suggestive of cavernous malformation with recent hemorrhage rather than a hemorrhagic mass.
- A lobar hemorrhage can obscure an underlying mass. Thus if the underlying cause is not identified on the initial MRI, and there is clinical concern for a primary or metastatic neoplastic process, a short-term follow-up MRI is recommended after resolution of the hemorrhage.
- SpH occurs in association with ischemic foci in neonates with cardiorespiratory failure, coagulopathy, or hypoxic ischemic encephalopathy.

Signs and Complications

The signs and complications are detailed in the preceding sections.

TABLE 4.1	Lobar Hemorrhage Differential Diagnosis
Cerebral amyloid angiopathy (older patients)	
Vascular malformation (younger patients)	
Aneurysm (saccular or mycotic)	
Venous sinus or cortical vein thrombosis	
Coagulation disorders or anticoagulation therapy	
Subpial hemorrhage (neonates)	
Others: tumor, vasculitis, autoimmune or infection	

Suggested Readings

Barreto ARF, Carrasco M, Dabrowski AK, et al: Subpial hemorrhage in neonates: what radiologists need to know, *AJR Am J Roentgenol* 216(4):1056–1065, 2021.

Brouwers HB, Battey TW, Musial HH, et al: Rate of contrast extravasation on computed tomographic angiography predicts hematoma expansion and mortality in primary intracerebral hemorrhage, *Stroke* 46(9): 2498–2503, 2015.

Cain DW, Dingman AL, Armstrong J, et al: Subpial hemorrhage of the neonate, *Stroke* 51(1):315–318, 2020.

Greenberg SM, Charidimou A: Diagnosis of cerebral amyloid angiopathy: evolution of the Boston criteria, *Stroke* 49(2):491–497, 2018.

Rodrigues MA, Samarasekera N, Lerpiniere C, et al: The Edinburgh CT and genetic diagnostic criteria for lobar intracerebral haemorrhage associated with cerebral amyloid angiopathy: model development and diagnostic test accuracy study, *Lancet Neurol* 17(3):232–240, 2018.

Roth P, Happold C, Eisele G, et al: A series of patients with subpial hemorrhage: clinical manifestation, neuroradiological presentation and therapeutic implications, *J Neurol* 255(7):1018–1022, 2008.

Yun TJ, Na DG, Kwon BJ, et al: A T1 hyperintense perilesional signal aids in the differentiation of a cavernous angioma from other hemorrhagic masses, *AJNR Am J Neuroradiol* 29(3):494–500, 2008.

5

Multifocal White Matter Lesions

CHAD WILLIAM FARRIS, MD, PHD

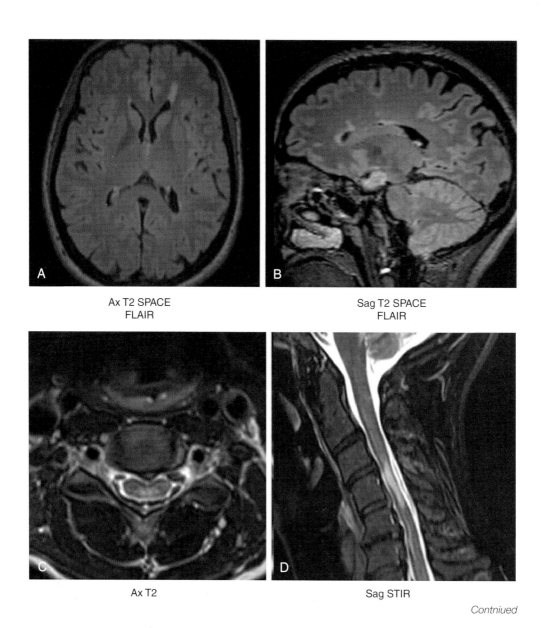

Ax T2 SPACE
FLAIR

Sag T2 SPACE
FLAIR

Ax T2

Sag STIR

Contniued

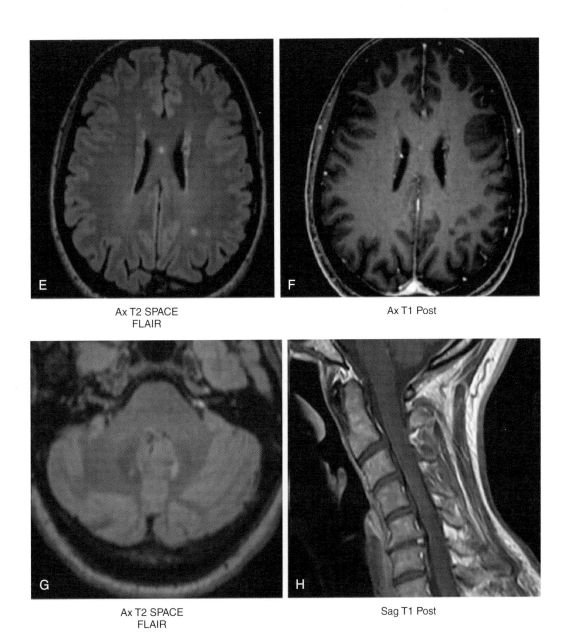

Ax T2 SPACE
FLAIR

Ax T1 Post

Ax T2 SPACE
FLAIR

Sag T1 Post

CASE A: A 37-year-old female who originally presented with right leg weakness and urinary urgency that resolved with subsequent bouts of optic neuritis and focal neurological deficits that also resolved. *Ax,* Axial; *FLAIR,* fluid-attenuated inversion recovery; *Sag,* sagittal; *space,* sampling perfection with application optimized contrasts using different flip angle evolution; *STIR,* short tau inversion recovery.

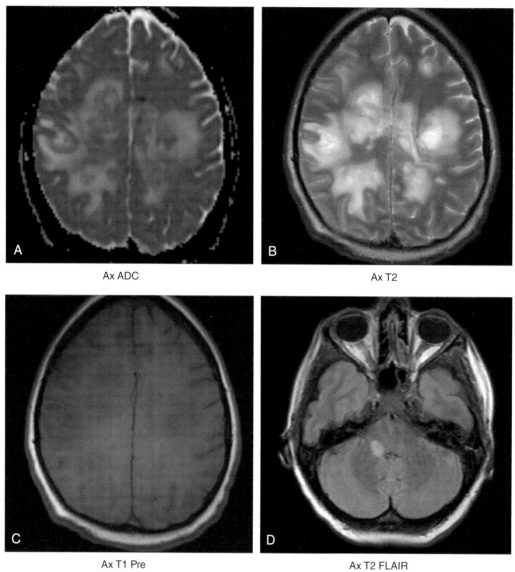

Ax ADC

Ax T2

Ax T1 Pre

Ax T2 FLAIR

Contniued

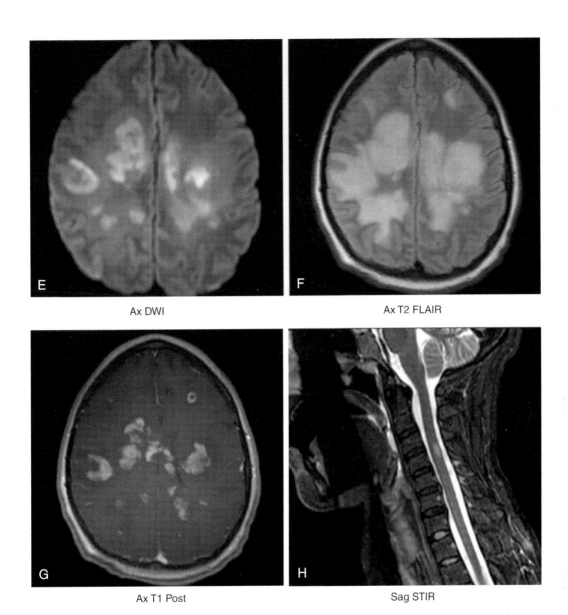

Ax DWI

Ax T2 FLAIR

Ax T1 Post

Sag STIR

CASE B A 29-year-old female with rapidly progressive multifocal neurological deficits over several weeks. *ADC,* Apparent diffusion coefficient; *Ax,* axial; *DWI,* diffusion-weighted imaging; *FLAIR,* fluid-attenuated inversion recovery; *Sag,* sagittal; *STIR,* short tau inversion recovery.

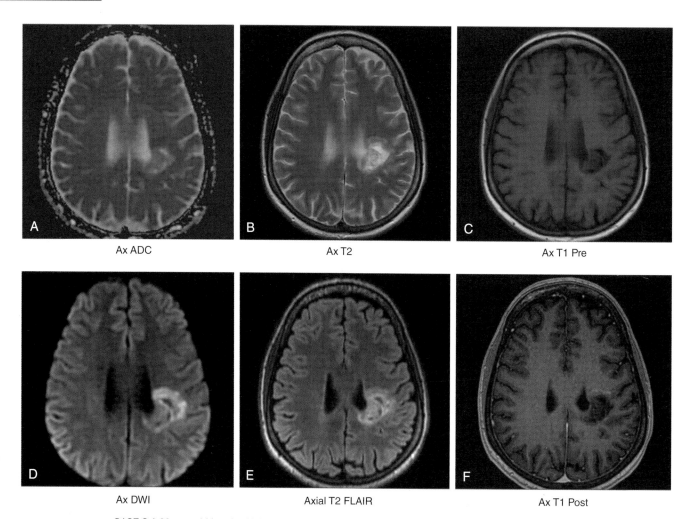

Ax ADC | Ax T2 | Ax T1 Pre
Ax DWI | Axial T2 FLAIR | Ax T1 Post

CASE C A 30-year-old female with left hemibody sensorimotor complaints. *ADC,* Apparent diffusion coefficient; *Ax,* axial; *DWI,* diffusion-weighted imaging; *FLAIR,* fluid-attenuated inversion recovery.

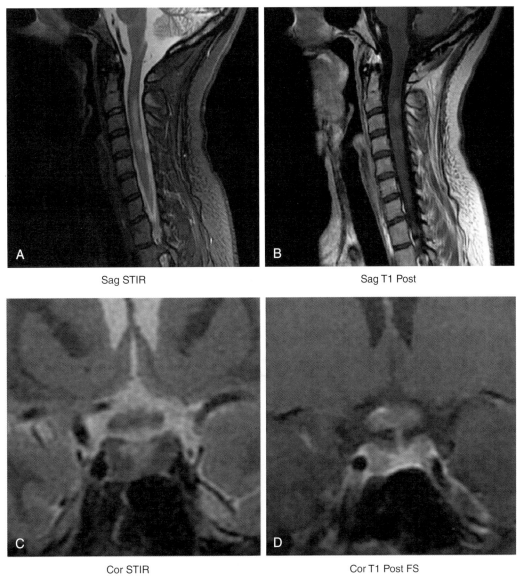

Sag STIR

Sag T1 Post

Cor STIR

Cor T1 Post FS

Contniued

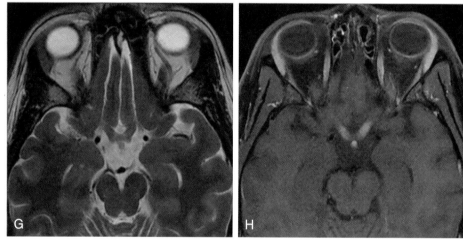

Cor T2 SPACE FLAIR

Cor T1 Post

Ax T2

Ax T1 Post FS

CASE D A 29-year-old female with 3 weeks of hemibody left-sided numbness and tingling and 2 weeks of blurry vision. *Ax,* Axial; *Cor,* coronal; *FLAIR,* fluid-attenuated inversion recovery; *FS,* fat saturated; *Sag,* sagittal; *SPACE,* sampling perfection with application optimized contrasts using different flip angle evolution; *STIR,* short tau inversion recovery.

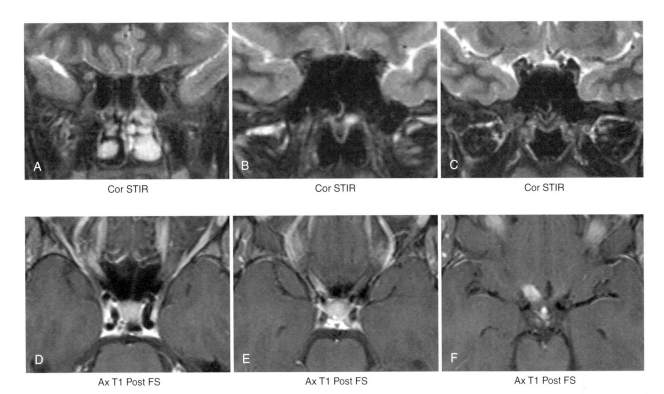

Cor STIR   Cor STIR   Cor STIR

Ax T1 Post FS   Ax T1 Post FS   Ax T1 Post FS

CASE E1 A 24-year-old female who developed right eye pain with eye movement and significant visual loss shortly thereafter. *Ax,* Axial; *Cor,* coronal; *FS,* fat saturated; *STIR,* short tau inversion recovery.

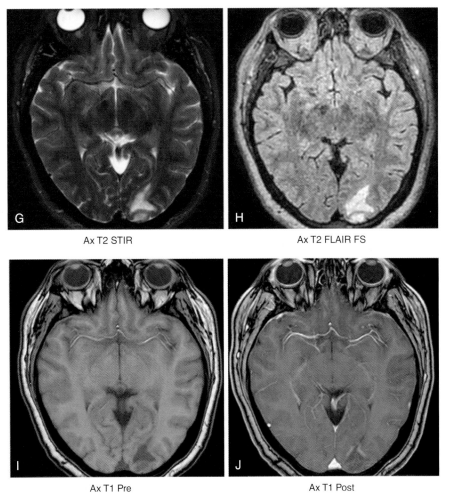

Ax T2 STIR   Ax T2 FLAIR FS

Ax T1 Pre   Ax T1 Post

Contniued

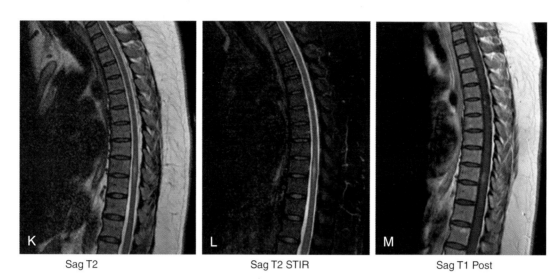

Sag T2   Sag T2 STIR   Sag T1 Post

CASE E2 A 49-year-old female with 2 weeks of progressive numbness of the bilateral lower extremities and pain. *Ax,* Axial; *FLAIR,* fluid-attenuated inversion recovery; *FS,* fat saturated; *Sag,* sagittal; *STIR,* short tau inversion recovery.

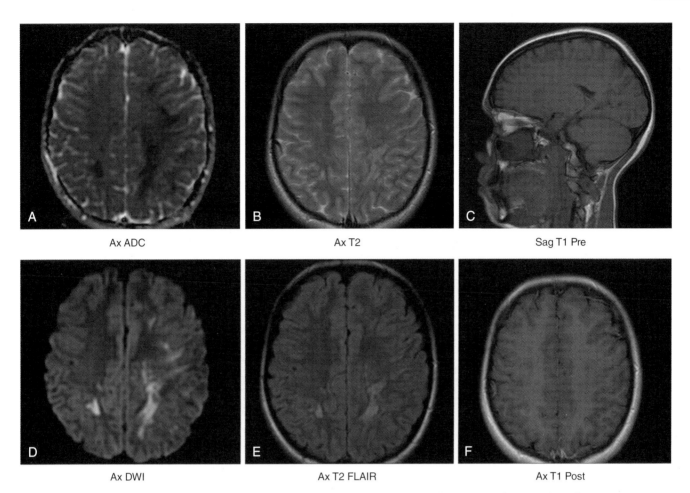

Ax ADC

Ax T2

Sag T1 Pre

Ax DWI

Ax T2 FLAIR

Ax T1 Post

CASE F An 18-year-old female presenting with brain fog, confusion, difficulty producing speech, and right arm and leg weakness 1 week after conjunctivitis. *ADC,* Apparent diffusion coefficient; *Ax,* axial; *DWI,* diffusion-weighted imaging; *FLAIR,* fluid-attenuated inversion recovery; *Sag,* sagittal.

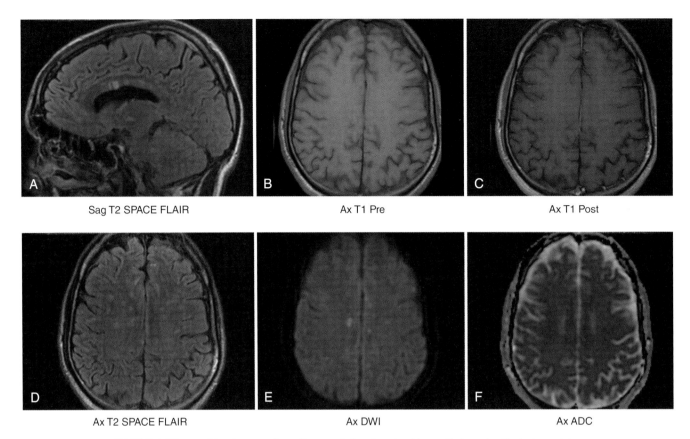

Sag T2 SPACE FLAIR   Ax T1 Pre   Ax T1 Post

Ax T2 SPACE FLAIR   Ax DWI   Ax ADC

CASE G A 32-year-old male presenting with encephalopathy, visual loss with branch retinal artery occlusions, and hearing loss. *ADC,* Apparent diffusion coefficient; *Ax,* axial; *DWI,* diffusion-weighted imaging; *FLAIR,* fluid-attenuated inversion recovery; *Sag,* sagittal; *SPACE,* sampling perfection with application optimized contrasts using different flip angle evolution.

DESCRIPTION OF FINDINGS

- Case A: There are multiple fluid-attenuated inversion recovery (FLAIR) hyperintense foci involving the periventricular white matter, subcortical white matter, corpus callosum, callososeptal interface, and bilateral cerebellar white matter. There is enhancement associated with a focus of T2/FLAIR hyperintensity within the corpus callosum. There are multiple short-segment (less than two vertebral body heights) foci of short tau inversion recovery (STIR) hyperintensity within the cervical spinal cord with the most prominent at the C4–C5 level where there is cord volume loss.
- Case B: There are extensive areas of T2/FLAIR hyperintensity throughout the supratentorial white matter that notably include involvement of the juxtacortical and periventricular white matter. There is also a focus of T2/FLAIR hyperintensity centered within the right middle cerebellar peduncle. There is reduced diffusion and enhancement associated with many of the T2/FLAIR hyperintense foci. Notably, some of the enhancing foci have an open ring appearance with the opening toward the cortex.
- Case C: The lesion centered in the left posterior left corona radiata is characterized by several concentric open rings with varying relatively normal to increased T2 and FLAIR signal. The rings demonstrate some reduced diffusion and some enhancement.
- Case D: There is a long segment (extending more than two vertebral body heights) of STIR hyperintensity within the central cervical spinal cord extending from the lower C2 level to the upper C5 level with associated patchy enhancement. There is also increased STIR signal and enhancement within the optic chiasm and adjacent prechiasmatic optic nerves as well as an enhancing, T2/FLAIR hyperintense lesion within the periventricular white matter along the body of the left lateral ventricle.
- Case E1: There is a long segment of STIR hyperintensity with associated enhancement involving the proximal aspect of the intraorbital segment, the intracanalicular segment, and the intracranial segment of the right optic nerve.
- Case E2: There is an area of T2/FLAIR hyperintensity within the juxtacortical and subcortical white matter of the left occipital lobe with associated patchy peripheral enhancement. There are also multiple short-segment STIR hyperintense lesions within the thoracic spinal cord with associated cord enhancement and some mild cord expansion with the larger cord lesions.
- Case F: There are multifocal areas of reduced diffusion in the left centrum semiovale and subcortical white matter of the bilateral cerebral hemispheres with associated T2 and FLAIR hyperintensity and no associated enhancement.
- Case G: There are multiple nonenhancing, FLAIR hyperintense foci within the corpus callosum, including several that involve the full thickness. There are additional small, nonenhancing FLAIR hyperintense foci within the subcortical white matter, with several demonstrating restricted diffusion.

Diagnosis

Case A: Multiple sclerosis

Case B: Marburg disease (Multiple sclerosis variant)

Case C: Baló concentric sclerosis (Multiple sclerosis variant)

Case D: Neuromyelitis optica spectrum disorder—aquaporin-4 antibody-positive

Case E1 and E2: Myelin oligodendrocyte glycoprotein antibody-associated disease

Case F: Acute disseminated encephalomyelitis

Case G: Susac syndrome (retinocochleocerebral vasculopathy)

Summary

The spectrum of disease processes that result in multifocal white matter lesions is very broad and includes inflammatory, demyelinating, autoimmune, toxic, and metabolic disorders, in addition to malignancy, microvascular disease, and sequelae of trauma. This chapter focuses on the important inflammatory and demyelinating disorders that commonly result in multifocal white matter lesions, including multiple sclerosis (MS) and its variants, neuromyelitis optica spectrum disorders (NMOSDs), acute disseminated encephalomyelitis (ADEM), and an autoimmune endotheliopathy, Susac syndrome, that is commonly misdiagnosed as MS.

Spectrum of Disease

MS is the most common acquired idiopathic inflammatory demyelinating disease with a peak age of onset between 20 and 40 years of age, a female predominance (2:1), and typical clinical presentation with sensory and motor disturbances. MS is diagnosed according to the McDonald criteria. Based on the 2017 revision of the McDonald criteria, MS is based on clinical symptoms and imaging findings that demonstrate dissemination of the disease in time and space. An MS lesion based on these criteria is an area of hyperintensity on a T2-weighted or proton-density-weighted image that is at least 3 mm in long axis. Lesions must be present in at least two of four characteristic locations to meet criteria for dissemination in space: (1) juxtacortical white matter, (2) periventricular white matter, (3) an infratentorial structure brainstem (typically near the surface), cerebellar peduncles, or cerebellum), and (4) the spinal cord. Dissemination in time is demonstrated on imaging by simultaneous presence of enhancing and nonenhancing lesions on a single scan, or new lesions developing on a subsequent scan. Lesions along the callososeptal interface that are perivenular in location (Dawson fingers) are also very characteristic of MS. Marburg disease is an acute fulminant form of MS most commonly seen in young adults that typically demonstrates a monophasic relentless progression with death usually occurring within 1 year of onset. Lesions are typically characterized by edema, enhancement, and restricted diffusion. Baló concentric sclerosis is an atypical MS variant that is notable for its very characteristic appearance on imaging of concentric rings that is described as an "onion ring" or "whorled" appearance created by alternating layers of demyelination and preservation of myelin. Baló concentric sclerosis usually presents acutely with rapid clinical deterioration and a variable prognosis, with some cases having a relatively benign course and others proving lethal. Baló concentric sclerosis is also notable for commonly presenting with nonspecific features such as headache and seizures.

Neuromyelitis optica spectrum disorder (NMOSD) is a severe acute autoimmune inflammatory demyelinating process with typical clinical features of longitudinally extensive transverse myelitis and optic neuritis. Approximately 70% of cases are associated with the aquaporin-4 antibody that targets astrocytes. NMOSD has a very strong female predominance of 8–9:1 over males. Intracranial lesions occur predominantly in periependymal regions in the distribution of aquaporin-4 and have a smooth confluent configuration in contradistinction to Dawson fingers associated with MS. A marbled appearance of the corpus callosum punctate deep white matter lesions, extensive longitudinal corticospinal tract lesions, and rare larger intracranial lesions have also been described. NMOSDs in general have a worse prognosis than MS, with 85% to 90% of patients having reoccurrence with progressive deficits.

Myelin oligodendrocyte glycoprotein antibody–associated disease (MOGAD) refers to inflammatory demyelinating disorders characterized by antibodies to myelin oligodendrocyte glycoprotein (MOG). Imaging features more typical of MOGAD compared to NMOSD and MS include: (1) optic nerve involvement, typically bilateral, in over 80% with frequent perineural enhancement, (2) lesions similar to those described in the following paragraph for ADEM predominantly in children, and (3) large ill-defined supratentorial lesions, predominantly in adults. Spinal lesions typically involve the central and peripheral cords and can be short or long segments. Leptomeningeal enhancement is common while it is rare with MS and NMOSD.

ADEM is the second most common acquired idiopathic inflammatory demyelinating disorder and is usually seen in the setting of a recent prior viral infection or after a recent immunization. Imaging features usually include multifocal T2/FLAIR hyperintense lesions that can have a "cotton ball"–like appearance and asymmetrically involve the supratentorial white matter. Basal ganglia and infratentorial lesions are common. Additionally, the lesions can demonstrate reduced diffusion in the acute phase and highly variable enhancement (from essentially none to marked enhancement). There is a seasonal variance in occurrence rates, with fall and spring being the most common, and there is no sex predominance. There is an association between children with ADEM and MS, with about 10% to 25% of children with ADEM going on to develop MS. ADEM is usually monophasic, but about 25% relapse in the same location (recurrent ADEM) or in a new location (multiphasic ADEM), which is associated with antimyelin oligodendrocyte glycoprotein antibodies. Overall, the majority of patients fully recover with only 20% having some residual functional impairment and with a mortality rate of only 1% to 2%.

Susac syndrome is an autoimmune endotheliopathy with microvascular infarcts. Typical imaging findings are multifocal T2 and FLAIR hyperintense white matter lesions, including full-thickness corpus callosum lesions that very characteristically involve the central corpus callosum much more than the call26ososeptal interfaces, which is a differentiating feature from MS. Susac syndrome is commonly mistaken for MS, which is likely due to both diseases having multifocal white matter lesions and both occurring most commonly in similar populations, women in their 20sto 40s (Susac syndrome has a 3–5:1 female-to-male predominance). The classic clinical triad of Susac syndrome is subacute encephalopathy, sensorineural hearing loss, and branch retinal artery occlusion, but many patients do not present with all three classic features. The disease process is usually self-limited, but the clinical course is unpredictable.

Differential Diagnosis

Multiple Sclerosis a space (MS)
Marburg disease
Baló concentric sclerosis
Neuromyelitis optica spectrum disorder (NMOSD), 70% with aquaporin-4 antibody-positive disease
Myelin oligodendrocyte glycoprotein antibody-associated disease (MOGAD)
Acute disseminated encephalomyelitis
Susac syndrome
Small vessel disease
Cerebral autosomal dominant arteriopathy with subcortical infarcts and leukoencephalopathy (CADASIL)
Marchiafava-Bignami syndrome
Glioma
Lymphoma
Vasculitis
Traumatic/diffuse axonal injury

Pearls

- Key features for supporting a diagnosis of MS by imaging are dissemination of white matter lesions by space and time. The requirement of dissemination in space by MRI is satisfied by having lesions in two or more of the following locations: juxtacortical, periventricular, infratentorial, and within the spinal cord. The requirement of dissemination in time by MRI is satisfied by simultaneous presence of enhancing and nonenhancing lesions on a single scan, or new lesions developing on a subsequent scan.
- Marburg disease is a variant of MS that demonstrates rapid progression with death commonly occurring within 1 year.
- Baló concentric sclerosis is a variant of MS with a very characteristic imaging appearance of concentric rings that has also been described as "onion ring" or "whorled."
- NMOSDs include both antibody-positive disease (anti-aquaporin-4 in 70%) and antibody-negative disease with typical clinical features including longitudinally extensive transverse myelitis and optic neuritis. The presence of anti-aquaporin-4 is 90% specific and 70% to 75% sensitive for an NMOSD and is almost always negative in MS.
- MOGAD is characterized by bilateral optic neuritis, short or long segment transverse myelitis, brain lesions similar to those associated with ADEM, and leptomeningeal enhancement.
- Recent history of viral illness or immunization should raise concern for ADEM or MOGAD.

Susac syndrome is commonly mistaken for MS on imaging. Susac syndrome typically presents with bilateral sensorineural hearing monocular visual impairment (due to branch retinal artery occlusions) and acute or subacute encephalopathy. Involvement of the corpus callosum in Susac syndrome is characteristically full thickness or central, while involvement with

MS tends to be small partial thickness lesions that frequently involve the genu and body.

Signs and Complications

Differentiating features for MS, ADEM, NMOSD, and MOGAD based on lesion location:
- Temporal pole white matter—MS (common) > ADEM, MOGAD > NMOSD (uncommon)
- Corpus callosum—MS and NMOSD (very common to common) > ADEM, MOGAD (uncommon)
- Subcortical U-fiber involvement—MS, ADEM, and MOGAD (common) > NMO (not commonly involved)
- Basal ganglia—ADEM, MOGAD (common) > MS and NMO (uncommon)
- Optic nerves—MS, NMOSD, and MOGAD (common) > ADEM (uncommon)

Features of white matter lesions in MS, ADEM, NMOSDs, and MOGAD significantly overlap and no pattern of lesions is diagnostic of a particular disease process. However, certain imaging features can favor one process over the others.
- Unilateral short-segment optic neuritis, short-segment (less than 2 vertebral body heights) peripheral lateral and dorsal involvement of the cervical cord, infratentorial lesions with involvement of the intrapontine trigeminal nerve nucleus, and supratentorial involvement of the juxtacortical and periventricular white matter, and callososeptal interfaces favor MS.
- Long segment optic neuritis with involvement of the optic chiasm, long segment cervicothoracic spinal cord involvement that is central or central and peripheral with greater than 50% cord circumference involved, involvement of the periependymal white matter, and involvement of the corticospinal tracts favor aquaporin-4 antibody-positive disease.
- Long segment anterior optic neuritis with perineural enhancement, conus medullaris and thoracolumbar cord involvement that is commonly central and peripheral in a long and/or short-segment pattern, in combination with ADEM-like lesions involving the subcortical white matter, basal ganglia, and infratentorial white matter as well as leptomeningeal enhancement favor MOGAD.
- Fluffy "cotton ball"–like subcortical white matter lesions as well as deep gray nuclei, pontine, and other infratentorial lesions are typical of ADEM.
- Unlike the demyelinative processes, Susac syndrome is typically characterized by white matter lesions with little to no edema as well as full-thickness corpus callosum lesions.

Suggested Readings

Dutra BG, da Rocha AJ, Nunes RH, et al: Neuromyelitis optica spectrum disorders: spectrum of MR imaging findings and their differential diagnosis, *Radiographics* 38(1):169–193, 2018.

Osborn AG, Hedlund GL, Salzman, KL: Demyelinating and inflammatory diseases. In Osborn's brain: imaging, pathology, and anatomy, Salt Lake City, UT, 2018, Elsevier, Inc.

Sarbu N, Oleaga L, Shih RY, et al: White matter diseases with radiologic-pathologic correlation, *Radiographics* 36(5):1426–1447, 2016.

Sarbu N, Shih RY, Oleaga L, et al: RadioGraphics update: white matter diseases with radiologic-pathologic correlation, *Radiographics* 40(3): E4–E7, 2020.

Thompson AJ, Banwell BL, Barkhof F, et al: Diagnosis of multiple sclerosis: 2017 revisions of the McDonald criteria, *Lancet Neurol* 17(2):162–173, 2018.

6

Multiple Small Diffuse-Weighted Imaging Hyperintensities

HAMID RAJEBI, MD

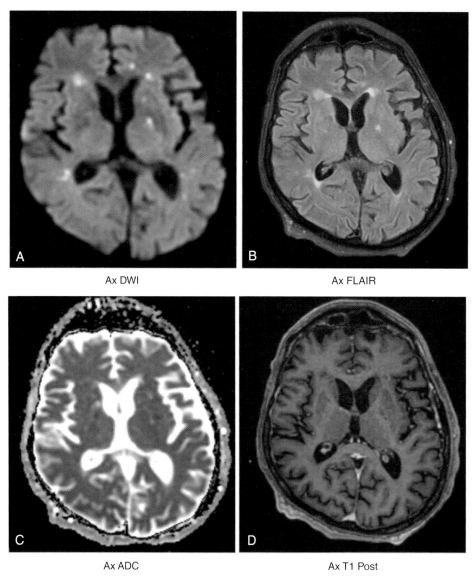

Ax DWI

Ax FLAIR

Ax ADC

Ax T1 Post

CASE A: A 75-year-old male with past medical history of atrial fibrillation presenting with altered mental status. *ADC*, Apparent diffusion coefficient; *Ax*, Axial; *DWI*, diffusion-weighted imaging; *FLAIR*, fluid attenuated inversion recovery.

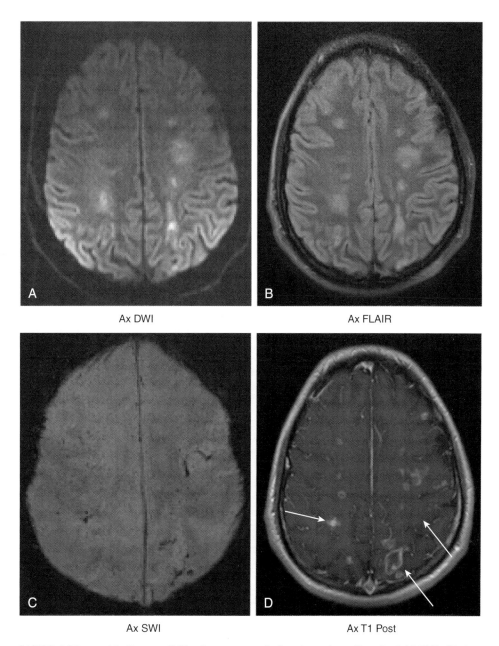

Ax DWI

Ax FLAIR

Ax SWI

Ax T1 Post

CASE B: A 33-year old with group B Streptococcus prosthetic valve endocardities. *Ax,* Axial; *DWI,* diffusion-weighted imaging; *FLAIR,* fluid attenuated inversion recovery; *SWI,* susceptibility- weighted imaging.

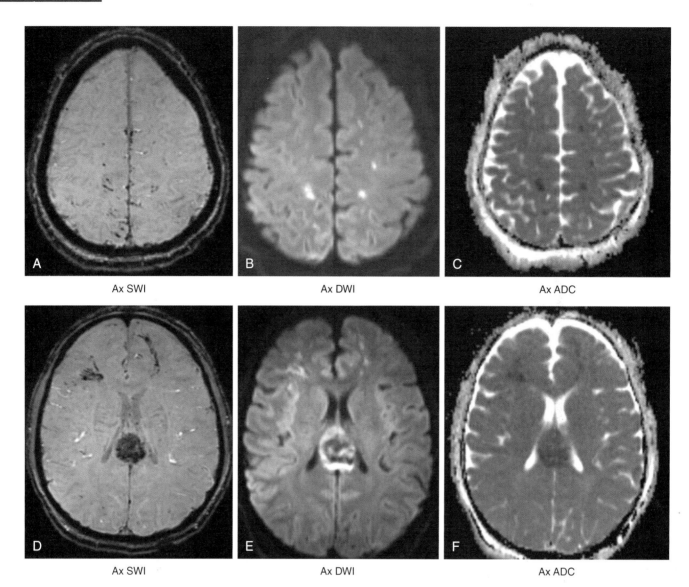

Ax SWI   Ax DWI   Ax ADC

Ax SWI   Ax DWI   Ax ADC

CASE C: A 32-year-old male with history of motor vehicle accident. *ADC,* Apparent diffusion coefficient; *Ax,* Axial; *DWI,* diffusion-weighted imaging; *SWI,* susceptibility- weighted imaging.

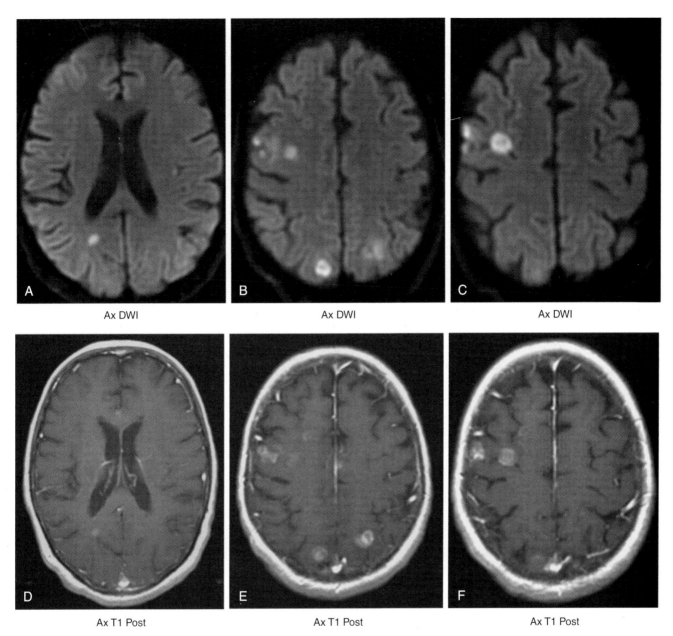

CASE D: Patient with a history of small cell lung carcinoma. *Ax,* Axial; *DWI,* diffusion-weighted imaging.

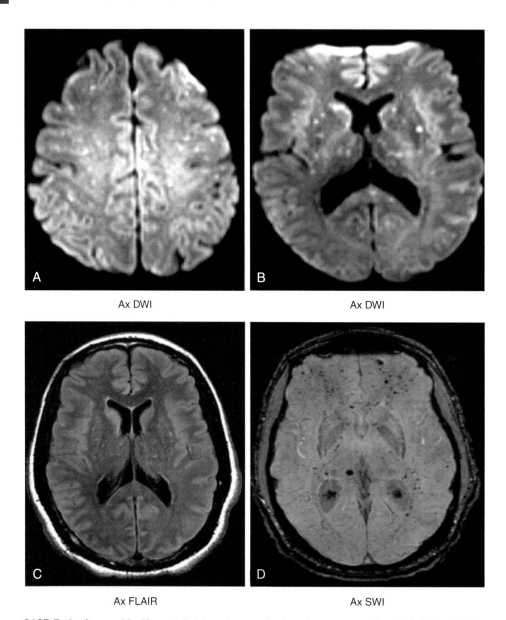

Ax DWI

Ax DWI

Ax FLAIR

Ax SWI

CASE E: A 42-year old with mental status change after long bone surgery. *Ax,* Axial; *DWI,* diffusion-weighted imaging; *FLAIR,* fluid attenuated inversion recovery; *SWI,* susceptibility- weighted imaging.

DESCRIPTION OF FINDINGS

Magnetic resonance (MR) images from five patients with multiple small foci with restricted diffusion.

- Case A: There are multiple foci of restricted diffusion scattered bilaterally throughout the brain parenchyma, involving multiple vascular territories. There are also prominent white matter chronic small-vessel ischemic changes.
- Case B: There are multiple diffusion-weighted imaging (DWI), hyperintense/apparent diffusion coefficient (ADC), hypointense (not shown), and fluid-attenuated inversion recovery (FLAIR) hyperintense lesions. Some of the lesions have associated foci of susceptibility, consistent with hemorrhage. Some of the lesions have rim enhancement (arrows).
- Case C: There are multiple DWI hyperintense/ADC hypointense foci with associated foci of susceptibility (susceptibility-weighted imaging [SWI] images) involving the gray-white matter junctions and splenium/posterior body of the corpus callosum.
- Case D: There are multiple DWI hyperintense/ADC (not shown) hypointense, enhancing lesions involving predominantly the gray-white matter junctions of both cerebral hemispheres.
- Case E: There are multiple foci of restricted diffusion scattered throughout the white matter and deep gray nuclei. The lesions have subtle associated FLAIR abnormality. SWI images demonstrate too numerous to count, predominantly white matter microhemorrhages.

Diagnosis

Case A: Cardioembolic stroke, embolic shower
Case B: Septic-embolic encephalitis
Case C: Traumatic axonal injury
Case D: Small-cell lung carcinoma metastases
Case E: Fat emboli

Summary

There is a wide spectrum of diseases that cause multiple small foci of DWI hyperintensity in the brain parenchyma. Although often a diagnostic challenge for the neuroradiologist, some magnetic resonance (MR) imaging characteristics of these lesions as well as clinical presentation can help in establishing an appropriate differential diagnosis.

Cardioembolic stroke accounts for 14% to 30% of ischemic strokes with patients being prone to early and long-term stroke recurrence. Certain clinical features are suggestive of cardioembolic infarction, including sudden onset, decreased level of consciousness at onset, Wernicke aphasia or global aphasia without hemiparesis, a Valsalva maneuver at the time of stroke onset, and co-occurrence of cerebral and systemic emboli. The common risk factors include atrial fibrillation, recent myocardial infarction, mechanical prosthetic valve, dilated myocardiopathy, and mitral rheumatic stenosis. In-hospital mortality in cardioembolic stroke is highest as compared with other subtypes of cerebral infarction, and thus, in general, it is a severe clinical condition.

Typical imaging features are multiple foci of restricted diffusion, consistent with acute strokes in multiple vascular territories or in border zones.

Septic-embolic encephalitis, also known as septic-embolic brain abscess, refers to a focal or diffuse brain infection, as a result of infective thromboembolism from any part of the body. It is usually caused by bacterial endocarditis. CNS involvement during the course of infective endocarditis occurs in ~30% (range 20% to 40%) of cases. Risk factors include rheumatic heart disease, mitral valve prolapse, prosthetic heart valves, congenital heart disease, intravenous drug abuse, immunocompromised patients, central venous catheter placement, and arteriovenous shunts. Ischemic stroke is the most common mode of presentation of patients with septic-embolic encephalitis. In almost 90% of cases this occurs in the distribution of the middle cerebral artery, and rarely in the posterior circulation. Typical imaging features include multiple foci of restricted diffusion in multiple vascular territories, consistent with acute strokes and or microabscesses. The microabscesses demonstrate rim enhancement. Vasogenic edema may be present. Microhemorrhages, with a predilection for cortex, are also a common feature. Less commonly, mycotic aneurysms may occur. They may regress spontaneously under clinical treatment, with persistent aneurysms warranting surgical or endovascular treatment.

Cerebral metastases have a variable appearance on MRI and may have facilitated or restricted diffusion and may be solid or have central necrosis with rim enhancement. Cerebral metastases with restricted diffusion have been reported in patients with lung cancer, breast cancer, colon cancer, testicular cancer, and renal cancer. Restricted diffusion may be due to dense cell packing or proteinaceous material associated with necrosis. When they are disseminated, they may mimic cardioembolic infarctions. Unlike acute infarctions, metastases enhance and they frequently also have surrounding edema.

Diffuse axonal injury, or traumatic axonal injury (TAI), is a severe form of traumatic brain injury due to shearing forces. Classically, patients with TAI present with low Glasgow Coma Scale (GCS) starting at the moment of impact and may have persistent severe neurological impairment. Typical imaging features of TAI include numerous FLAIR hyperintense lesions, frequently with restricted diffusion, located at gray-white matter junctions, in the splenium of the corpus callosum and in the brainstem. T2*-weighted sequences and SWI may detect hemorrhage associated with these lesions as well as additional lesions not seen on FLAIR or DWI sequences.

Fat emboli syndrome is usually seen in association with long bone fractures and orthopedic prosthetic surgeries, but rarely occurs from bone marrow necrosis and fat embolism associated with a sickle cell crisis. Fat emboli can disseminate to any organ but are most evident in the brain, lungs, and skin. Symptoms typically occur at 24 to 48 hours following the fracture or surgery and include shortness of breath, a petechial rash and confusion, drowsiness, seizures, or coma. Typical imaging features include symmetric foci of restricted diffusion in the subcortical white matter as well as within the corpus callosum and internal capsule, referred to as the "starry sky appearance." Similar to small cardiac emboli, fat emboli may occur in a border zone distribution. Fat emboli incite an inflammatory response with increased vascular permeability and profuse white matter microhemorrhages, best delineated on SWI.

Spectrum of Disease

Although multiple small, disseminated brain lesions, that are characterized by restricted diffusion on DWI, typically indicate acute or hyperacute cardioembolic infarcts, they can also be due to hypercellular metastases, small brain abscesses, brain demyelinating lesions, TAI, intravascular lymphoma, fat emboli, or Rocky Mountain spotted fever. History, clinical presentation, underlying risk factors, and follow-up imaging will play a pivotal role in categorizing the differential diagnosis, treatment, and prognosis of these conditions.

Differential Diagnosis

Cardioembolic infarcts, embolic shower
Septic-embolic encephalitis
Metastatic disease
Traumatic axonal injury
Fat emboli
Lymphoma
Rocky Mountain spotted fever
Demyelinating lesions

Pearls

- Although often a diagnostic challenge for the neuroradiologist, some MRI characteristics of numerous DWI hyperintense lesions as well as clinical presentation, history, and follow-up studies can help in establishing an appropriate diagnosis.
- Cases of cerebral metastases with diffusion restriction have occurred in patients with lung cancer, breast cancer, colon cancer, testicular cancer, and renal cancer.
- Fat emboli should be suspected in the setting of long bone fracture, sickle cell crisis, shortness of breath, and/or petechial rash.
- Cardioembolic infarcts should be considered in patients with atrial fibrillation, myocardial infarction, valvular disease, and endocarditis.

- TAI frequently occurs in association with high-speed motor vehicle accidents.
- TAI, fat emboli, septic emboli, and Rocky Mountain spotted fever DWI hyperintense lesions are usually accompanied by microhemorrhages. Hemorrhages are less common with metastases, cardioembolic infarcts, lymphoma, and demyelination.
- Lesions in the splenium and brainstem are more common with TAI, lymphoma, demyelinative lesion, fat emboli, and Rocky Mountain spotted fever.
- The starry sky appearance on DWI is typical of fat emboli and Rocky Mountain spotted fever.
- Edema and enhancement are more common with metastases, lymphoma, demyelination, Rocky Mountain spotted fever, and septic emboli.
- Demyelinative lesions with restricted diffusion and/or enhancement are usually seen in the setting of numerous additional nonenhancing periventricular, callosal, juxtacortical, and brainstem lesions that do not show restricted diffusion.

Signs and Complications

- A low GCS in a patient who has experienced trauma is suggestive of TAI.
- In a patient with long bone fracture, petechial rash, shortness of breath, and altered mental status, fat emboli syndrome should be considered.
- Sudden onset of neurologic deficit, especially in the presence of known cardiac risk factors is suggestive of cardioembolic strokes. In-hospital mortality in cardioembolic stroke is the highest as compared with other subtypes of cerebral infarction, and thus, in general it is a severe clinical condition; hence, a prompt diagnosis is necessary.
- CNS involvement during the course of infective endocarditis occurs in ~30% (range 20% to 40%) of cases. Presence of mycotic aneurysm and history of known bacterial endocarditis may suggest septic-embolic encephalitis.
- Presence of an underlying malignancy, especially if hypercellular, raises the concern for an intracranial metastatic disease and warrants follow-up studies to confirm stability or progression of the disease.
- A history of optic neuritis and/or other prior neurologic deficits such as numbness, weakness, and fatigue suggest a demyelinative process.
- Intravascular lymphoma should be considered in older patients who have CNS and systemic symptoms without signs of an infectious or inflammatory process (Fig. 6.1).
- Rocky Mountain spotted fever is a bacterial disease transmitted by ticks. Headache, fever, and rash are typical presenting symptoms.

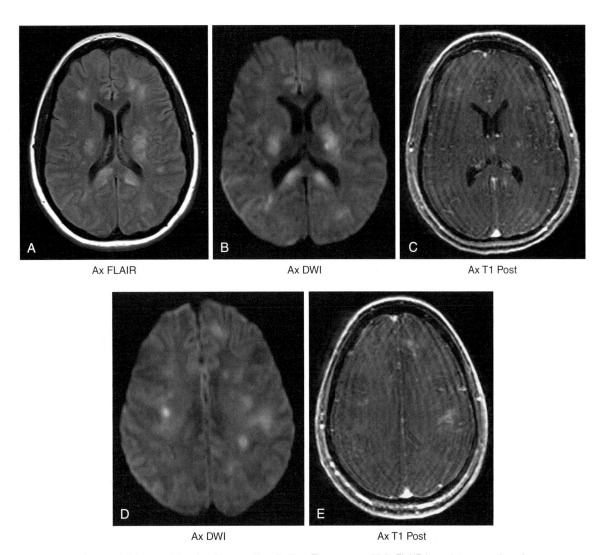

Ax FLAIR   Ax DWI   Ax T1 Post

Ax DWI   Ax T1 Post

• **Fig. 6.1** A 64-year-old male with cognitive decline. There are multiple FLAIR hyperintense, enhancing lesions with restricted diffusion in the periventricular, deep, and subcortical white matter, typical of intravascular lymphoma. *Ax,* Axial; *DWI,* diffusion-weighted imaging; *FLAIR,* fluid attenuated inversion recovery.

Suggested Readings

Arboix A, Alió J. Cardioembolic stroke: clinical features, specific cardiac disorders and prognosis, *Curr Cardiol Rev* 6(3):150–161, 2010.

Gofton TE, Young GB. Sepsis-associated encephalopathy, *Nat Rev Neurol* 8(10):557–566, 2012.

Hayashida Y, Hirai T, Morishita S, et al: Diffusion-weighted imaging of metastatic brain tumors: comparison with histologic type and tumor cellularity, *AJNR Am J Neuroradiol* 27(7):1419–1425, 2006.

Hergan K, Schaefer PW, Sorensen AG, et al: Diffusion-weighted MRI in diffuse axonal injury of the brain, *Eur Radiol* 12(10):2536–2541, 2002.

Hess A, Klein I, Iung B, et al: Brain MRI findings in neurologically asymptomatic patients with infective endocarditis, *AJNR AM J Neuroradiol* 34(8):1579–1584, 2013.

Loureiro BMC, Reis F, Pereira GF, et al: Rocky Mountain spotted fever: brain imaging findings, *Braz J Infect Dis* 22(2):153–154, 2018.

Momota H, Narita Y, Miyakita Y, et al: Intravascular lymphoma of the central nervous system presenting as multiple cerebral infarctions, *Nagoya J Med Sci* 74(3–4):353–358, 2012.

Ryu CW, Lee DH, Kim TK, et al: Cerebral fat embolism: diffusion-weighted magnetic resonance imaging findings, *Acta Radiol* 46(5): 528–533, 2005.

Sarbu N, Shih RY, Oleaga L, et al: RadioGraphics update: white matter diseases with radiologic-pathologic correlation. *Radiographics* 40(3): E4–E7, 2020.

7

Cortical Restricted Diffusion

YUH-SHIN CHANG, MD, PHD AND PAMELA W. SCHAEFER, MD

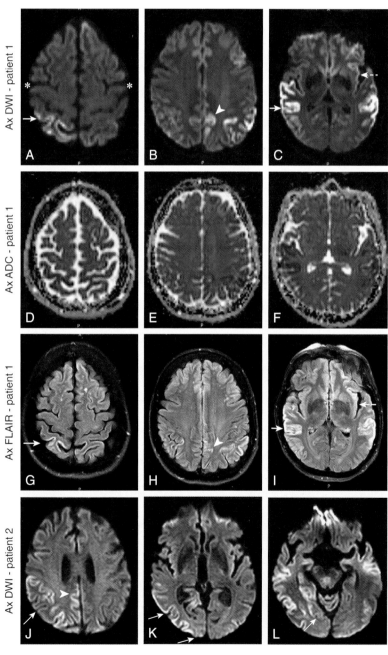

CASE A: (A–I) A 65-year-old female with rapidly progressive dementia, word finding difficulties and dyscalculia. (J–L) A 78-year-old male with 1 week-history of progressive limb apraxia, optic ataxia, agraphesthesia, visuospatial problems. *ADC,* Apparent diffusion coefficient; *Ax,* axial; *DWI,* diffusion-weighted imaging; *FLAIR,* fluid-attenuated inversion recovery.

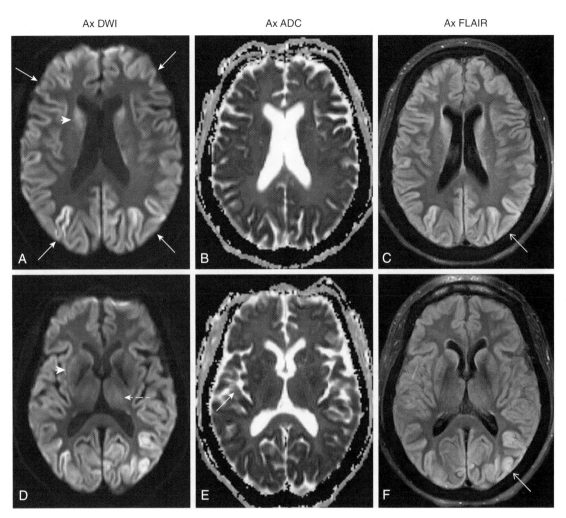

Ax DWI   Ax ADC   Ax FLAIR

CASE B: A 78-year-old female who was revived after cardiac arrest. *ADC,* Apparent diffusion coefficient; *Ax,* axial; *DWI,* diffusion-weighted imaging; *FLAIR,* fluid-attenuated inversion recovery.

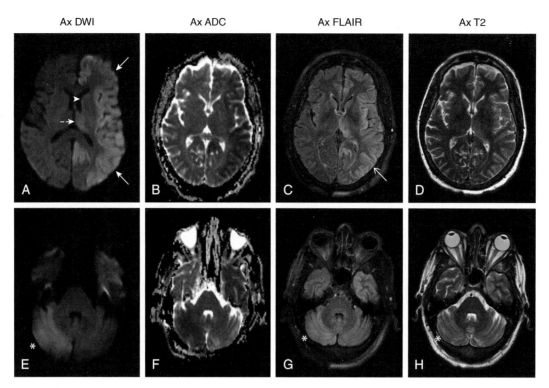

CASE C: A 53-year-old male with alcohol use disorder who was found with left gaze preference, right-sided hemiparesis, and EEG findings of ongoing seizure. *ADC,* Apparent diffusion coefficient; *Ax,* axial; *DWI,* diffusion-weighted imaging; *FLAIR,* fluid-attenuated inversion recovery.

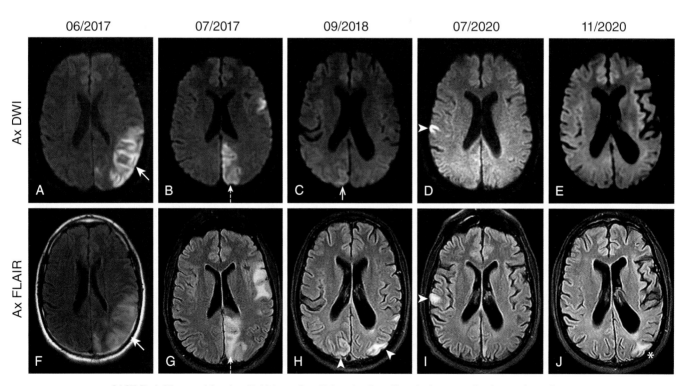

CASE D: A 29-year-old male with history of multiple episodes of headache, paresthesias, and transient vision loss. *Ax,* Axial; *DWI,* diffusion-weighted imaging; *FLAIR,* fluid-attenuated inversion recovery.

Ax DWI   Ax ADC   Ax FLAIR   Ax T2

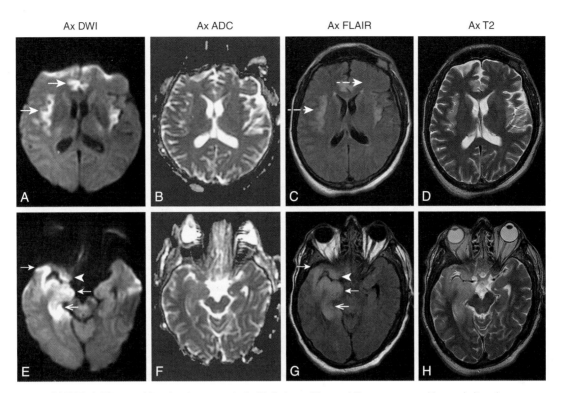

CASE E: A 59-year-old male who presented with 3 days of fever, chills, nausea, vomiting and altered consciousness. *ADC,* Apparent diffusion coefficient; *Ax,* axial; *DWI,* diffusion-weighted imaging; *FLAIR,* fluid-attenuated inversion recovery.

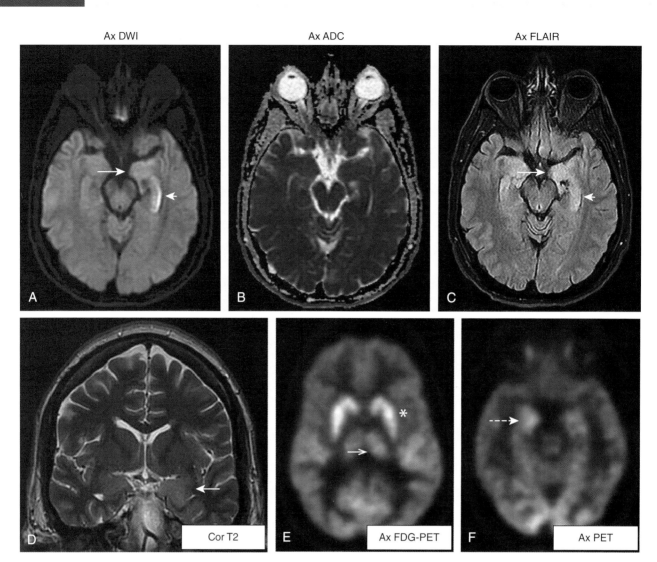

Ax DWI · Ax ADC · Ax FLAIR · Cor T2 · Ax FDG-PET · Ax PET

CASE F: A 56-year-old male with history of faciobrachial dystonic seizures and cognitive impairment.
ADC, Apparent diffusion coefficient; *Ax,* axial; *DWI,* diffusion-weighted imaging; *FLAIR,* fluid-attenuated inversion recovery ; cor T2, coronal T2-weighted imaging; FDG-PET, [18F]Fluorodeoxyglucose.

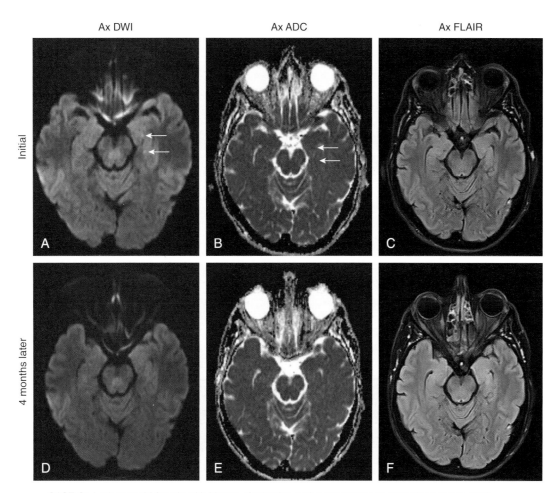

| | Ax DWI | Ax ADC | Ax FLAIR |

CASE G: A 72-year-old female with history of migraine and acute onset anterograde amnesia. *ADC,* Apparent diffusion coefficient; *Ax,* axial; *DWI,* diffusion-weighted imaging; *FLAIR,* fluid-attenuated inversion recovery.

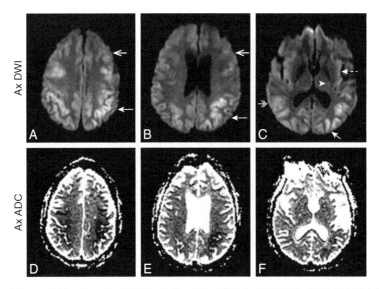

CASE H: A 33-year-old female with diabetes mellitus type I (DM I), presented with right facial droop, hemiparesis, and slurred speech, and found to be in diabetic ketoacidosis. Became unresponsive after insulin administration. *ADC,* Apparent diffusion coefficient; *Ax,* axial; *DWI,* diffusion-weighted imaging.

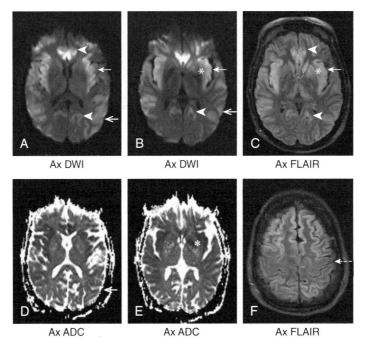

CASE I: A 57-year-old female with liver failure from secondary biliary cirrhosis, with progressive altered mental status. *ADC,* Apparent diffusion coefficient; *Ax,* axial; *DWI,* diffusion-weighted imaging; *FLAIR,* fluid-attenuated inversion recovery.

DESCRIPTION OF FINDINGS

MRI scans from eight patients that demonstrate cortical restriction diffusion.

- Case A: Axial diffusion-weighted imaging (DWI) (A–C) and ADC (D–F) MR demonstrate bilateral relatively symmetric cortical diffusion restriction in the parietal and temporal lobes (arrows) and, to a lesser extent, in the left insula (dashed arrow) and posterior left cingulate gyrus (arrowhead). Other areas of subtle diffusion restriction include both thalami and anterior lentiform nuclei. The perirolandic regions are spared (*). (G–I) The cortex with restricted diffusion is hyperintense on fluid-attenuated inversion recovery (FLAIR) images (arrows), but there is no gyral swelling or sulcal effacement. (J–L) MR imaging in a different patient demonstrates bilateral asymmetric cortical diffusion restriction predominantly in the parietal, temporal, and occipital lobes (arrows), right greater than left posterior cingulate gyri (arrowhead). Subcortical structures are not affected.
- Case B: (A–F) Axial DWI and FLAIR show extensive symmetric cortical diffusion restriction and FLAIR hyperintensity in both cerebral hemispheres (arrows), not conforming to vascular territories. The basal ganglia (arrowhead) and thalami (dashed arrow) are also involved. There is mild mass effect with effacement of sulci (open arrow) consistent with diffuse cortical edema.
- Case C: (A–D) DWI MRI demonstrates extensive cortical diffusion restriction involving most of the left cerebral hemisphere (arrow), left caudate nucleus (arrowhead), left medial, and posteromedial thalamus (dashed arrow). There is associated gyral swelling with sulcal effacement (open arrow) and hyperperfusion (not shown). (E–H) There is also diffuse restricted diffusion and T2/FLAIR hyperintense edema in the contralateral right cerebellar hemisphere (*) as well as hyperperfusion (not shown), consistent with crossed cerebellar diaschisis.
- Case D: Axial DWI and FLAIR images from multiple MR studies over 3 years demonstrate areas of cortical T2/FLAIR hyperintensity, in some instances with diffusion restriction, in a migratory pattern. (A, F) Initial axial DWI and FLAIR images show cortical diffusion restriction and cortical/subcortical FLAIR hyperintensity with edema predominantly in the lateral left parietal lobe (arrow). (B, G) Follow-up axial MR images 1 month later show resolution of the signal abnormality in the lateral left parietal lobe and new areas of cortical diffusion restriction in the left frontal operculum, and paramedian left parietal lobe (dashed arrow). There is associated cortical/subcortical FLAIR hyperintensity and edema. (C, H) MR imaging 1 year later shows resolution of the changes seen on 07/2017 and new areas of subtle cortical diffusion restriction in the right paramedian parietal lobe and cortical/subcortical FLAIR hyperintensity in the left parietal lobe and right paramedian parietal lobe (open arrow) with mild gyral swelling (arrowhead). (D, I) Two years later, the axial DWI shows resolution of the findings seen on 09/2018, new cortical diffusion restriction, FLAIR hyperintensity and gyral swelling in the lateral right precentral gyrus (arrowhead), and a FLAIR hyperintense focus in the left paramedian parietal lobe with no DWI signal abnormality. (E, J) Follow-up MRI 4 months later shows resolution of the diffusion restriction findings seen in (D, I) and a new small FLAIR hyperintense area in the left posterior parietal lobe (*).
- Case E: (A–D) There is symmetric DWI hyperintensity with no apparent diffusion coefficient (ADC) hypointensity and T2/FLAIR hyperintensity with mild edema in both insular cortices and cingulate gyri (arrows). There is associated cortical and subcortical FLAIR-hyperintense edema with relative sparing of the white matter (dashed arrow). (E–H) Asymmetric areas of T2/FLAIR hyperintensity and DWI hyperintensity with no ADC hypointensity in the right mesial temporal and anterior temporal lobe (arrows), right hippocampus (open arrow), and right inferior frontal lobe (arrowhead). There is marked edema in the right mesial temporal lobe (arrow) and hippocampus (open arrow). No hemorrhage or enhancement is noted.
- Case F: (A–C) Asymmetric left greater than right DWI and T2/FLAIR hyperintensity in both amygdala (arrow) and hippocampi (arrowhead). ADC values are slightly reduced in the corresponding areas. (D) Coronal T2 image shows T2 hyperintense edema in the left hippocampus. (E–F) Fluorodeoxyglucose positron emission tomography ((FDG-PET) shows

hypermetabolism in the caudate nuclei, putamen (*), thalami (open arrow), and mesial temporal lobes (dashed arrow) bilaterally.
- Case G: (A–C) MRI done at the time of presentation shows two faint punctate diffusion restricting foci in the left hippocampus (arrows) with no correlation on FLAIR. (D–F) Follow-up MRI performed 4 months later shows complete resolution of the DWI findings.
- Case H: (A–F) There is cortical diffusion restriction predominantly in the parietooccipital regions (arrow) and temporal lobes (double arrow), posterior limbs of the internal capsules (arrowhead), and to a lesser extent in the insulae (dashed arrow) and frontal lobes (open arrow).
- Case I: Imaging findings demonstrate bilateral swollen, T2/FLAIR hyperintense gyri (C, F) with diffusion restriction (A–B, D–E) most severely involving the insular cortex (arrow), cingulate gyri (arrowhead), and the left basal ganglia (*). (F) There is sparing of the perirolandic (dashed arrow) and occipital regions (not shown).

Diagnosis

Case A: Creutzfeldt–Jakob disease (CJD). (Top rows) Sporadic CJD. (Bottom row) Heidenhain phenotypic variant of sporadic CJD.

Case B: Global hypoxic-ischemic injury

Case C: Status epilepticus

Case D: Mitochondrial encephalomyopathy, lactic acidosis and stroke-like episodes (MELAS) syndrome

Case E: Herpes simplex type 1 encephalitis

Case F: Autoimmune encephalitis

Case G: Transient global amnesia

Case H: Hypoglycemia

Case I: Acute hepatic encephalopathy

Summary

The investigation of patients presenting with altered mental status includes neuroimaging with MRI, in particular when the initial CT imaging is unrevealing. In these patients, MRI often reveals small, previously unrecognized acute cerebral infarcts. Less frequently, patterns of restricted diffusion limited to the cerebral cortex are identified. Although uncommon, cortical restricted diffusion is seen in a limited number of clinical scenarios, and accurate interpretation is often an important step in reaching a definite diagnosis. In some instances, the evaluation of cortical diffusion restriction anomalies may guide clinical prognosis.

The presence of restricted diffusion is most often associated with acute cerebral ischemia. In this setting, the prevailing theory is that the biophysical process leading to restricted water diffusivity is secondary to cytotoxic edema caused by disruption of energy metabolism, failure of cellular ion pumps and structural changes at the level of intracellular organelles, each contributing to reduced water diffusivity. With its high metabolic demand, the cerebral cortex is uniquely sensitive to conditions affecting its energy metabolism, such as situations affecting the respiratory chain, e.g. hypoxia, hypoglycemia, or mitochondrial diseases. Other conditions associated with cytotoxic edema include hyperammonemia, infection, or seizures. In other instances, such as in transient global amnesia or in Creutzfeldt–Jakob disease, the mechanism underlying diffusion restriction remains speculative.

In the approach to the interpretation of cortical diffusion restriction, an important consideration is pattern distribution. A bilateral and symmetric pattern points to a defect in metabolic supply or metabolic disorder as the underlying cause. Alternatively, an asymmetric pattern suggests that focal processes, such as an infectious or neurodegenerative disorder, or a postictal state, are causative.

Spectrum of Disease

Creutzfeldt–Jakob Disease

Numerous studies have established the essential role of MRI in the diagnostic evaluation of patients suspected to have CJD. Current MRI imaging criteria require that restricted diffusion be present in the striatum, cingulate gyri, and/or neocortex. Imaging criteria based on diffusion restriction have proven to be highly specific and sensitive in the diagnosis of CJD, surpassing conventional tests such as electroencephalogram (EEG) and cerebrospinal fluid (CSF) protein biomarkers, and are comparable to values obtained using prion-based techniques such as real-time quaking induced conversion (RT-QuIC).

Typically, the pattern of cortical restricted diffusion is bilateral and asymmetric, and mainly involves the insula, cingulate gyrus, and gyri of the parietal and frontal lobes with relative sparing of the perirolandic area. Isolated involvement of limbic structures is not seen. The cerebral cortex and basal ganglia are affected in 70% of cases. Restricted diffusion predominates in the caudate nuclei, followed by the putamen and thalamus. The globus pallidus is relatively spared. Diffusion restriction limited to the cortex is identified in 24% of patients with CJD. The remaining cases show only striatal involvement. There is no contrast enhancement, and no cortical or subcortical edema is apparent on FLAIR/T2-weighed imaging.

The MRI diffusion restriction patterns have been found to differ depending on the clinical and genetic subtypes of CJD. The biophysical process underlying the restriction of diffusion in CJD remains uncertain. Vacuoles formed within neurons are thought to be an important factor restricting water displacement in affected areas.

HSV1 Encephalitis

Herpes simplex virus type 1 encephalitis (HSE) is the most commonly identified form of focal encephalitis. Involvement of the mesial temporal and orbitofrontal lobes, the insula, and the cingulate gyri are typical of HSE, while the basal ganglia are spared. Lesions can be unilateral or bilateral. In the latter situation, the lesions are often asymmetric. Cortical diffusion restriction abnormalities in these areas are an early finding and are secondary to the cytotoxic injury caused by neuronal viral infection. These anomalies can precede the identification of herpes simplex virus type 1 DNA in the CSF by polymerase chain reaction (PCR). Other imaging findings include edema of the affected structures with associated T2 and FLAIR hyperintensity, and hemorrhages. Once vasogenic edema has developed and diffusion increases, DWI hyperintense signal persists

due to T2 hyperintensity but the ADC hypointensity may no longer be present. Contrast enhancement is variable. In a large cohort of patients with temporal lobe encephalitis, bilateral temporal lobe involvement and lesions outside the temporal lobe, insula, or cingulate predicted lower odds of HSE. When present, extratemporal involvement in HSE is more often seen in pediatric or immunocompromised patients. Although restricted diffusion is a sensitive MRI finding early in the course of HSE, it should not be used to differentiate HSE from other causes of temporal lobe encephalitis.

Cortical restricted diffusion has additionally been described in other types of viral encephalitis. However, neuroimaging findings affecting extratemporal regions help to differentiate these cases from HSE.

Immune-mediated disorders are an increasingly recognized cause of temporal lobe encephalitis. Multiple autoantibodies have been identified, and varying clinical and MRI findings have been described depending on the antibody involved. Cortical restricted diffusion is however rare. Extratemporal involvement further distinguishes these cases from HSE.

Acute Hepatic Encephalopathy

Hyperammonemia from severe acute liver failure or from genetic metabolic disorders can cause cortical diffusion restriction preferentially involving the insular cortex and cingulate gyri, in a bilateral and symmetric pattern. Involvement of other cortical areas is variable. The occipital lobes and perirolandic region are relatively spared. T2 and FLAIR hyperintense signals and cortical swelling are often present. Contrast enhancement is variable. Diffusion restriction abnormalities are also present in the thalamus and other subcortical structures. Hyperammonemia appears to cause these MRI changes primarily through the osmotic effect of glutamine in astrocytes, resulting in cytotoxic edema. Symmetric involvement of the insular cortex and cingulate gyri suggests acute hepatic encephalopathy rather than hypoxic-ischemic encephalopathy.

Acute Hypoglycemic Encephalopathy

Cortical diffusion restriction can be seen in acute severe hypoglycemia. Signal abnormalities are usually bilateral and symmetric, and most commonly include gyriform T2/FLAIR hyperintensity and strong diffusion restriction in the parieto-occipital and temporal lobes. Other commonly involved areas include the internal capsules, basal ganglia, hippocampi, and amygdalae. In severe cases, the globus pallidus and striatum are involved. The thalami, brainstem, white matter, and cerebellum are typically spared, which differentiates the findings in hypoglycemia from those of hypoxic-ischemic encephalopathy. Thalamic involvement is one of the features differentiating status epilepticus from hypoglycemic encephalopathy. Hypoglycemia causes restricted diffusion because it leads to cellular energy failure, which results in sodium/potassium pump failure and cytotoxic edema. The patterns of diffusion restriction observed in hypoglycemic encephalopathy can be used for prognostic implications, with persistent lesions in the basal ganglia on follow-up imaging being associated with poor outcome.

Hypoxic-Ischemic Injury

In adults, hypoxic-ischemic injury is most often seen following cardiac arrest, drowning, or asphyxiation. Moderate-to-severe hypoxic-ischemic injury causes bilateral and symmetric diffusion restriction abnormalities in the perirolandic and occipital cortex. In more severe cases, the entire cerebral cortex may be affected. Other susceptible areas include the thalamus, cerebellum, cerebral white matter, caudate, and putamen. There is diffuse cerebral edema with gyral swelling and sulcal effacement, and affected structures appear hyperintense on T2-weighed and FLAIR images.

Apparent diffusion coefficient (ADC) changes appearing after a severe hypoxic-ischemic injury follow a different time course than during an acute stroke, and diffusion restriction may not be apparent in the initial hours after a hypoxic-ischemic event. Cortical diffusion restriction changes are most apparent between 3 and 5 days. Patients with less severe injuries may instead show normal or even increased diffusivity during this time period, due to vasogenic edema counterbalancing the effects of the cytotoxic edema. Following cardiac arrests in adults, the presence of diffusion restriction in cortical regions predicts an unfavorable patient outcome.

In neonates, the imaging findings of hypoxic-ischemic brain injury differ from that seen in adults. Two main patterns (peripheral and basal ganglia/thalamus) have been described in neonates, depending on brain maturity, duration, and severity of the insult.

Mitochondrial Encephalomyopathy, Lactic Acidosis and Stroke-Like Episodes Syndrome (MELAS)

This rare genetic syndrome is caused by mutations in the mitochondrial genome and affects children and young adults. Classically, patients present with a triad of lactic acidosis, focal or generalized seizures, and stroke-like episodes. Other clinical manifestations include sensorineural hearing loss, recurrent migraine-like headaches, short stature, diabetes, and muscle weakness. The stroke-like episodes are likely caused by angiopathy, secondary to mitochondrial dysfunction.

MR findings include diffusion restriction and/or T2/FLAIR hyperintense lesions in the cerebral cortex and, to a lesser extent, in the subcortical white matter, commonly of different ages, in a migratory and fluctuating pattern and not respecting vascular territories. There is a predilection for the parietooccipital and temporal lobes involving the primary visual cortex, the middle-third of the primary somatosensory cortex and primary auditory cortex. These acute cortical lesions are symmetric in half of the cases. Diffusion restriction in other cortical regions and in the thalamic nuclei and cerebellar hemisphere are less common.

Status Epilepticus

The role of neuroimaging in refractory seizures and status epilepticus lies in localizing the seizure focus and identifying an underlying structural abnormality. Estimates of the incidence of neuroimaging changes following seizures vary, but are evaluated to occur in between 5% and 30% of patients. These changes are more common following status epilepticus than after a single seizure or after a cluster of seizures. In the region of the epileptic discharge, the sustained ictal activity creates a situation where the cellular energy demands become greater than the supply. This energy deficit results in inactivation of ion pumps, leading to cytotoxic edema. Vasogenic edema secondary to alteration in cell membrane permeability and blood brain barrier breakdown is also present.

Status epilepticus–related MR findings in the acute phase include gyriform cortical diffusion restriction, rising greater than 1 hour after seizure onset, peaking between 1 and 2 days and resolving by day 7. The restricted diffusion and associated T2/FLAIR hyperintensity with gyral swelling are related to cytotoxic edema and can be seen in the cerebral cortex and/or subcortical white matter with possible additional involvement of the hippocampus, thalamus, or splenium of the corpus callosum. Its presence indicates more prolonged and permanent cell injury and worse prognosis and can resolve within days or persist for weeks. Findings on perfusion weighted imaging and PET differ with seizure activity. In the ictal phase, perfusion weighted imaging demonstrates increased relative cerebral blood flow and relative cerebral blood volume and PET demonstrates hypermetabolism. In the interictal phase, hypoperfusion and hypometabolism are demonstrated in the epileptogenic region. Gyriform or leptomeningeal enhancement may be present. MR spectroscopy shows an elevated lipid and/or lactate peak within 24 hours after seizure onset. Additional findings include T2 prolongation or restricted diffusion in the splenium of the corpus callosum or in the contralateral cerebellar hemisphere, termed crossed cerebellar diaschisis. In the chronic phase, focal atrophy in the affected brain parenchyma can be present.

Transient Global Amnesia

Hippocampal lesions are frequently identified on diffusion-weighted MRI in patients with transient global amnesia. There is typically a single lesion. These lesions are small, with a mean size of 4 mm. Lesions are more often left-sided, but can also be right-sided or bilateral. The lesions are detected in more than 90% of patients within a 12-to-24-hour time window. Imaging can be normal in the acute (0 to 12 h) period, and these lesions remain present on diffusion-weighed MRI for about a week. Surprisingly, 7T MRI performed within months after an episode of transient global amnesia shows no remaining structural abnormality at the site of the previous hippocampal lesion. The mechanism underlying these diffusion restriction abnormalities remains unclear, since ischemic lesions are larger and appear earlier after the onset of symptoms. In addition, a residual lesion would be expected after an ischemic injury.

Differential Diagnosis for Cortical Restricted Diffusion

- CJD
- Encephalitis
- Hyperammonemia
- Hypoglycemia
- Hypoxic-ischemic injury
- MELAS
- Seizures
- Transient global amnesia

Pearls

- Symmetry: An important consideration in evaluating cortical restricted diffusion is to determine whether the pattern of MRI findings is symmetric. A symmetric involvement strongly hints that the underlying disorder is either a defect in the energy supply to the brain, such as hypoxia or hypoglycemia, or an underlying metabolic disorder such as hyperammonemia. Alternatively, an asymmetric pattern of restricted diffusion is commonly seen with seizures, transient global amnesia, HSE, MELAS, and CJD.
- Distribution: In most cases, a quick and accurate interpretation of cortical restricted diffusion anomalies is possible, since each condition has a fairly typical distribution of imaging anomalies. Some of the more common imaging patterns are presented in the Figures (Cases A-I). Important features allowing the differentiation between these conditions are summarized in Table 7.1.
- Edema and contrast enhancement: Parenchymal edema and contrast enhancement are not features of CJD. If these

TABLE 7.1 **Imaging Features of Conditions Associated With Cortical Restricted Diffusion**

		CORTEX		SUBCORTICAL AREAS			
	Pattern	Affected	Spared	Affected	Spared	Edema/Contrast Enhancement	Clinical Context; Others
CJD	B/A	Insula, cingulate, parietal, frontal	Perirolandic	Caudate, putamen, thalamus	Globus pallidus	−/−	Rapidly progressive dementia; positive RT-QuIC (CSF, other)
Encephalitis (HSV-1)	U>B/A	Temporal, frontal, insula, cingulate	Rarely widespread (immune compromised)	Uncommon	Basal ganglia, thalamus	+/+	Fever, confusion, seizures; hemorrhages; positive HSV-1 PCR in CSF
Hyperammonemia	B/S	Insula, cingulate	Occipital, perirolandic; rarely widespread	Thalamus, periventricular white matter, brainstem	Other areas not reported	+/ID	Hepatic failure (90%); laboratory confirmation (NH_3)
Hypoglycemia	B/S	Parieto-occipital and temporal lobes; hippocampus	Can be widespread	Basal ganglia, internal capsule	Thalamus, cerebellum, brainstem	+/+	Insulin/hypoglycemic agent; laboratory confirmation
Hypoxic/ischemic injury	B/S	Perirolandic and occipital	Can be widespread	Thalamus, cerebellum, striatum, white matter (can be delayed)	Can be widespread	+/+	Cardiac arrest
MELAS	B/S (50%)	Occipital, parietal, temporal	All lobes can be affected	Subcortical white matter, thalamus, cerebellum, brainstem	Cerebral deep white matter	+/+	Stroke in young adult; encephalomalacia, cerebral atrophy
Seizures	U>B/A	Temporal (75%)	All lobes can be affected	Thalamus, splenium of corpus callosum, contralateral cerebellum, basal ganglia, claustrum	Other areas not reported	+/+	Seizures, unresponsiveness
TGA	U (left)>B/A	Hippocampus (>97%)	–	–	–	−/−	Amnestic event; small (4 mm) often unique lesion

A, Asymmetric; *B,* bilateral; *CSF,* cerebrospinal fluid; *HSV-1,* herpes simplex virus type 1; *ID,* insufficient data; *RT-QuIC,* real-time quaking induced conversion; *S,* symmetric; *U,* unilateral.

features are detected on MRI, alternative diagnoses should be considered.

- History and laboratory findings: Most of the conditions associated with cortical restricted diffusion are acute, and the history and laboratory findings should provide important clues toward reaching the diagnosis. In contrast, patients affected with CJD present with a subacute and unrelenting cognitive decline.
- Multiple etiologies may be present: Rarely, there may be more than one cause to explain the pattern of cortical diffusion restriction observed in a patient. For example, seizures are common following a prolonged cardiac arrest, or in patients with severe hypoglycemia or hyperammonemia, and some radiologic overlap may be identified.

Future Developments

Although morphological imaging data from MRI can be used to predict functional outcome after an ischemic stroke, its use in predicting the outcome in other types of cerebral injury has been limited. There is, however, an important need to develop precise tools to predict outcome in patients with severe neurological injury, because of the limited sensitivity of current prognostic tools that are based on clinical evaluation. In patients surviving a cardiac arrest, quantitative diffusion-weighed MRI has been shown to be both specific and sensitive in identifying poor outcome patients. Eventually, quantitative diffusion-weighed MRI analysis may be commonly used as a tool to facilitate outcome prediction following a cardiac arrest. Additionally, quantitative diffusion-weighed MRI may be used as a prognostic tool in other conditions in which there is severe cortical injury, for example, in determining the prognosis of patients with prolonged status epilepticus.

Suggested Readings

Bhatia KD, Krishnan P, Kortman H, et al: Acute cortical lesions in MELAS syndrome: Anatomic distribution, symmetry, and evolution, *AJNR Am J Neuroradiol* 41(1):167–173, 2020.

Chow FC, Glaser CA, Sheriff H, et al: Use of clinical and neuroimaging characteristics to distinguish temporal lobe herpes simplex encephalitis from its mimics, *Clin Infect Dis* 60(9):1377–1383, 2015.

Ghei SK, Zan E, Nathan JE, et al: MR imaging of hypoxic-ischemic injury in term neonates: Pearls and pitfalls, *Radiographics* 34(4):1047–1061, 2014.

Goncalves FG, Alves CAPF, Heuer B, et al: Primary mitochondrial disorders of the pediatric central nervous system: neuroimaging findings, *Radiographics* 40:2042–2067, 2020.

Guerriero RM, Gaillard WD: Imaging modalities to diagnose and localize status epilepticus, *Eur J Epilepsy* 68:46–51, 2019.

Hermann P, Appleby B, Brandel JP, et al: Biomarkers and diagnostic guidelines for sporadic Creutzfeldt-Jakob disease: *Lancet Neurol* 20(3):235–246, 2021.

Hershman M, Carmody R, Udayasankar UK: Case 252: Acute hyperammonemic encephalopathy resulting from late-onset ornithine transcarbamylase deficiency: *Radiology* 287(1):353–359, 2018.

Hirsch KG, Fischbein N, Mlynash M, et al: Prognostic value of diffusion-weighted MRI for post-cardiac arrest coma: *Neurology* 95(4):e335–e341, 2020.

Kang EG, Jeon SJ, Choi SS, et al: Diffusion MR imaging of hypoglycemic encephalopathy, *AJNR Am J Neuroradiol* 31(3):559–564, 2010.

Paech D, Kuder TA, Roßmanith C, et al: What remains after transient global amnesia (TGA)? An ultra-high field 7 T magnetic resonance imaging study of the hippocampus, *Eur J Neurol* 27(2):406–409, 2020.

Rennebaum F, Kassubek J, Pinkhardt E, et al: Status epilepticus: clinical characteristics and EEG patterns associated with and without MRI diffusion restriction in 69 patients, *Epilepsy Res* 120:55–64, 2016.

Rosenbloom MH, Tartaglia MC, Forner SA, et al: Metabolic disorders with clinical and radiologic features of sporadic Creutzfeldt-Jakob disease, *Neurol Clin Pract* 5(2):108–115, 2015.

Schaefer PW, Grant PE, Gonzalez RG: Diffusion-weighted MR imaging of the brain, *Radiology* 217(2):331–345, 2000.

White ML, Zhang Y, Helvey JT, et al: Anatomical patterns and correlated MRI findings of non-perinatal hypoxic-ischaemic encephalopathy, *Br J Radiol* 86(1021):20120464, 2013.

8

Ring-Enhancing Lesions

JUAN E. SMALL, MD, MSC

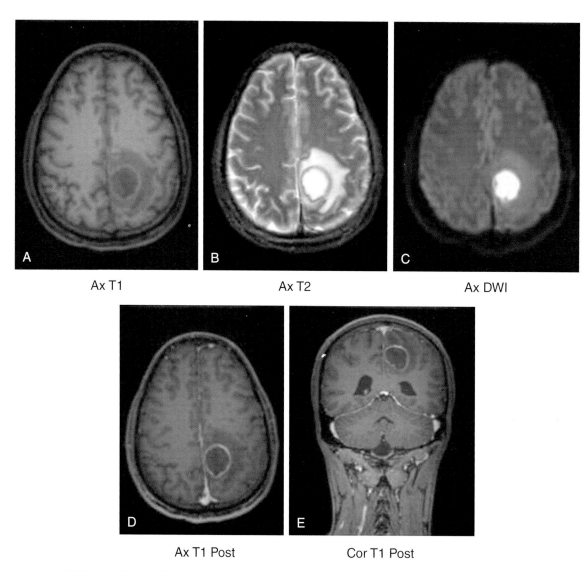

Ax T1

Ax T2

Ax DWI

Ax T1 Post

Cor T1 Post

CASE A: A 39-year-old who had a dental procedure several weeks earlier now presenting with right leg numbness and weakness. *Ax*, Axial; *Cor*, coronal; *DWI*, diffusion-weighted imaging.

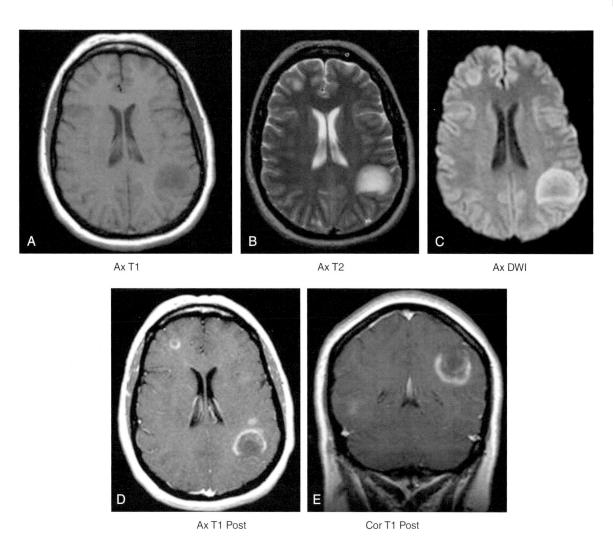

Ax T1

Ax T2

Ax DWI

Ax T1 Post

Cor T1 Post

CASE B: A 37-year-old with a 1-month history of right-sided numbness presenting with a 3-day history of right-sided weakness. *Ax*, Axial; *Cor*, coronal; *DWI*, diffusion-weighted imaging.

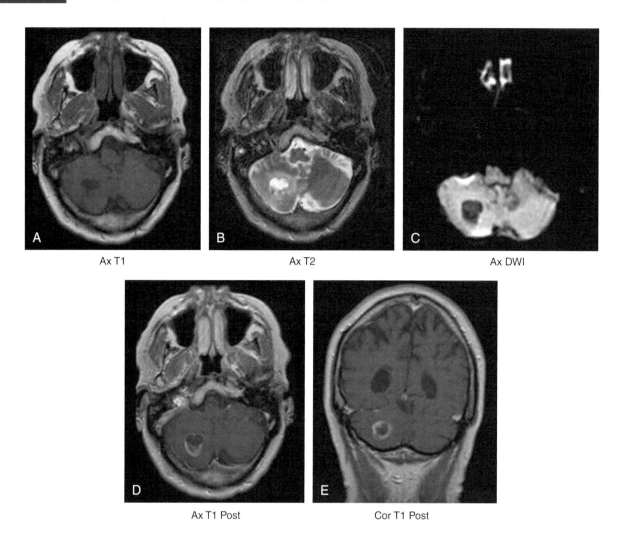

Ax T1   Ax T2   Ax DWI

Ax T1 Post   Cor T1 Post

CASE C: A 70-year-old smoker presenting with shortness of breath and headache of 3 weeks' duration. *Ax*, Axial; *Cor*, coronal; *DWI*, diffusion-weighted imaging.

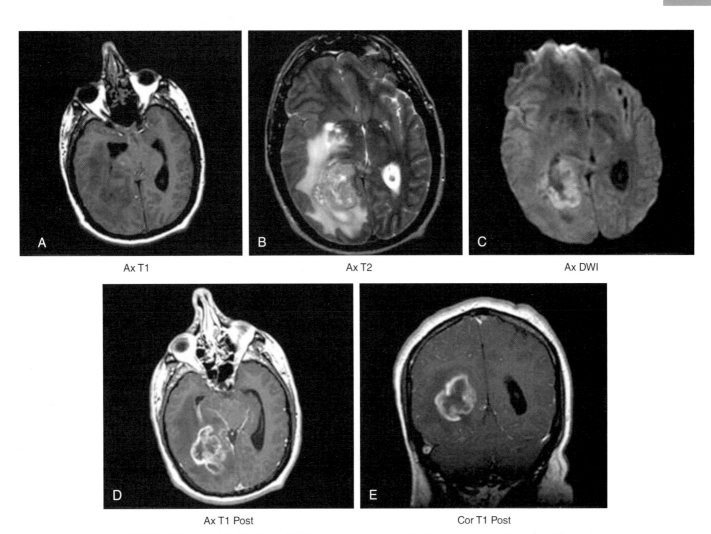

Ax T1

Ax T2

Ax DWI

Ax T1 Post

Cor T1 Post

CASE D: A 41-year-old with a 3-week history of recurrent sinus infections now presenting with rapid onset of headache and confusion. *Ax*, Axial; *Cor*, coronal; *DWI*, diffusion-weighted imaging.

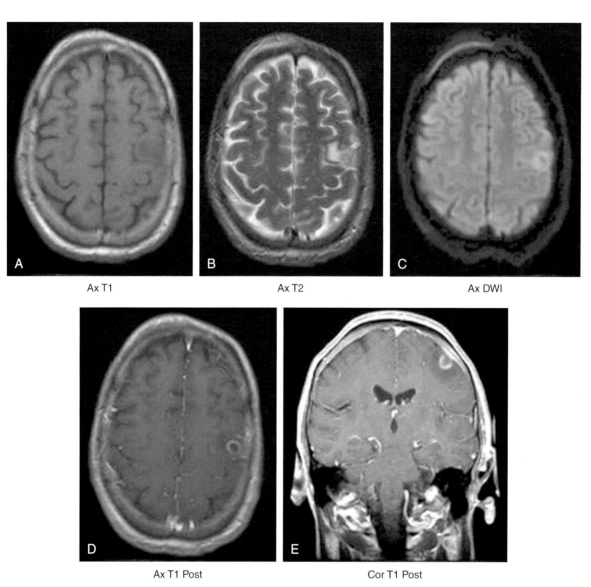

Ax T1

Ax T2

Ax DWI

Ax T1 Post

Cor T1 Post

CASE E: A 36-year-old with a history of chronic renal disease who had two kidney transplants now presenting after a generalized seizure. *Ax*, Axial; *Cor*, coronal; *DWI*, diffusion-weighted imaging.

DESCRIPTION OF FINDINGS

- Case A: There is a 3-cm left parietal lesion with a thin, T2 hypointense peripheral rim, smooth enhancement, prominent surrounding edema, and central restricted diffusion. Of note, the ring of peripheral enhancement is slightly thicker toward its cortical margin.
- Case B: There are multiple supratentorial white matter T2 hyperintense lesions. The largest lesion in the left parietal lobe measures 2.7 cm and demonstrates a thin, smooth, incomplete rim of enhancement. Despite the size of this lesion, a paucity of surrounding edema and mass effect is noted. There is restricted diffusion in the periphery of the lesion but not in the center. Lesions in the right frontal and right occipital lobe also enhance.
- Case C: A 2.2-cm right cerebellar ring-enhancing lesion without associated restricted diffusion is identified. Of note, there is an enhancing internal septation as well as irregularity, nodularity, and varying thickness of the enhancing wall.
- Case D: A 5-cm, heterogeneous right occipital mass demonstrates a thick and nodular rim of enhancement. No internal restricted diffusion is noted. However, DWI hyperintensity associated with the enhancing rim suggests hypercellularity. Subtle ependymal enhancement is noted along the walls of the temporal horn of the right lateral ventricle. Marked surrounding edema and mass effect are noted.
- Case E: This patient was receiving long-term immunosuppression. There is a 1.1-cm ring-enhancing lesion centered in the posterior left middle frontal gyrus with surrounding edema. There is mildly restricted diffusion in the rim of the lesion but not in the center. There is minimal surrounding linear enhancement along perivascular spaces as well as overlying dural enhancement.

Diagnosis

Case A: Abscess
Case B: Multiple sclerosis
Case C: Metastasis
Case D: Glioblastoma multiforme
Case E: Lymphoma (large B-cell lymphoma consistent with posttransplant lymphoproliferative disorder)

Summary

Several important imaging characteristics of ring-enhancing lesions often can lead to a more specific diagnosis:
1. Multiplicity
2. Thin versus a thick/irregular rim of enhancement
3. A thicker outer margin of rim enhancement
4. An incomplete rim of enhancement
5. The presence of adjacent perivascular enhancement
6. A T2 hypointense rim
7. Central restricted diffusion
8. The degree of perilesional edema

A solitary ring-enhancing lesion is usually due to a neoplastic process, infection, or demyelination. In decreasing order of frequency, solitary ring-enhancing lesions represent gliomas, metastases, abscesses, or demyelinating lesions.

Multiplicity, on the other hand, in decreasing order of frequency, suggests metastases, pyogenic abscesses, demyelinating lesions, or opportunistic infections.

In an adult patient, a heterogeneous lesion with a thick, irregular, and nodular rim of enhancement suggests a necrotic neoplastic lesion, such as glioblastoma multiforme or metastasis.

An abscess often presents with specific clues to the diagnosis, including homogeneous central restricted diffusion, an often T2 hypointense peripherally enhancing rim, considerable surrounding edema, and a thicker wall toward the cortex/periphery. Because abscesses tend to grow away from the well-vascularized gray matter, thinning of the medial wall is seen. Hematogenous abscesses (in the setting of endocarditis, cardiac shunts, and pulmonary arteriovenous malformations) are usually multiple and present at gray/white matter junctions. Perilesional edema is usually quite prominent.

Ring enhancement associated with demyelination is often incomplete or open. Open-ring enhancement (i.e., crescent-like enhancement) greatly increases the likelihood that the lesion represents demyelination (the likelihood ratio is 5 times greater than that of a neoplasm and 17 times greater than that of infection). Nevertheless, because of the higher incidence of neoplasms and infection, these entities still remain considerations with this pattern of enhancement. Further support for this diagnosis comes in the form of multiple white matter lesions seen in a typical distribution for demyelination, such as at the callosal-septal interface, and oriented perpendicularly to the ventricular surface.

Primary central nervous system (CNS) lymphoma is a rare form of extranodal non-Hodgkin lymphoma. Primary CNS lymphoma has a distinct imaging appearance because of its hypercellularity and high nuclear/cytoplasmic ratio, as well as the disruption of the blood-brain barrier. Masses are commonly hyperdense to isodense on computed tomography and demonstrate dense homogeneous enhancement. On magnetic resonance imaging, lesions are commonly hypointense to gray matter on T1-weighted images and isointense to hyperintense on T2-weighted images, with the hypercellular nature of these lesions resulting in DWI hyperintensity and apparent diffusion coefficient (ADC) hypointensity. Although avid homogenous enhancement is usually seen in immunocompetent patients, imaging tends to be more variable in immunocompromised patients, and lesions may be heterogeneously enhancing or ring enhancing. Importantly, linear enhancement at the margins of the lesion tracking along Virchow-Robin perivascular spaces is highly specific. Hemorrhage, calcification, and necrosis are rare prior to treatment. In immunocompetent patients, intracranial lesions are solitary 70% of the time, whereas in immunocompromised patients, lesions are equally likely to be multiple versus solitary. Approximately 85% of lesions are supratentorial, with more than 60% of intracranial lesions occurring in a periventricular location and 12% of lesions involving the corpus callosum. The identification of a "transspatial" lesion (i.e., a lesion involving both the intraaxial and extraaxial space) often can be an important clue for the diagnosis of intracranial lymphoma. Transspatial lesions typically have intraparenchymal enhancement with adjacent dural enhancement.

Spectrum of Disease

The spectrum of disease is detailed in the preceding section.

Differential Diagnosis

The differential diagnosis is provided in Table 8.1.

Pearls

- A thick, nodular, or irregular rim of enhancement suggests a tumor.

TABLE 8.1	Solitary vs. Multiple Ring-Enhancing Lesions	
	Solitary Ring-Enhancing Lesion	Multiple Ring-Enhancing Lesions
Common	Metastases, glioblastoma multiforme, abscess, subacute intracerebral hematoma, subacute cerebral infarction, radiation necrosis	Metastases, multiple sclerosis, neurocysticercosis, abscesses
Less common	Tumefactive demyelinating lesion, neurocysticercosis, lymphoma, toxoplasmosis, tuberculoma	Acute disseminated encephalomyelitis, opportunistic infections, tuberculosis, lymphoma, neurosarcoidosis, glioblastoma multiforme
Rare	Subacute lacunar infarction, fungal infection, parasitic infection	Vasculitis, Lyme disease, intravascular lymphoma, parasitic infections

- A lesion demonstrating homogeneous central restricted diffusion, a T2 hypointense, smoothly enhancing rim thicker toward the brain periphery and considerable surrounding edema, suggests an abscess.
- An incomplete rim of enhancement suggests a demyelinative lesion.
- The presence of hypointense ADC associated with the areas of enhancement, as well as adjacent perivascular enhancement, suggests lymphoma in an immunocompromised patient. Transspatial lesions also suggest lymphoma.

Signs and Complications

Signs and complications are predominantly related to mass effect and the specific location of the lesion.

Suggested Readings

Eichler AF, Batchelor TT: Primary central nervous system lymphoma: presentation, diagnosis and staging, *Neurosurg Focus* 21(5):E16, 2006.

Masdeu JC, Quinto C, Olivera C, et al: Open-ring imaging sign: highly specific for atypical brain demyelination, *Neurology* 54(7):1427–1433, 2000.

Schwartz KM, Erickson BJ, Lucchinetti C: Pattern of T2 hypointensity associated with ring-enhancing brain lesions can help to differentiate pathology, *Neuroradiology* 48(3):143–149, 2006.

Smirniotopoulos JG, Murphy FM, Rushing EJ, et al: Patterns of contrast enhancement in the brain and meninges, *Radiographics* 27(2):525–551, 2007.

9

Punctate and Curvilinear Enhancing Foci

KATHARINA EIKERMANN-HAERTER, MD

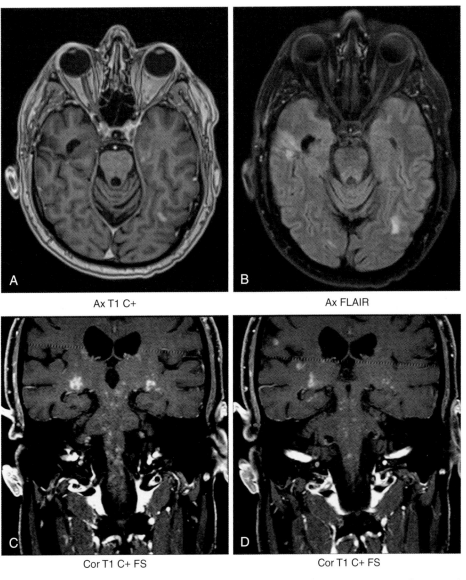

CASE A: A 56-year-old with history of treated CNS lymphoma and worsening gait. *Ax,* Axial; *Cor,* coronal; *FLAIR,* fluid-attenuated inversion recovery; *FS,* fat saturated.

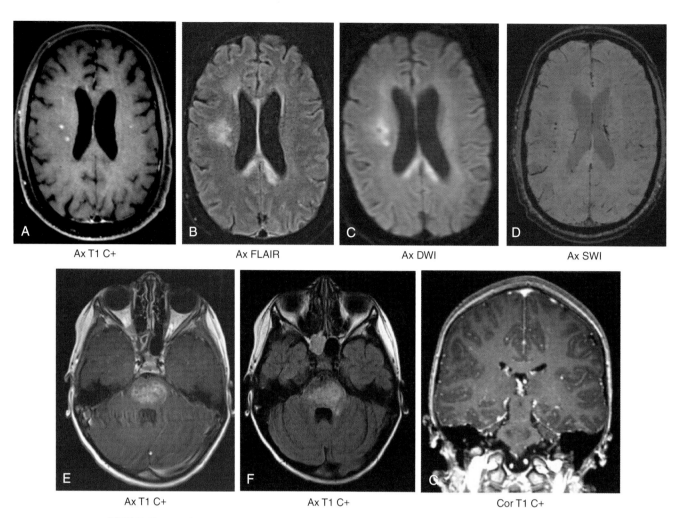

Ax T1 C+ Ax FLAIR Ax DWI Ax SWI

Ax T1 C+ Ax T1 C+ Cor T1 C+

CASE B: Row 1—A 51-year-old with progressive fatigue, cognitive changes, and unsteady gait.
Row 2—A 7-year-old with ataxia and weakness. *Ax,* Axial; *Cor,* coronal; *WI,* diffusion-weighted imaging;
FLAIR, fluid-attenuated inversion recovery; *SWI,* susceptibility-weighted imaging.

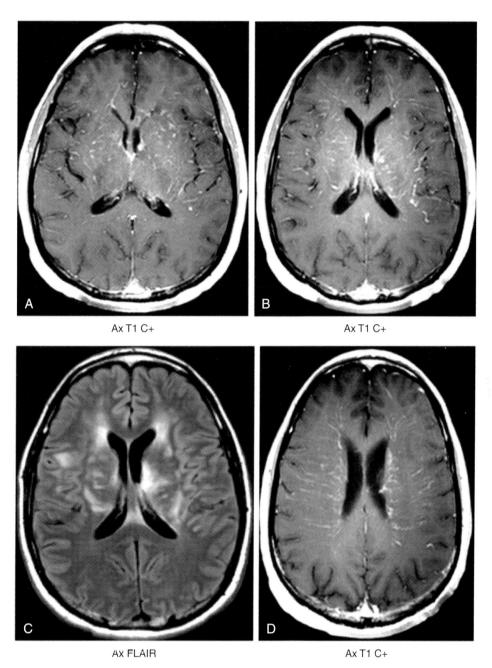

Ax T1 C+   Ax T1 C+

Ax FLAIR   Ax T1 C+

CASE C: A 23-year-old with aphasia. *Ax,* Axial; *FLAIR,* fluid-attenuated inversion recovery.

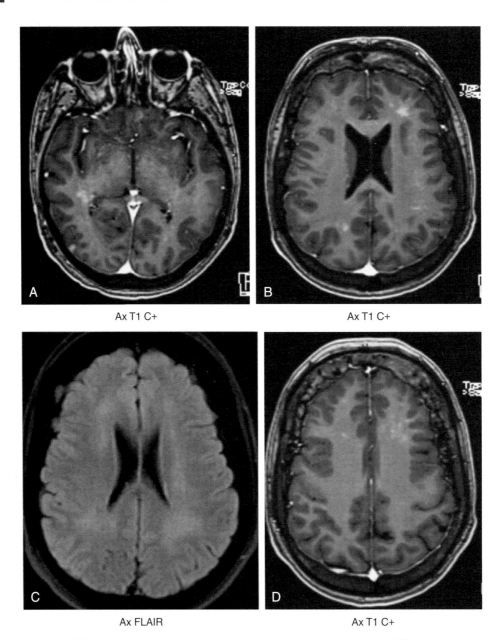

Ax T1 C+

Ax T1 C+

Ax FLAIR

Ax T1 C+

CASE D: A 64-year-old on pembrolizumab for metastatic melanoma. *Ax,* Axial; *FLAIR,* fluid-attenuated inversion recovery.

DESCRIPTION OF FINDINGS

CT and MR images from four patients with different patterns of enhancing punctate or curvilinear foci.

- Case A: There are punctate enhancing foci throughout the upper cervical cord, medulla, pons, and midbrain. There are also punctate and curvilinear foci of enhancement in the temporal lobes, right inferior frontal lobe, and basal ganglia. Some lesions have associated edema. There is no associated mass effect or abnormality on diffusion or susceptibility sequences.
- Case B, row 1: There are multifocal punctate enhancing foci in the periventricular and deep white matter. There are confluent fluid-attenuated inversion recovery T2/FLAIR hyperintense regions with restricted diffusion in the right corona radiata and splenium of the corpus callosum and punctate foci of susceptibility in the right corona radiata. High-resolution 3T vessel wall imaging in this patient (not shown) revealed characteristic long-segmental smooth concentric wall enhancement affecting multiple distal vessels. Row 2: There are multifocal punctate enhancing foci in the pons with associated FLAIR abnormality and there are multifocal punctate enhancing foci in the supratentorial white matter.
- Case C: There are multifocal punctate and linear foci of parenchymal enhancement in the basal ganglia, internal capsules, corona radiata, and subcortical white matter. Some of the lesions are associated with FLAIR hyperintensity, consistent with associated edema. There is the suggestion of associated nodular leptomeningeal enhancement.
- Case D: There is nodular enhancement throughout the periventricular and subcortical white matter with patchy hyperintensity on FLAIR images, consistent with mild edema.

Diagnosis

Case A: Chronic lymphocytic inflammation with pontine perivascular enhancement responsive to steroids (CLIPPERS)

Case B: Central nervous system (CNS) vasculitis

Case C: Sarcoidosis

Case D: Checkpoint inhibitor (pembrolizumab) toxicity

Summary

Punctate and curvilinear enhancing foci reflect either blood-brain barrier breakdown or the presence of one or more lesions within or surrounding vessels. MR imaging utilizing dedicated sequences, such as vessel wall imaging can aid in establishing an appropriately weighted differential diagnosis.

CLIPPERS may initially present as an isolated enhancing mass in the pons/cerebellar peduncle before exhibiting the characteristic pattern of "peppering" pontocerebellar lesions, typically measuring less than 3 mm in size. There may be involvement of the basal ganglia, hemispheric white matter, midbrain, medulla, or spinal cord. Mean age at onset is 50 years, and males are more commonly affected than females. Clinical presentation is usually subacute relapsing-remitting pontocerebellar dysfunction with marked clinical and imaging response to corticosteroids. Of note, there is a variant that is clinically, radiologically, and pathologically similar to CLIPPERS but isolated to supratentorial locations, called SLIPPERS.

Primary CNS vasculitis is characterized by nonatheromatous inflammation and necrosis of blood vessel walls, involving second- or third-order arteries and/or veins. When very small vessels are involved, a nodular and linear pattern with or without associated edema, subcortical and deep white matter ischemia, and microhemorrhages is seen. With this pattern, no significant abnormalities on angiography are seen. When larger arteries are involved, multifocal stenoses are seen on digital subtraction angiography (DSA), magnetic resonance angiography (MRA), and CT angiography (CTA), and conventional MRI may show infarcts of multiple ages with restricted diffusion associated with acute infarcts, gyriform enhancement associated with subacute infarcts, and encephalomalacia associated with more chronic infarcts. With this pattern, the infarcts are typically in multiple vascular distributions, and are at times associated with hemorrhage. High-resolution vessel wall imaging may show long-segmental smooth concentric wall enhancement. Leptomeningeal enhancement is another manifestation of primary CNS vasculitis. Rarely, a tumefactive pattern with a solitary tumor-like enhancing mass occurs.

Neurosarcoidosis belongs to a multisystem chronic inflammatory disease spectrum characterized by noncaseating epithelioid cell granulomas that may infiltrate along perivascular spaces into brain. CNS involvement is rare in 5% to 10% of cases, with preferential involvement of the basal cisterns. One-third of patients have multiple parenchymal enhancing lesions, one-third have leptomeningeal enhancement, and 10% have a solitary enhancing parenchymal intraaxial mass. There may also be diffuse or focal dural thickening, cranial nerve enhancement, pituitary stalk thickening, infiltration of the choroid plexus, or small vessel vasculitis in white matter with engorged corkscrew enhancing deep medullary veins. Lacunar infarcts may occur, and 50% of patients show periventricular T2 hyperintensities. Two-thirds of cases are clinically monophasic; one-third is chronic remitting-relapsing. MR imaging resolution lags clinical symptom resolution.

Immune checkpoint inhibitors are an important cornerstone of cancer therapy, by targeting regulatory steps of T-cell activation, resulting in an enhanced endogenous antitumor immune response. Undesired neurologic autoimmunity occurs in 4% of patients receiving monotherapy and up to 14% of patients treated with combination of CTLA4 and PD1/PDL1 inhibitors, frequently manifesting as neuromuscular dysfunction. Most common CNS manifestations are encephalopathy, followed by cerebellar ataxia, and hyperkinetic movement disorders. Ninety-five percent of these patients have abnormal cerebrospinal fluid (CSF) results; neural specific autoantibodies can be identified in 54% of the patients; and 61% exhibit MRI abnormalities that include localized FLAIR/T2 hyperintensities with possible parenchymal and leptomeningeal enhancement, frequently involving the mesiotemporal lobes and basal ganglia. Another common adverse effect of immune checkpoint inhibitors is hypophysitis. Advanced cases can show focal atrophy, such as involving the cerebellum.

Spectrum of Disease: There is a wide spectrum of diseases that can cause punctate and curvilinear enhancing foci. Possible disease entities include inflammatory, autoimmune, toxic, neoplastic, and infectious. Features narrowing the differential diagnoses include the clinical/demographic factors (patient's age, comorbidities, therapies), recognition of disease spread

TABLE 9.1 **Imaging Features of Conditions Associated With Multifocal Nodular +/– Curvilinear Enhancement**

Disease	Demographics	Clinical Presentation	Additional Imaging Findings	Other Tests
CLIPPERS	Middle age	Posterior fossa symptoms – ataxia, dizziness	Spinal cord lesions SLIPPERS is the supratentorial variant Mediastinal adenopathy	Spine MRI
Neurosarcoidosis	Young adults African American	Headache, cranial nerve palsies, systemic symptoms	Spinal cord lesions, dural and leptomeningeal disease, hypothalamic pituitary axis lesions, bone lesions, pulmonary involvement	Chest CT, bronchoalveolar lavage
Primary CNS vasculitis	Middle age	Headache, focal neurologic deficits	Microhemorrhages Multifocal infarcts in different vascular distributions	DSA, biopsy, VWI with concentric enhancement
Checkpoint inhibitor toxicity	Older adults with metastatic disease	Encephalopathy, ataxia, hyperkinetic movement disorder	Hypophysitis Cerebellar atrophy	Checkpoint inhibitor regimen
Non-Hodgkin lymphoma	Older age	Headache, encephalopathy	Leptomeningeal spinal cord and cranial nerve enhancement	CSF sampling PET CT
GFAP encephalomyelitis	Middle age	Encephalomyelitis	Leptomeningeal enhancement	CSF Anti-GFAP Serum GFAP - IgG
Erdheim-Chester	Older adults	Confusion, fatigue, strokes, bone pain, proptosis, cardiac tamponade, shortness of breath, abdominal pain, dysuria	Orbital masses, dural lesions, long bone metaphyseal lesions, pericardial, renal capsular and pleural infiltration, interstitial lung disease	CD68(+), CD1a(−) histiocytes on biopsy, long bone, chest and abdomen CT and MR imaging
Tuberculosis	Children, young adults	Headache, focal neurologic deficit	Thick nodular leptomeningeal enhancement; nodules are T2 hypointense, pulmonary involvement	CSF sampling PCR Chest CT
Fungal infections	Immunocompromised and endemic areas	Meningismus, headache, encephalopathy	Leptomeningeal enhancement, microhemorrhages with candida, pulmonary involvement	CSF culture Chest CT
Metastases	Elderly Primary is usually lung CA	Headache, focal neurologic deficit	Leptomeningeal enhancement, pulmonary involvement	CSF – malignant cells PET CT
PML-IRIS	immunocompromised	Patients receiving HAART with rising CD4 cell count and falling HIV-1-RNA level with worsening clinical course despite optimal antimicrobial treatment	Marked edema, evidence of prior PML	CSF – PCR JC Virus, Rising CD4 cell count and falling HIV-1-RNA

along perivascular spaces, leptomeningeal enhancement, presence of hemorrhagic lesions, specific lesion location or systemic/spinal cord involvement. Disease entities and differentiating factors are outlined in Table 9.1.

Differential Diagnosis

Non-Hodgkin lymphoma
CLIPPERS/SLIPPERS
Neurosarcoidosis
Vasculitis (primary, secondary)
Erdheim-Chester disease (non-Langerhans cell histiocytosis)
Fungal infections (Candida, histoplasmosis)

Immune reconstitution inflammatory syndrome (IRIS) (Fig. 9.1)
Tuberculosis
Glial fibrillary acidic protein (GFAP) meningoencephalomyelitis

Pearls

• Posterior fossa involvement should suggest CLIPPERS, which is characterized by a peppered appearance of pontomesencephalic structures that is responsive to steroids.
• Vasculitis typically affects second- and third-order branches and long segments. The linear and nodular pattern is frequently associated with microhemorrhages. When larger vessels are involved, multifocal stenoses are seen on

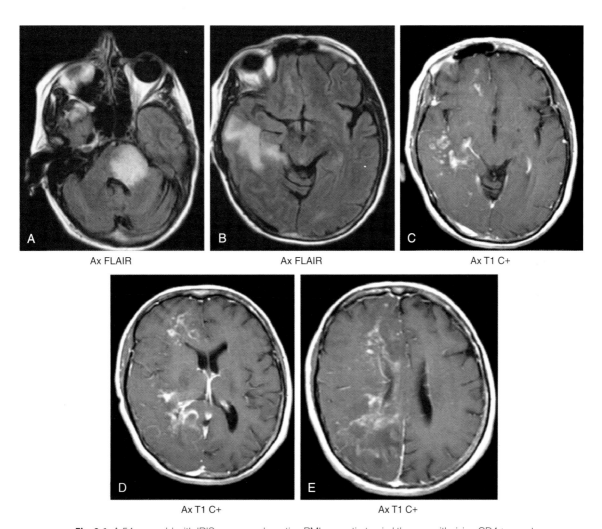

• Fig. 9.1 A 54-year-old with IRIS, presumed pontine PML on antiretroviral therapy with rising CD4+ count and decreasing HIV RNA. There is expansile pontine FLAIR hyperintensity, consistent with PML unchanged from a prior MRI scan obtained 6 months earlier (not shown). There is FLAIR hyperintensity, consistent with edema in the right temporal lobe. There is linear and nodular enhancement in the right temporal, frontal, and parietal periventricular and subcortical white matter with extension into the corpus callosum. There is associated mass effect with effacement of sulci, partial effacement of the right lateral ventricle, and midline shift to the left by approximately 3 mm. *Ax,* Axial; *FLAIR,* fluid-attenuated inversion recovery; *MRI,* magnetic resonance imaging; *PML,* progressive leukoencephalopathy.

angiography, smooth concentric enhancement is identified on vessel wall imaging, and multiple vascular distribution infarcts are seen. Brain biopsy may be necessary to confirm vasculitis, requiring presence of inflammation and necrosis for diagnosis.

- Neurosarcoid most frequently affects small arterial perforators. The linear and nodular pattern is frequently accompanied by leptomeningeal or dural enhancement. An abnormal chest radiograph is common.
- Immune checkpoint inhibitor toxicity parenchymal foci of enhancement may be associated with hypophysitis.
- Age of the patient helps differentiate lesions.
  - In the elderly adult, consider lymphoma, metastases, and Erdheim-Chester disease.
  - In the child, consider TB cerebritis and meningitis.
- In immunocompromised patients, consider fungal infections, IRIS.

- Hemorrhagic lesions are suggestive of vasculitis and fungal infections.
- Meningeal enhancement is seen with metastatic disease, neurosarcoidosis, CNS lymphoma, and infectious diseases.
- Spinal cord involvement is seen with neurosarcoidosis, CLIPPERS, GFAP, and lymphoma.
- Bone lesions can be seen with infections and sarcoidosis.
- History of primary malignancy should raise suspicion for metastatic disease.

Signs and Complications

The clinical presentation of multifocal small nodular and linear enhancing lesions is highly variable, and depends on the lesion location, but often includes headache, encephalopathy, ataxia, and focal neurologic deficits. Stroke and intracranial microhemorrhages resulting from vascular inflammation are the most frequent complications. Vasculitis, neurosarcoidosis, checkpoint inhibitor toxicity, CLIPPERS, lymphoma, progressive leukoencephalopathy (PML)-IRIS, and GFAP encephalomyelitis are responsive to steroids. Immunocompromised patients with fungal infections tend to have progressive disease in spite of optimal antifungal treatment. Patients with metastatic disease and Erdheim-Chester disease also usually have progressive disease.

Suggested Readings

Bathla G, Watal P, Gupta S, et al: Cerebrovascular manifestations of neurosarcoidosis: an underrecognized aspect of the imaging spectrum. *AJNR Am J Neuroradiol* 39(7):1194–1200, 2018.

Bot JCJ, Mazzai L, Hagenbeek RE, et al: Brain miliary enhancement. *Neuroradiology* 62(3):283–300, 2020.

Corrêa DG, Hygino da Cruz LC, Jr.: High-resolution vessel wall MR imaging as an alternative to brain biopsy. *AJNR Am J Neuroradiol* 40:E17–E18, 2019.

Eiden S, Beck C, Venhoff N, et al: High-resolution contrast-enhanced vessel wall imaging in patients with suspected cerebral vasculitis: prospective comparison of whole-brain 3D T1 SPACE versus 2D T1 black blood MRI at 3 Tesla. *PLoS One* 14(3):e0213514, 2019.

Kurokawa R, Ota Y, Gonoi W, et al: MRI findings of immune checkpoint inhibitor-induced hypophysitis: possible association with fibrosis. *AJNR Am J Neuroradiol* 41(9):1683–1689, 2020.

Li Z, Jiang Z, Ouyang S, et al: CLIPPERS, a syndrome of lymphohistiocytic disorders. *Mult Scler Relat Disord* 42:102063, 2020.

Sechi E, Markovic SN, McKeon A, et al: Neurologic autoimmunity and immune checkpoint inhibitors: autoantibody profiles and outcomes. *Neurology* 95(17):e2442–e2452, 2020.

Stern BJ, Royal W, 3rd, Gelfand JM, et al: Definition and consensus diagnostic criteria for neurosarcoidosis: from the Neurosarcoidosis Consortium Consensus Group. *JAMA Neurol* 75(12):1546–1553, 2018.

Taieb G, Mulero P, Psimaras D, et al: CLIPPERS and its mimics: evaluation of new criteria for the diagnosis of CLIPPERS. *J Neurol Neurosurg Psychiatry* 90(9):1027–1038, 2019.

Turnquist C, Pretorius PM, DeLuca GC, et al: CLIPPERS: a case report with radiology, three serial biopsies and a literature review. *Clin Neuropathol* 39(1):19–24, 2020.

10
Leptomeningeal Enhancement

JUAN E. SMALL, MD, MSC

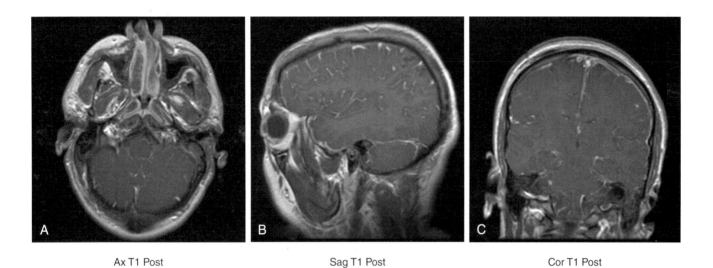

Ax T1 Post   Sag T1 Post   Cor T1 Post

CASE A: A 44-year-old who had upper respiratory infection symptoms 4 weeks earlier, now presenting with severe headache, purulent otorrhea, irritability, and progressive decline of mental status. *Ax*, Axial; *Cor*, coronal; *Sag*, sagittal.

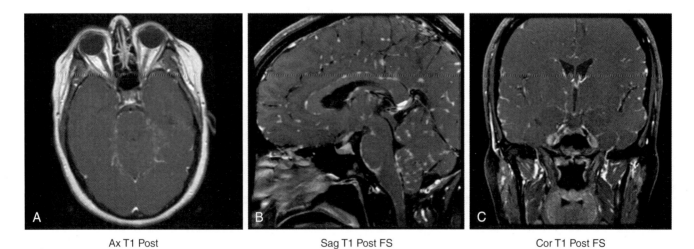

Ax T1 Post   Sag T1 Post FS   Cor T1 Post FS

CASE B: A 38-year-old with a history of diabetes insipidus and hyperprolactinemia presenting with a complex partial seizure. *Ax*, Axial; *Cor*, coronal; *Sag*, sagittal.

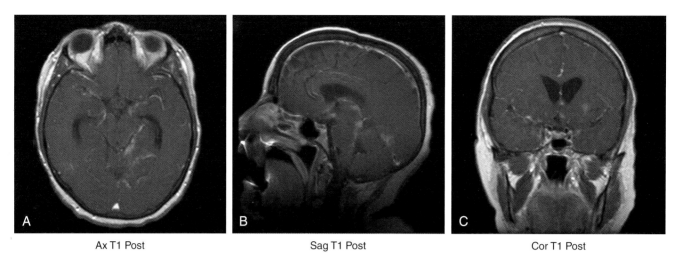

Ax T1 Post   Sag T1 Post   Cor T1 Post

CASE C: A 58-year-old with 5-week history of fever and headache now presenting with increasing confusion, vomiting, and lethargy. *Ax*, Axial; *Cor*, coronal; *Sag*, sagittal.

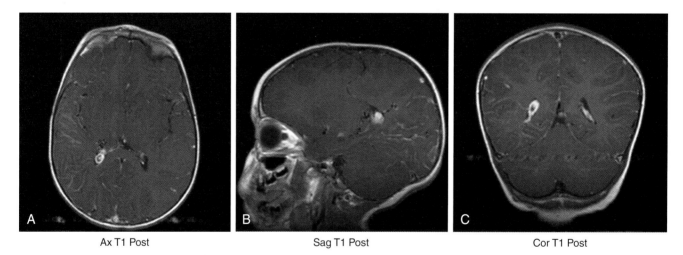

Ax T1 Post   Sag T1 Post   Cor T1 Post

CASE D: A 2-year-old with a history of seizures presenting with a decline in language function. *Ax*, Axial; *Cor*, coronal; *Sag*, sagittal.

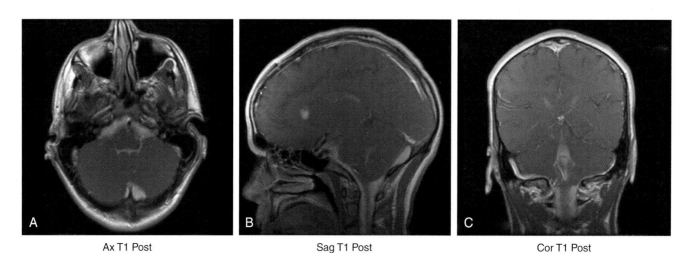

Ax T1 Post   Sag T1 Post   Cor T1 Post

CASE E: A 22-year-old recently diagnosed with communicating hydrocephalus of unknown cause now presenting with intractable headaches, lightheadedness, and episodes of near syncope. *Ax*, Axial; *Cor*, coronal; *Sag*, sagittal.

DESCRIPTION OF FINDINGS

- Case A: There is a thin, smooth pattern of leptomeningeal enhancement with left mastoiditis evident as the source of infection.
- Case B: There is a markedly nodular pattern of leptomeningeal enhancement slightly more prominent in the basal cisterns and the hypothalamic region. There is also bilateral trigeminal nerve involvement. Thoracic imaging (not shown) demonstrated mediastinal and pulmonary sarcoidosis.
- Case C: There is a thick and nodular pattern of leptomeningeal enhancement predominantly involving the basilar cisterns.
- Case D: A thin, smooth pattern of right temporal parietal leptomeningeal enhancement is evident. There is associated cortical atrophy, ipsilateral choroid plexus hypertrophy, and a prominent medullary vein. A port-wine stain was seen on physical examination.
- Case E: There is a very thick, smooth leptomeningeal enhancement predominantly involving the basilar cisterns.

Diagnosis

Case A: Bacterial meningitis
Case B: Neurosarcoidosis
Case C: Tuberculous meningitis
Case D: Sturge-Weber syndrome
Case E: Leptomeningeal gliomatosis

Summary

The most common causes of leptomeningeal (pia-arachnoid) enhancement are bacterial and fungal meningitis, leptomeningeal carcinomatosis, and neurosarcoidosis. Less common etiologies include vasculitis, gliomatosis, Sturge-Weber syndrome, and moyamoya disease. Rare causes include Wegener granulomatosis, Lyme disease, dural arteriovenous fistula, meningioangiomatosis, and neurocutaneous melanosis. Leptomeningeal gliomatosis is very rare.

Unfortunately, most causes of leptomeningeal enhancement have similar appearances. However, two key factors often can help narrow the differential diagnosis. The easiest is determined first by attempting to differentiate infectious from noninfectious entities, a prospect often aided by a suggestive clinical history or imaging findings suggesting the source of infection. Second, the pattern of enhancement can help tailor the differential diagnosis. Uncomplicated bacterial meningitis typically demonstrates thin, smooth leptomeningeal enhancement. Entities classically presenting with thick, nodular, basal-predominant enhancement include tuberculous meningitis, fungal meningitis, neurosarcoidosis, pyogenic meningitis, and neurosyphilis. Entities with more diffuse nodular leptomeningeal enhancement include meningeal carcinomatosis, lymphomatous meningitis, and leukemia. Very thick, smooth, basilar leptomeningeal enhancement can suggest the unlikely diagnosis of leptomeningeal gliomatosis in the setting of a chronic aseptic meningitis pattern of presentation.

Spectrum of Disease

As previously indicated, most causes of leptomeningeal enhancement can have a similar appearance, and it is important to realize that entities that typically present with thin/smooth, nodular, or basilar enhancement can have an atypical appearance (e.g., meningeal carcinomatosis that presents with a thin rather than a nodular pattern of enhancement).

Differential Diagnosis

The differential diagnosis of leptomeningeal (pia-arachnoid) enhancement can be summarized broadly into infectious, inflammatory, vascular, neoplastic, and traumatic etiologies (Box 10.1).

Infectious meningitis results in leptomeningeal enhancement because of the breakdown of the blood-brain barrier. Uncomplicated bacterial meningitis usually results in thin, smooth enhancement.

Tuberculous and fungal forms of meningitis are often basilar predominant and confluent. In addition, fungal and tuberculous meningitis may produce thicker nodular enhancement in contrast to the typical bacterial meningitis enhancement pattern.

Leptomeningeal carcinomatosis is typically nodular or mass-like and more diffuse. However, it is important to note that carcinomatous meningitis can appear as thin and smooth.

Neurosarcoidosis often demonstrates a nodular pattern with basilar predominance, and cranial nerve involvement often is present.

Sturge-Weber syndrome typically demonstrates thin, smooth leptomeningeal enhancement associated with cortical atrophy with gyriform calcification, as well as ipsilateral choroid plexus hypertrophy. In addition, prominent medullary and ependymal veins can be visible.

Moyamoya disease demonstrates enhancement of multiple engorged pial and parenchymal collateral vessels due to slow flow. The internal carotid, proximal middle cerebral, and anterior cerebral artery flow voids are absent or small. There frequently are associated acute and chronic hemorrhages and/or infarctions.

Meningioangiomatosis is a rare hamartomatous cortical and leptomeningeal malformation usually appearing as a calcified cortical mass with a linear, granular, and/or gyriform cortical and leptomeningeal enhancement pattern.

Neurocutaneous melanosis may demonstrate diffuse leptomeningeal enhancement.

Primary diffuse leptomeningeal gliomatosis is an exceedingly rare neoplastic condition of meningeal glial cell infiltration without evidence of a primary parenchymal tumor. This condition should be considered in the differential diagnosis of

---

• BOX 10.1 Types of Differential Diagnoses

Infectious: Bacterial meningitis, viral meningitis, tuberculous meningitis, fungal meningitis, neurosyphilis
Inflammatory: Langerhans cell histiocytosis, sarcoidosis, Wegener granulomatosis, chemical meningitis (ruptured dermoid)
Neoplastic: Leptomeningeal gliomatosis, melanoma, sarcoma, lymphoma; cerebrospinal fluid spread of tumor such as medulloblastoma, germinoma, and pineoblastoma; and metastatic carcinomatosis (breast, leukemia/lymphoma, lung, melanoma, gastrointestinal carcinoma, genitourinary carcinoma)
Traumatic: Old subarachnoid hemorrhage, surgical scarring from a prior craniotomy, the sequela of a lumbar puncture, or contrast leakage

chronic aseptic meningitis. Although very rare, imaging features include a very thick, smooth, basilar predominant leptomeningeal pattern of enhancement.

Pearls

The following entities typically present with thin, smooth leptomeningeal enhancement:
- Bacterial meningitis

The following entities can present with basal-predominant nodular enhancement:
- Tuberculous meningitis
- Fungal meningitis
- Neurosarcoidosis
- Pyogenic meningitis
- Neurosyphilis

The following entities typically have more diffuse nodular leptomeningeal enhancement:
- Meningeal carcinomatosis
- Lymphomatous meningitis
- Leukemia

Signs and Complications

When considering infectious etiologies, look carefully for a possible source of infection, areas of parenchymal infarction or hemorrhage due to arterial or venous sinus thrombosis, intracranial collections of pus, or abscesses.

Suggested Readings

Jicha GA, Glantz J, Clarke MJ, et al: Primary diffuse leptomeningeal gliomatosis, *Eur Neurol* 62(1):16–22, 2009.

Smirniotopoulos JG, Murphy FM, Rushing EJ, et al: Patterns of contrast enhancement in the brain and meninges, *Radiographics* 27(2): 525–551, 2007.

11
Dural Enhancement

REZA FORGHANI, MD, PHD

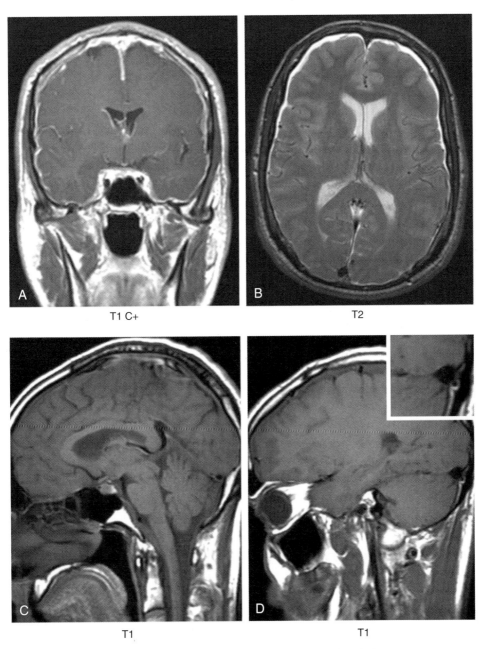

CASE A: A 45-year-old man with new-onset postural headache.

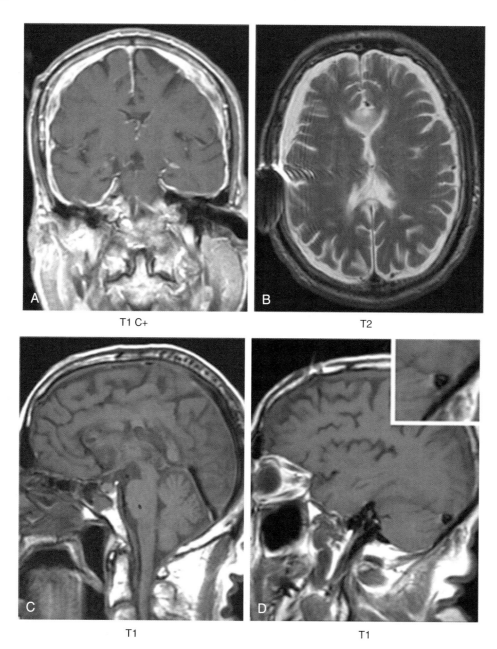

T1 C+

T2

T1

T1

CASE B: A 72-year-old man, history withheld.

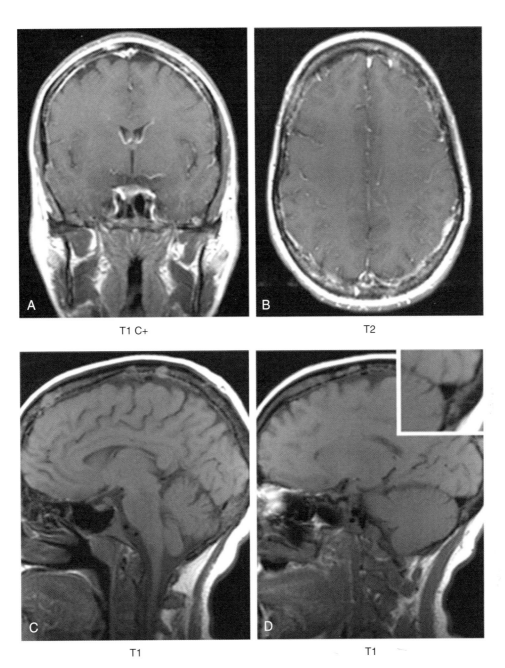

A   T1 C+

B   T2

C   T1

D   T1

CASE C: A 39-year-old woman with breast cancer.

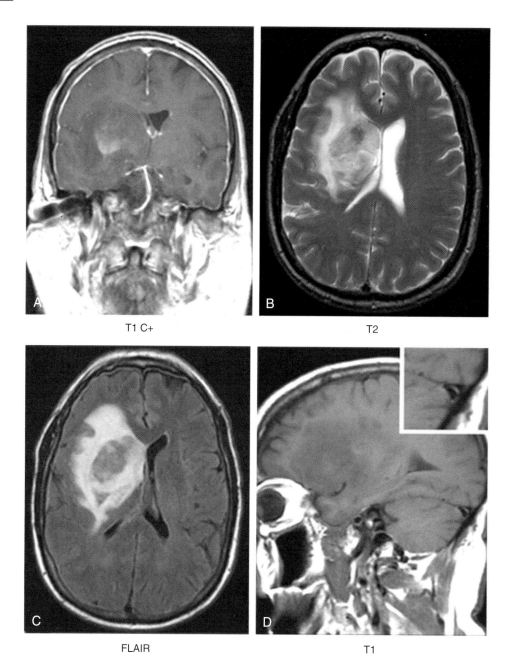

T1 C+

T2

FLAIR

T1

CASE D: A 63-year-old man with a history of kidney transplantation. *FLAIR*, fluid attenuated inversion recovery.

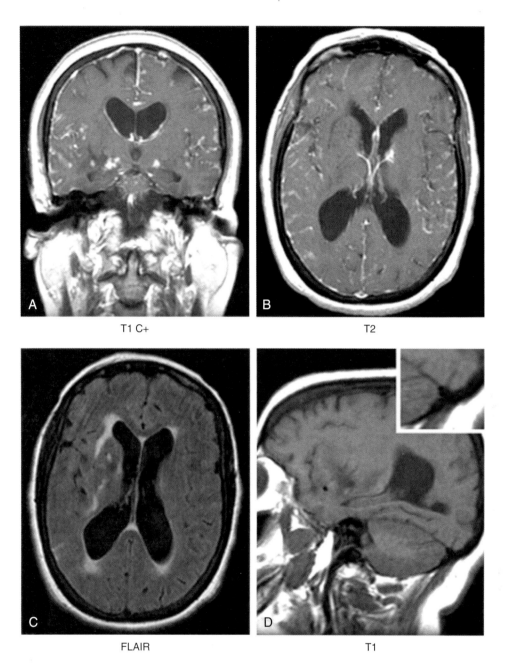

T1 C+

T2

FLAIR

T1

CASE E: A 55-year-old woman, history withheld. *FLAIR,* fluid attenuated inversion recovery.

DESCRIPTION OF FINDINGS

MRI scans from five patients demonstrate diffuse pachymeningeal enhancement.

- Case A: There are diffuse smooth pachymeningeal enhancement, small subdural effusions, caudal displacement of supratentorial structures, low-lying cerebellar tonsils, prominence of the pituitary gland with the pituitary protruding beyond the margins of the sella, and a prominent transverse sinus with a convex inferior border (known as venous distention sign [VDS]). Note the absence of leptomeningeal enhancement or pachymeningeal nodularity.
- Case B: There are marked diffuse thickening and enhancement of the pachymeninges, a positive VDS sign, small subdural effusions, and mild prominence of the pituitary gland, along with a ventricular shunt with its tip in the frontal horn of the right lateral ventricle and slit-like ventricles (also note the artifact from the shunt apparatus outside the calvarium). The brain does not have a sunken appearance despite the marked pachymeningeal thickening.
- Case C: There is pachymeningeal enhancement with areas of nodularity, unlike the other cases shown in which the pachymeningeal enhancement is smooth. Closer inspection of the images reveals multiple skull lesions. Also, note the concave inferior border of the transverse sinus (a negative VDS sign), unlike in cases A and B.
- Case D: There is diffuse smooth pachymeningeal enhancement in addition to a heterogeneously enhancing mass centered in the right basal ganglia. A negative VDS sign is noted.
- Case E: There is mild diffuse pachymeningeal enhancement in addition to extensive nodular leptomeningeal enhancement. Nonspecific areas of FLAIR hyperintensity also are noted, along with a negative VDS sign.

Diagnosis

Case A: Spontaneous (primary) intracranial hypotension (IH) (imaging and clinical criteria); improved after treatment with an epidural blood patch

Case B: Chronic shunting for aqueductal stenosis with pachymeningeal thickening that has been stable over many years

Case C: Disseminated breast cancer with biopsy-proven osseous metastases

Case D: Posttransplant B-cell lymphoproliferative disorder (proven by a biopsy of a mass centered in the basal ganglia)

Case E: Neurosarcoidosis, based on negative neoplastic and infectious workup, biopsy of mediastinal nodes consistent with sarcoidosis, and central nervous system findings stable for many years on imaging

Summary

Intracranial Hypotension/Hypovolemia— Primary and Secondary

The syndrome of IH or hypovolemia encompasses a broad spectrum of clinical and imaging findings related to cerebrospinal fluid (CSF) leaks. The leak may be primary (also known as spontaneous IH) or secondary. Primary IH is believed to occur from a combination of weakness in the dural sac and minor trauma, with the leak usually occurring in the spine, whereas secondary IH results from breaching of the dura from iatrogenic manipulation, such as a lumbar puncture or cranial or spinal surgery. The classic clinical syndrome is that of a postural headache that is aggravated in the standing position and relieved in the recumbent position. However, IH has many clinical presentations that may range from atypical headaches or focal neurologic deficits to coma, highlighting the importance of imaging in making an accurate diagnosis.

The most important imaging modality for the diagnosis of IH is MRI. The classic finding on MRI of the brain is diffuse smooth pachymeningeal thickening and enhancement without nodularity or evidence of leptomeningeal disease. In one report, pachymeningeal thickening was detectable on FLAIR in 74% of cases. Although some studies report close to 100% sensitivity of diffuse smooth pachymeningeal enhancement on MRI for IH, up to 20% of IH may have normal cranial MRI according to some reports. Engorgement of the venous sinuses and cerebral veins in patients with IH may be seen on conventional MRI and magnetic resonance angiography. On sagittal T1-weighted images, there is a convex contour of the undersurface of the dominant transverse sinus, known as the VDS. Serial imaging, if available, may also change over time in the engorgement of dural venous sinuses. The combination of diffuse pachymeningeal enhancement and a positive VDS sign has a high accuracy for the diagnosis of IH. Many other ancillary signs of IH exist that are not always present, but when combined with the aforementioned signs, they further support the diagnosis of IH. These ancillary signs include subdural collections that are usually small and are frequently hygromas but may be hemorrhagic. Caudal displacement of the supratentorial structures resulting in draping of the optic chiasm over the sella and tonsillar herniation mimicking a Chiari I malformation may be present. In addition, the pituitary gland may be enlarged. The latter finding is often difficult to determine with certainty given the relatively small size of the gland and normal variations in gland size based on the patient's age and sex. However, pituitary enlargement may be suggested if extension of the gland above the margins of the sella is observed. There have also been descriptions of associated reduction of CSF (subarachnoid) spaces along the optic nerve sheath complexes, restored to their normal state on serial follow-up examination after treatment. IH should also be considered when encountering extradural CSF collections on spine imaging.

A mild degree of linear pachymeningeal enhancement can frequently be observed after a recent lumbar puncture as a transient finding reflecting the same physiological processes discussed earlier (a common iatrogenic cause in contradistinction with "spontaneous" forms of IH). Chronic shunting may present with features of IH, likely as part of the continuum of the same pathophysiologic process. However, the implications are different because some imaging findings of IH, such as pachymeningeal enhancement, can represent an expected finding in a patient with a shunt and, in isolation, does not warrant any intervention. Case B is an example of chronic shunting. Different hypotheses have been proposed to explain why some patients with chronic shunting and pachymeningeal enhancement are asymptomatic and do not have a sunken appearance of the supratentorial structures; these hypotheses are beyond the scope of this text. It is noteworthy that the case presented is an extreme example of pachymeningeal thickening and enhancement and a wide spectrum of findings may be seen with shunting, ranging from minimal enhancement to prominent enhancement with marked thickening.

Although diffuse pachymeningeal enhancement is a sensitive sign of IH, it is not a specific sign in isolation, and it is imperative that the images be evaluated carefully for additional signs suggesting alternate diagnoses. The presence of nodularity or any leptomeningeal enhancement argues against IH and mandates consideration of a neoplastic process. Even without any leptomeningeal enhancement, pachymeningeal enhancement can be seen with metastatic disease, especially in the presence of skull metastases, as in Case C. Such pachymeningeal thickening and enhancement does not necessarily represent neoplastic invasion of the dura and can represent an inflammatory reaction. Presumably, such enhancement may be seen with metastases from any primary malignancy, but common extracranial sources include breast and prostate metastases. Pachymeningeal enhancement also can be seen with hematologic malignancies, usually in association with parenchymal lesions, as in Case D.

A variety of inflammatory and infectious conditions also can present with pachymeningeal thickening and enhancement, although many are readily distinguishable from IH based on their pattern and distribution. Neurosarcoidosis and granulomatosis with polyangiitis (Wegener granulomatosis) are included in these conditions, among others. Patients with neurosarcoidosis usually have pachymeningeal disease associated with leptomeningeal disease, as shown in Case E, along with parenchymal lesions, which allow this condition to be distinguished from IH. In addition, VDS and other ancillary findings seen in patients with IH are absent. Rare conditions such as IgG4-related hypertrophic pachymeningitis also can manifest as diffuse pachymeningeal enhancement. IgG4 is a fibroinflammatory disease characterized by infiltration of multiple tissues with lymphocytes and IgG4 secreting plasma cells with the development of fibrosis. The pachymengitis, similar to granulomatosis with polyangiitis and, at times, sarcoidosis, tends to be markedly hypointense on T2-weighted images. Brain, head, and neck findings, in addition to pachymeningitis, include IgG4-related orbital disease, hypophysitis, sialadenitis, and thyroiditis.

Spectrum of Disease

The most sensitive and widely reported sign of IH is diffuse smooth pachymeningeal enhancement. Otherwise unexplained appearance of subdural effusions should also prompt consideration of IH. Some studies also suggest that the VDS can be a highly accurate sign of IH. Additional but less specific signs described earlier can be seen in a subset of cases, and when combined, they further support the diagnosis of IH.

Differential Diagnosis

Postlumbar puncture dural enhancement
Chronic shunting and cranial or spinal surgery (likely representing a similar pathophysiologic process)

Neoplasm (most commonly metastases from breast, prostate, or hematologic malignancies)
Inflammatory and infectious processes, such as sarcoidosis, granulomatosis with polyangiitis, IgG4-related hypertrophic pachymeningitis, and tuberculosis

Pearls

- The combination of diffuse smooth pachymeningeal enhancement and a positive VDS is highly suggestive of IH. However, the use of the VDS requires familiarity with the appearance of the transverse sinus on unenhanced scans. Care must be taken to use the middle two-thirds of the dominant transverse sinus for determination of the VDS. Evaluation of the sinus too far medially or laterally may result in erroneous interpretation.
- Look for other signs of IH when encountering unexplained subdural collections, including rarely along the clivus or when encountering extradural CSF collections on spine imaging.
- If gadolinium-enhanced images are not available, look for pachymeningeal thickening on FLAIR and the VDS sign on sagittal T1-weighted images.
- Exercise caution in diagnosing IH in patients with chronic surgical shunts or recent cranial or spinal surgery.
- Mild transient pachymeningeal enhancement can be seen after an uncomplicated lumbar puncture, and information regarding such procedures is important for image interpretation. Always inquire about a history of recent lumbar puncture as a potential cause for the imaging findings.
- When considering treatment of IH with an epidural blood patch, recommend spinal imaging for identification of the site of the CSF leak.

Signs and Complications

Occasionally, subdural hygromas or hematomas may be large enough to cause significant mass effect and clinical decompensation requiring surgical evacuation.

Many reports have been made of IH with atypical clinical presentation, including atypical headache patterns, focal neurologic deficits, or even rare cases of coma. A high index of suspicion is required for accurate diagnosis of this treatable condition.

Suggested Readings

Alvarez-Linera J, Escribano J, Benito-León J, et al: Pituitary enlargement in patients with intracranial hypotension syndrome. *Neurology* 55(12):1895–1897, 2000.

Atkinson JL, Weinshenker BG, Miller GM, et al: Acquired Chiari I malformation secondary to spontaneous spinal cerebrospinal fluid leakage and chronic intracranial hypotension syndrome in seven cases. *J Neurosurg* 88(2):237–242, 1998.

Baryshnik DB, Farb RI: Changes in the appearance of venous sinuses after treatment of disordered intracranial pressure. *Neurology* 62(8):1445–1446, 2004.

Bond KM, Benson JC, Cutsforth-Gregory JK, et al: Spontaneous intracranial hypotension: atypical radiologic appearances, imaging mimickers, and clinical look-alikes. *AJNR Am J Neuroradiol* 41(8):1339–1347, 2020.

D'Antona L, Jaime Merchan MA, Vassiliou A, et al: Clinical presentation, investigation findings, and treatment outcomes of spontaneous intracranial hypotension syndrome: a systematic review and meta-analysis. *JAMA Neurol* 78(3):329–337, 2021.

Farb RI, Forghani R, Lee SK, et al: The venous distension sign: a diagnostic sign of intracranial hypotension at MR imaging of the brain. *AJNR Am J Neuroradiol* 28(8):1489–1493, 2007.

Forghani R, Farb RI: Diagnosis and temporal evolution of signs of intracranial hypotension on MRI of the brain. *Neuroradiology* 50(12): 1025–1034, 2008.

Guermazi A: Consecutive bilateral cranial subdural fluid collections in misdiagnosed SIH. *Eur Radiol* 12(10):2606–2610, author reply 2610, 2002.

Hadizadeh DR, Kovács A, Tschampa H, et al: Postsurgical intracranial hypotension: diagnostic and prognostic imaging findings. *AJNR Am J Neuroradiol* 31(1):100–105, 2010.

Kremer S, Taillandier L, Schmitt E, et al: Atypical clinical presentation of intracranial hypotension: coma. *J Neurol* 252(11):1399–1400, 2005.

Marangoni S, Argentiero V, Tavolato B: Neurosarcoidosis. Clinical description of 7 cases with a proposal for a new diagnostic strategy. *J Neurol* 253(4):488–495, 2006.

Mokri B: Headaches caused by decreased intracranial pressure: diagnosis and management. *Curr Opin Neurol* 16(3):319–326, 2003.

Nowak DA, Widenka DC: Neurosarcoidosis: a review of its intracranial manifestation. *J Neurol* 248(5):363–372, 2001.

Nowak DA, Rodiek SO, Zinner J, et al: Broadening the clinical spectrum: unusual presentation of spontaneous cerebrospinal fluid hypovolemia. Case report. *J Neurosurg* 98(4):903907, 2003.

River Y, Schwartz A, Gomori JM, et al: Clinical significance of diffuse dural enhancement detected by magnetic resonance imaging. *J Neurosurg* 85(5):777–783, 1996.

Roll JD, Larson TC 3rd, Soriano MM: Cerebral angiographic findings of spontaneous intracranial hypotension. *AJNR Am J Neuroradiol* 24(4):707–708, 2003.

Schievink WI, Atkinson JL: Spontaneous intracranial hypotension. *J Neurosurg* 84(1):151–152, 1996.

Schievink WI, Jacques L: Recurrent spontaneous spinal cerebrospinal fluid leak associated with "nude nerve root" syndrome: case report. *Neurosurgery* 53(5):1216–1218, discussion 1218–1219, 2003.

Schievink WI, Maya MM, Moser FG, et al: Spectrum of subdural fluid collections in spontaneous intracranial hypotension. *J Neurosurg* 103(4):608–613, 2005.

Schievink WI, Maya MM, Louy C: Cranial MRI predicts outcome of spontaneous intracranial hypotension. *Neurology* 64(7):1282–1284, 2005.

Schievink WI: Misdiagnosis of spontaneous intracranial hypotension. *Arch Neurol* 60(12):1713–1718, 2003.

Schievink WI, Gordon OK, Tourje J: Connective tissue disorders with spontaneous spinal cerebrospinal fluid leaks and intracranial hypotension: a prospective study. *Neurosurgery* 54(1):65–70, discussion 70–71, 2004.

Schievink WI: Spontaneous intracranial hypotension. *N Engl J Med.* 385(23):2173–2178, 2021.

Schievink WI: Spontaneous spinal cerebrospinal fluid leaks and intracranial hypotension. *JAMA* 295(19):2286–2296, 2006.

Zajicek JP, Scolding NJ, Foster O, et al: Central nervous system sarcoidosis—diagnosis and management. *QJM* 92(2):103–1017, 1999.

12

Lesions Containing Fat

HILLARY R. KELLY, MD

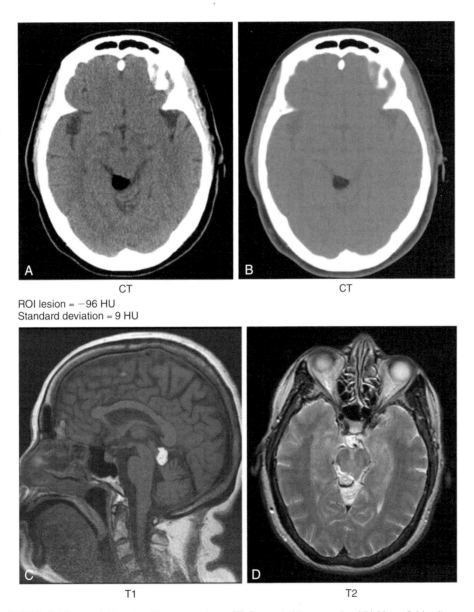

ROI lesion = −96 HU
Standard deviation = 9 HU

CASE A: A 65-year-old female with memory loss. *CT,* Computed tomography; *HU,* Hounsfield units; *ROI,* region of interest.

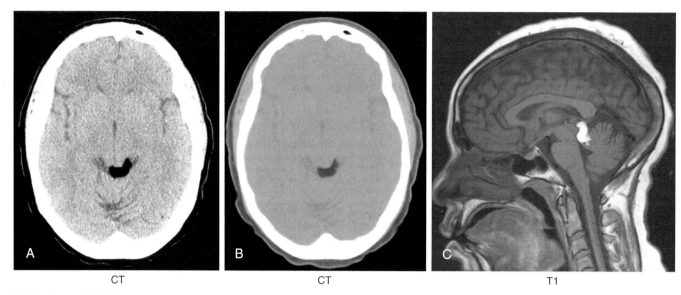

CT   CT   T1

ROI lesion = −106 HU
Standard deviation = 4 HU

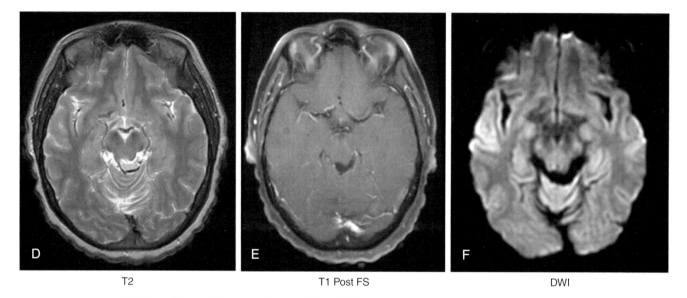

T2   T1 Post FS   DWI

CASE B: A 45-year-old female with a headache. *CT,* Computed tomography; *DWI,* diffusion-weighted imaging; *FS,* fat saturated; *HU,* Hounsfield units; *ROI,* region of interest.

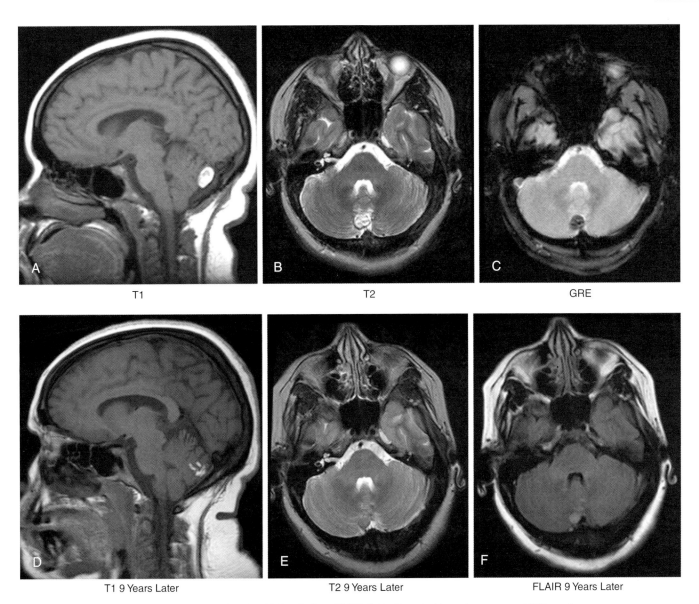

T1

T2

GRE

T1 9 Years Later

T2 9 Years Later

FLAIR 9 Years Later

CASE C: A 29-year-old female with headaches. *FLAIR,* fluid attenuated inversion recovery; *GRE,* gradient refocused echo.

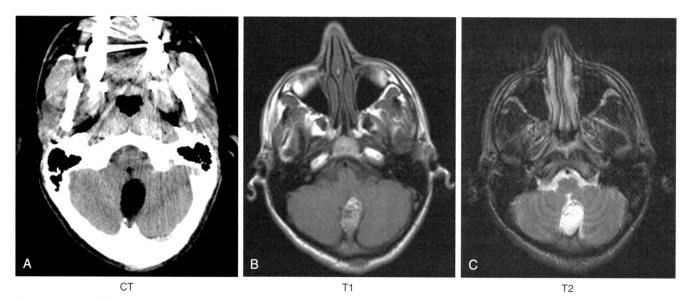

CT

T1

T2

ROI lesion = −35 HU
Standard deviation = 11 HU

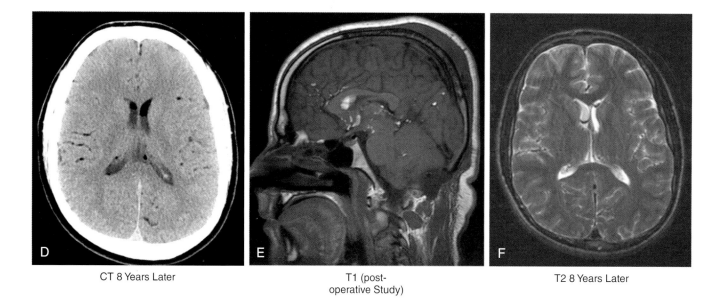

CT 8 Years Later

T1 (post-
operative Study)

T2 8 Years Later

CASE D: A 19-year-old male with severe suboccipital neck pain. *CT,* Computed tomography;
HU, Hounsfield units; *ROI,* region of interest.

DESCRIPTION OF FINDINGS

- Case A: CT demonstrates a fat density lesion in the right quadrigeminal plate cistern. The lesion measured −96 Hounsfield units (HU) with a standard deviation of 9 HU. The lesion is markedly hyperintense on T1-weighted imaging. The lesion also is hyperintense on T2-weighted imaging, and chemical shift artifact is noted.
- Case B: CT demonstrates a fat density lesion in the left quadrigeminal plate cistern. The lesion measured −106 HU with a standard deviation of 4 HU. The lesion is markedly hyperintense on T1-weighted imaging and hyperintense on T2-weighted imaging, with chemical shift artifact. The lesion does not enhance and is hypointense on the fat-saturated T1 postcontrast sequence. No restricted diffusion is noted within the lesion.
- Case C: A markedly T1 hyperintense lesion abuts the posterior aspect of the cerebellar vermis. The lesion demonstrates heterogeneous signal on T2-weighted imaging, with areas of both hypointensity and hyperintensity and subtle chemical shift artifact. Susceptibility artifact is associated with the lesion on the gradient echo sequence. On follow-up imaging for a severe headache 9 years later, multiple foci of T1 hyperintense signal are now seen in the subarachnoid space adjacent to the posterior right vermis. The T2 signal within these foci is now more homogeneous and isointense to the adjacent parenchyma. Subtle fluid-attenuated inversion recovery (FLAIR) hyperintense signal is noted within these foci.
- Case D: A fat density lesion abuts the inferior vermis. This lesion had a density of approximately −35 HU with a standard deviation of 11 HU. On MRI, this lesion is heterogeneously T1 hyperintense and is predominantly hyperintense on the T2 sequence, with linear areas of hypointensity. A head CT scan obtained 8 years later for an episode of severe pain demonstrates fat density droplets in the subarachnoid space and within the ventricles anteriorly. The patient underwent surgery for resection, and a postoperative MRI study demonstrates the residual T1 hyperintense fat droplets throughout the subarachnoid space and ventricles. The T2 sequence demonstrates the chemical shift artifact associated with these foci of fat.

Diagnosis

Case A: Presumed lipoma
Case B: Presumed lipoma
Case C: A dermoid cyst that ruptured 9 years after initial presentation
Case D: A ruptured dermoid cyst

Summary

Intracranial lesions that contain fat include lipomas, dermoid cysts, and teratomas. Teratomas are usually heterogeneous, often contain calcification and soft tissue density in addition to lipid, and usually are in the pineal region. Dermoids and lipomas can appear similar on both CT and MRI examinations.

Intracranial dermoid cysts are benign ectodermal inclusion cysts that arise from inclusion of cutaneous elements at the time of neural tube closure. These cysts are rare, accounting for less than 0.5% of intracranial tumors. On imaging, dermoids are round or lobulated unilocular cystic masses with well-circumscribed margins. They typically occur at or near midline and are most commonly found in the suprasellar, parasellar, or frontonasal regions. They also can occur in the posterior fossa, typically adjacent to the vermis or within the fourth ventricle. A fistulous connection to the skin (dermal sinus) may be present with spinal, anterior, or posterior fossa lesions. On CT, dermoids typically are low in density, demonstrating negative HU because of internal liquid cholesterol. Up to 20% have capsular calcifications. On MRI, dermoid cysts typically are T1 hyperintense but demonstrate variable signals on T2-weighted imaging ranging from hypointense to hyperintense. Fat suppression sequences will confirm the presence of lipid elements. Dermoid cysts do not enhance, although the capsule may demonstrate minimal linear enhancement.

Intracranial lipomas are congenital malformations rather than true neoplasms or hamartomas. They are thought to arise from abnormal persistence and maldifferentiation of the meninx primitiva, a mesenchymal derivative of the neural crest. Like dermoid cysts, intracranial lipomas tend to occur at or near midline. Lipomas often occur in the subarachnoid spaces, including the dorsal pericallosal, quadrigeminal, ambient, interpeduncular, and chiasmatic cisterns. On CT, lipomas are lobulated fat density masses that can encase vessels and cranial nerves. Dermoid cysts tend to be less lobulated than lipomas and will displace blood vessels and nerves rather than encase them. Capsular calcification can vary from none to extensive but typically is seen only with pericallosal interhemispheric lipomas and occurs less commonly than with dermoid cysts. On MRI, lipomas are hyperintense on T1-weighted images and are hyperintense with chemical shift artifacts on T2-weighted images. These lesions will become hypointense on fat-suppressed images and do not enhance.

In addition to location and MRI signal characteristics, reports in the neurosurgical literature suggest that CT density can be helpful in differentiating dermoid cysts from lipomas. Dermoids typically demonstrate higher average Hounsfield units when compared with lipomas. This observation may be due to the presence of sebaceous lipid in dermoids rather than mesodermal (adipose) fat or could reflect the greater heterogeneity of dermoids because of the presence of additional ectodermal elements (such as hair follicles, apocrine glands, and proteinaceous debris). Case series reports from the neurosurgical literature report that dermoids typically measure between −20 and −40 HU compared with −50 to −100 HU for lipomas. These reports also conclude that because of their more homogeneous contents, lipomas will have small standard deviations in Hounsfield units on histogram analysis (<10 HU), whereas dermoids tend to have larger standard deviations, typically greater than 20 HU.

Spectrum of Disease

Occasionally a dermoid cyst can be confused with an epidermoid cyst. Although epidermoids typically follow cerebrospinal fluid (CSF) density on CT and CSF intensity on MR, with the exception of FLAIR and diffusion-weighted images, a dermoid cyst can mimic an epidermoid if it is composed primarily of nonfatty contents. Both epidermoids and dermoids can demonstrate restricted diffusion, although this finding is typically described with epidermoid cysts (see Fig. 12.1). Whereas epidermoids are lined solely by squamous epithelium, dermoid cysts contain dermal elements, including hair follicles and sebaceous and sweat glands. Their etiology is similar, but epidermoids are thought to occur slightly later in embryogenesis and typically are found off of midline. Dermoids are four to nine times less

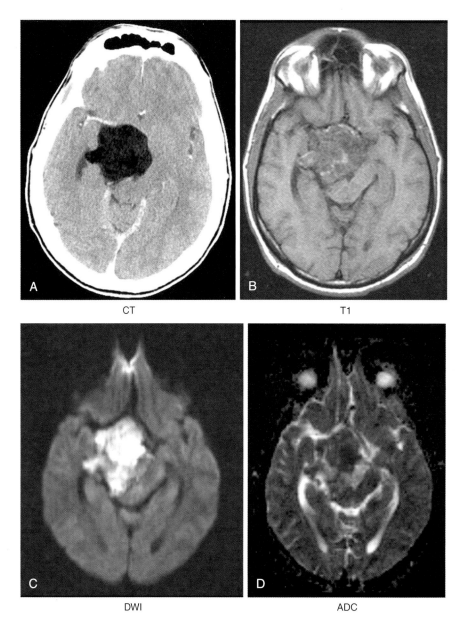

• **Fig. 12.1** Dermoid cyst. (A and B) Computed tomography *(CT)* imaging demonstrates a large, low-density lesion centered in the suprasellar cistern. The density measured approximately −15 HU with a standard deviation of 8 HU. (C and D) Magnetic resonance imaging reveals that the lesion has only minimal linear foci of T1 hyperintense signal centrally. Restricted diffusion also was noted. Initially this lesion was thought to be an epidermoid cyst, but at surgery it was found to be a dermoid. *ADC,* Apparent diffusion coefficient; *DWI,* diffusion-weighted imaging; *HU,* Hounsfield units.

common than epidermoid cysts. Because epidermoids by definition only contain squamous epithelium and keratin, the presence of any fat within a lesion should suggest the alternative diagnosis of a dermoid cyst (Fig. 12.2).

Rarely, dermoid cysts can demonstrate very high density on CT, referred to as "dense" or "white" dermoids. These lesions tend to occur almost exclusively in the cerebellum and are thought to have high protein concentrations. These lesions will be T1 hyperintense because of the protein content, but extremely hypointense on T2-weighted imaging.

Dermoid cysts can rupture, with subarachnoid and intraventricular spread of contents. On CT, fat density droplets are seen in the subarachnoid space, and fat fluid levels are seen layering antidependently in the ventricles. Extensive leptomeningeal enhancement is seen in the setting of rupture in patients with chemical meningitis.

Associated abnormalities can be seen with lipomas, most commonly corpus callosum anomalies (Fig. 12.3); additional associated congenital malformations include cephaloceles and closed spinal dysraphism. Interhemispheric/pericallosal lipomas can occur in two subtypes, which are named according to their morphology. The tubulonodular subtype tends to occur anteriorly and can demonstrate rim calcification. The curvilinear subtype is typically posterior, curving around the callosal body and splenium. Lipomas of the sylvian fissure can be associated with aneurysms of the middle cerebral arteries.

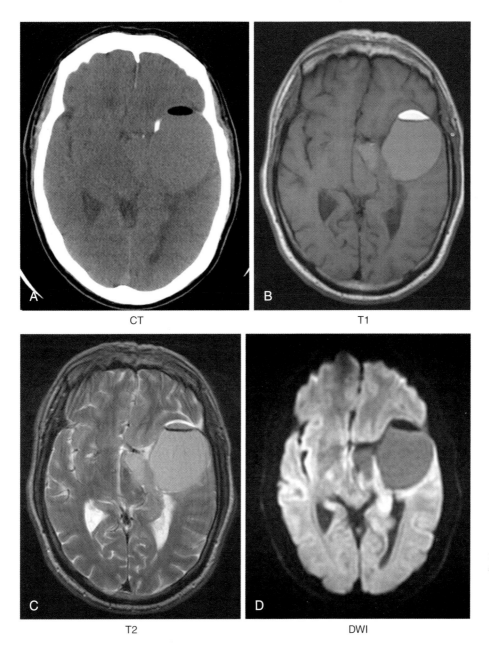

CT

T1

T2

DWI

• **Fig. 12.2** Dermoid cyst. (A) Computed tomography *(CT)* imaging demonstrates a large, slightly hyperdense lesion centered in the left middle cranial fossa with a fat fluid level anteriorly and foci of rim calcification. (B) Magnetic resonance imaging reveals T1 hyperintense signal within the fat fluid level and (C) chemical shift artifact on T2-weighted images associated with the fatty component of the lesion. (D) No restricted diffusion is seen. *DWI,* diffusion-weighted imaging.

Differential Diagnosis

Lipoma
Dermoid cyst
Teratoma
Epidermoid cyst
Craniopharyngioma

Pearls

• Location: Both dermoids and lipomas tend to occur at or near midline. Whereas dermoids typically are frontobasal,

suprasellar, parasellar, vermian, or fourth ventricular lesions, lipomas most frequently are located in the region of the corpus callosum, as well as near the tuber cinereum, the quadrigeminal plate, and the ambient cistern.

• Morphology: Dermoid cysts tend to be less lobulated than lipomas. Lipomas encase and engulf vessels and nerves, whereas dermoid cysts displace them.

• CT density: Average HU measurements and histogram analysis with standard deviations can be helpful in differentiating dermoid cysts from lipomas, although considerable overlap exists. Dermoids tend to be more heterogeneous, with higher HU and greater standard deviations compared

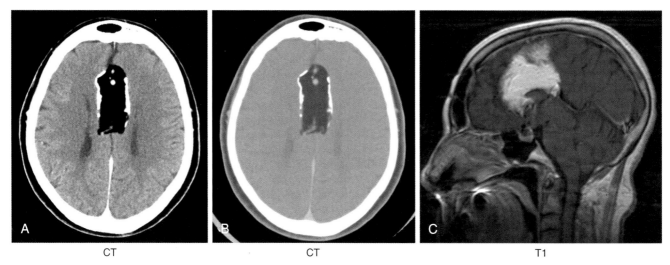

CT   CT   T1

ROI lesion = −91 HU
Standard deviation = 5 HU

• **Fig. 12.3** Partial agenesis of the corpus callosum with a callosal lipoma, tubulonodular subtype. A fat density lesion with peripheral calcification centered in the interhemispheric fissure is partially imaged. Magnetic resonance imaging reveals a lobulated, markedly T1 hyperintense lesion abutting the superior margin of the corpus callosum. *CT,* Computed tomography; *HU,* Hounsfield units; *ROI,* region of interest.

with lipomas. Lipomas demonstrate CT density in the −50 to −100 HU range, with standard deviations less than 10 HU, whereas dermoids can range up to −20 to −40 HU, with standard deviations greater than 20 HU.

• Calcification: Capsular calcifications are more common in dermoid cysts (up to 20%). The tubulonodular subtype of pericallosal interhemispheric lipomas can have rim calcification, but this finding is rare in parasellar and posterior fossa lesions.

• T2-weighted imaging: Whereas lipomas are homogeneously T2 hyperintense, dermoids tend to be more heterogeneous and can vary from hyperintense to hypointense. Lipomas also tend to show striking chemical shift artifact, which often is less apparent with dermoid cysts.

• Rupture: Fatty droplets throughout the subarachnoid space and fat fluid levels in the lateral ventricles are seen in the setting of a ruptured dermoid cyst.

Signs and Complications

The most common presenting symptom with unruptured dermoid cysts is headache, although seizures and symptoms related to mass effect also can occur. Intracranial lipomas typically are found incidentally when imaging is performed. Both dermoids and lipomas of the sylvian fissure have been reported to have a higher association with seizures. Dermoids enlarge slowly over time by progressive cell division, desquamation, and secretion of dermal elements into the cystic cavity. Spontaneous, traumatic, or iatrogenic rupture can occur, with dissemination of the cyst contents into the CSF spaces. Cyst rupture can lead to chemical meningitis, hydrocephalus, seizures, and cranial nerve deficits.

Treatment of dermoid lesions is surgical. Complete excision is essential to prevent recurrence. Preoperative differentiation of dermoid cysts from lipomas is important because lipomas are nonsurgical lesions. Lipomas tend to be highly vascular with adherent fibrous capsules, which, combined with the intricate involvement of traversing vessels and/or cranial nerves, can make complete surgical excision extremely difficult and dangerous. High surgical morbidity and mortality rates have been reported with attempted excisions of intracranial lipomas.

Suggested Readings

Barkovich AJ, Raybaud C. Congenital malformations of the brain and skull. *Pediatric neuroimaging,* ed 6, Philadelphia, 2019, Wolters Kluwer/Lippincott Williams & Wilkins.

Feldman RP, Marcovici A, LaSala PA: Intracranial lipoma of the sylvian fissure, *J Neurosurg* 94:515–519, 2001.

Kazner E, Stochdorph O, Wende S, et al: Intracranial lipoma. Diagnostic and therapeutic considerations, *J Neurosurg* 52(2):234–245, 1980.

Li ZJ, Miao YX, Sun P, et al: Unusual CT hyperattenuating dermoid cyst of cerebellum: a new case report and literature review, *Cerebellum* 10:536–539, 2011.

Orakcioglu B, Halatsch ME, Fortunati M, et al: Intracranial dermoid cysts: variations of radiological and clinical features, *Acta Neurochir (Wien)* 150(12):1227–1234, 2008.

Osborn AG, Preece MT: Intracranial cysts: radiologic-pathologic correlation and imaging approach, *Radiology* 239(3):650–664, 2006.

Smirniotopoulos JG, Chiechi MV: Teratomas, dermoids, and epidermoids of the head and neck, *Radiographics* 15(6):1437–1455, 1995.

Warakaulle DR, Anslow P: Differential diagnosis of intracranial lesions with high signal on T1 or low signal on T2-weighted MRI, *Clin Radiol* 58:922–933, 2003.

Yildiz H, Hakyemez B, Koroglu M, et al: Intracranial lipomas: importance of localization, *Neuroradiology* 48:1–7, 2006.

13

Dural-Based Extraaxial Lesions

JUAN E. SMALL, MD, MSC

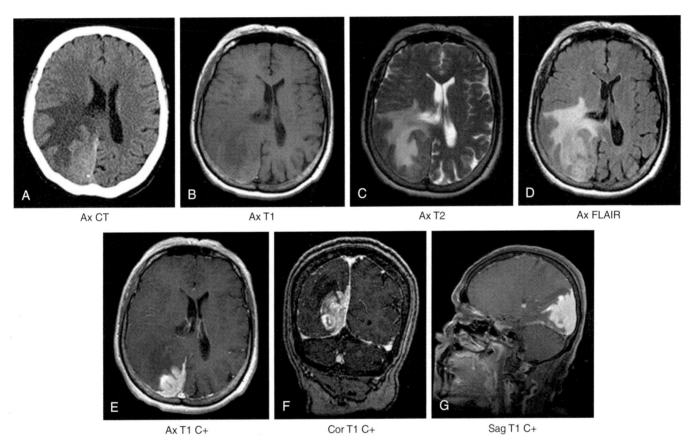

Ax CT   Ax T1   Ax T2   Ax FLAIR

Ax T1 C+   Cor T1 C+   Sag T1 C+

CASE A: A 75-year-old presenting with ataxia. *Ax*, Axial; *Cor*, coronal; *CT*, Computed tomography; *FLAIR*, fluid attenuated inversion recovery; *Sag*, sagittal.

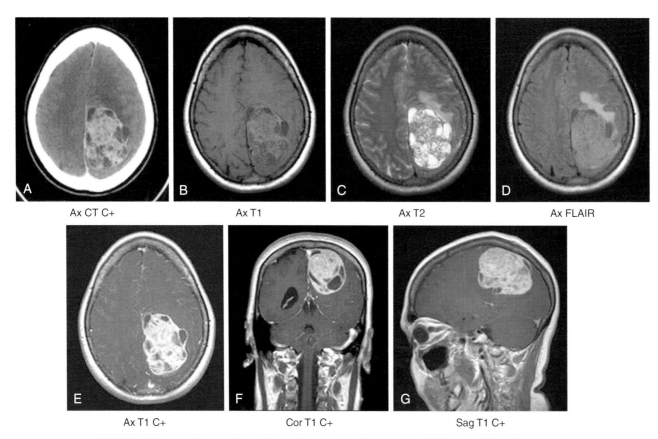

Ax CT C+   Ax T1   Ax T2   Ax FLAIR

Ax T1 C+   Cor T1 C+   Sag T1 C+

CASE B: A 51-year-old presenting with headaches and weakness of the right leg. *Ax,* Axial; *Cor,* coronal; *CT,* Computed tomography; *FLAIR,* fluid attenuated inversion recovery; *Sag,* sagittal.

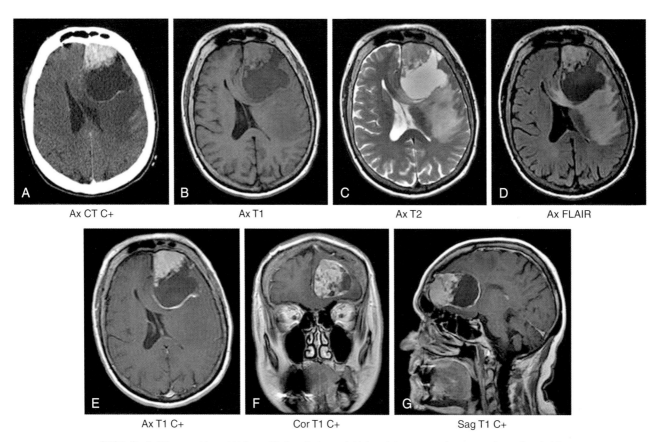

Ax CT C+   Ax T1   Ax T2   Ax FLAIR

Ax T1 C+   Cor T1 C+   Sag T1 C+

CASE C: A 73-year-old presenting with headaches, right hand tremor, and memory loss. *Ax,* Axial; *Cor,* coronal; *CT,* Computed tomography; *FLAIR,* fluid attenuated inversion recovery; *Sag,* sagittal.

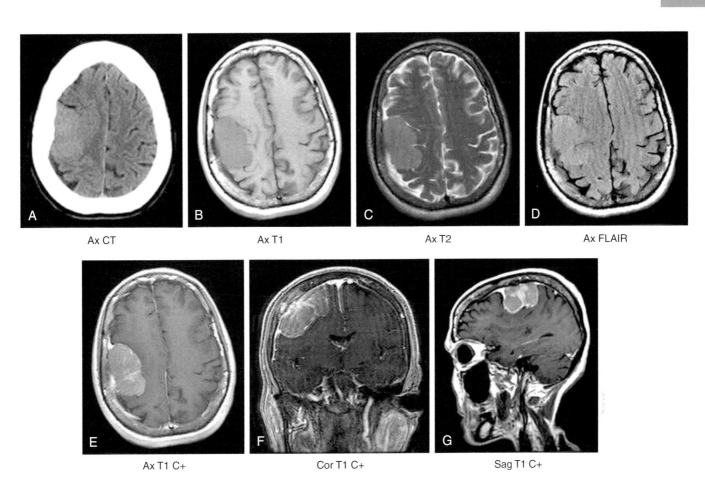

Ax CT | Ax T1 | Ax T2 | Ax FLAIR

Ax T1 C+ | Cor T1 C+ | Sag T1 C+

CASE D: A 72-year-old presenting with weakness of the left arm. *Ax,* Axial; *Cor,* coronal; *CT,* Computed tomography; *FLAIR,* fluid attenuated inversion recovery; *Sag,* sagittal.

DESCRIPTION OF FINDINGS

- Case A: A CT relatively hyperdense, T2 isointense, avidly enhancing extraaxial parasagittal right parietal lesion with thick dural enhancement, extensive surrounding white matter edema, and adjacent brain parenchymal enhancement, indicating parenchymal invasion.
- Case B: A large parasagittal left parietal extraaxial lesion with heterogeneous enhancement and cystic changes. Mild white matter edema is present anterior to the lesion without parenchymal enhancement.
- Case C: A large, densely enhancing left frontal extraaxial lesion with a large posterior cystic component. A large amount of parenchymal edema is present without parenchymal enhancement. A small cerebrospinal fluid cleft separating the lesion from the parenchyma is visible on the T2-weighted image.
- Case D: A large, T2 hypointense, densely enhancing right frontoparietal extraaxial lesion with a dural tail, adjacent hyperostosis, and patchy enhancement of the overlying bone.

Diagnosis

Case A: Malignant meningioma
Case B: Hemangiopericytoma
Case C: Typical cystic meningioma
Case D: Typical meningioma with intraosseous extension

Summary

Statistically speaking, the overwhelming majority of enhancing, dural-based, extraaxial lesions are meningiomas. A meningioma is an extraaxial neoplasm that generally is a slowly growing, well-circumscribed, dural-based, homogeneously and intensely enhancing mass. Linear thickening and enhancement of the dura adjacent to the meningioma has been termed the "dural tail," which is somewhat similar in appearance to the tail on a bell-shaped curve. Although a dural tail is characteristic of meningiomas, it is important to note that a dural tail is not always seen on imaging and may be seen with several dural masses other than meningiomas. Meningiomas may exhibit a plaque-like growth pattern or, rarely, may grow in an intraventricular location (most commonly in the trigones of the lateral ventricles). At times, adjacent cerebral parenchymal edema is noted. Other characteristics are calcification of the mass (>20%) and adjacent calvarial hyperostosis (20% to 40%). Because meningiomas are usually well-vascularized lesions, flow voids may be identified. The mass itself generally is T1 isointense to hypointense and T2 isointense to hyperintense compared to gray matter. On computed tomography, a meningioma generally is slightly hyperdense compared with normal brain tissue. Occasionally, necrosis and cystic components can be seen. At times, meningiomas cause adjacent venous sinus compression or invasion as well as arterial encasement and narrowing.

Meningiomas are commonly diagnosed in middle-aged and elderly patients (the peak incidence is during the seventh decade of life). A female predilection is noted; the female to male ratio is 2:1 intracranially and 4:1 in the spinal canal. Female predominance and occasional accelerated growth during pregnancy suggest a hormonal role. Meningiomas arise from the meningeal coverings of the brain and spinal cord. Specifically, they probably arise from arachnoid cap cells, which are concentrated in arachnoid villi. Because arachnoid villi are most numerous in the parasagittal region, the cerebral convexities, and along the skull base, meningiomas tend to present at these locations. Ionizing radiation has been established as a clear cause of meningiomas. Another clear cause is mutations in the neurofibromatosis type 2 (NF2) gene. Therefore meningiomas (along with schwannomas and ependymomas) are hallmarks of NF2.

Considering their generally slow growth over extended periods, simple meningiomas typically are monitored with imaging. However, it is important to note that both benign and more aggressive lesions remain within the differential diagnosis of enhancing dural-based lesions. With this factor in mind, the imaging interpreter must have a clear understanding of the features that suggest a benign versus an aggressive or malignant lesion. In addition, one also must understand the imaging features that are common to both types of lesions and therefore are not helpful in tailoring the differential diagnosis.

Lesion stability or minimal growth appears to be the most important feature to differentiate lesions across this spectrum. Adjacent hyperostosis or heavy calcification are suggestive of a typical meningioma. Rapid growth, on the other hand, is not typical of a benign lesion. Although most meningiomas are benign, several histologic subsets have been identified (Table 13.1). Some histologic subsets are associated with a higher risk of recurrence, and even more rarely, some histologic subsets exhibit malignant behavior.

Unfortunately, a considerable amount of overlap exists in the imaging appearance of typical, atypical, and malignant meningiomas. The most important imaging finding to be ascertained is that of parenchymal invasion because it is the one imaging sign that most specifically suggests an aggressive lesion, such as an aggressive atypical meningioma, malignant meningioma, or other aggressive dural-based lesion. Of note, other imaging findings, such as the presence of a dural tail, heterogeneous enhancement, cystic changes, bone involvement, and the degree of brain edema (even when quite prominent), are not specific and may be seen throughout the entire spectrum of dural-based lesions (Fig. 13.1). Cerebral edema in relation to simple meningiomas is poorly understood (Fig. 13.2). Meningioma size, location,

TABLE 13.1	World Health Organization Meningioma Classification	
Classification	**Recurrence Rates**	**Histologic Types**
Grade I (~80%)	5% at 5 years	Meningothelial, fibroblastic, transitional, angiomatous, microcystic, secretory, lymphoplasmacytic metaplastic, and psammomatous
Atypical grade II (5%–20%)	~40% at 5 years	Clear cell and chordoid variants
Anaplastic (malignant) grade III (1%–2%)	50%–80%, with median survival of <2 years	Rhabdoid and papillary variants; usually have large zones of necrosis

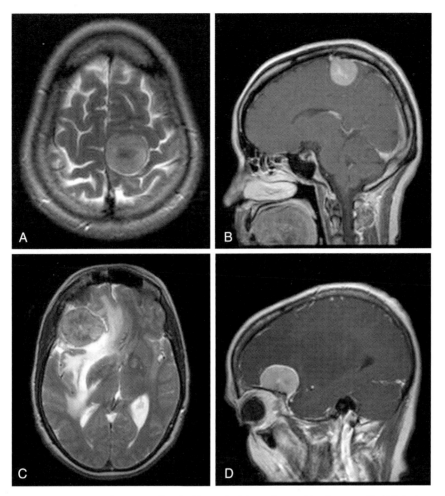

• **Fig. 13.1** Parenchymal edema associated with meningiomas does not imply a specific histologic grade. Axial T2 (**A**) and sagittal T1 (**B**) postcontrast images in a 33-year-old right-handed patient with a pathologically proven atypical meningioma demonstrate a benign-appearing extraaxial enhancing left frontal mass without adjacent edema. In contrast, axial T2 (**C**), and sagittal T1 (**D**) contrast-enhanced images in a 58-year-old with a pathologically proven simple/benign meningioma demonstrate a similar-sized right frontal enhancing extraaxial mass with a large amount of associated parenchymal edema and mass effect.

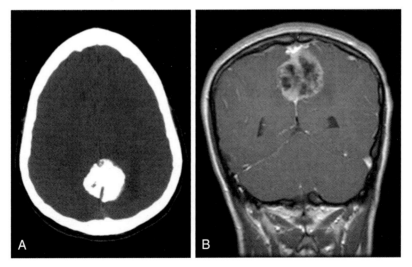

• **Fig. 13.2** Densely calcified typical/benign meningioma. A 19-year-old with a history of neurofibromatosis type 2 returned to the clinic for follow-up. Axial computed tomography (**A**) and coronal T1 (**B**) contrast-enhanced images demonstrate a densely calcified, partially enhancing extraaxial midline falcine mass consistent with a meningioma. Mild associated adjacent edema is present.

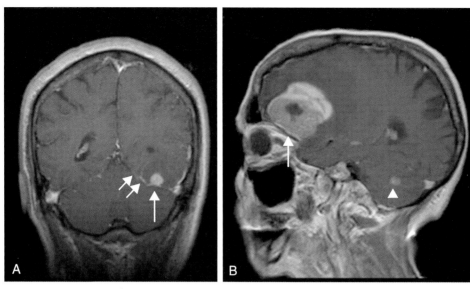

• **Fig. 13.3** Dural metastases. (**A**) A 62-year-old with history of metastatic malignant melanoma presented with a change in mental status. The coronal contrast-enhanced T1 image demonstrates a pathologically proven dural-based tentorial metastasis *(long arrow)* with adjacent leptomeningeal enhancement *(short arrows)*. (**B**) A 77-year-old with a history of lung cancer presented with altered mental status and memory difficulties. The sagittal contrast-enhanced T1 image demonstrates a large, heterogeneously enhancing frontal metastasis *(arrow)* and a smaller cerebellar metastasis *(arrowhead)*. A history of a primary neoplasm, the presence of multiple lesions, and leptomeningeal enhancement suggest the diagnosis of metastases.

venous compression, and secretion of vasoactive products all have been implicated in the literature.

Differential considerations should include dural metastasis (Fig. 13.3), hemangiopericytoma, and lymphoma in adult patients. Hemangiopericytomas tend to be lobular, heterogeneously and avidly enhancing masses without calcification and without adjacent hyperostosis. Cystic or necrotic areas are common. In patients with a known malignancy or multiple lesions (outside the spectrum of meningiomatosis or multiple meningiomas in the setting of NF2), meningeal metastases or lymphoma are more likely pathologies. Unfortunately, the imaging appearance can be difficult or impossible to differentiate from meningioma.

Spectrum of Disease

See Figs. 13.1, 13.2, and 13.3.

Differential Diagnosis of an Enhancing Dural-Based Mass

Typical/benign meningioma
Atypical meningioma
Malignant meningioma
Meningeal metastasis
Lymphoma
Hemangiopericytoma (rare, may be indistinguishable from classic meningiomas)
Langerhans cell histiocytosis (in a pediatric patient)

IgG4-related disease
Granulomatosis with polyangiitis
Neurosarcoidosis

Pearls

Location

- Confirm that the lesion is extraaxial by clearly separating it from the adjacent parenchyma with the help of signs indicating that a mass is an extraaxial lesion: meniscus sign/cerebrospinal fluid cleft sign, cortical ribbon sign/buckling gray matter, and displacement of subarachnoid veins.

Imaging Appearance

- Significant overlap exists between benign and malignant entities.
- Characteristic imaging features of meningiomas are calcification, hyperostosis, a dural tail, and intense homogeneous enhancement.
- A heavily calcified dural-based lesion favors a diagnosis of meningioma.
- Although a dural tail is characteristic of a meningioma, a dural tail also may be seen with several other dural masses.
- Rapid growth is uncharacteristic of a typical meningioma, no matter how homogenous the lesion appears.
- Meningiomas (even typical ones) may invade the dura, venous sinuses, skull, and extraaxial compartments—characteristics that do not necessarily imply an atypical or malignant variant.

However, brain invasion implies at least an atypical or anaplastic meningioma.

- Dural-based masses associated with granulomatosis with polyangiitis, sarcoidosis, and IgG4-related disease are typically markedly hypointense on T2-weighted images.
- Dural-based lymphomas may have restricted diffusion.
- Hemangiopericytomas frequently contain multiple cysts.

Complications

Complications generally are related to encasement and narrowing of arteries (Fig. 13.4) and/or invasion of venous sinuses (Fig. 13.5).

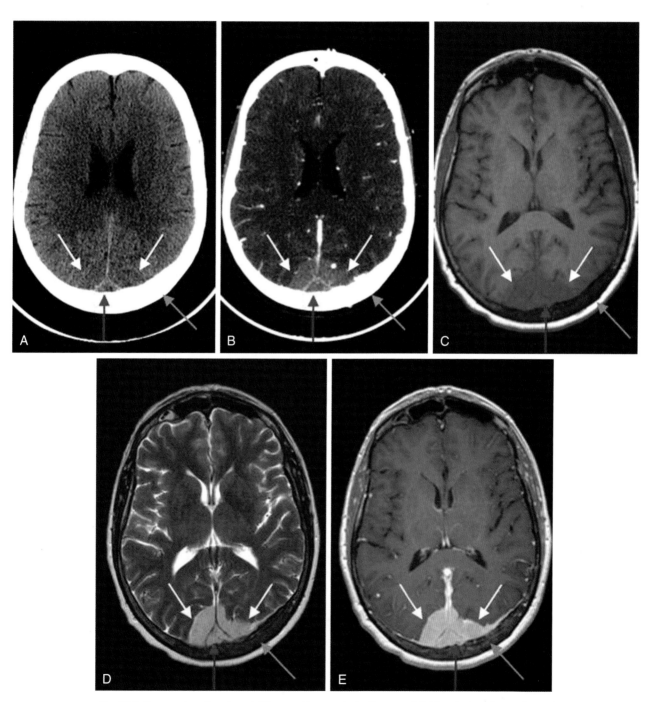

• **Fig. 13.4** Venous sinus invasion. A 69-year-old presented with an occipital headache of several years' duration, which worsened recently. Axial computed tomography (**A**), axial contrast-enhanced computed tomography (**B**), axial T1 (**C**), axial T2 (**D**), and axial T1 (**E**) contrast-enhanced images demonstrate a large posterior parasagittal enhancing extraaxial meningioma *(white arrows)* with adjacent hyperostosis *(gray arrows)* that is invading, expanding, and occluding the adjacent superior sagittal venous sinus *(red arrows)*.

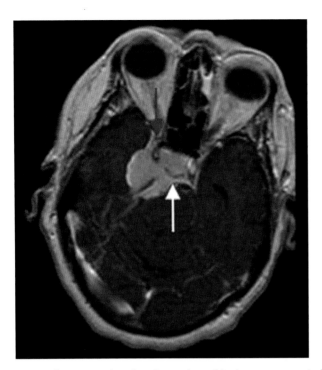

• **Fig. 13.5** Cavernous sinus invasion and carotid artery encasement. A 79-year-old with a known meningioma. The axial T1 contrast-enhanced image demonstrates an avidly enhancing meningioma that is invading the sella turcica *(white arrow)* and right cavernous sinus and encasing and narrowing the right internal carotid artery *(red arrow)*.

Suggested Readings

Black PM, Morokoff AP, Zauberman J: Surgery for extra-axial tumors of the cerebral convexity and midline, *Neurosurgery* (SHC suppl 3):SHC1115–SHC1123, 2008.

Buetow MP, Buetow PC, Smirniotopoulos JG: Typical, atypical, and misleading features in meningioma, *Radiographics* 11:1087–1106, 1991.

Casasco A, Mani J, Alachkar F, et al: Peritumoral edema in intracranial meningiomas. Angiographic and computerized tomographic correlations [in French], *Neurochirurgie* 32(4):296–303, 1986.

Nägele T, Petersen D, Klose U, et al: The "dural tail" adjacent to meningiomas studied by dynamic contrast-enhanced MRI: a comparison with histopathology, *Neuroradiology* 36(4):303–307, 1994.

Prayson RA: *Neuropathology*, St Louis, 2005, Saunders Elsevier.

Riemenschneider MJ, Perry A, Reifenberger G: Histological classification and molecular genetics of meningiomas, *Lancet Neurol* 5(12): 1045–1054, 2006.

Simon M, Boström JP, Hartmann C: Molecular genetics of meningiomas: from basic research to potential clinical applications, *Neurosurgery* 60(5):787–798, 2007.

Takeguchi T, Miki H, Shimizu T, et al: The dural tail of intracranial meningiomas of fluid-attenuated inversion-recovery images, *Neuroradiology* 46:130–135, 2004.

Zhang HX, Rodiger LA, Shen T, et al: Perfusion MRI for differentiation of benign and malignant meningiomas, *Neuroradiology* 50(6): 525–530, 2008.

14

Bilateral Central Gray Matter Abnormality

JUAN E. SMALL, MD, MSC

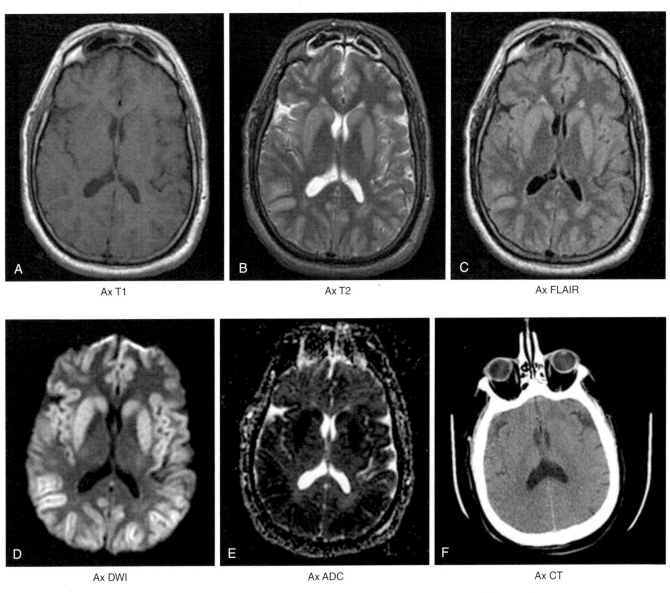

Ax T1

Ax T2

Ax FLAIR

Ax DWI

Ax ADC

Ax CT

CASE A: A 50-year-old with a history of chronic obstructive pulmonary disease and hypertension was found unresponsive. *ADC,* Apparent diffusion coefficient; *Ax,* axial; *CT,* Computed tomography; *DWI,* diffusion-weighted imaging; *FLAIR,* fluid attenuated inversion recovery.

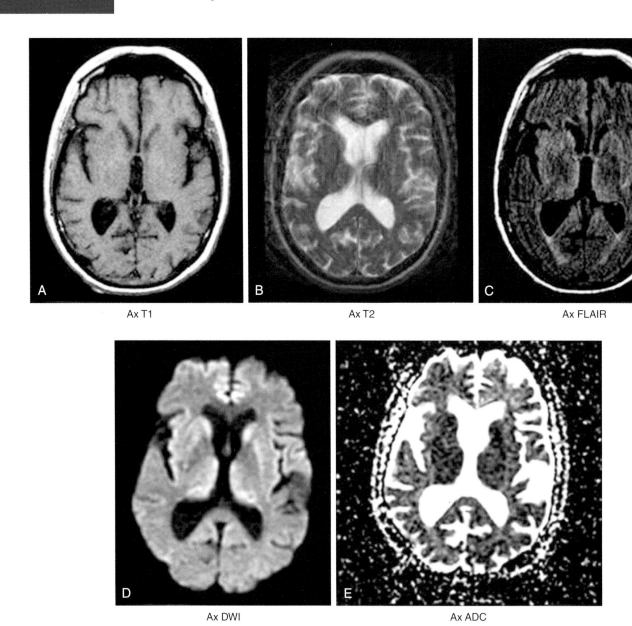

Ax T1

Ax T2

Ax FLAIR

Ax DWI

Ax ADC

CASE B: A 67-year-old presenting with ataxia, rapidly progressive deterioration in mental status, and myoclonus. *ADC,* Apparent diffusion coefficient; *Ax,* axial; *DWI,* diffusion-weighted imaging; *FLAIR,* fluid attenuated inversion recovery.

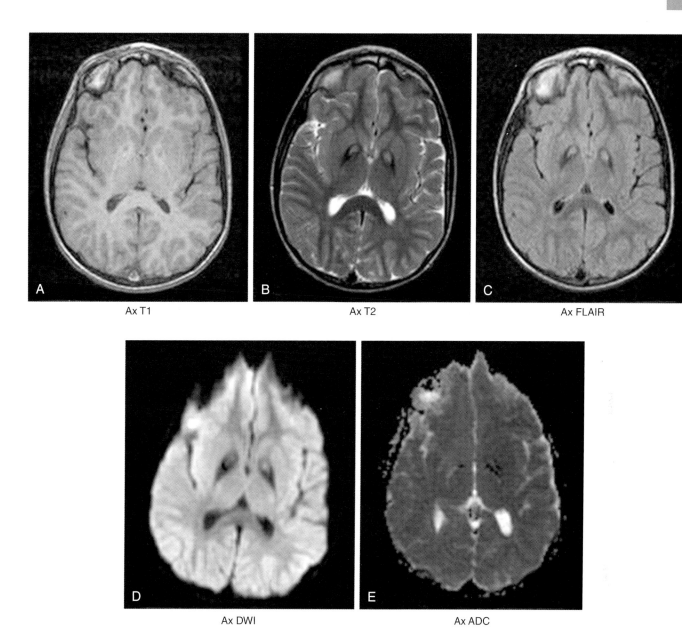

Ax T1   Ax T2   Ax FLAIR

Ax DWI   Ax ADC

CASE C: An 11-year-old with chronic progressive neurologic symptoms since the age of 9 years. *ADC,* Apparent diffusion coefficient; *Ax,* axial; *DWI,* diffusion-weighted imaging; *FLAIR,* fluid attenuated inversion recovery.

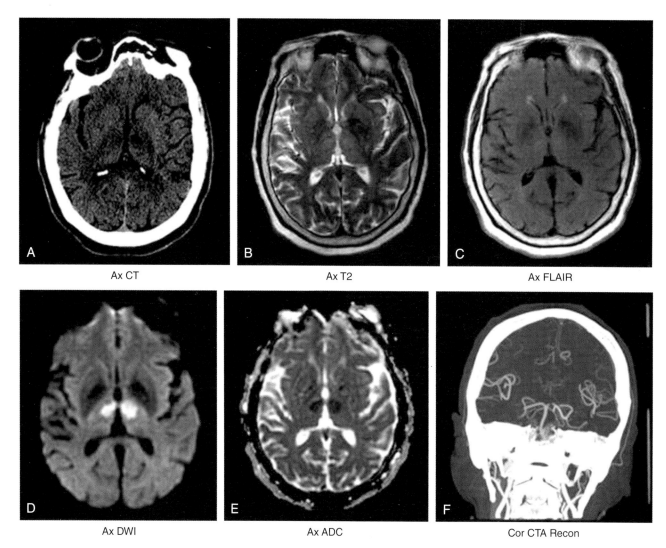

Ax CT

Ax T2

Ax FLAIR

Ax DWI

Ax ADC

Cor CTA Recon

CASE D: A 72-year-old with a history of coronary artery bypass grafting who was unable to be aroused in the morning. *ADC,* Apparent diffusion coefficient; *Ax,* axial; *Cor,* coronal; *CT,* Computed tomography; *CTA,* CT angiography; *DWI,* diffusion-weighted imaging; *FLAIR,* fluid attenuated inversion recovery; *Recon,* reconstruction.

- Case A: Uniform, bilateral restricted diffusion is noted involving the caudate nuclei, putamina, and cerebral cortex. These structures are hyperintense on fluid attenuated inversion recovery (FLAIR) and T2-weighted images and hypodense on noncontrast CT. Swelling of the ischemic structures also is noted.
- Case B: Patchy, asymmetric areas of restricted diffusion and FLAIR hyperintensity involve the cerebral cortex (including the cingulate gyri). Symmetric areas of restricted diffusion and FLAIR hyperintensity involve the caudate nuclei and putamina. Bilateral symmetric involvement of the thalamic pulvinar and dorsomedial thalamic nuclei is also present (consistent with a "hockey stick" sign).
- Case C: Prominent, symmetric, bilateral globus pallidus central FLAIR and T2 hyperintensity is present with surrounding hypointensity consistent with the "eye of the tiger" sign. The lesions have central hypointensity on T1-weighted images.
- Case D: Bilateral anterior thalamic CT hypodensity and restricted diffusion consistent with bilateral thalamic infarction are present. The infarctions are mildly hyperintense on FLAIR and T2-weighted images. Coronal CT angiography reconstruction demonstrates a focal unilateral occlusion of the left P1 segment at the expected site of thalamoperforators.

Diagnosis

Case A: Hypoxic-ischemic encephalopathy (HIE)

Case B: Creutzfeldt-Jakob disease (CJD)

Case C: Neurodegeneration with brain iron accumulation (NBIA) (formerly Hallervorden-Spatz disease) resulting from *PANK2* mutation

Case D: Bilateral thalamic infarcts resulting from occlusion of the artery of Percheron

Summary

A wide range of insults, including systemic, toxic, metabolic, vascular, infectious, hereditary, and degenerative disorders, may result in bilateral symmetric basal ganglia and thalamic imaging abnormalities. A few key imaging characteristics may yield a specific diagnosis. In addition, careful inspection of other sites of involvement, including the cerebral cortex, white matter, and brainstem, can narrow the differential diagnosis. Differentiating an acute, subacute, or chronic process based on history also is often quite valuable.

Assessing whether a specific subset or most of the basal ganglia nuclei and/or thalami are involved in the disease process is the first step in assessment. Some processes that typically involve any combination or all of the deep gray nuclei include HIE, CJD, toxic exposures, hyperglycemia, hypoglycemia, liver disease (T1 hyperintensity), Wilson disease, osmotic myelinolysis, and deep venous thrombosis. Some processes that classically or preferentially involve a subset of the deep gray nuclei include diseases primarily affecting the caudate nuclei, such as Huntington disease; the putamen, such as methanol toxicity, cyanide poisoning, and Leigh disease; the globus pallidus, such as NBIA (formerly Hallervorden-Spatz disease) and carbon monoxide poisoning (preferentially involves the globus pallidus early, but all structures may become involved); and the thalamus, such as infarction of the artery of Percheron. Lastly,

the identification of specific imaging signs, such as the eye of the tiger sign (NBIA), hockey stick sign (CJD), or pulvinar sign (CJD), can markedly limit the diagnostic considerations.

Basal Ganglia/Thalamic and Cortical Involvement

Attention to involvement of sites other than the deep gray nuclei, such as the cerebral cortex, is important. The high metabolic rate of the basal ganglia and cortex makes these sites particularly susceptible to hypoxemia/anoxia. Both Cases A and B demonstrate involvement of the basal ganglia and cerebral cortex, with one representing HIE and the other CJD. Although the findings can be quite similar to those of HIE, cortical involvement tends to be asymmetric in persons with CJD versus symmetric in persons with HIE, and edema is often present in acute cases of HIE but not CJD.

Severe HIE prominently affects the gray matter structures, that is, the cerebral cortex, basal ganglia, thalami, and hippocampi. Swelling usually is seen 24 hours or more after the initial insult. Imaging findings are highly variable and depend on the severity of insult and timing of the evaluation.

CJD is a prion-mediated, transmissible, neurodegenerative disorder. Four main subtypes have been described: familial, sporadic, iatrogenic, and variant. Approximately 90% of cases are classified as sporadic. A rapidly progressive dementia with myoclonus, ataxia, and multifocal neurologic dysfunction is the characteristic presenting history. Although generalized periodic sharp wave complexes on an electroencephalogram and the detection of the 14-3-3 proteins within cerebrospinal fluid are required for noninvasive diagnosis, a brain biopsy or autopsy is required for definitive diagnosis. Characteristic imaging features of sporadic CJD include restricted diffusion and T2/FLAIR hyperintensity involving the basal ganglia and the cerebral cortex. Cortical abnormalities may be unilateral or bilateral and focal or diffuse. Signal abnormality may involve the cerebral cortex only. Typical imaging features of variant CJD are bilateral FLAIR/T2 hyperintense lesions in the pulvinar of the thalami described as the pulvinar sign. The hockey stick sign represents contiguous high FLAIR/T2 hyperintense signal involving the pulvinar and dorsomedial thalamic nuclei. Basal ganglia involvement may be focal or diffuse, and the caudate nucleus is most often involved.

Acute Versus Chronic Symptomatology

Acute symptomatology suggests differential considerations, including HIE, vascular insults, toxin/drug exposure, and hypoglycemia, among other considerations. Acute causes of HIE, such as cardiac or respiratory arrest, often are known at the time of presentation, which makes imaging interpretation straightforward. Unfortunately, the presenting history is not always clear, as in cases of coma of unknown etiology, and a differential diagnosis must be entertained.

Exposures to toxins such as carbon monoxide, cyanide, or methanol (i.e., cellular respiratory toxins affecting mitochondrial function) may predominantly affect the basal. Methanol exposure may present with optic neuritis as the initial symptom. Although laboratory/toxicology results yield the specific diagnosis, imaging documents the extent of damage. Carbon monoxide toxicity most commonly involves the globus pallidus (Fig. 14.1), although the entire basal ganglia may be affected in more severe cases. In addition, the putamen, caudate, and thalamus may be involved without globus pallidus involvement. The white matter also may be involved, although less commonly. Cyanide and methanol poisoning may result in hemorrhagic necrosis of the putamen.

Specific Sites of Involvement

When confronted with a case demonstrating bilateral basal ganglia or thalamic abnormalities, it often is helpful to find a focal site of involvement to tailor the differential diagnosis.

Selective caudate atrophy is the hallmark of Huntington disease, an autosomal dominant neurodegenerative process. Ex-vacuo dilation of the adjacent frontal horns of the lateral ventricles gives them their typical squaring or "boxcar" appearance, as seen in Fig. 14.2. Of note, juvenile Huntington disease

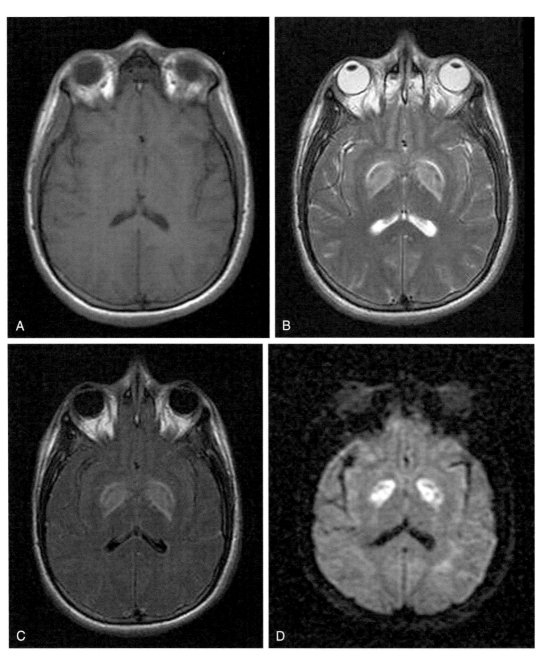

• **Fig. 14.1** Globus pallidus involvement in carbon monoxide poisoning. (**A**) Axial T1, (**B**) axial T2, (**C**) axial fluid attenuated inversion recovery, and (**D**) axial diffusion-weighted imaging images in a 23-year-old known to have carbon monoxide poisoning demonstrate symmetric, bilateral, restricted diffusion and edema of the globus pallidi.

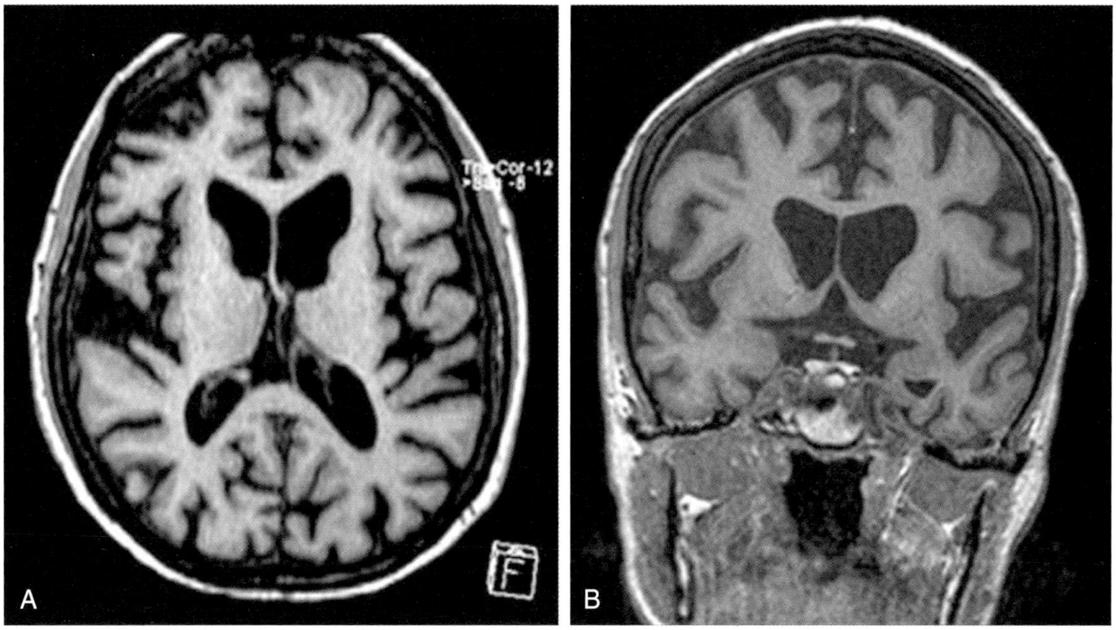

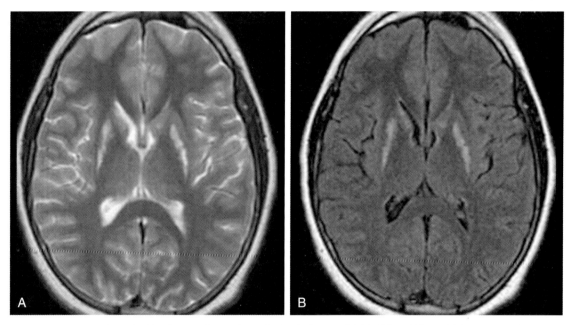

• **Fig. 14.2** Caudate involvement in Huntington disease. (**A**) Axial and (**B**) coronal T1 images demonstrate bilateral severe caudate head atrophy with adjacent ex-vacuo dilation of the frontal horns leading to squaring or a "boxcar" appearance of the anterior lateral ventricles.

• **Fig. 14.3** Putaminal involvement in a patient with Leigh disease. (**A**) Axial T2 and (**B**) axial fluid attenuated inversion recovery images in a 13-year-old patient with a history of Leigh disease demonstrate predominant putaminal involvement with T2/FLAIR hyperintensity and volume loss. *FLAIR,* Fluid attenuated inversion recovery.

presents with hyperintense signal in the caudate nucleus and putamen.

Focal putaminal involvement may be seen with specific disease processes such as Leigh disease (subacute necrotizing encephalomyelopathy), an inherited autosomal recessive mitochondrial disorder of cellular respiratory metabolism (Fig. 14.3). Although Leigh disease most commonly presents with symmetric involvement of the corpora striata (putamen more than caudate), signal abnormality may be seen in the globus pallidi, as well as the thalami, periventricular white matter, periaqueductal gray matter, brainstem, spinal cord, and cerebral peduncles. Spectroscopy reveals high lactate levels in the basal ganglia, which, in conjunction with elevated serum and cerebrospinal fluid lactate levels, establish the diagnosis.

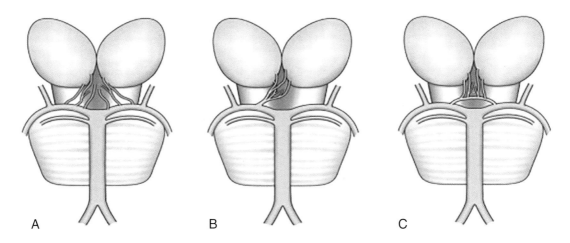

• **Fig. 14.4** Variations of the paramedian thalamic-mesencephalic arterial supply according to Percheron. (**A**) The most common variation with many small perforating arteries arising from the P1 segments. (**B**) A single perforating vessel arising from a unilateral P1 segment supplying the bilateral thalami is named the artery of Percheron. (**C**) Another variant with a bridging arcade of perforating branches arising from both P1 segments of both posterior cerebral arteries. (Modified from Matheus MG, Castillo M: Imaging of acute bilateral paramedian thalamic and mesencephalic infarcts, *AJNR Am J Neuroradiol* 24(10):2005–2008, 2003.)

Prominent signal abnormality centered in the globus pallidus is seen with processes such as NBIA, a group of disorders characterized by cerebral degeneration and iron deposition. Pantothenate kinase–associated neurodegeneration (PKAN, previously known as Hallervorden-Spatz disease) is one such disorder in this group. Although not present in all cases, the *PANK2* gene mutation is present in a substantial portion of both the classic early-onset and atypical late-onset cases. Case C clearly demonstrates the virtually pathognomonic imaging feature of *PANK2* mutation cases—the eye of the tiger sign—in which a T2 hyperintense center is surrounded by a T2 hypointense rim, correlating with excessive iron accumulation.

Venous and arterial abnormalities may result in bilateral basal ganglia and thalamic abnormalities. In particular, deep cerebral venous thrombosis (internal cerebral vein, vein of Galen, and/or straight sinus) may result in venous hypertension and cerebral edema involving the basal ganglia, thalami, and deep white matter with or without associated hemorrhagic conversion. Arterial occlusion, including basilar tip occlusion, may result in bilateral thalamic infarcts. In addition, occlusion of the rare artery of Percheron anatomic variant, in which a single common trunk arises from a proximal posterior cerebral artery to supply the bilateral thalami and midbrain, also may result in bilateral thalamic infarcts, as demonstrated in Case D. Fig. 14.4 demonstrates variations of the paramedian thalamic-mesencephalic arterial supply according to Percheron.

Specific Signal Characteristics

Intrinsic T1 hyperintensity also may point to specific differential considerations such as hepatic encephalopathy, parenteral nutrition/hyperalimentation, hypermagnesemia, and Wilson disease. Magnetic resonance imaging findings in patients with

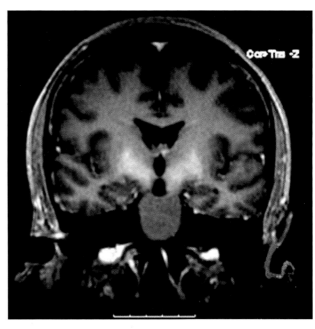

• **Fig. 14.5** T1 basal ganglia hyperintensity in a patient with hepatic encephalopathy. Coronal T1 image in an adult patient with liver failure demonstrates bilateral T1 hyperintensity involving the globus pallidi and midbrain.

liver dysfunction (Fig. 14.5) include bilateral T1 hyperintense signal abnormality involving the globus pallidus and substantia nigra.

Spectrum of Disease

Variable imaging findings can be seen in cases of HIE depending on the duration and severity of brain insult, timing of imaging, and the age of the patient.

CJD imaging findings may be variable depending on the individual, the timing of imaging, the severity of involvement, and the type of CJD (Fig. 14.6).

Differential Diagnosis

1. Toxic exposures: carbon monoxide, methanol, cyanide
2. Metabolic disorders: hepatic encephalopathy/liver disease, hyperammonemia, hyperglycemia, hypoglycemia, HIE, Wilson disease, Leigh disease, osmotic myelinolysis, Wernicke encephalopathy
3. Vascular disease: arterial occlusion, artery of Percheron occlusion, deep cerebral vein thrombosis
4. Degenerative disorders: CJD, NBIA, Fahr disease
5. Inflammatory/infectious disease: toxoplasmosis, viral infections, Behçet syndrome
6. Neoplastic: lymphoma, thalamic glioma, type 1 neurofibromatosis

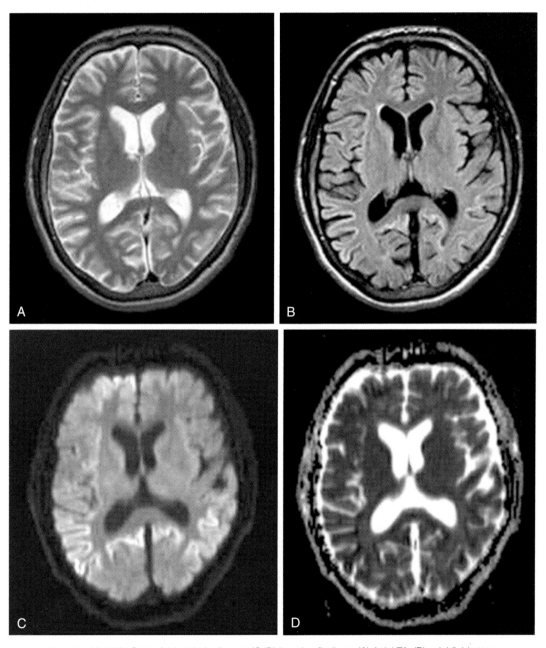

• **Fig. 14.6** Variable Creutzfeldt-Jakob disease (CJD) imaging findings. (**A**) Axial T2, (**B**) axial fluid attenuated inversion recovery, (**C**) axial diffusion-weighted imaging, and (**D**) axial apparent diffusion coefficient images in a 44-year-old presenting with rapidly progressive cognitive decline, including memory loss, and myoclonus demonstrate patchy, asymmetric areas of predominantly cortical restricted diffusion with only subtle caudate head involvement. As noted previously, cortical abnormalities in persons with CJD may be unilateral or bilateral and focal or diffuse, and signal abnormality may involve just the cerebral cortex. Basal ganglia involvement in persons with CJD may be focal or diffuse, with the caudate nucleus most often involved. In addition, the imaging appearance of CJD may vary with respect to the type of CJD in question.

Pearls

- Location:
- Caudate: Huntington disease
- Putamen: Leigh disease, cyanide, methanol
- Globus pallidus: NBIA, carbon monoxide
- Thalamus: artery of Percheron infarction
- Basal ganglia, thalamic and cortical restricted diffusion: HIE, CJD; cortical involvement tends to be asymmetric in persons with CJD, and edema is often present in acute cases of HIE; the history is most often strongly suggestive of one versus the other
- Intrinsic T1 hyperintensity may point to specific differential considerations, such as hepatic encephalopathy, parenteral nutrition/hyperalimentation, hypermagnesemia, and Wilson disease

Signs and Complications

- Eye of the tiger: NBIA
- Hockey stick sign: variant CJD
- Pulvinar sign: variant CJD

Suggested Readings

Beltz EE, Mullins ME: Radiological reasoning: hyperintensity of the basal ganglia and cortex on FLAIR and diffusion-weighted imaging, *AJR Am J Roentgenol* 195(3 suppl):S1–S8, 2010.

Hayflick SJ, Hartman M, Coryell J, et al: Brain MRI in neurodegeneration with brain iron accumulation with and without PANK2 mutations, *AJNR Am J Neuroradiol* 27(6):1230–1233, 2006.

Hegde AN, Mohan S, Lath N, et al: Differential diagnosis for bilateral abnormalities of the basal ganglia and thalamus, *Radiographics* 31(1):5–30, 2011.

Huang BY, Castillo M: Hypoxic-ischemic brain injury: imaging findings from birth to adulthood, *Radiographics* 28(2):417–439, 2008.

Lim CC: Magnetic resonance imaging findings in bilateral basal ganglia lesions, *Ann Acad Med Singapore* 38(9):795–798, 2009.

Macfarlane RG, Wroe SJ, Collinge J, et al: Neuroimaging findings in human prion disease, *J Neurol Neurosurg Psychiatry* 78(7):664–670, 2007.

Matheus MG, Castillo M: Imaging of acute bilateral paramedian thalamic and mesencephalic infarcts, *AJNR Am J Neuroradiol* 24(10):2005–2008, 2003.

Ukisu R, Kushihashi T, Tanaka E, et al: Diffusion-weighted MR imaging of early-stage Creutzfeldt-Jakob disease: typical and atypical manifestations, *Radiographics* 26(suppl 1):S191–S204, 2006.

15
Temporal Lobe Lesions

HENRY SU, MD, PHD

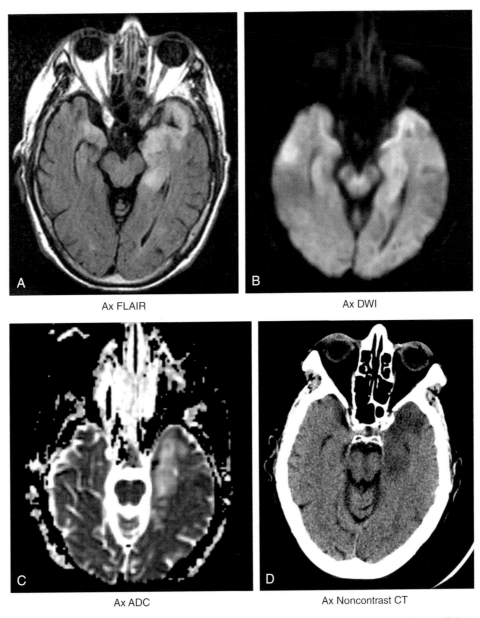

Ax FLAIR

Ax DWI

Ax ADC

Ax Noncontrast CT

CASE A: An 80-year-old with headache and speech changes. *ADC,* Apparent diffusion coefficient; *Ax,* axial; *CT,* Computed tomography; *DWI,* diffusion-weighted imaging; *FLAIR,* fluid attenuated inversion recovery.

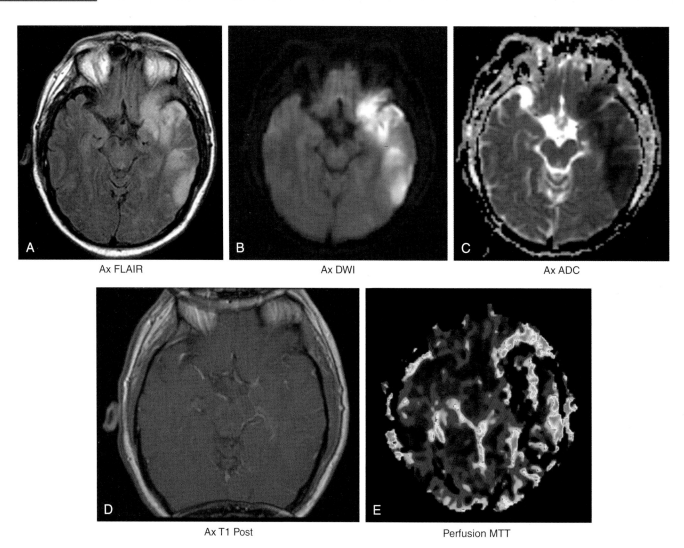

Ax FLAIR   Ax DWI   Ax ADC

Ax T1 Post   Perfusion MTT

CASE B: A 59-year-old with hypertension and poor medical compliance was found down and unable to speak, presenting with dense right hemiplegia. *ADC,* Apparent diffusion coefficient; *Ax,* axial; *DWI,* diffusion-weighted imaging; *FLAIR,* fluid attenuated inversion recovery; *MTT,* mean transit time.

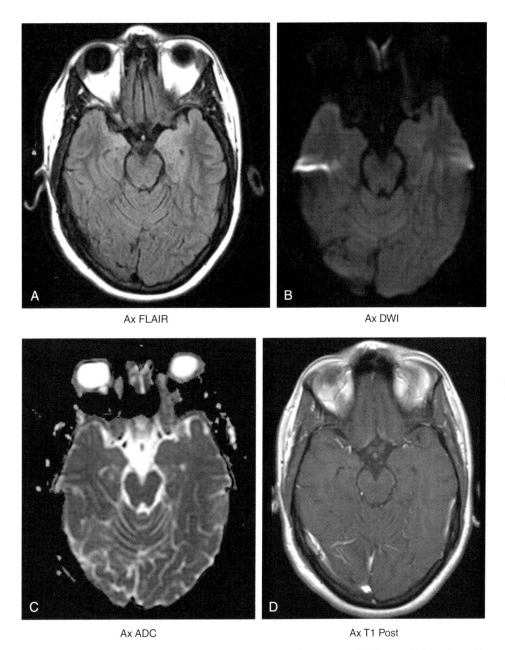

Ax FLAIR

Ax DWI

Ax ADC

Ax T1 Post

CASE C: A 28-year-old with hallucinations and amnesia. *ADC*, Apparent diffusion coefficient; *Ax*, axial; *DWI*, diffusion-weighted imaging; *FLAIR*, fluid attenuated inversion recovery.

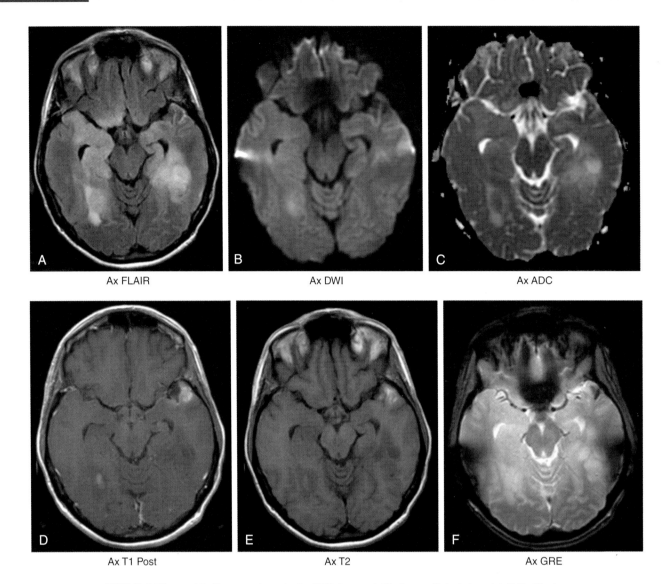

Ax FLAIR

Ax DWI

Ax ADC

Ax T1 Post

Ax T2

Ax GRE

CASE D: A 53-year-old with expressive aphasia. *ADC,* Apparent diffusion coefficient; *Ax,* axial; *DWI,* diffusion-weighted imaging; *FLAIR,* fluid attenuated inversion recovery; *GRE,* gradient refocused echo.

DESCRIPTION OF FINDINGS

- Case A: There are temporal lobe FLAIR hyperintense lesions (greater on the left than the right) with mild mass effect. There is mild hyperintensity on DWI due to T2 effects and hyperintensity, consistent with elevated diffusion, on the ADC maps. Corresponding hypodensity is seen on noncontrast head CT.
- Case B: A left temporal and inferior frontal FLAIR abnormality with mild mass effect in the middle cerebral artery (MCA) vascular territory without associated enhancement is seen. Restricted diffusion is present with DWI hyperintensity and ADC hypointensity. MR perfusion imaging demonstrates prolonged mean transit time in the abnormal left temporal lobe. Not shown is involvement of a significant portion of the MCA territory, including the perirolandic region.
- Case C: There are left larger than right medial temporal lobe FLAIR hyperintense lesions. The lesions do not enhance and have normal diffusion.
- Case D: Bilateral temporal and right inferior frontal FLAIR hyperintense lesions have mild mass effect and normal-to-elevated diffusion. The left anterior temporal lobe has a T1 hyperintense focus that demonstrates blooming, consistent with hemorrhage, on the gradient echo susceptibility sequence. In the right posterior mesial temporal lobe there is a small focus of enhancement. On subsequent imaging several months later, there was marked progression of enhancement to involve both temporal lobes.

Diagnosis

Case A: Herpes simplex virus (HSV) encephalitis confirmed by CSF polymerase chain reaction

Case B: Temporal lobe infarct

Case C: Nonneoplastic limbic encephalitis or autoimmune encephalitis (confirmed by positive antibodies against voltage-gated potassium channels)

Case D: Anaplastic astrocytoma grade 3

Summary

The imaging characteristics of HSV encephalitis are nonspecific, but the presence of T2/FLAIR signal abnormality in the temporal lobes should raise concern for this disease entity because the associated morbidity is particularly high if treatment is not initiated early. HSV encephalitis involves the limbic system; it typically demonstrates asymmetric, bilateral mesial temporal FLAIR hyperintense signal with additional involvement of the inferior frontal lobes, insular cortex, and/or cingulate gyrus. The acute phase typically has restricted diffusion. Petechial hemorrhage, gyriform enhancement, marked swelling, and normal or elevated diffusion are more common in the subacute phase. On CT, hypodensity is more prominent in the subacute phase due to the increasing edema. Although cerebrospinal fluid (CSF) polymerase chain reaction is the definitive diagnostic test, initiation of antiviral treatment often is begun after imaging findings.

Other types of autoimmune encephalitis are categorized into paraneoplastic and nonparaneoplastic causes. The clinical course is helpful in trying to differentiate them from HSV because they are more indolent in presentation. Imaging findings are nonspecific and can look similar to HSV but are rarely associated with hemorrhage. These entities can be either unilateral or bilateral. History of existing primary malignancy, such as lung cancer, helps order the differential diagnosis.

Nonparaneoplastic causes of autoimmune encephalitis are rarer; if there is clinical suspicion, antibody tests are performed to help detect the specific subtype because there is prognostic value regarding response to treatment (often steroids).

Distinguishing the above entities from temporal lobe infarctions is important. Unilateral involvement, a lesion within a single vascular distribution (MCA, anterior choroidal or posterior cerebral artery) and very low ADC values should raise the suspicion for ischemia. Clinical history of an acute change in a patient with known vasculopathy is also helpful. In the subacute infarct phase—when ADC has normalized and there is gyral enhancement, increasing FLAIR abnormality and mass effect—differentiation from HSV and autoimmune encephalitis can be challenging, and the evolution of radiographic findings may be helpful for delineation.

Primary glial neoplasms also can involve the temporal lobes; they usually are unilateral but can be bilateral. When the neoplasms are nonenhancing, they have mass effect, FLAIR hyperintensity, and elevated diffusion and can mimic HSV and autoimmune encephalitis. Persistent signal abnormality and mass effect after antiviral treatment suggest the presence of tumor. Glioblastomas can have ring enhancement, which would be atypical for other entities. Advanced MR imaging, such as perfusion or MR spectroscopy, may be helpful for further evaluation, although biopsy offers definitive diagnosis.

Repeated seizures can cause FLAIR hyperintense lesions with restricted diffusion in the temporal lobes. The lesions usually have a gyriform appearance and can resolve once seizures are controlled.

Differential Diagnosis

HSV encephalitis
Autoimmune encephalitis (paraneoplastic and nonparaneoplastic)
Primary central nervous system (CNS) infiltrating neoplasms
Infarctions
Seizures

Pearls

- Herpes encephalitis should always be considered with mesial temporal lobe FLAIR abnormalities because early treatment is critical. Bilateral asymmetric involvement of the limbic system is typical. Gyriform enhancement and petechial hemorrhage are fairly common but not always seen.
- Autoimmune encephalitides can have a similar appearance, and the clinical timing is helpful in distinguishing them (more indolent) from HSV (more fulminant).
- Unilateral involvement, a lesion within a single vascular distribution (MCA, anterior choroidal or posterior cerebral artery), very low ADC values, and acute symptom onset should raise the suspicion for ischemia.
- Primary CNS neoplasms can have similar imaging characteristics. Clinical history may be helpful, as well as advanced imaging, such as MR perfusion (with increased cerebral blood flow [CBF] and cerebral blood volume [CBV]) or MR spectroscopy (with a high choline peak). These lesions do not respond to antiviral therapy.

- Seizure-related lesions usually have gyriform FLAIR hyperintensity and restricted diffusion. They typically decrease when seizures are controlled.
- Hemorrhage most often occurs with HSV but can be seen with infarctions and high-grade tumors.

Signs and Complications

The common pathway for infectious, inflammatory, and ischemic lesions is tissue loss with gliosis. Hemorrhage can worsen the outcome in patients with HSV and ischemic lesions. Infiltrative neoplasms typically are not resectable and continue to spread.

Suggested Readings

Anderson NE, Barber PA: Limbic encephalitis—a review, *J Clin Neurosci* 15(9):961–971, 2008.

Baringer JR: Herpes simplex infections of the nervous system, *Neurol Clin* 26(3):657–674, 2008.

Barnett GH: *High grade gliomas*, Totowa, NJ, 2007, Humana Press.

Duckworth JL, Hawley JS, Riedy G, et al: Magnetic resonance restricted diffusion resolution correlates with clinical improvement and response to treatment in herpes simplex encephalitis, *Neurocrit Care* 3(3):251–253, 2005.

Küker W, Nägele T, Schmidt F, et al: Diffusion-weighted MRI in herpes simplex encephalitis: a report of three cases, *Neuroradiology* 46(2): 122–125, 2004.

Landy HJ, Lee TT, Potter P, et al: Early MRI findings in high grade glioma, *J Neurooncol* 47(1):65–72, 2000.

Steiner I, Budka H, Chaudhuri A, et al: Viral meningoencephalitis: a review of diagnostic methods and guidelines for management, *Eur J Neurol* 17(8):999–e57, 2010.

Urbach H, Soeder BM, Jeub M, et al: Serial MRI of limbic encephalitis, *Neuroradiology* 48(6):380–386, 2006.

16

Temporal Lobe Cystic Lesions

HILLARY R. KELLY, MD

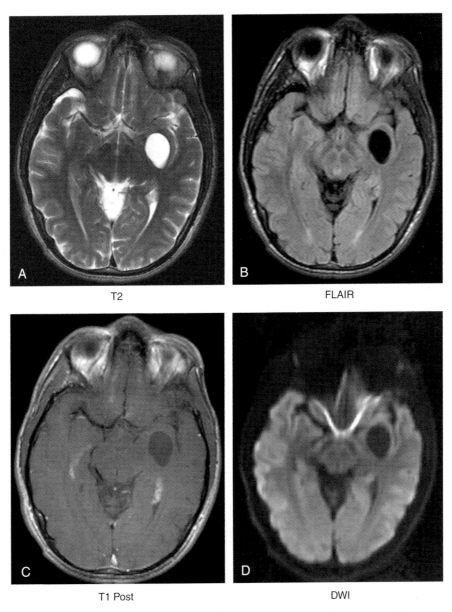

T2   FLAIR

T1 Post   DWI

CASE A: A 16-year-old male with "abnormal head computed tomography" after a minor head trauma. *DWI,* Diffusion-weighted imaging; *FLAIR,* fluid attenuated inversion recovery.

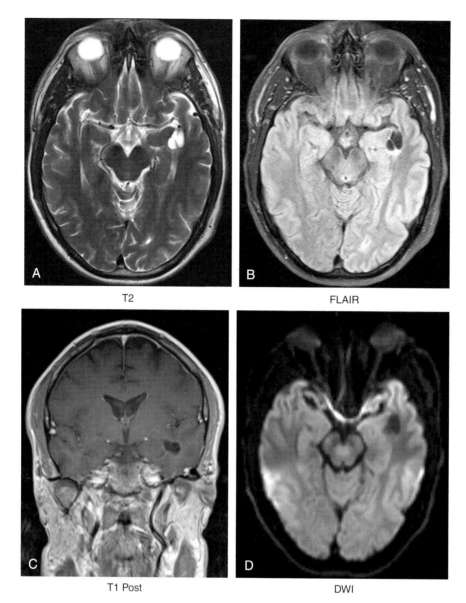

T2

FLAIR

T1 Post

DWI

CASE B: A 49-year-old male with postconcussive syndrome after a bicycle accident. *DWI,* Diffusion-weighted imaging; *FLAIR,* Fluid attenuated inversion recovery.

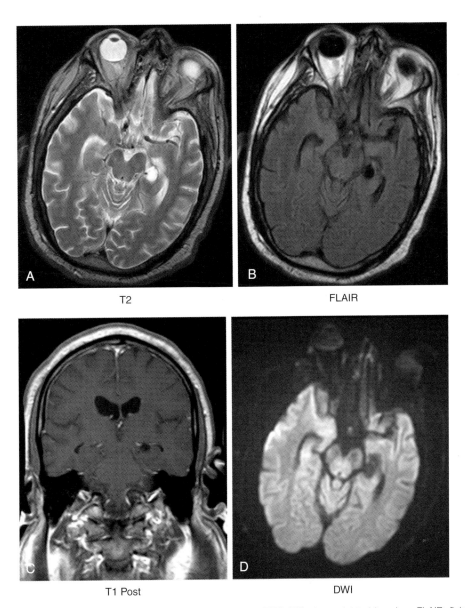

CASE C: A 50-year-old male with altered mental status. *DWI*, Diffusion-weighted imaging; *FLAIR*, fluid attenuated inversion recovery.

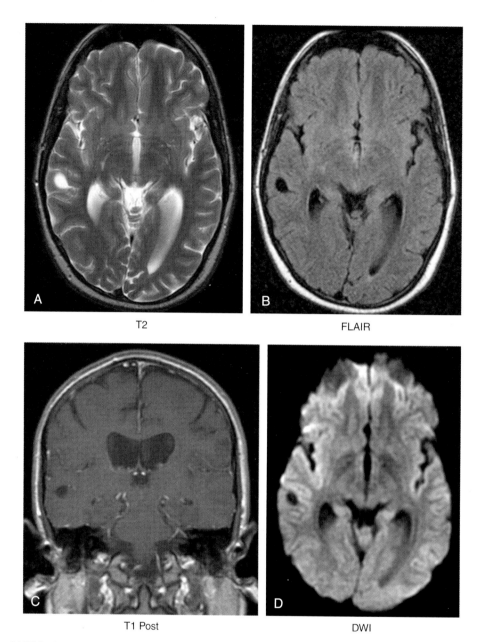

T2

FLAIR

T1 Post

DWI

CASE D: A 24-year-old male with adrenoleukodystrophy. *DWI,* Diffusion-weighted imaging; *FLAIR,* fluid attenuated inversion recovery.

DESCRIPTION OF FINDINGS

- Case A: MRI of the brain demonstrates a T2 hyperintense cystic lesion in the left temporal lobe and subinsular region. This lesion is hypointense on FLAIR and DWI, follows cerebrospinal fluid (CSF) signal on all sequences, and does not enhance on postcontrast T1-weighted images. No abnormal signal is noted in the surrounding brain parenchyma.
- Case B: MRI of the brain demonstrates a T2 hyperintense multiseptated cystic lesion in the left mesial and anterior temporal lobe. This lesion is hypointense on FLAIR and DWI, follows CSF signal on all sequences, and does not enhance on postcontrast T1-weighted images. A thin rim of FLAIR hyperintense signal is noted in the surrounding brain parenchyma.
- Case C: MRI of the brain demonstrates a T2 hyperintense cystic lesion in the left mesial temporal lobe that appears to be centered within the choroidal fissure on the coronal T1-weighted postcontrast images. This lesion is hypointense on FLAIR and DWI and follows CSF signal on all sequences.
- Case D: MRI of the brain demonstrates a T2 hyperintense cystic lesion in the right superior temporal gyrus with a small tail extending to the adjacent subarachnoid space. This lesion is hypointense on FLAIR and DWI, follows CSF signal on all sequences, and does not enhance on postcontrast T1-weighted imaging. No abnormal signal is noted in the surrounding brain parenchyma.

Diagnosis

Case A: Neuroglial cyst versus arachnoid cyst versus enlarged perivascular space

Case B: Enlarged perivascular space versus neuroglial cyst

Case C: Neuroglial cyst versus arachnoid cyst of the choroidal fissure

Case D: Neuroglial cyst versus arachnoid cyst

Summary

Unilocular, simple cystic lesions of the temporal lobe may be intraaxial or extraaxial, and include neuroglial cysts, arachnoid cysts, and enlarged perivascular spaces. Definitive diagnosis of these lesions by imaging often is not possible given the lack of distinguishing radiologic features and minimal radiologic and pathologic correlation in the literature.

Neuroglial cysts are fluid-filled cavities lined by epithelium of ependymal or choroidal origin or both. Many names have been used to describe these lesions, including neuroepithelial cysts, ependymal cysts, and glioependymal cysts. When the lesions are intraventricular or paraventricular, the term *ependymal cyst* is typically used. Neuroglial cysts can arise at any location in the central nervous system and can be intraaxial or extraaxial. They are thought to arise from abnormal sequestration of neuroectodermal tissue during embryogenesis. It is believed that intraparenchymal neuroglial cysts are most common in the frontal lobes. These lesions typically take the form of smooth, round, unilocular cavities within the hemispheric white matter, although they can abut the pial surface with only a thin wall separating the cyst from a ventricle or the subarachnoid space. Neuroglial cysts are isodense to CSF on CT. On MRI, they follow CSF signal on all sequences, including fluid attenuated inversion recovery (FLAIR), diffusion-weighted imaging (DWI), and apparent diffusion coefficient. They demonstrate no peripheral enhancement and minimal to no surrounding FLAIR hyperintense signal abnormality.

Arachnoid cysts are extraaxial intraarachnoidal cavities containing CSF that do not communicate with the ventricle.

These cysts lack an epithelial lining and have walls composed of vascular connective tissue lined by flattened arachnoidal cells. The exact mechanism for the formation of congenital arachnoid cysts is unknown; proposed mechanisms include splitting or a diverticulum of the developing arachnoid, or failure of the embryonic meninges to merge during embryogenesis. The middle cranial fossa is the most common location for an arachnoid cyst. Upon imaging, these lesions typically are sharply marginated extraaxial cysts that displace or deform the adjacent brain parenchyma. Classically, these cysts follow CSF signal intensity on all MRI sequences and do not demonstrate contrast enhancement.

Enlarged perivascular spaces (also known as Virchow-Robin spaces) are fluid-filled interstitial cavities that accompany penetrating arteries and veins. They are pial lined but do not communicate directly with the subarachnoid space. These spaces frequently are seen at the inferior aspect of the basal ganglia and clustering around the anterior commissure. They are isodense to CSF on CT, follow CSF signal intensity on all MRI sequences, and do not enhance on postcontrast images. A characteristic finding in this entity is multiple similar lesions in the subinsular region adjacent to the anterior commissure or within the inferior basal ganglia. The surrounding brain parenchyma usually is normal in appearance, although a small rim of hyperintense T2 or FLAIR signal can be seen in up to 25% of cases.

Spectrum of Disease

Cysts at the level of the choroid fissure are often referred to as choroidal fissure cysts or choroid fissure cysts based on the imaging appearance. However, this is simply an anatomic description rather than a distinct pathologic entity. Neuroglial and arachnoid cysts in this location can appear identical on imaging. Often only histopathologic examination can distinguish between these two entities in the choroid fissure; however, tissue diagnosis is rare as they are benign and require no treatment. Abnormal evagination of the primitive neuroepithelium is thought to occur along the line of the choroid fissure at the junction of the differentiating ependyma and choroid plexus, thus explaining the mixture of these two tissue elements in the lining of many neuroglial cysts. Arachnoid cyst formation is thought to occur most often in the middle cranial fossa as the primitive frontal and temporal meninges (endomeninx) fail to merge as the sylvian and choroid fissures form.

Simple cysts that appear to be within the temporal lobe parenchyma are more likely to be neuroglial cysts or enlarged perivascular spaces, although a small connection to the subarachnoid space may be missed by imaging. Although most arachnoid cysts are easily identifiable as extraaxial lesions, in some cases a small cyst may appear to be enveloped by the surrounding parenchyma.

Simple cysts in the temporal lobe can be confused with more aggressive neoplastic processes, especially if abnormal signal is noted in the surrounding brain parenchyma. The greater degree of mass effect and abnormal FLAIR signal in the surrounding brain parenchyma should help distinguish the previously described simple cystic lesions from a neoplasm. The signal within the cystic components of tumors often will not follow CSF on FLAIR and/or DWI (Fig. 16.1). Postcontrast

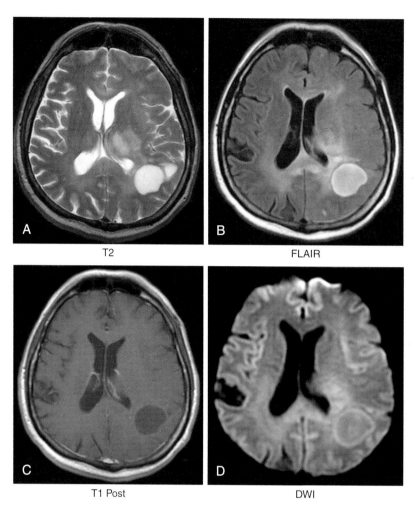

• **Fig. 16.1** Anaplastic astrocytoma. Magnetic resonance images demonstrate a partially cystic mass lesion in the left temporoparietal region with marked surrounding fluid attenuated inversion recovery *(FLAIR)* hyperintense signal abnormality. The cystic component of the mass lesion does not follow cerebrospinal fluid signal, with hyperintense signal on the FLAIR sequence and slightly hypointense signal on the diffusion-weighted imaging *(DWI)* sequence.

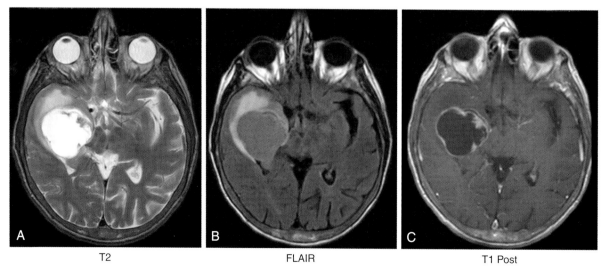

• **Fig. 16.2** Metastatic ovarian carcinoma. Magnetic resonance imaging of the brain demonstrates a cystic lesion in the right temporal lobe with marked mass effect and surrounding fluid attenuated inversion recovery *(FLAIR)* hyperintense signal abnormality. The irregular wall of the cyst is well demonstrated on the T2-weighted image. Corresponding peripheral nodular enhancement is seen on the postcontrast T1-weighted image. The cyst is also hyperintense to cerebrospinal fluid on the FLAIR image.

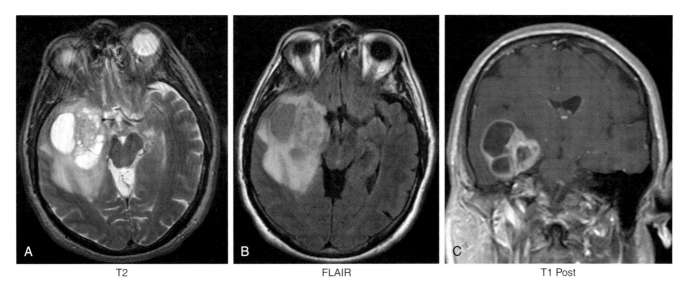

T2 FLAIR T1 Post

• **Fig. 16.3** Glioblastoma. Magnetic resonance imaging of the brain demonstrates a cystic and solid lesion in the right temporal lobe with extensive surrounding fluid attenuated inversion recovery *(FLAIR)* hyperintense signal abnormality and marked mass effect. The signal within the cystic components of the mass is hyperintense to cerebrospinal fluid on the FLAIR image. Thick peripheral enhancement is noted on the postcontrast T1-weighted image.

imaging also is helpful when trying to exclude malignancy (Figs. 16.2 and 16.3). If neoplasm persists as a clinical concern, repeat imaging also may be indicated. Neuroglial cysts, arachnoid cysts, and enlarged perivascular spaces may enlarge slightly with time but should appear grossly stable on follow-up imaging, whereas increased size and signal abnormality are more often seen with neoplastic entities.

Differential Diagnosis

Neuroglial cyst
Arachnoid cyst
Enlarged perivascular space
Cystic neoplasm
Lacunar infarct
Porencephalic cyst
Infectious cyst

Pearls

- Morphology: Benign cystic lesions in the temporal lobe are typically round with smooth margins and a thin wall. They also are typically unilocular, although multiple adjacent enlarged perivascular spaces can give the appearance of a multiloculated or multiseptated lesion.
- Internal signal characteristics: Neuroglial cysts, arachnoid cysts, and enlarged perivascular spaces should demonstrate internal signal identical to that of CSF on all MRI sequences.
- Effect on the adjacent brain parenchyma: Neuroglial cysts and arachnoid cysts may displace the adjacent brain parenchyma, but little if any abnormal parenchymal signal should be noted on T2 or FLAIR sequences.
- Enhancement: Lack of contrast enhancement is characteristic of benign cysts in the temporal lobe.

Signs and Complications

Temporal lobe cystic lesions are largely asymptomatic and are often found incidentally. They are nearly always benign and often require no further intervention. Neuroglial cysts have rarely been associated with headaches, seizures, and neurologic deficits and can be treated by surgical drainage or fenestration. Arachnoid cysts have been associated with headaches, dizziness, and seizures, among other symptoms, depending on their location. Arachnoid cysts also are associated with subdural hematomas, especially in the middle cranial fossa. Enlarged perivascular spaces are considered a normal variant, but in rare cases they may become so large that they cause local mass effect or hydrocephalus. In these cases, they often are referred to as *giant* or *tumefactive* perivascular spaces.

Suggested Readings

de Jong L, Thewissen L, van Loon J, et al: Choroidal fissure cerebrospinal fluid-containing cysts: case series, anatomical correlation, and review of the literature, *World Neurosurg* 75(5-6):704–708, 2011.

Hall A, White MAJ, Myles L: Spontaneous subdural haemorrhage from an arachnoid cyst: a case report and literature review, *Br J Neurosurg* 31(5):607–610, 2017.

Ironside JW, et al: Neuroglial cysts. In *Diagnostic pathology of nervous system tumours*, London, 2002, Churchill Livingstone.

Ironside JW, et al: Congenital arachnoidal cysts. In *Diagnostic pathology of nervous system tumours*, London, 2002, Churchill Livingstone.

Mathias J, Koessler L, Brissart H, et al: Giant cystic widening of Virchow-Robin spaces: an anatomofunctional study, *AJNR Am J Neuroradiol* 28:1523–1525, 2007.

Osborn AG, Preece MT: Intracranial cysts: radiologic-pathologic correlation and imaging approach, *Radiology* 239(3):650–664, 2006.

Sherman JL, Camponovo E, Citrin CM: MR imaging of CSF-like choroidal fissure and parenchymal cysts of the brain, *AJR Am J Roentgenol* 155:1069–1075, 1990.

17
Multicystic Lesions

SIMONE MONTOYA, MD

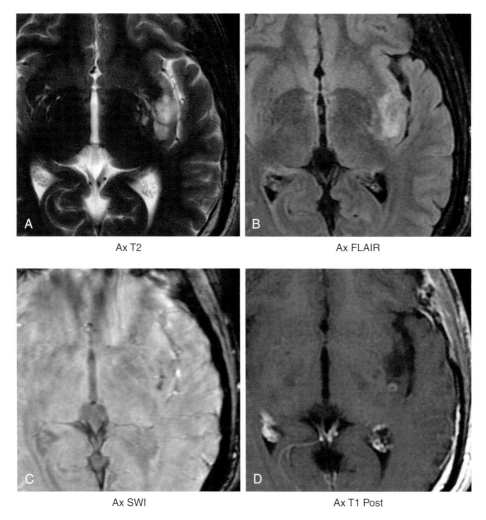

Ax T2

Ax FLAIR

Ax SWI

Ax T1 Post

CASE A: A 25-year-old male with worsening epilepsy. *Ax*, Axial; *FLAIR*, fluid attenuated inversion recovery; *SWI*, susceptibility-weighted imaging.

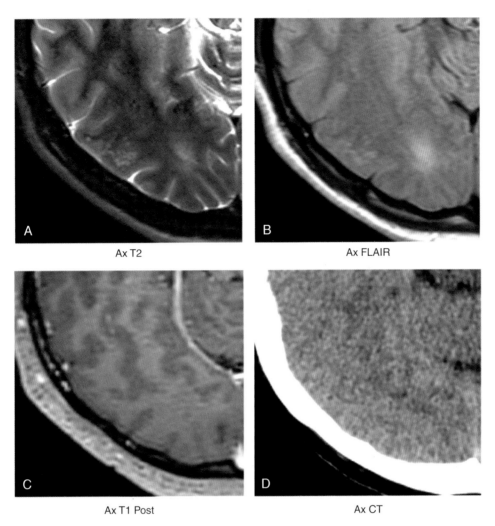

Ax T2

Ax FLAIR

Ax T1 Post

Ax CT

CASE B: A 39-year-old male with incidental finding on workup for neck pain after motor vehicle crash. *Ax,* Axial; *CT,* Computed tomography; *FLAIR,* fluid attenuated inversion recovery.

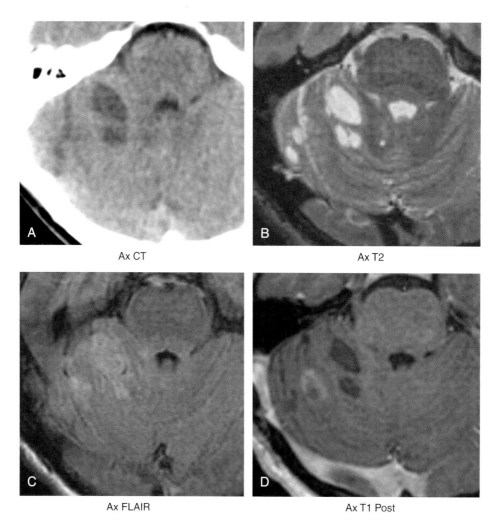

Ax CT

Ax T2

Ax FLAIR

Ax T1 Post

CASE C: A 28-year-old male with headaches. *Ax*, Axial; *CT*, Computed tomography; *FLAIR*, fluid attenuated inversion recovery.

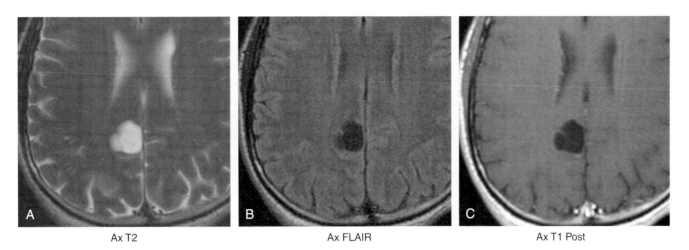

Ax T2 Ax FLAIR Ax T1 Post

CASE D: A 58-year-old male with intermittent imbalance and dizziness. *Ax*, Axial; *FLAIR*, fluid attenuated inversion recovery.

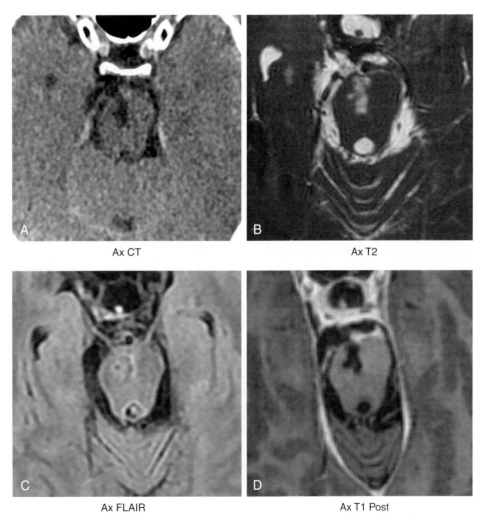

Ax CT Ax T2

Ax FLAIR Ax T1 Post

CASE E: A 47-year-old male (immigrant) with intermittent headaches precipitated by bending and lifting/straining. *Ax*, Axial; *CT*, Computed tomography; *FLAIR*, fluid attenuated inversion recovery.

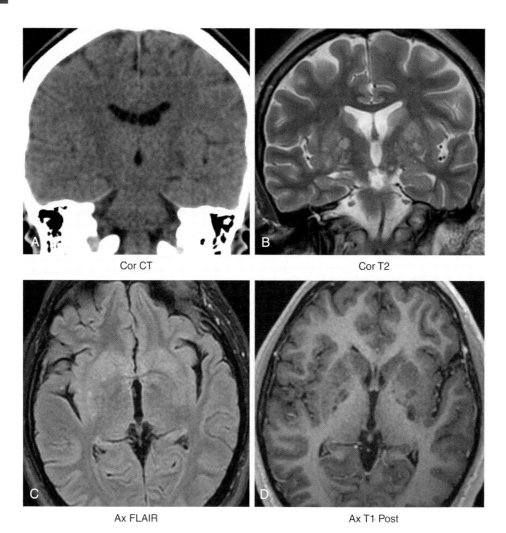

Cor CT

Cor T2

Ax FLAIR

Ax T1 Post

CASE F: A 24-year-old male presenting with seizure and subsequently diagnosed with HIV/AIDS. *Ax*, Axial; *Cor*, coronal; *CT*, Computed tomography; *FLAIR*, fluid attenuated inversion recovery.

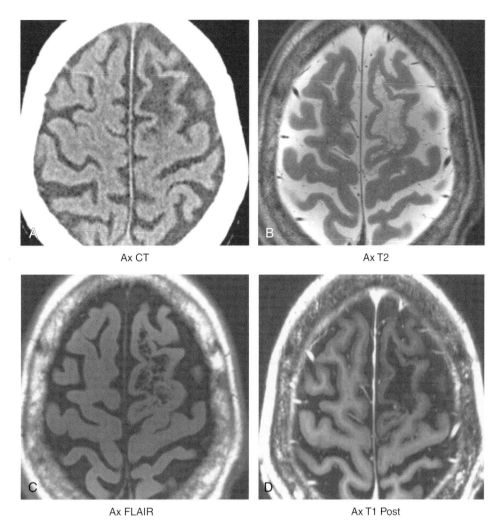

Ax CT Ax T2

Ax FLAIR Ax T1 Post

CASE G: A 70-year-old male with incidental finding on workup for encephalopathy and adenocarcinoma. *Ax*, Axial; *CT*, Computed tomography; *FLAIR*, fluid attenuated inversion recovery.

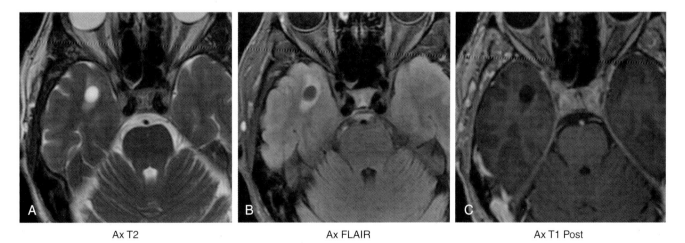

Ax T2 Ax FLAIR Ax T1 Post

CASE H: A 61-year-old female with episodic confusion, question of partial complex seizure. *Ax*, Axial; *FLAIR*, fluid attenuated inversion recovery.

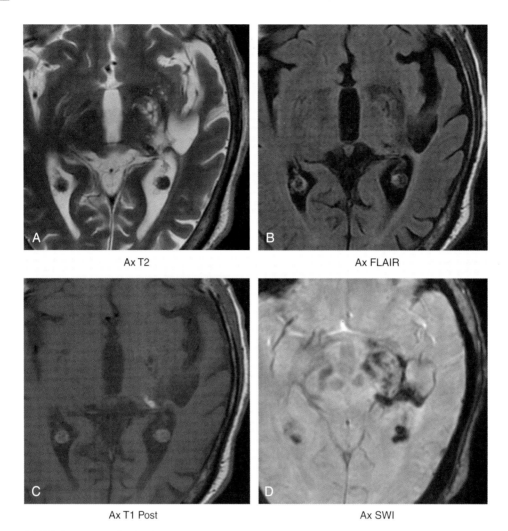

Ax T2

Ax FLAIR

Ax T1 Post

Ax SWI

CASE I: A 69-year-old male with seizures, hypertension, and prior stroke. *Ax*, Axial; *FLAIR*, fluid attenuated inversion recovery; *SWI*, susceptibility-weighted imaging.

DESCRIPTION OF FINDINGS

CT and MR images from nine patients with multicystic parenchymal lesions.

- Case A: An expansile lesion comprised of multiple cysts is located in the left insula and subinsular region. There is mild effacement of the left Sylvian fissure. The contents are T2 hyperintense with incomplete suppression on FLAIR imaging. There is a rim of FLAIR hyperintensity, no significant susceptibility effect, and a small focus of enhancement posteriorly.
- Case B: Several tiny cystic foci are clustered subcortically at the lateral right temporo-occipital junction. There is no discrete mass lesion or mass effect. Some of the lesions are hyperintense on FLAIR images. There is no associated enhancement. The foci are not well seen on CT images.
- Case C: Multiple cystic lesions are located in the right cerebellar hemisphere. The cystic lesions exert mild local mass effect, including effacement of the adjacent folia and subtle deviation of the fourth ventricle. The internal contents are T2 hyperintense with incomplete signal suppression on FLAIR imaging. One of the cystic lesions demonstrates slightly nodular peripheral enhancement.
- Case D: An expansile cystic lesion is centered within the medial right parietal lobe. The internal contents are T2 hyperintense and fully suppressed on FLAIR imaging. There is no surrounding FLAIR hyperintensity or enhancement of the wall or septae.
- Case E: A cluster of cysts is located in the right ventral pons. There is minimal surrounding FLAIR hyperintensity and no appreciable enhancement. Not shown are several septations within several of the basal cisterns and other subarachnoid spaces, which are expanded.
- Case F: Several subcentimeter foci of hypoattenuation are located within the basal ganglia bilaterally. There is corresponding T2/FLAIR hyperintensity, but no appreciable mass effect or enhancement.
- Case G: Several cystic foci occupy a geographic region of the left frontal lobe, many in a parallel orientation. The cortex of the left superior frontal gyrus appears thinned and stretched around these foci; however, there is no real mass effect or volume loss as the adjacent cerebrospinal fluid (CSF) spaces are neither effaced nor enlarged. On FLAIR imaging, there is complete suppression of internal signal and no surrounding signal abnormality. There is no appreciable enhancement.
- Case H: a discrete T2 hyperintense focus is located within the right temporal pole. On FLAIR imaging, there is complete suppression of internal signal and a small amount of surrounding hyperintensity. There is no perceivable wall, associated mass effect, or appreciable enhancement.
- Case I: several foci of T2 hyperintensity involving the left thalamus and subinsular region are accompanied by volume loss. There is intrinsic marginal T1 hyperintensity posteriorly, surrounding FLAIR hyperintensity, and amorphous susceptibility effect also involving the adjacent white matter.

Diagnosis

Case A: Dysembryoplastic neuroepithelial tumor
Case B: Multinodular and vacuolating neuronal tumor
Case C: Rosette-forming glioneuronal tumor
Case D: Neuroglial cyst
Case E: Neurocysticercosis
Case F: Cryptococcus
Case G: Bizarre/tumefactive perivascular space
Case H: Anterior temporal perivascular space
Case I: Encephalomalacia (stroke)

Summary

Lesions presenting as multiple cysts in the parenchyma are diverse and include developmental, neoplastic, infectious, and vascular etiologies. While some lesions have a characteristic appearance, there can be significant overlap in presentation, and clinical context may not be discriminatory. Providing an appropriate differential diagnosis is important to guide surveillance, as many of these lesions are not examined pathologically.

Dysembryoplastic neuroepithelial tumors (DNETs) are benign WHO grade I neoplasms of mixed glioneuronal origin. People with these lesions tend to be young and neurologically normal, with refractory epilepsy and partial seizures. Most DNETs are cortically based, usually in the temporal lobe, and do not have significant edema or mass effect. Classically, these lesions were described as having a "bubbly" T2 hyperintense appearance with mixed/incomplete suppression on FLAIR imaging. Calcification and hemorrhage are uncommon. Pathologically, the specific glioneuronal element (SGNE) is characteristic and stains positively for glial fibrillary acidic protein (GFAP), although the nonspecific histologic form does not contain SGNE. Although the vast majority of these lesions do not grow or undergo malignant degeneration, surgical resection may be performed if seizures cannot be otherwise managed.

Multinodular and vacuolating neuronal tumors (MVNTs) of the cerebrum are a newly recognized entity–provisionally designated by the WHO central nervous system (CNS) tumor classification system as a pattern of gangliocytoma; however, it is unclear if this is a neoplastic or a dysplastic process. Its characteristic appearance is of a subcortical cluster of "bubbly" nodules of varying sizes that are T2 hyperintense, and the majority does not suppress on FLAIR imaging. There is usually no enhancement or mass effect. Leading considerations in the differential diagnosis are DNET and focal cortical dysplasia. It is thought that many lesions identified as either of these entities may in fact be MVNTs. Many are asymptomatic, and case series describe little if any change over an extended period of time, suggesting that they are most often a "don't touch" lesion. Some may be associated with seizures, however, and those that are epileptogenic and amenable to surgical resection do not recur. Given its recent recognition, often incidental detection, and lack of pathologic confirmation, along with the fact that many detected prior to 2016 have likely been misdiagnosed, the true incidence of this lesion is unknown.

Rosette-forming glioneuronal tumors (RF-GNTs) are another entity previously classified as DNET. RG-GNTs are most often found in the posterior fossa, specifically in close proximity to the fourth ventricle. Aside from location, RF-GNTs and DNETs can look identical on imaging. Pathologically, they can be distinguished from DNET by pseudorosette formation that stain positively for synaptophysin and can also have a histological component of pilocytic astrocytoma.

Neuroglial cysts (also known as neuroepithelial or glioependymal cysts) are benign non-neoplastic parenchymal lesions that comprise fewer than 1% of all intracranial cysts. They are fluid-filled, glial-lined lesions that develop as a result of sequestered neural tube embryonic elements, can occur anywhere throughout the neuraxis, and are usually unilocular (at least on CT). The borders are round and smooth, and the internal contents typically follow CSF signal on all sequences. There is no enhancement and no/minimal surrounding FLAIR hyperintense signal abnormality. Symptoms, if any, depend on size and location. These cysts often demonstrate long-term stability.

Encephalomalacia, a pathologic term meaning "brain softening," is used radiographically to describe the loss of brain parenchyma due to liquefactive necrosis. The inciting insult may be ischemic, hemorrhagic, traumatic, inflammatory, or other etiology, with the end result of tissue loss. CSF fills the space left behind, so encephalomalacic lesions follow CSF signal on all sequences; gliosis is often also present and is characterized by T2/FLAIR hyperintensity. The morphology of encephalomalacia can vary by extent and location of injury; if there is incomplete tissue loss, the lesion may have a reticular or cystic appearance due to preservation of intervening tissue. Lacunar infarcts involve the deep penetrating vessels (e.g., lenticulostriates and thalamic and pontine perforators) and occur in characteristic locations (e.g., basal ganglia, internal capsules, thalami, and central pons). These lesions appear as defined "holes" surrounded by gliosis. Multicystic encephalomalacia is a specific subtype that occurs in neonates after hypoxic-ischemic encephalopathy.

Dilated perivascular spaces (PVS), colloquially known as Virchow-Robin spaces occur within the interstitium along perforating vessels. Typical locations include the basal ganglia, thalami, pons, and centrum semiovale. In dilated PVS, the normal perivascular space is expanded, filled with fluid, and lined by pia (as opposed to epithelium/ependyma in a true cyst). Dilated PVS typically occur in clusters and tend to follow CSF signal on all sequences, although depending on fluid composition they may not completely suppress on FLAIR imaging. The main differential diagnosis is lacunar infarcts, since these entities tend to occur at the same locations; however, dilated PVS tend not to be surrounded by T2/FLAIR hyperintensity. Anterior temporal dilated PVS are an exception; these lesions are often unilocular with surrounding T2/FLAIR hyperintensity and thus can be confused for a cyst or cystic tumor.

CNS cryptococcosis is caused by disseminated hematogenous spread of the *Cryptococcus neoformans* yeast-like fungus after primary pulmonary infection. While the meningitic and parenchymal forms can be seen in immunocompetent hosts (often with bird exposure), the perivascular form is seen almost exclusively in immunocompromised patients. In this form, a mucinous exudate accumulates within PVS, particularly within the basal ganglia, and forms gelatinous pseudocysts. Signal will not follow CSF on all sequences, differentiating these lesions from dilated PVS. Depending on the protein content, gelatinous pseudocysts may be hypointense or intermediate on T1-weighted imaging, not quite as bright as CSF on T2-weighted imaging, have incomplete or no suppression on FLAIR imaging, and have either facilitated or restricted diffusion. In addition, gelatinous pseudocysts do not exert mass effect. Perivascular CNS cryptococcosis used to be a common initial presentation of HIV/AIDS, but now is rarely seen due to improved detection and treatment.

Neurocysticercosis is caused by the pork tapeworm *Taenia solium*, endemic to Central and South America, Africa, and Asia. Infection occurs after ingestion of food or drink contaminated with *T. solium* eggs and progresses to extraintestinal disease, including dissemination into the CNS. The cysts of neurocysticercosis are the actual encapsulated parasites; the scolex (attachment end) of the tapeworm may be visible inside. Cysts can be located virtually anywhere in the CNS. They can be parenchymal (usually at the gray-white junction), intraventricular, or subarachnoid. In the racemose form, which most often occurs within the basal cisterns, cysts clump together and appear similar to a bunch of grapes. Both solitary and racemose lesions can block CSF flow. Symptoms include seizures from cortical irritation, headaches from increased intracranial pressure, hydrocephalus from CSF obstruction, and focal neurologic deficit depending on lesion location.

Spectrum of Disease

Multicystic lesions are generally hypoattenuating on CT and hyperintense on MRI T2-weighted images, although appearance may vary with proteinaceous or otherwise complex internal contents. The cysts are often well-demarcated from the surrounding parenchyma; surrounding T2/FLAIR hyperintensity may be due to perilesional gliosis and/or vasogenic edema. Smaller lesions may look like a cluster of cystic foci (e.g., MVNT), while larger lesions can have a more coalescent appearance (e.g., DNET or RF-GNT), or look like a large cyst with multiple septations or locules. Location is often characteristic: tumors may have a lobar predominance, perivascular spaces occur along vascular structures, and encephalomalacia will develop in areas of prior injury.

Subcortical arteriosclerotic encephalopathy, also known as small vessel dementia or Binswanger disease, is a type of vascular dementia specifically affecting the white matter. On FLAIR/T2-weighted images, there is typically periventricular and subcortical white matter hyperintensity and multiple lacunar infarcts.

Dilated PVS and lacunar infarcts are found in the same locations and can be difficult to differentiate and they may be present concurrently. Etat criblé is used to describe when dilated PVS are numerous and extensive, appearing like a colander. These can have a similar appearance to multiple lacunar infarcts (état lacunaire). Dilated PVS may also take on unusual appearances, as in tumefactive PVS or giant PVS, which are very large and bizarre in shape and can be mistaken as tumors or encephalomalacia.

Neurocysticercosis has four stages: vesicular, colloidal vesicular, granular nodular, and nodular calcified. In the asymptomatic vesicular stage, the worm is still viable, and the cyst membrane is intact. The lesion is similar in attenuation/signal to CSF, the scolex may be seen as an eccentrically located hyperattenuating/T1 hyperintense focus, and there will be no edema or enhancement. In the colloidal vesicular stage, the worm dies and the cyst membrane breaks down, eliciting an inflammatory response; the cyst becomes hyperattenuating and T1 hyperintense due to fluid turbidity, and there is peripheral enhancement and surrounding edema. In the granular nodular stage, the scolex is no longer identifiable, and inflammation decreases as the cysts retract. In the terminal nodular calcified stage, inflammation and hence, edema and enhancement should be resolved, and there are foci of hyperdensity and T2/T2* signal dropout due to calcification.

Differential Diagnosis

Perivascular spaces
Encephalomalacia
Neuroglial cyst
Neuroglial tumor
Cystic infection
Cystic metastases (more often multiple lesions rather than a single multicystic lesion)

Pearls

- A subcortical cluster of bubbles is characteristic of MVNT, while a cortically based "bubbly" lesion is more likely DNET. RF-GNT may appear similar to MVNT or DNET, but occurs predominantly in the cerebellum.
- The presence or absence of surrounding gliosis can differentiate a lacunar infarct from dilated PVS. For larger lesions, adjacent sulcal prominence and ex-vacuo ventricular dilatation may be seen with encephalomalacia, but not with PVS. Cryptococcal gelatinous pseudocysts do not typically follow CSF in all sequences, thereby differentiating them from dilated PVS.
- Parenchymal expansion and thinning associated with tumefactive PVS may give the appearance of a space-occupying lesion, however, there should not be true mass effect. Radial orientation of cystic spaces along vessel pathways will be another clue.

Signs and Complications

The DNET "bright rim sign" on T2-weighted FLAIR imaging is due to glioneuronal elements tightly packed along the tumor margins; the ring may be either complete or incomplete.

The "cyst with dot" sign of neurocysticercosis represents the scolex contained eccentrically within the cyst and can be seen during the vesicular and colloidal vesicular stages on both CT and MRI. Aside from different imaging presentations, these stages can also be distinguished by the absence or presence of symptoms due to CNS irritation.

RF-GNT and neurocysticercosis can both be complicated by hydrocephalus—the former due to compression of the fourth ventricle and the latter due to intraventricular and extraaxial lesions obstructing CSF flow. Neurocysticercosis is a leading cause for Brun syndrome, which is episodic sudden onset of symptoms related to increased intracranial pressure, brought on by acute hydrocephalus secondary to ball valve effect, and precipitated by abrupt head movements.

Suggested Readings

Alsufayan R, Alcaide-Leon P, Noel de Tilly L, et al: Natural history of lesions with the MR imaging appearance of multinodular and vacuolating neuronal tumor, *Neuroradiology* 59:873–883, 2017.

Das A, Kesavadas C, Radhakrishnan VV, et al: Teaching NeuroImages: Bruns syndrome caused by intraventricular neurocysticercosis, *Neurology* 73:e34, 2009.

Fernandez C, Girard N, Paz Paredes A, et al: The usefulness of MR imaging in the diagnosis of dysembryoplastic neuroepithelial tumor in children: a study of 14 cases, *Am J Neuroradiol* 24:829–834, 2003.

Hsu C, Kwan G, Lau Q, et al: Rosette-forming glioneuronal tumour: imaging features, histopathological correlation and a comprehensive review of literature, *Br J Neurosurg* 26:668–673, 2012.

Johnson DR, Guerin JB, Giannini C, et al: 2016 updates to the WHO brain tumor classification system: what the radiologist needs to know, *Radiographics* 37:2164–2180, 2017.

Koeller KK, Henry JM: Superficial gliomas: radiologic-pathologic correlation, *Radiographics* 21:1533–1556, 2001.

Lerner A, Shiroishi MS, Zee CS, et al: Imaging of neurocysticercosis, *Neuroimag Clin N Am* 22:659–676, 2012.

Naidich TP, Chakera TMH: Multicystic encephalomalacia: CT appearance and pathological correlation, *J Comput Assist Tomogr* 8:631–636, 1984.

Nunes RH, Hsu CC, da Rocha AJ, et al: Multinodular and vacuolating neuronal tumor of the cerebrum: a new "leave me alone" lesion with a characteristic imaging pattern, *Am J Neuroradiol* 38:1899–1904, 2017.

Osborn AG, Preece MT: Intracranial cysts: radiologic-pathologic correlation and imaging approach, *Radiology* 239:650–664, 2006.

Parmar HA, Hawkins C, Ozelame R, et al: Fluid-attenuated inversion recovery ring sign as a marker of dysembryoplastic neuroepithelial tumors, *J Comput Assist Tomogr* 31:348–353, 2007.

18
Cerebellopontine Angle Cisterns

HUI J. JENNY CHEN, MD

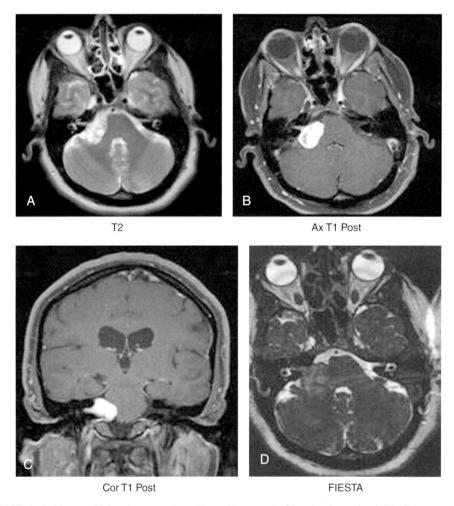

A — T2

B — Ax T1 Post

C — Cor T1 Post

D — FIESTA

CASE A: A 47-year-old female presenting with sudden onset of hearing loss. *Ax*, Axial; *Cor*, coronal; *FIESTA*, fast imaging employing steady-state acquisition.

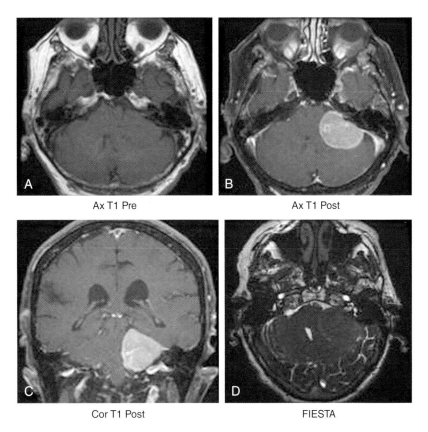

CASE B: A 75-year-old male presenting with progressive left hearing loss, left facial numbness, and worsening balance. *Ax,* Axial; *Cor,* coronal; *FIESTA,* fast imaging employing steady-state acquisition.

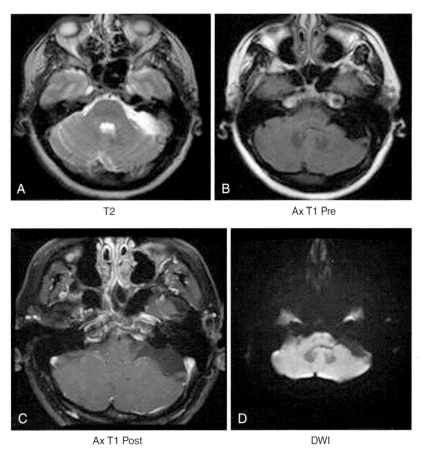

CASE C: A 52-year-old female presenting with new onset of coordination disturbance, worsening headache, and dizziness. *Ax,* Axial; *DWI,* diffusion-weighted imaging.

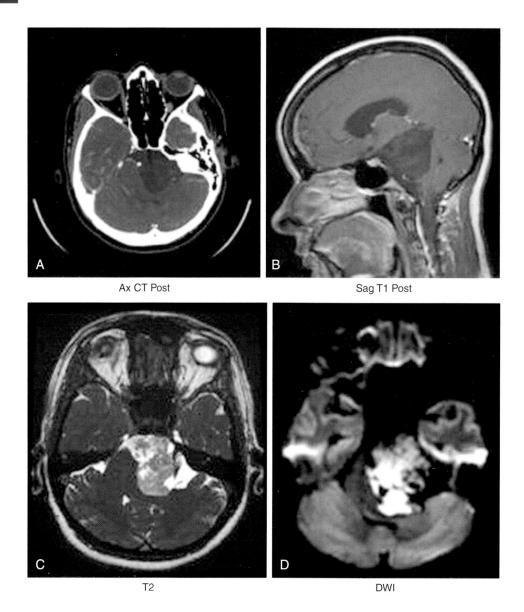

Ax CT Post

Sag T1 Post

T2

DWI

CASE D: A 32-year-old female presenting with gait imbalance, falls, and blurred vision. *Ax,* Axial; *CT,* Computed tomography; *DWI,* diffusion-weighted imaging; *Sag,* sagittal.

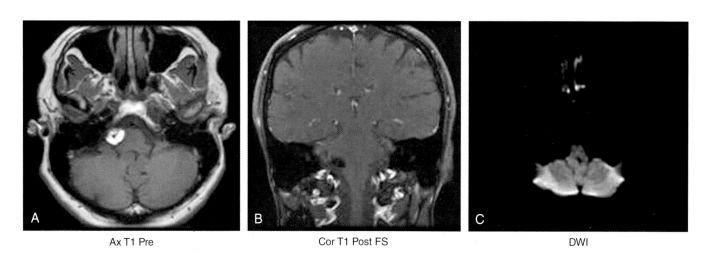

Ax T1 Pre

Cor T1 Post FS

DWI

CASE E: Incidental finding in a 58-year-old female. *Ax,* Axial; *Cor,* coronal; *DWI,* diffusion-weighted imaging; *FS,* fat saturated.

DESCRIPTION OF FINDINGS

MRI scans demonstrate five typical cerebellopontine angle (CPA) pathologies with mass effect on the adjacent brainstem and cerebellum.

- Case A: The images show a T2 heterogeneously hyperintense and avidly enhancing mass with cystic components in the CPA with mass effect on the adjacent right cerebellum, middle cerebellar peduncle, and the pons. The mass extends into and expands the internal auditory canal (IAC).
- Case B: The images demonstrate a T1 isointense, T2 isointense, and homogeneously enhancing mass with a dural tail in the left CPA, without obvious extension into the IAC.
- Case C: It features a nonenhancing extraaxial CPA mass with mild mass effect on adjacent structures. The signal intensity of this mass follows the cerebrospinal fluid (CSF) signal on all sequences, including DWI.
- Case D: It features an ill-defined nonenhancing extraaxial left CPA mass insinuating around the nerves and vessels. On the postcontrast axial CT image, the mass is shown to encase the adjacent basilar artery. On the axial T2 image, the mass is shown to encase the traversing left trigeminal nerve. Although the mass is heterogeneously T2 bright and T1 dark, it does not follow CSF signal intensity. The mass is markedly hyperintense on the DWI image.
- Case E: It features a T1 hyperintense nonenhancing mass in the right CPA. Suppression of signal is noted on the fat-saturated sequence. The mass encases the visualized anterior inferior cerebellar artery. The mass is hypointense on DWI.

Diagnosis

Case A: Vestibular schwannoma with cystic components
Case B: Meningioma with a typical dural tail
Case C: Arachnoid cyst
Case D: Epidermoid cyst encasing the basilar artery and trigeminal nerve
Case E: Lipoma encasing the anterior inferior cerebellar artery

Summary

Vestibular Schwannoma—Cerebellopontine Angle Lesions

The clinical presentation of CPA pathology is often nonspecific, and the differential diagnosis is broad. MRI is the study of choice for a definitive diagnosis. The typical imaging strategy includes obtaining 2- to 3-mm-thick images through the CPA and IAC. Sequences should include axial noncontrast T1-weighted images, coronal and axial postcontrast T1-weighted images with fat saturation, axial T2-weighted images, FIESTA images, and DWI. The most important imaging features used to make the diagnosis quickly include contrast enhancement pattern, location, intrinsic T1 signal, and DWI hyperintensity (Fig. 18.1).

Vestibular schwannoma accounts for 70% to 80% of all CPA lesions and usually presents with hearing loss. It originates from the Schwann cell sheath of the superior division of the vestibular nerve in the IAC (posterior superior location in the IAC). It grows slowly into the typical "ice cream cone" pattern by having both an IAC component, with remodeling of the posterior edge of the porus acusticus, and a CPA cistern component. Purely intracisternal schwannoma exists but is much less common. These lesions usually grow to a large size before symptoms occur due to mass effect on the

adjacent cerebellum, brainstem, and/or fourth ventricle. Vestibular schwannomas are typically T1 isointense and T2 hyperintense to brain parenchyma. They have homogeneous or heterogeneous enhancement and may have cystic components. Lesions larger than 25 mm tend to grow faster and have a less favorable surgical outcome in terms of facial nerve preservation.

A common differential diagnosis for an enhancing CPA mass is meningioma, which is the second most common CPA lesion (10% to 15% of all CPA lesions). Typically, meningiomas are isointense to cerebral cortex on T1 and T2 sequences with avid contrast enhancement. They arise from arachnoid meningothelial cells. Meningiomas usually are centered anterior or posterior to the IAC. They can extend into the IAC but do not expand the porus acusticus. They are dense on CT in 70% of cases. Other differentiating features include the presence of a dural tail, intrinsic calcification, mild diffusion restriction, and hyperostosis of the adjacent skull.

A less common but important differential diagnosis for an enhancing CPA mass is metastasis. The most common malignancies to metastasize to the CPA are lung, breast, melanoma, and lymphoma. When bilateral enhancing CPA lesions are seen in adults, metastases should be suspected in patients without known neurofibromatosis type 2.

The third most common CPA lesion is an epidermoid cyst, which is a congenital lesion arising from the accidental inclusion of ectodermal epithelial tissue during neural tube closure in the first weeks of embryogenesis. These lesions become symptomatic only when they are large because of their insinuating growth pattern. On CT, they are hypodense with occasional calcified margins. On MRI, they have a cauliflower-like irregular outer surface. Because of their softness, epidermoid cysts frequently are observed to surround and even stretch traversing nerves and vessels, as demonstrated in Case D. They can cause trigeminal neuralgia, and on rare occasions they can even cause posterior circulation ischemia.

In contrast, arachnoid cysts tend to have a more rounded contour and displace adjacent neural and vascular structures. They also result in smooth deformity of adjacent brain parenchyma and scalloping of adjacent bones because of a slow remodeling process.

Arachnoid cysts are isodense to CSF on CT and are isointense to CSF on all MRI sequences. Epidermoid cysts usually have signal intensity close to that of CSF on T1- and T2-weighted sequences. On fluid attenuated inversion recovery (FLAIR) sequences, epidermoid cysts are hyperintense to CSF and hypointense to brain parenchyma. On DWI sequences, epidermoid cysts demonstrate marked hyperintensity compared with CSF and brain parenchyma. On apparent diffusion coefficient (ADC) sequences, epidermoid cysts are hypointense compared to CSF and isointense compared to brain parenchyma.

Lipoma is another common nonenhancing CPA mass that can be easily differentiated by its high intrinsic T1 signal and signal suppression on fat-saturated sequences. It often encases adjacent neural and vascular structures. Unlike supratentorial lipomas, posterior fossa lipomas usually are not associated with congenital malformations.

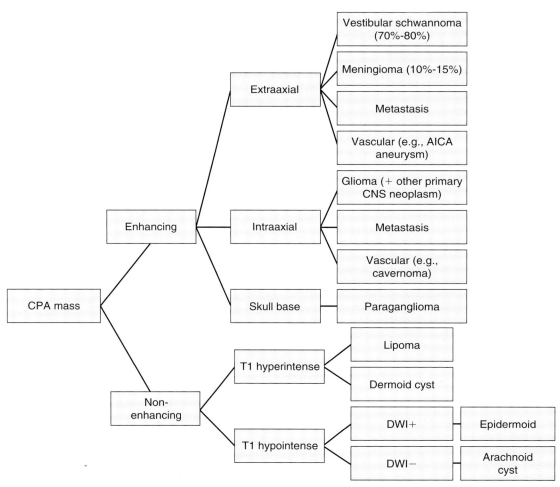

• **Fig. 18.1** Diagnostic algorithm for cerebellopontine angle *(CPA)* masses. *AICA,* Anterior inferior cerebellar artery; *CNS,* central nervous system; *DWI,* diffusion-weighted imaging.

Spectrum of Disease

The best approach to differentiating CPA lesions is to consider their prevalence, enhancement pattern, and location (Fig. 18.1). Schwannomas, which constitute 70% to 80% of all CPA lesions, and meningiomas, which constitute 10% to 15% of all CPA lesions, are the two most common CPA masses. The imaging features that are most typical of a schwannoma are its ice cream cone appearance, with its filling and expanding of the IAC and extension into the CPA, T2 hyperintensity, and enhancement. Meningiomas do not expand the IAC. They are typically T2 isointense, eccentric to the IAC. They may or may not have calcification (Fig. 18.2), have homogeneous enhancement, and may have adjacent skull base hyperostosis. Rarely, a schwannoma and a meningioma may coexist, typically in the setting of neurofibromatosis type 2 (Fig. 18.3). Bilateral enhancing IAC lesions in adults are suspicious for leptomeningeal metastatic disease. Paragangliomas (glomus jugulotympanicum lesions) can extend up into the IAC. Primary and secondary bone malignances also can involve the IAC. Rarely, intraaxial lesions such as gliomas, metastases, and cavernous malformations are exophytic and can extend into the IAC.

In addition to schwannomas arising from the superior vestibular nerve, schwannomas originating from the trigeminal and facial nerves also can occur in the CPA.

Nonenhancing lesions are usually arachnoid cysts (isointense to CSF on all MRI sequences with smooth margins and displacement of neurovascular structures) or epidermoid cysts (hyperintense to CSF on FLAIR and DWI sequences with lobulated margins and encasement of neurovascular structures). Lipomas are hyperintense on T1-weighted sequences.

Differential Diagnosis

Fig. 18.1 provides a brief diagnostic approach to a CPA lesion based on conventional MRI features.

Vestibular schwannoma (70% to 80%)
Meningioma (10% to 15%)
Epidermoid cyst (5%)
Vascular lesions (3% to 4%)
Arachnoid cyst (<1%)
Lipoma (<1%)
Metastasis

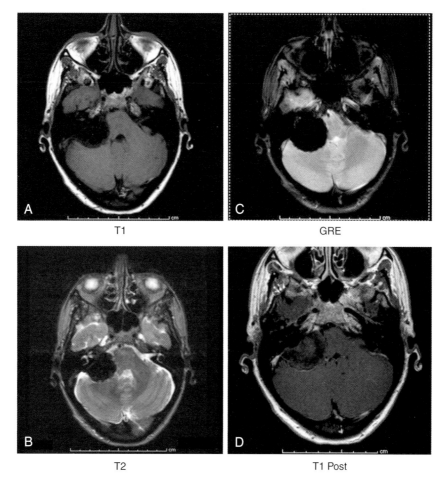

• **Fig. 18.2** Multiple images through the internal auditory canal demonstrate a right cerebellopontine angle meningioma. Because of extensive calcification, the mass is markedly T1 and T2 hypointense, susceptibility is present on the gradient echo sequence, and the mass enhances less avidly than does a noncalcified meningioma. *GRE,* Gradient refocused echo.

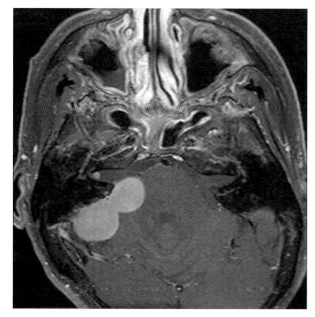

• **Fig. 18.3** An axial T1 postcontrast image shows a bilobed homogeneously enhancing mass in the right cerebellopontine angle with a dural tail consistent with a meningioma. An additional small homogeneously enhancing mass consistent with a vestibular schwannoma is seen in the ipsilateral internal auditory canal.

Pearls

- Schwannomas are centered on the IAC and expand the IAC. They have an "ice cream cone" appearance.
- Schwannomas with cystic components tend to grow faster and have a less favorable surgical outcome in terms of preservation of facial nerve function.
- Description of CPA schwannomas should include the following features because they will be important to surgical approaches (e.g., subtemporal, retrosigmoid, translabyrinthine approach)
  - Tumor dimensions in terms of both the cisternal and intracanalicular components
  - Lateral extent of the tumor within the IAC, especially if the tumor has extended up to the cochlear aperture
  - If an associated cyst is present, the size of the cyst should be described
- The following are some of the major surgical approaches based on the imaging features:
  - The subtemporal middle cranial fossa approach is used predominantly for small, mainly IAC masses
  - The retrosigmoid approach is used for schwannomas with a large CPA component

- The translabyrinthine approach often results in complete hearing loss and is reserved for tumors that extend far laterally within the IAC
- A combination of translabyrinthine and retrosigmoid approaches is used for large, complicated masses involving both the CPA and IAC
- Other treatment options include observation for asymptomatic lesions, microsurgery, and Gamma Knife radiosurgery.
- Meningiomas may have prominent dural tails, calcification in 20%, and adjacent bone hyperostosis.
- FLAIR and DWI will clearly distinguish epidermoid from arachnoid cysts. Arachnoid cysts follow CSF on all sequences. Epidermoids are hyperintense to CSF on FLAIR and DWI sequences.
- T1 and fat-saturation sequences will differentiate lipoma from the other nonenhancing CPA lesions.

Signs and Complications

Most clinical symptoms from CPA lesions are due to mass effect and include tinnitus, vertigo, hearing loss, and cranial nerve palsies. Purely intracisternal schwannomas may remain asymptomatic until reaching a large size. Epidermoid cysts tend to insinuate among the nerves and vessels and are associated with trigeminal neuralgia when they extend into Meckel cave. Brainstem stroke, due to stretching of the basilar artery branches by CPA masses, rarely occurs. Spontaneous or traumatic intracystic hemorrhage can complicate arachnoid cysts, but occurs rarely. Rare acute hemorrhagic expansion of a schwannoma also may result in the sudden onset of vertigo or emesis.

Suggested Readings

Bonneville F, Savatovsky J, Chiras J: Imaging of cerebellopontine angle lesions: an update. Part 1: enhancing extra-axial lesions, *Eur Radiol* 17(10):2472–2482, 2007.

Bonneville F, Savatovsky J, Chiras J: Imaging of cerebellopontine angle lesions: an update. Part 2: intra-axial lesions, skull base lesions that may invade the CPA region, and non-enhancing extra-axial lesions, *Eur Radiol* 17(11):2908–2920, 2007.

Lakshmi M, Glastonbury CM: Imaging of the cerebellopontine angle, *Neuroimaging Clin N Am* 19:393–406, 2009.

19

Lateral Ventricular Lesions

JOHN M. FAGNOU, MD

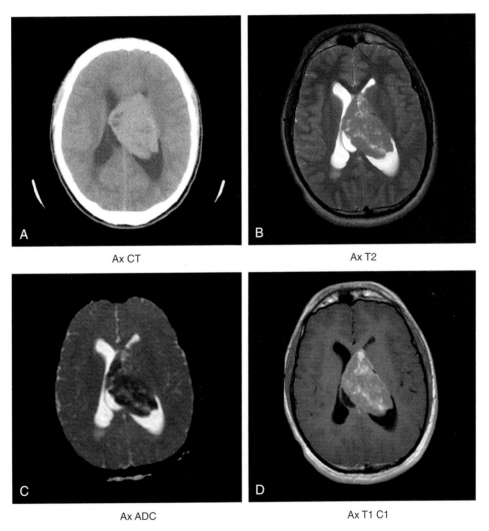

Ax CT

Ax T2

Ax ADC

Ax T1 C1

CASE A: A 20-year-old man presenting with a 2-month history of a worsening headache. *ADC,* Apparent diffusion coefficient; *Ax,* axial; *CT,* Computed tomography.

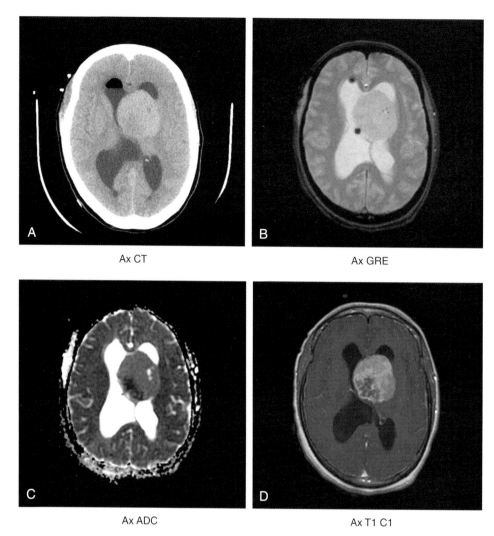

Ax CT

Ax GRE

Ax ADC

Ax T1 C1

CASE B: A 25-year-old woman presenting with a 2-week history of confusion (magnetic resonance imaging after a ventriculostomy for hydrocephalus). *ADC,* Apparent diffusion coefficient; *Ax,* axial; *CT,* Computed tomography; *GRE,* gradient refocused echo.

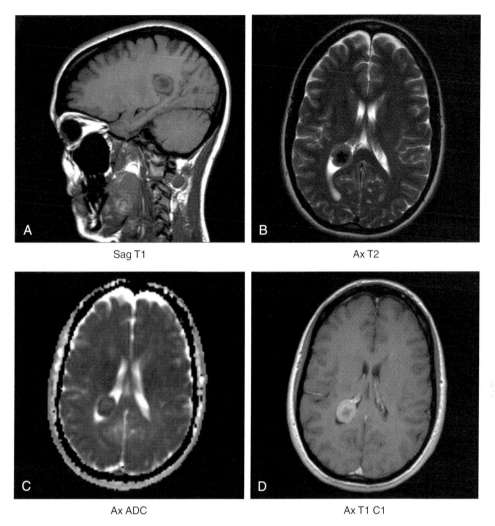

CASE C: A 34-year-old woman presenting with a 2-week history of headache. *ADC,* Apparent diffusion coefficient; *Ax,* axial; *Sag,* sagittal.

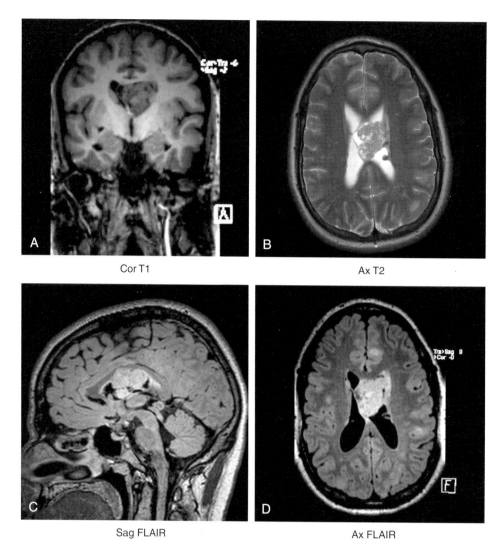

Cor T1

Ax T2

Sag FLAIR

Ax FLAIR

CASE D: A 17-year-old male adolescent with chronic seizures. *Ax,* Axial; *Cor,* coronal; *FLAIR,* fluid attenuated inversion recovery; *Sag,* sagittal.

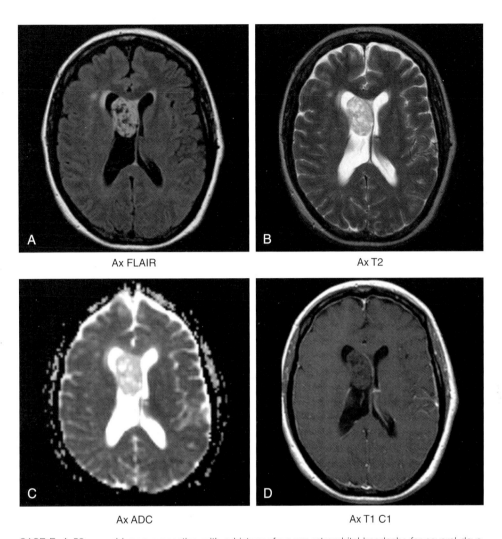

Ax FLAIR

Ax T2

Ax ADC

Ax T1 C1

CASE E: A 58-year-old man presenting with a history of severe retroorbital headache for several days. *ADC*, Apparent diffusion coefficient; *Ax*, axial; *FLAIR*, fluid attenuated inversion recovery.

DESCRIPTION OF FINDINGS

- Case A: A large, heterogeneously enhancing intraventricular mass containing small areas of intratumoral cystic change and abutting the septum pellucidum with early hydrocephalus. Note CT hyperdensity and mildly restricted diffusion.
- Case B: A hyperdense, avidly enhancing intraventricular mass with a few tiny foci of susceptibility artifact consistent with intratumoral hemorrhage or calcification. There is also a small focus of air in the frontal horn of the right lateral ventricle and hydrocephalus.
- Case C: An avidly enhancing T2 hypointense mass in the atrium of the right lateral ventricle with peripheral restricted diffusion.
- Case D: An intraventricular mass with multiple associated cortical/subcortical foci of T2/FLAIR signal hyperintensity and subependymal nodules.
- Case E: A nonenhancing intraventricular mass with small areas of intratumoral cystic change.

Diagnosis

Case A: Central neurocytoma
Case B: Ependymoma
Case C: Meningioma
Case D: Subependymal giant cell astrocytoma (presumptive based on location and confirmed diagnosis of tuberous sclerosis [TS])
Case E: Subependymoma

Summary

When evaluating a lateral intraventricular mass in an adult, the differential diagnosis most commonly includes meningioma, central neurocytoma, subependymoma, ependymoma, and metastasis. Rare diagnostic considerations include neurocysticercosis, neurosarcoidosis, cavernous malformation, and epidermoid or dermoid cysts. Meningiomas are usually low-grade (World Health Organization [WHO] grade I), surgically treated lesions. Central neurocytomas, which were misclassified as oligodendrogliomas prior to 1982, also are low-grade (WHO II), surgically treated lesions unless their size precludes gross total resection, in which case adjuvant radiotherapy can be used. Subependymomas are low-grade (WHO I), often incidental lesions that are treated conservatively or surgically. Lateral ventricular ependymomas are WHO grade II or III lesions that may be periventricular or intraventricular and are managed with surgery, radiation, and/or chemotherapy. Metastases are rare but can be seen in persons with advanced systemic malignancies or central nervous system (CNS) neoplasms with a propensity to spread through the cerebrospinal fluid (CSF).

In the pediatric age group, the differential diagnosis most commonly includes choroid plexus papilloma (CPP) and choroid plexus carcinoma (CPC), subependymal giant cell astrocytoma (SEGA), and, less commonly, the aforementioned adult differential considerations. Choroid plexus papillomas (WHO I) and carcinomas (WHO III) are surgically treated lesions that cannot be reliably distinguished radiologically. Patients with choroid plexus carcinomas can receive adjuvant chemotherapy and/or radiotherapy. SEGAs are WHO I lesions for which annual/biannual screening is prescribed throughout childhood in patients with tuberous sclerosis.

Key imaging features that help differentiate these lesions are provided in the following sections.

Spectrum of Disease

CPPs and CPCs occur in the lateral (most commonly in the atrium), fourth, and third ventricles 50%, 40%, and 10% of the time, respectively. Eighty percent present with hydrocephalus. Seventy-five percent are CT isodense to hyperdense, and 24% have calcification. On an MRI, virtually all CPPs and CPCs avidly enhance, and more than half show evidence of hemorrhage (55%) or flow voids (55%).

Central neurocytomas almost always occur in the lateral ventricles. They usually are anterior (77%) and located along the septum pellucidum, with extension into the third ventricle in 26%. On CT, 51% have calcification. On MRI, they demonstrate moderate to strong enhancement with cystic change (85%) and flow voids (69%).

Intraventricular meningiomas are hyperattenuating, with calcification in 50%. On MRI, they tend to be isointense to gray matter on T1- and T2-weighted images. They usually avidly enhance and can show restricted diffusion. They are typically located in the atrium of the lateral ventricle.

Subependymomas usually occur in the lateral (55%) or fourth ventricles (45%). On MRI, 55% show mild (36%) to moderate (21%) enhancement. They typically are T1 isointense and T2 hyperintense compared with brain parenchyma. Calcification and perilesional edema are rare.

Ependymomas usually occur in the fourth ventricle in children and in the lateral and third ventricles in adults. On CT, 40% to 80% have calcification. On MRI, ependymomas typically demonstrate avid enhancement and frequently demonstrate cystic change and intratumoral hemorrhage (best seen on T2*-weighted images).

Subependymal giant cell astrocytomas (SEGAs) occur near the foramen of Monro in the setting of tuberous sclerosis and usually are centered in the lateral ventricle but can be centered in the anterior third ventricle. Interval growth is the most useful diagnostic feature in distinguishing SEGAs from subependymal nodules. They exhibit variable enhancement and signal characteristics.

Intraventricular metastases are rare. They typically grow rapidly and enhance and can invade adjacent ependyma and brain parenchyma.

Differential Diagnosis

CPPs and CPCs are most commonly seen in the atria of the lateral ventricles in the pediatric age group (median age, 1.5 years). They cannot be reliably differentiated radiologically. These tumors often demonstrate concomitant hydrocephalus and may seed the CSF, even with benign histology (CPP).

Central neurocytomas are tumors of young adults (age 20 to 40 years), usually with broad-based apposition to the septum pellucidum. They usually are well circumscribed and have a heterogeneous "bubbly" appearance (i.e., demonstrating cystic change) with heterogeneous enhancement.

Intraventricular meningiomas typically occur in middle-aged (age 30 to 60 years) females (female/male, 2:1) in the atrium of the lateral ventricle. Imaging characteristics often reflect high lesion cellularity (CT hyperdense, T2 hypointense, mildly restricted diffusion and dense, homogeneous enhancement).

Subependymomas often are discovered incidentally in middle-aged to elderly males. They grow slowly and frequently demonstrate little or no enhancement and have intratumoral cystic changes.

Ependymomas are more commonly periventricular (70%) than truly intraventricular (30%) when arising supratentorially; therefore they require close scrutiny for parenchymal origin. Lateral ventricular lesions most commonly occur in the 18- to 24-year age range. They can metastasize through the CSF, especially if anaplastic (WHO grade III).

SEGAs occur almost exclusively in the setting of tuberous sclerosis in the first or second decades of life. Interval growth allows confident diagnosis of a SEGA, whereas enhancement and size do not reliably differentiate SEGAs from subependymal nodules.

Intraventricular metastases have a heterogeneous imaging appearance. The most common primary tumors are bronchogenic and renal cell carcinomas. Other primary tumors that metastasize to the lateral ventricles are melanoma, gastric carcinoma, colon carcinoma, and lymphoma. CNS neoplasms with a propensity for CSF spread include CPP and CPC, medulloblastoma, ependymoma, germ cell neoplasms, and embryonal tumors with multilayered rosettes.

Pearls

- CPPs and CPCs are avidly enhancing pediatric atrial masses.
- A central neurocytoma is a heterogeneously enhancing large, bubbly mass broadly apposed to the septum pellucidum in a young adult.
- A meningioma is a cellular (T2 and apparent diffusion coefficient hypointense), avidly enhancing atrial mass in an adult woman.
- A subependymoma is a mildly enhancing or nonenhancing, small (<2 cm), incidental mass in an elderly man.
- An ependymoma is a periventricular or intraventricular, avidly enhancing mass, demonstrating evidence of calcification and/or hemorrhage in a young adult.

- A SEGA is an enlarging mass near the foramen of Monro in a pediatric patient with known tuberous sclerosis or other imaging stigmata thereof.
- Metastasis is a new enhancing mass in the setting of advanced systemic cancer or a CNS neoplasm with a propensity for CSF spread.

Signs and Complications

Noncommunicating hydrocephalus may complicate any of these lesions and often is noted at presentation. CSF seeding may occur in the setting of CPP/CPC, ependymoma, and metastases. Screening of the entire spine with contrast-enhanced MRI is indicated with these lesions.

Suggested Readings

Furie DM, Provenzale JM: Supratentorial ependymomas and subependymomas: CT and MR appearance, *J Comput Assist Tomogr* 19(4): 518–526, 1995.

Goh S, Butler W, Thiele EA: Subependymal giant cell tumors in tuberous sclerosis complex, *Neurology* 63(8):1457–1461, 2004.

Kerkovský M, Zitterbart K, Svoboda K, et al: Central neurocytoma: the neuroradiological perspective, *Childs Nerv Syst* 24(11):1361–1369, 2008.

Koeller KK, Sandberg GD: Armed Forces Institute of Pathology: from the archives of the AFIP. Cerebral intraventricular neoplasms: radiologic-pathologic correlation, *Radiographics* 22(6):1473–1505, 2002.

McDermott MW: Intraventricular meningiomas, *Neurosurg Clin North Am* 14(4):559–569, 2003.

Morrison G, Sobel DF, Kelley WM, et al: Intraventricular mass lesions, *Radiology* 153(2):435–442, 1984.

Ragel BT, Osborn AG, Whang K, et al: Subependymomas: an analysis of clinical and imaging features, *Neurosurgery* 58(5):881–890, 2006.

Rushing EJ, Cooper PB, Quezado M, et al: Subependymoma revisited: clinicopathological evaluation of 83 cases, *J Neurooncol* 85(3): 297–305, 2007.

Shogan P, Banks KP, Brown S: AJR teaching file: intraventricular mass, *AJR Am J Roentgenol* 189(6 suppl):S55–S57, 2007.

Wolff JE, Sajedi M, Brant R, et al: Choroid plexus tumours, *Br J Cancer* 87(10):1086–1091, 2002.

Zhang D, Wen L, Henning TD, et al: Central neurocytoma: clinical, pathological and neuroradiological findings, *Clin Radiol* 61(4): 348–357, 2006.

20
Third Ventricular Lesions

JOHN M. FAGNOU, MD

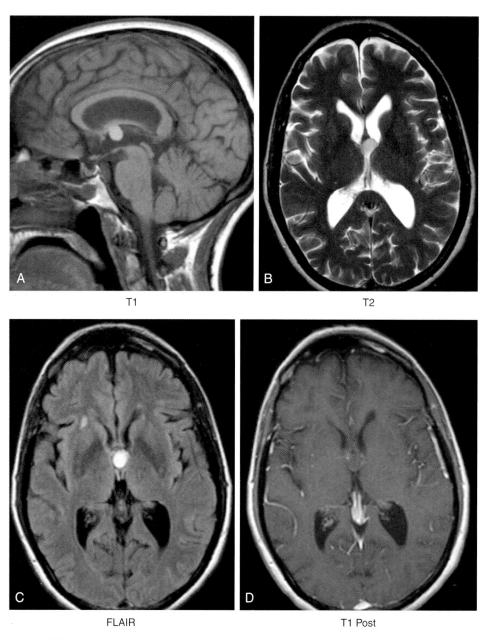

T1

T2

FLAIR

T1 Post

CASE A: A 54-year-old asymptomatic female. *FLAIR*, Fluid attenuated inversion recovery.

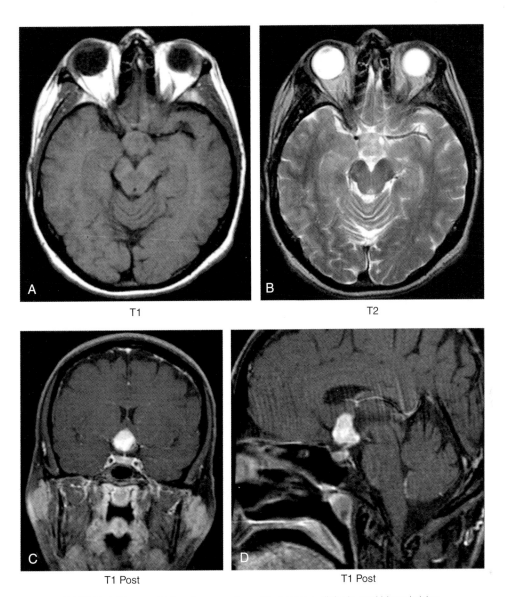

T1

T2

T1 Post

T1 Post

CASE B: A 53-year-old female presenting with dizziness, diplopia, and blurred vision.

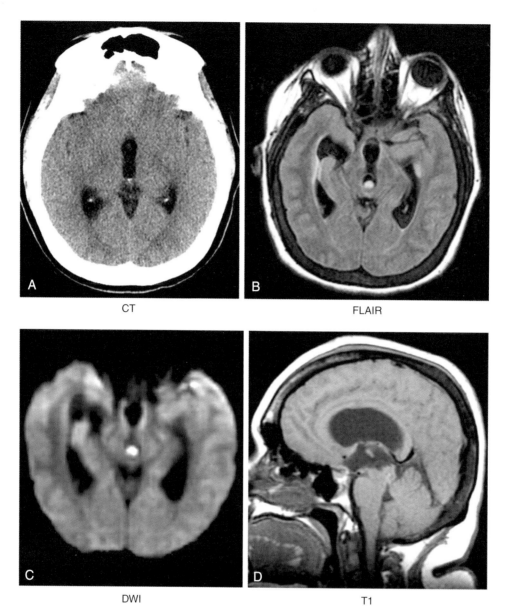

CT

FLAIR

DWI

T1

CASE C: A 32-year-old Latin American female presenting with a severe headache. *CT*, Computed tomography; *DWI*, diffusion-weighted imaging; *FLAIR*, fluid attenuated inversion recovery.

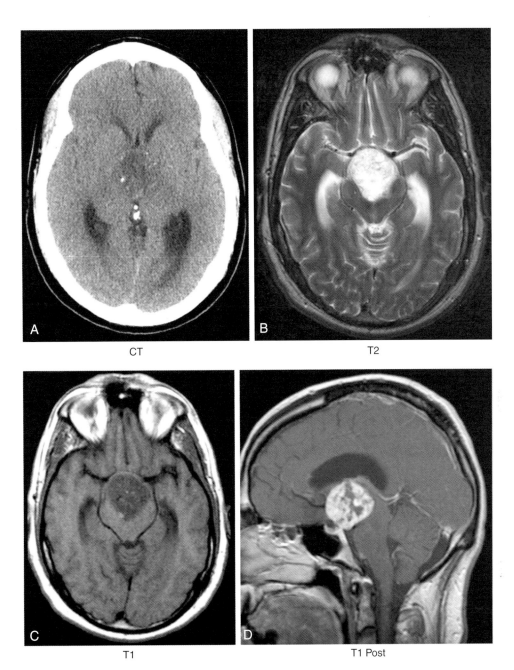

CASE D. A 37-year-old male presenting with a 1 year history of headaches, fatigue, and memory loss. *CT,* Computed tomography.

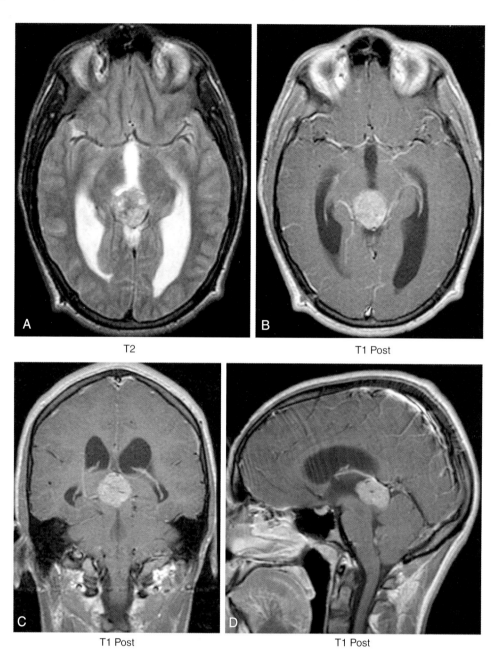

T2

T1 Post

T1 Post

T1 Post

CASE E: A 17-year-old boy presenting with a history of chronic headaches.

DESCRIPTION OF FINDINGS

- Case A: A small, T1 and FLAIR/T2 hyperintense, nonenhancing, anterior, third ventricular mass.
- Case B: A homogeneously enhancing, T2 isointense mass in the anterior floor of the third ventricle containing small cystic foci.
- Case C: A small T1 and FLAIR/T2 hyperintense cystic lesion with a focus of mural calcification in the posteroinferior third ventricle obstructing the cerebral aqueduct and causing hydrocephalus.
- Case D: A large heterogeneously enhancing third ventricular mass containing punctate calcifications and scattered small areas of intrinsic T1 hyperintensity.
- Case E: A predominantly T2 isointense, homogeneously enhancing posterior third ventricular mass with small internal cysts.

Diagnosis

Case A: Colloid cyst (presumptive; 14-year imaging stability)
Case B: Chordoid glioma (proven by pathology)
Case C: Intraventricular neurocysticercosis (IVNCC) (presumptive; positive serology in an immigrant from Latin America)
Case D: Craniopharyngioma (proven by pathology)
Case E: Germinoma (proven by pathology)

Summary

True third ventricular masses are rare, with the colloid cyst representing the only primary lesion of the third ventricle that can be termed "common." The recently described chordoid glioma represents a rare primary tumor that arises exclusively in the third ventricle.

In addition to colloid cysts and chordoid gliomas, other rare differential considerations that may occur as primary to the third ventricle (but more commonly elsewhere) include choroid plexus papilloma (CPP) and choroid plexus carcinoma (CPC), neurocysticercosis (NCC), and ependymoma. Metastases are a differential consideration in the setting of a central nervous system neoplasm with a propensity for CSF spread or in persons with advanced systemic malignancies. Furthermore, masses that arise from the suprasellar and pineal regions often appear to be arising from the third ventricle.

Spectrum of Disease

Colloid Cyst

The vast majority of colloid cysts occur in the anterior third ventricle (rarely in the lateral ventricle or fourth ventricle). Colloid cysts are 3 to 40 mm in diameter and usually are hyperdense on CT. On MRI, approximately 50% are T1 hyperintense and most are T2 hypointense secondary to high protein content. A thin rim of enhancement may be present.

Chordoid Glioma

Chordoid gliomas, which occur only in the third ventricle, typically are hyperdense on CT. On MRI, they are usually T1 isointense and T2 isointense to slightly hyperintense compared to brain parenchyma with avid homogeneous enhancement. Rarely, chordoid gliomas have small cystic areas and vasogenic edema along the optic pathways.

Choroid Plexus Papilloma and Carcinoma

Ten percent of CPPs and CPCs occur in the third ventricle, with 40% occurring in the fourth ventricle and 50% occurring in the atrium of the lateral ventricle. Eighty percent present with hydrocephalus. These tumors are typically (75%) isodense to hyperdense on CT, with calcification occurring in 24%. On MRI, these tumors almost always avidly enhance. The majority also show evidence of hemorrhage (~55%) or flow voids (~55%).

Neurocysticercosis

IVNCC occurs in 7% to 20% of cases (vs. 60% to 92% for parenchymal NCC). CT detects intraventricular lesions in only 10% of cases, whereas MRI detects intraventricular lesions in nearly 100% of cases. Fifty percent of cases demonstrate parenchymal calcifications on CT and 97% demonstrate hydrocephalus at presentation. IVNCC cysts occur most frequently in the fourth ventricle (70%). Enhancement is identified in 55% of cases imaged with MRI. CISS (constructive interference in steady state) sequences improve detection of small lesions.

Ependymomas

Ependymomas typically arise from the ependymal lining of the lateral ventricle in children and young adults, but rarely arise in the third ventricle. The solid components usually densely enhance. Cysts, calcification, and hemorrhage are common.

Differential Diagnosis

Colloid Cyst

Colloid cysts are rare lesions of obscure origin (likely endodermal) that most commonly present with headache. Their location in the anterior third ventricle predisposes them to obstruction of the foramina of Monro and acute hydrocephalus (which may be intermittent), with rare cases of sudden death reported.

Chordoid Glioma

Discovered in 1998 and named for its microscopic resemblance to chordomas, nearly all chordoid glioma lesions described to date have been located in the third ventricle. Chordoid gliomas typically occur in middle-aged females (~75%). Despite its low pathologic grade (World Health Organization II), prognosis is poor because of its tight adherence to important regional structures (e.g., the hypothalamus and optic chiasm), precluding complete surgical resection.

Choroid Plexus Papilloma and Carcinoma

CPPs and CPCs are avidly enhancing masses that usually occur in the atria of the lateral ventricles in children and the fourth ventricle in adults. Third ventricular involvement is uncommon. Papillomas and carcinomas cannot be reliably differentiated by imaging. These tumors often demonstrate concomitant hydrocephalus and may seed the CSF, even when they are histologically benign.

Neurocysticercosis

IVNCC cysts usually present with headache, nausea, and vomiting in contradistinction to parenchymal NCC cysts, which usually present with seizures. The intraventricular form often manifests as a solitary cystic lesion, which may attach to the choroid plexus or ventricular wall, causing a granular ependymitis and hydrocephalus that is often asymmetric. The cyst also may be mobile within the ventricular system and migrate between examinations.

Ependymomas

Ependymomas can occur anywhere in the ventricular system. However, they rarely occur in the third ventricle. They usually densely enhance and frequently have cysts, calcification, and hemorrhage.

Other Differential Diagnoses

Masses that arise from the suprasellar and pineal regions often appear to be arising from the third ventricle. Craniopharyngiomas and germinomas should be considered in the differential diagnosis when an anterior third ventricular mass is visualized. Pineal region tumors and germinomas should be considered when a posterior third ventricular mass is visualized.

Pearls

- A CT hyperdense and T1 hyperintense, anterior third ventricular cyst is nearly pathognomonic of colloid cyst, but beware of the NCC mimic!
- An intraventricular cyst with a calcified scolex is diagnostic of NCC.
- Homogeneously enhancing masses in middle-aged women suggest chordoid gliomas, although a suprasellar or pineal region germinoma can have a similar appearance.
- CPPs and CPCs have a frond-like appearance with microcysts, calcification, and hemorrhage.
- Ependymomas have larger cysts along with calcification and hemorrhage.

Signs and Complications

Frequent complications are noncommunicating hydrocephalus and visual (optic pathway) or endocrinologic (hypothalamus) symptoms at presentation. CSF seeding may occur in the setting of CPP/CPC, and screening contrast-enhanced spinal MRI is indicated.

Suggested Readings

Armao D, Castillo M, Chen H, et al: Colloid cyst of the third ventricle: imaging-pathologic correlation, *AJNR Am J Neuroradiol* 21(8):1470–1477, 2000.

Cuetter AC, Andrews RJ: Intraventricular neurocysticercosis: 18 consecutive patients and review of the literature, *Neurosurg Focus* 12(6):e5, 2002.

Koeller KK, Sandberg GD: Armed Forces Institute of Pathology: from the archives of the AFIP. Cerebral intraventricular neoplasms: radiologic-pathologic correlation, *Radiographics* 22(6):1473–1505, 2002.

Meyers SP, Khademian ZP, Chuang SH, et al: Choroid plexus carcinomas in children: MRI features and patient outcomes, *Neuroradiology* 46(9):770–780, 2004.

Wolff JE, Sajedi M, Brant R, et al: Choroid plexus tumours, *Br J Cancer* 87(10):1086–1091, 2002.

21
Fourth Ventricular Lesions

JOHN M. FAGNOU, MD

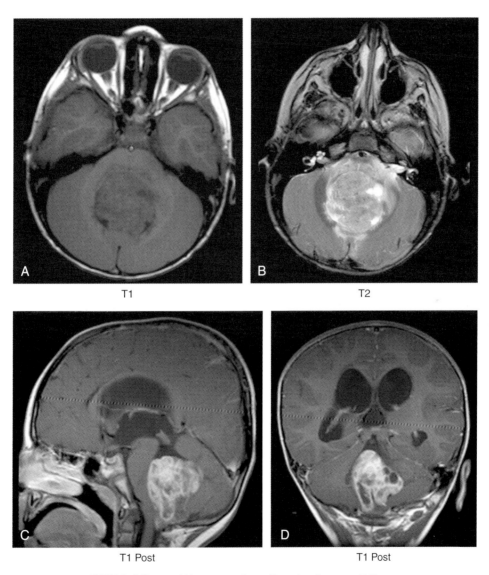

T1

T2

T1 Post

T1 Post

CASE A: A 2-year-old boy presenting with unsteadiness and lethargy.

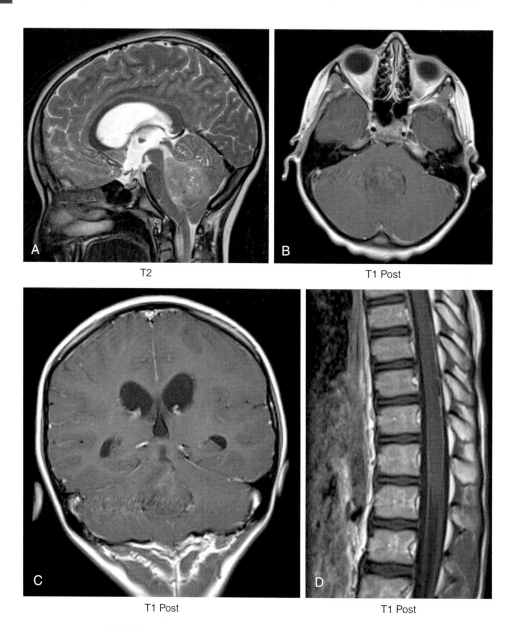

T2

T1 Post

T1 Post

T1 Post

CASE B: An 8-year-old boy presenting with emesis and headache.

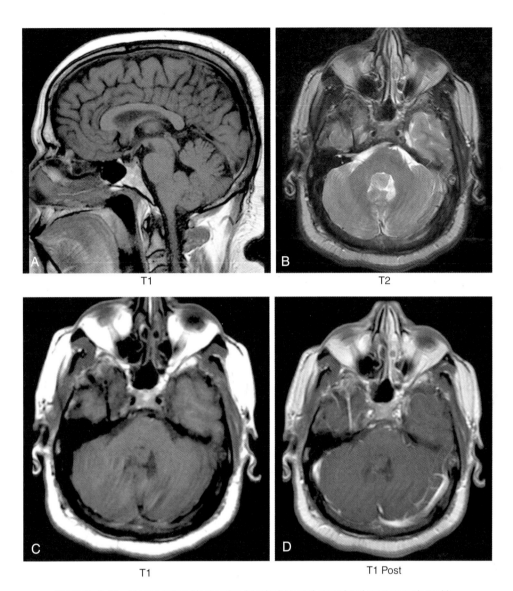

CASE C: A 45-year-old man with morning headaches and occasional nausea and vomiting.

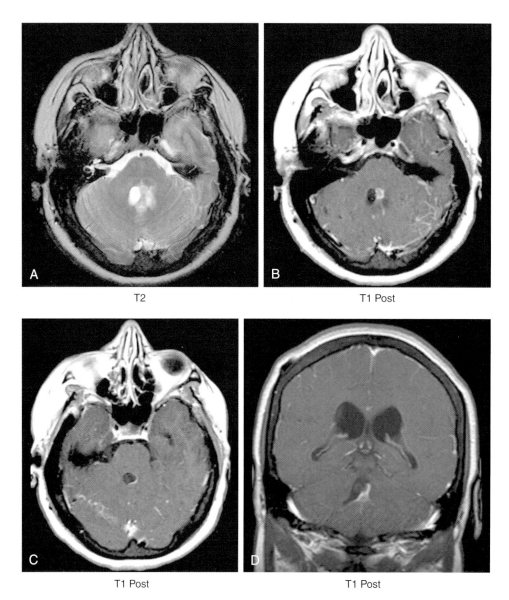

T2

T1 Post

T1 Post

T1 Post

CASE D: A 32-year-old Latin American woman presenting with a severe headache.

DESCRIPTION OF FINDINGS

- Case A: A large T2 hyperintense heterogeneously enhancing, intraventricular mass with internal cystic components and extrusion through the foramen of Magendie.
- Case B: A T2 isointense, minimally enhancing, intraventricular mass with leptomeningeal enhancement along the spinal cord consistent with spinal drop metastases.
- Case C: A small, T1 and T2 isointense, minimally enhancing fourth ventricular mass.
- Case D: A solid and cystic, partially enhancing fourth ventricular mass with mild periventricular edema.

Diagnosis

Case A: Ependymoma (proven by pathology)
Case B: Medulloblastoma (proven by pathology)
Case C: Subependymoma (proven by pathology)
Case D: Intraventricular neurocysticercosis (IVNCC) (presumptive; positive serology in an immigrant from Latin America)

Summary

Fourth ventricular masses are much more common in the pediatric population than in adults. In children, medulloblastomas and ependymomas are the most common masses found in the fourth ventricle. Other pediatric posterior fossa primary neoplasms, including pilocytic astrocytoma and brainstem glioma, occasionally may grow exophytically into the fourth ventricle and mimic a mass of ventricular origin.

In adults, primary neoplasms also may occur in the fourth ventricle, including subependymomas and choroid plexus papillomas (CPPs). Although a hemangioblastoma rarely arises within the fourth ventricle, it should be considered in the setting of von Hippel Lindau disease. Metastases that occur both via cerebrospinal fluid (CSF) spread (central nervous system neoplasms) and hematogenous spread (systemic neoplasms) also must be considered.

IVNCC, although rare, most commonly occurs in the fourth ventricle and should be considered in the setting of a cystic fourth ventricular lesion in the appropriate clinical history.

Spectrum of Disease

Medulloblastoma

Most medulloblastomas are hyperdense on CT (~89%), isointense to hypointense on T1-weighted MRI, and isointense on T2-weighted MRI. They show variable enhancement. While some medulloblastomas are homogeneous, some are heterogeneous due to calcification, cyst formation, and necrosis. Restricted diffusion (low apparent diffusion coefficient) is typical because of high tumor cellularity.

Ependymoma

Approximately 70% of brain ependymomas are infratentorial (i.e., fourth ventricular). Calcifications on CT appear in 40% to 80% of brain ependymomas. The MRI signal is typically heterogeneous, but overall T1 hypointense and T2 hyperintense. Cysts and foci of hemorrhage are common. Avid enhancement of solid components is usually seen. Areas of restricted diffusion may be present. Extension through the foramina of Magendie (~60%) and Luschka (~15%) frequently occurs.

Subependymoma

Subependymomas usually are found in the fourth ventricle (55% of cases) or lateral ventricle (45% of cases). They typically occur in middle-aged to elderly men (mean age, 50 years). Mild-to-moderate enhancement is present in up to 55% of cases. Subependymomas are most frequently T1 isointense and T2 hyperintense. Surrounding edema is rare (13% of cases). Subependymomas are often small (<2 cm), but mean lesion size is approximately 4 cm in symptomatic patients with hydrocephalus.

Choroid Plexus Papilloma and Carcinoma

Choroid plexus tumors occur in the lateral ventricle (50% of cases), fourth ventricle (40% of cases), and third ventricle (10% of cases). Eighty percent of choroid plexus tumors present with hydrocephalus. On CT they typically are isodense to hyperdense, with calcification in 24%. On MRI, virtually all choroid plexus tumors avidly enhance, and they frequently show evidence of hemorrhage (55%) or flow voids (55%).

Neurocysticercosis

IVNCC occurs in 7% to 20% of patients with neurocysticercosis. Intraventricular cysts are identified on CT in only 10% of cases in which MRI identifies a cyst. Approximately 50% also demonstrate parenchymal calcifications on CT. IVNCC most frequently occurs in the fourth ventricle (70%) followed by the third ventricle (15%) and lateral ventricle (15%). At presentation, 97% demonstrate hydrocephalus. On MRI, enhancement is seen in 55% of cases.

Differential Diagnosis

Medulloblastoma

Arising from the roof of the fourth ventricle, most medulloblastomas (77%) present in the pediatric age group, with a mean age of 7.3 years at diagnosis. In adults, a desmoplastic/nodular medulloblastoma or medulloblastoma with extensive nodularity (MBEN) located in the cerebellar hemispheric location is more common; this finding is thought to be related to the superolateral migration of undifferentiated cells with oncogenic potential originating in the posterior medullary velum.

Ependymoma

The mean age at presentation of fourth ventricular ependymomas is 6 years. Ependymomas are differentiated from medulloblastomas by a higher likelihood of demonstrating calcifications, hemorrhage (T2 imaging), higher diffusivity, and "plastic" tumor behavior with extrusion through the foramina of Magendie and Luschka. Ependymomas may disseminate through the CSF, especially if they are anaplastic (World Health Organization grade III), but they disseminate less frequently than do medulloblastomas.

Subependymoma

Thought to arise from subependymal glia, subependymomas are benign (World Health Organization grade I), often incidental tumors that are most commonly seen in middle-aged or elderly men. Approximately 10% demonstrate an admixture of ependymoma on histopathologic examination. Modern microsurgical techniques yield good outcomes, even with subtotal resection.

Choroid Plexus Papilloma and Carcinoma

Choroid plexus tumors occur most commonly in young adults (median age, 23 years) when they appear in the fourth ventricle. Relative to CPP, choroid plexus carcinoma (CPC) is less common in the fourth ventricle. CPP treatment is surgical, with adjuvant chemotherapy or radiation therapy reserved for CPC. CPP may rarely metastasize through the CSF in spite of a benign histology.

Neurocysticercosis

Approximately half of patients also demonstrate parenchymal evidence of neurocysticercosis (NCC), adding diagnostic specificity. IVNCC has a more aggressive behavior than does parenchymal NCC, with the host inflammatory response causing ependymitis and symptomatic hydrocephalus. Parenchymal NCC, by contrast, usually presents with seizures.

Pearls

- In the pediatric population, identifying calcifications, evidence of hemorrhage, and "plastic" tumor behavior favor

ependymoma, while high tumor cellularity (diffusion restriction), favors medulloblastoma.
- In adults, age, enhancement, and clinical history must be used in concert to differentiate choroid plexus tumors (young adults, avid enhancement), subependymomas (older males, frequently do not enhance), and metastases (history of primary malignancy and multiple lesions.)
- A cystic lesion with a calcified scolex is pathognomonic for IVNCC. In less clear-cut cases, a careful search for parenchymal or cisternal disease will increase diagnostic specificity. Constructive interference in steady state (CISS) images improve detection and delineation of disease.

Signs and Complications

Noncommunicating hydrocephalus may complicate any of these lesions and often is noted at presentation. CSF seeding may occur in the setting of medulloblastoma, CPP/CPC, and ependymoma; screening-enhanced spinal MRI is indicated with these lesions.

Suggested Readings

Cuetter AC, Andrews RJ: Intraventricular neurocysticercosis: 18 consecutive patients and review of the literature, *Neurosurg Focus* 12(6):e5, 2002.

Koeller KK, Rushing EJ: Armed Forces Institute of Pathology: From the archives of the AFIP: medulloblastoma: a comprehensive review with radiologic-pathologic correlation, *Radiographics* 23(6):1613–1637, 2003.

Koeller KK, Sandberg GD: Armed Forces Institute of Pathology: From the archives of the AFIP: cerebral intraventricular neoplasms: radiologic-pathologic correlation, *Radiographics* 22(6):1473–1505, 2002.

Ragel BT, Osborn AG, Whang K, et al: Subependymomas: an analysis of clinical and imaging features, *Neurosurgery* 58(5):881–890, 2006.

Rushing EJ, Cooper PB, Quezado M, et al: Subependymoma revisited: clinicopathological evaluation of 83 cases, *J Neurooncol* 85(3):297–305, 2007.

Wolff JE, Sajedi M, Brant R, et al: Choroid plexus tumours, *Br J Cancer* 87(10):1086–1091, 2002.

Yuh EL, Barkovich AJ, Gupta N: Imaging of ependymomas: MRI and CT, *Childs Nerv Syst* 25(10):1203–1213, 2009.

22

Suprasellar Cystic Lesions

JUAN E. SMALL, MD, MSC

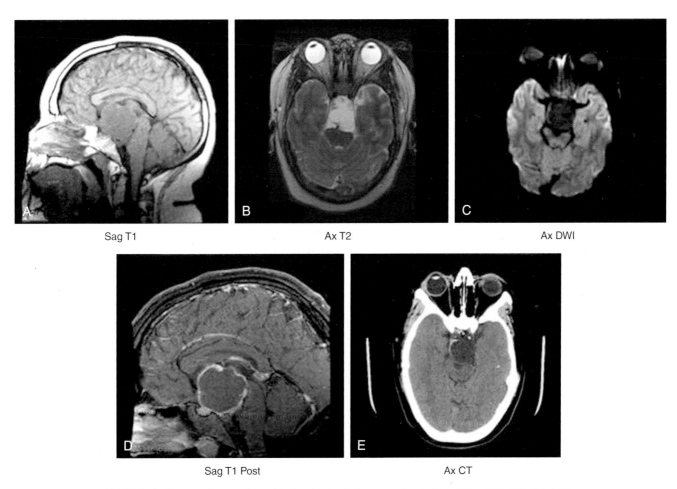

Sag T1	Ax T2	Ax DWI
Sag T1 Post	Ax CT	

CASE A: A 19-year-old presenting with chronic visual changes, amenorrhea, and weight gain. *Ax,* Axial; *CT,* Computed tomography; *DWI,* diffusion-weighted imaging; *Sag,* sagittal.

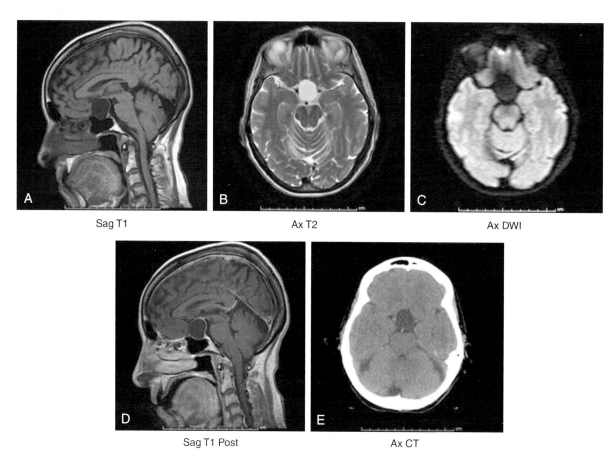

Sag T1   Ax T2   Ax DWI

Sag T1 Post   Ax CT

CASE B: A 70-year-old presenting after sustaining trauma. *Ax,* Axial; *CT,* Computed tomography; *DWI,* diffusion-weighted imaging; *Sag,* sagittal.

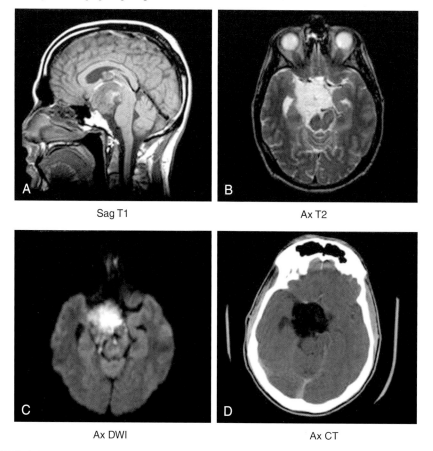

Sag T1   Ax T2

Ax DWI   Ax CT

CASE C: A 41-year-old presenting with headaches. *Ax,* Axial; *CT,* Computed tomography; *DWI,* diffusion-weighted imaging; *Sag,* sagittal.

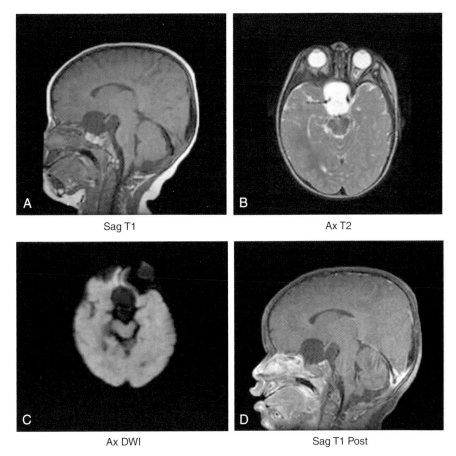

CASE D: A 19-month-old with anisocoria. *Ax,* Axial; *DWI,* diffusion-weighted imaging; *Sag,* sagittal.

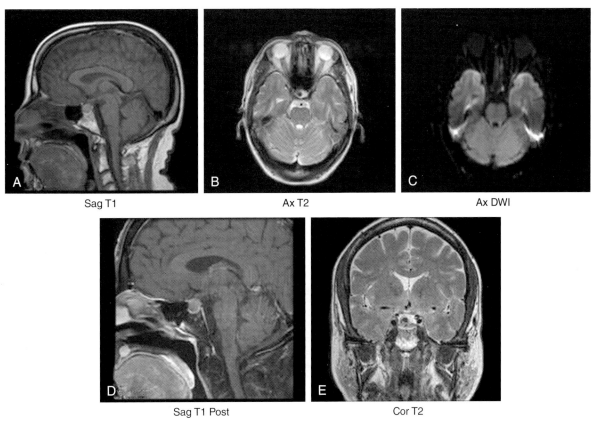

CASE E: A 60-year-old with a history of left tonsil squamous cell carcinoma and a sellar/suprasellar lesion incidentally noted on a neck computed tomography scan. *Ax,* Axial; *Cor,* coronal; *DWI,* diffusion-weighted imaging; *Sag,* sagittal.

DESCRIPTION OF FINDINGS

- Case A: A predominantly cystic suprasellar mass with mild T1 hypointensity and marked T2 hyperintensity and without associated restricted diffusion. A sagittal postcontrast fat-saturated image demonstrates an irregular, mildly thickened, and mildly nodular rim of enhancement. Close inspection of the axial CT image demonstrates a few associated peripheral punctuate calcifications that are most prominent anteriorly.
- Case B: A sellar and suprasellar, ovoid, smoothly contoured, homogeneous lesion with cerebrospinal fluid (CSF)-like signal on T1, T2, DWI diffusion-weighted imaging (DWI), and gadolinium-enhanced T1-weighted sequences and CSF-like density on axial CT with a thin rim of peripheral enhancement. No associated calcification is noted.
- Case C: A suprasellar, nonenhancing, lobulated, cystic-appearing mass that is mildly hyperintense compared to CSF on T1-weighted images, slightly hypointense compared to CSF on T2-weighted images, markedly hyperintense compared to CSF and brain parenchyma on DWI, and has similar hypodensity compared to CSF on contrast-enhanced axial CT.
- Case D: A suprasellar, nonenhancing, mildly lobulated smooth-walled, cystic lesion that is isointense compared to CSF on T1, T2, DWI, and gadolinium-enhanced T1-weighted sequences and that distorts the infundibulum.
- Case E: A sellar/suprasellar, noncalcified, ovoid, smoothly contoured, nonenhancing, cystic lesion with intrinsically T1 hyperintense signal suggesting proteinaceous content. T2 images demonstrate mild hyperintensity with a hypointense intracystic module. The lesion does not have restricted diffusion.

Diagnosis

Case A: Craniopharyngioma
Case B: Rathke cleft cyst
Case C: Epidermoid cyst
Case D: Arachnoid cyst
Case E: Rathke cleft cyst

Summary

A number of cystic lesions can present within the suprasellar cistern, the extraaxial space between the sella and the floor of the third ventricle. Although solid or vascular lesions related to the optic nerves or chiasm, the circle of Willis, the hypothalamus, or pituitary infundibulum present at this site, the identification of a cystic-appearing lesion significantly narrows the differential diagnosis. Cystic-appearing suprasellar lesions include arachnoid cysts, Rathke cleft cysts, epidermoid and dermoid cysts, adamantinomatous craniopharyngiomas, and juvenile pilocytic astrocytomas.

When evaluating a cystic suprasellar lesion, the presence of nodular or frankly solid enhancing components suggests a neoplastic lesion, the most common of which is an adamantinomatous craniopharyngioma. Craniopharyngiomas may be sellar and suprasellar, exclusively suprasellar, or purely intrasellar. They demonstrate a bimodal distribution, with two-thirds of them presenting in childhood/adolescence and a second smaller peak generally presenting in middle to late adulthood. Childhood craniopharyngiomas tend to be adamantinomatous and present as predominantly cystic or solid and cystic lobulated masses with hemorrhage and calcification. Adult craniopharyngiomas tend to be papillary and present more often as predominantly solid or mixed solid and cystic masses. As noted, careful inspection for the presence of nodular or frankly solid enhancing components should be performed. Nodular or rim-like calcification involving cyst walls or solid components is highly suggestive of this diagnosis. Because MRI is insensitive to calcification, CT often is particularly valuable. The hallmark characteristics of predominantly cystic craniopharyngiomas are calcification, cyst formation, and nodular and/or rim enhancement. However, a craniopharyngioma may not have all or any of these characteristics. Furthermore, other less common neoplastic lesions that typically present as cystic and solid masses, such as hypothalamic/optic pathway juvenile pilocytic astrocytomas, should be considered in the appropriate clinical setting.

Rathke cleft cysts are congenital, nonneoplastic sellar/suprasellar cysts that arise from remnants of Rathke pouch. Approximately 80% of these lesions are seen between the anterior and posterior pituitary lobes. Although usually intrasellar, these lesions may rarely be purely suprasellar. On imaging, they typically appear as smoothly contoured, spherical or ovoid, nonenhancing lesions, although a thin rim of peripheral enhancement occasionally can be present. However, solid or nodular enhancement, such as that seen in craniopharyngiomas, should not be present. The variable MR signal intensity of Rathke cleft cysts depends on the content of the cyst (e.g., protein, hemosiderin, cholesterol). Despite the variable signal intensity of different lesions, the signal intensity is generally homogeneous. Importantly, in up to 40% of lesions the homogenous signal intensity is disrupted by the presence of an intracystic T2 hypointense nodule (protein and cellular debris), the identification of which is particularly suggestive of this diagnosis. Rathke cleft cysts tend to be less than 0.3 cm in size, and craniopharyngiomas tend to have a tumor diameter greater than 2 cm. Rathke cleft cysts generally do not contain calcification, a finding that, as previously noted, is one of the hallmarks of craniopharyngiomas. Various studies in the literature note that between 42% and 87% of craniopharyngiomas exhibit calcification, whereas 0% to 13% of Rathke cleft cysts exhibit calcification.

Arachnoid cysts are smooth-walled, nonenhancing, noncalcified cystic lesions exhibiting signal characteristics isointense compared to CSF on all sequences. Although they occur anywhere along the neuraxis, 10% to 15% present in the suprasellar region.

Epidermoid cysts can readily be distinguished from arachnoid cysts based on fluid attenuated inversion recovery (FLAIR) and DWI. An epidermoid is markedly hyperintense compared to CSF and brain parenchyma on DWI due to marked T2 hyperintensity and diffusion similar to that of normal brain parenchyma. On FLAIR images, epidermoids are heterogeneously hyperintense compared to CSF and slightly hypointense compared to brain parenchyma. Epidermoids also are slightly hyperintense compared to CSF on T1-weighted images and slightly hypointense compared to CSF on T2-weighted images. The morphology of these lesions provides further distinguishing features from arachnoid cysts. Epidermoids generally exhibit lobulated, crenulated, and irregular margins compared, while arachnoid cysts have smooth walls. As slowly growing lesions, epidermoids tend to insinuate themselves into the subarachnoid space and sulci encasing adjacent structures such as nerves or blood vessels. Arachnoid cysts, by contrast, tend to displace nerves and blood vessels.

Other midline developmental lesions to consider are lipomas and dermoids. The identification of fat density components on

CT or of T1 and T2 hyperintense fat components on MRI generally renders the correct diagnosis. Dermoids typically are much more complex, heterogeneous lesions that contain squamous epithelium, hair follicles, and sebaceous components. Because the fatty/sebaceous internal components of dermoids are fluid at normal body temperature, fat fluid levels can be apparent, in contrast to the "solid" fat of lipomas.

Although the diagnosis of a giant aneurysm on postcontrast images generally does not pose a diagnostic dilemma, a thrombosed aneurysm may mimic a cystic lesion. Generally, the contiguity of the aneurysm with the parent vessel clinches the diagnosis. Peripheral rim-like calcification, concentric lamellation (layers of thrombus of different ages), susceptibility

blooming, or the presence of pulsation artifact are important and helpful clues to this diagnosis.

Spectrum of Disease

An intrinsically T1 hyperintense and T2 hypointense nonenhancing cystic-appearing sellar/suprasellar Rathke cleft cyst is shown in Fig. 22.1. Variable MRI signal intensity of Rathke cleft cysts is dependent on the content of the cyst (protein, hemosiderin, or cholesterol). Despite the variable signal intensity of different lesions, a homogenous signal intensity is generally evident.

A partially thrombosed suprasellar aneurysm (Fig. 22.2) may pose diagnostic difficulties in the absence of a

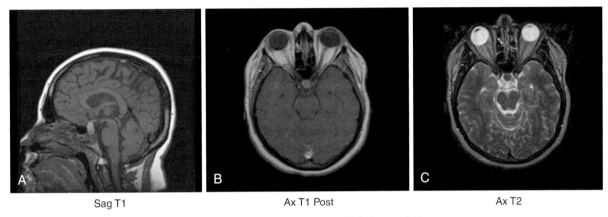

Sag T1   Ax T1 Post   Ax T2

• **Fig. 22.1** Rathke cleft cyst. *Ax,* Axial; *Sag,* sagittal.

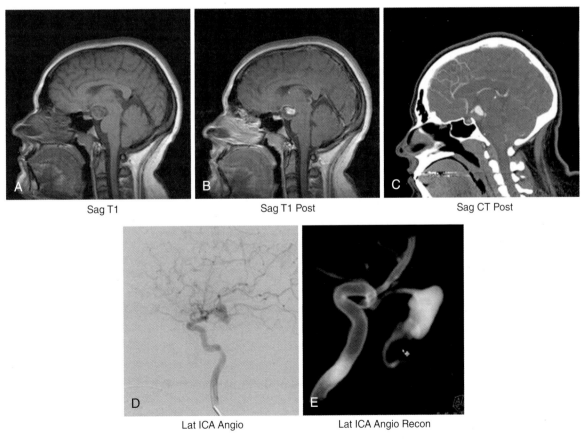

Sag T1   Sag T1 Post   Sag CT Post

Lat ICA Angio   Lat ICA Angio Recon

• **Fig. 22.2** Aneurysm. *Angio,* Angiogram; *CT,* Computed tomography; *ICA,* internal coronary artery; *Lat,* lateral; *Recon,* reconstruction; *Sag,* sagittal.

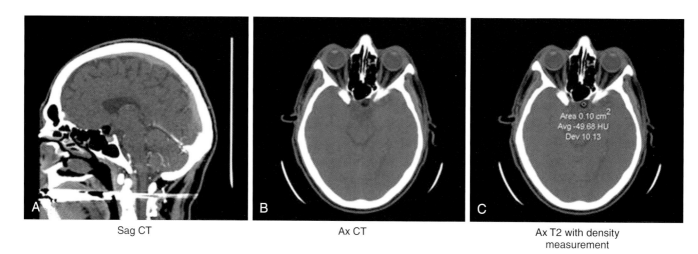

Sag CT   Ax CT   Ax T2 with density measurement

• **Fig. 22.3** Lipoma. *Ax*, Axial; *CT*, Computed tomography; *Sag*, sagittal.

contrast-enhanced study. Generally, the contiguity of the aneurysm with the parent vessel clinches the diagnosis. Angiographic images nicely demonstrate this posterior communicating artery aneurysm.

A small hypodense suprasellar lesion (Fig. 22.3) may be diagnosed incorrectly as a cystic lesion if the density of the lesion is not inspected. Identification of homogeneous fat-density components on CT (approximately –50 HU [Hounsfield units] in this case), or identification lipoma.

Differential Diagnosis

Craniopharyngioma
Rathke cleft cyst
Arachnoid cyst
Epidermoid cyst
Dermoid cyst
Aneurysm
Pilocytic astrocytoma

Pearls

Pearls are provided in Tables 22.1 and 22.2.

Signs and Complications

When a sellar/suprasellar mass is large enough, it may exert a mass effect on the important contents of the suprasellar cistern, including the optic chiasm and optic tracts, the anterior third ventricle, the tuber cinereum/hypothalamus, and the pituitary stalk. Many of these complications are either suggested in the history or evident in the images of unknown cases.

In Fig. 22.4, a large arachnoid cyst in a child is seen effacing the suprasellar cistern, hypothalamus, and third ventricle, resulting in noncommunicating hydrocephalus with marked enlargement of the lateral ventricles.

TABLE 22.1 Craniopharyngioma vs. Rathke Cleft Cyst

	Craniopharyngioma	Rathke Cleft Cyst
Diameter	Generally >2 cm	Generally <0.3 cm
Contours	Lobulated	Spherical/ovoid
Enhancement	Solid or nodular	No or thin peripheral rim
Calcification	Classically present (42%–87%)	Very rarely present (0%–13%)
Special features	Bimodal age distribution	T2 hypointense internal nodule

TABLE 22.2 Arachnoid vs. Epidermoid Cysts

	Arachnoid Cyst	Epidermoid Cyst
Restricted diffusion	–	+
Fluid attenuated inversion recovery	Completely suppresses	Internal heterogeneity
Contours	Smooth	Irregular/lobulated
Nerves/vessels	Displaces them	Often encases them

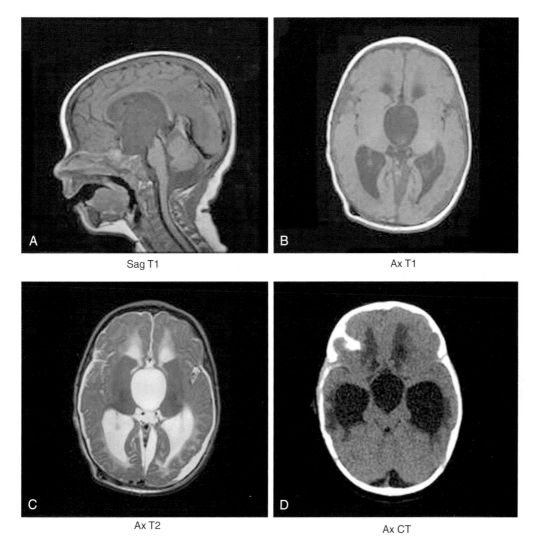

Sag T1

Ax T1

Ax T2

Ax CT

• **Fig. 22.4** Arachnoid cyst resulting in noncommunicating hydrocephalus. *Ax*, Axial; *CT*, computed tomography; *Sag*, sagittal.

Suggested Readings

Byun WM, Kim OL, Kim D: MR imaging findings of Rathke's cleft cysts: significance of intracystic nodules, *AJNR Am J Neuroradiol* 21(3):485–488, 2000.

Rao VJ, James RA, Mitra D: Imaging characteristics of common suprasellar lesions with emphasis on MRI findings, *Clin Radiol* 63(8):939–947, 2008.

Zada G, Lin N, Ojerholm E, et al: Craniopharyngioma and other cystic epithelial lesions of the sellar region: a review of clinical, imaging, and histopathological relationships, *Neurosurg Focus* 28(4):E4, 2010.

23
Pineal Region

ROBERT CHUN CHEN, MD AND MELISSA SHUHUI LEE, MBBS, FRCR

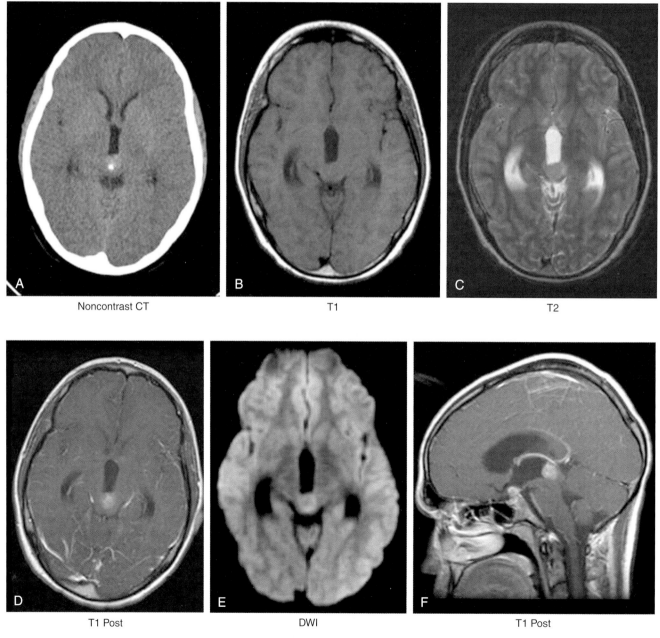

Noncontrast CT	T1	T2
T1 Post	DWI	T1 Post

CASE A: A 19-year-old Asian man presenting with headaches and visual difficulties. *CT,* Computed tomography; *DWI,* diffusion-weighted imaging.

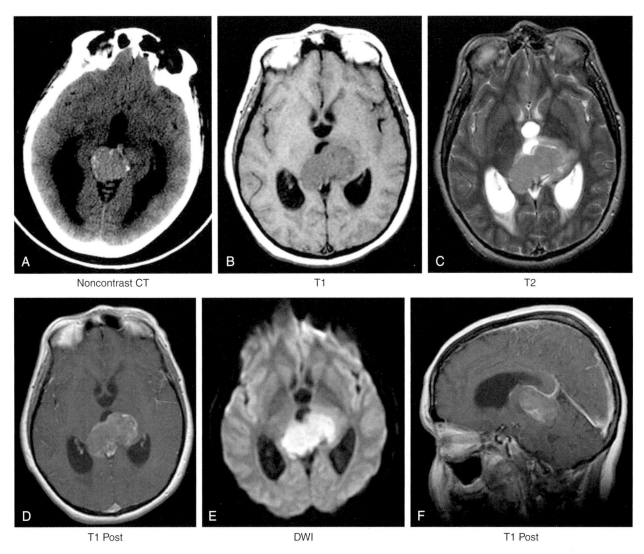

CASE B: A 55-year-old woman presenting with headaches, nausea, and vomiting. *CT*, Computed tomography; *DWI*, diffusion-weighted imaging.

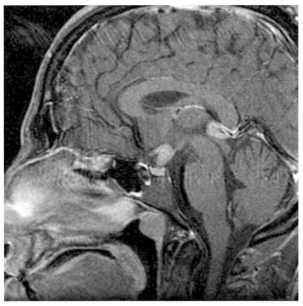

T1 Post FS

CASE C: A 24-year-old man presenting with excessive thirst. *FS*, fat saturated.

DESCRIPTION OF FINDINGS

- Case A: A CT scan demonstrates a well-defined mass in the pineal region that is intrinsically hyperdense to brain parenchyma and has centrally positioned "engulfed" calcification. MRI confirms a homogeneously enhancing pineal region mass located directly beneath the internal cerebral veins that nearly follows the signal intensity of gray matter on T1- and T2-weighted images, infiltrates the margins of the thalamus, and demonstrates restricted diffusion. There is associated obstructive hydrocephalus.
- Case B: A CT scan demonstrates a lobulated pineal region mass that is intrinsically hyperdense to brain parenchyma and has peripheral "exploded" calcification. It nearly follows the signal intensity of gray matter on T1- and T2-weighted images, enhances after the administration of contrast material, and demonstrates restricted diffusion. There is mild edema in the contiguous bilateral thalami. There is associated obstructive hydrocephalus.
- Case C: A sagittal postcontrast T1-weighted image demonstrates abnormal thickening and enhancement of the pituitary stalk extending into the optic chiasm, as well as a synchronous enhancing mass lesion within the pineal region.

Diagnosis

Case A: Germinoma
Case B: Pineoblastoma
Case C: A synchronous germinoma affecting the pineal and suprasellar regions

Summary

Pineal region masses are an important group of lesions that may be overlooked. Tumors in this region account for less than 1% of all adult intracranial neoplasms and 3% to 8% of pediatric intracranial neoplasms. They are much more common in the Asian than the White population, representing 10% of intracranial pediatric neoplasms in Asia, while accounting for only 2% to 4% of intracranial pediatric neoplasms in North America and Europe. Fortunately, the close confines of the pineal region facilitate early clinical detection. Pineal masses easily compromise the adjacent aqueduct of Sylvius and tectum, resulting in obstructive hydrocephalus and Parinaud syndrome, respectively. When pineal region masses become large, it may be difficult to discern where the mass arises. It is useful to note the displacement of the internal cerebral veins, which will be elevated with pineal region masses and depressed with masses that originate from the splenium of the corpus callosum.

Pineal region lesions can be divided into several main categories: nonneoplastic lesions such as pineal cysts; neoplastic lesions such as germ cell tumors, pineal parenchymal neoplasms, tumors arising from the supporting stroma (e.g., tectal gliomas, meningiomas, lymphoma), and metastases; congenital lesions; and finally, vascular lesions of the pineal region (aneurysms, vein of Galen malformations, cavernous malformations).

The pineal region cyst is by far the most common pineal region mass, seen in 2% to 40% of autopsy specimens, and should be considered when a peripherally enhancing lesion demonstrates isointensity to CSF on T1- and T2-weighted images. Pineal cysts have no detectable internal matrix and rarely cause clinical symptoms from hydrocephalus or result in Parinaud syndrome unless they are large or undergo pineal apoplexy with

intracystic hemorrhage. If a pineal region mass demonstrates more nodular enhancement or has an internal matrix, other entities, such as neoplastic processes, should be considered. Although several of the neoplastic entities occurring within this region have nonspecific imaging characteristics, taking into account the imaging appearance, demographic information (particularly age, sex, and race), and serum/CSF tumor markers will help formulate a reasonable differential diagnosis.

Germ cell tumors are the most common neoplasms arising from the pineal region. Two-thirds of pineal neoplasms are germ cell tumors, two-thirds of intracranial germ cell neoplasms are germinomas, and two-thirds of intracranial germinomas occur in the pineal region. Germinomas are much more common in people of Asian descent within their second and third decades of life, with males affected 10 times more frequently than females. On imaging, they classically engulf calcification, enhance avidly, and demonstrate intrinsic hyperdensity on CT and isointensity to gray matter on most MRI sequences. Because they are histologically unencapsulated, they sometimes invade the adjacent thalamus or tectum and disseminate via the CSF. For this reason, imaging of the entire neural axis for detection of metastases is vital during the initial workup. Pure germinomas are very radiosensitive, and patients typically have an excellent prognosis with a 90% to 95% long-term remission rate.

The remainder of germ cell tumors are nongerminomatous and include teratomas, choriocarcinomas, embryonal cell carcinomas, and endodermal sinus tumors. Teratomas possess unique imaging characteristics because of fat and calcium, and choriocarcinomas may hemorrhage; these characteristics help identify these entities. The remainder of the nongerminomatous germ cell tumors have no unique imaging characteristics that can be used to confidently distinguish them. However, serum and CSF markers can aid in the diagnosis. Germinomas typically secrete placental alkaline phosphatase, choriocarcinomas secrete beta-human chorionic gonadotropin, endodermal sinus tumors secrete alpha-fetoprotein, and embryonal carcinomas secrete a mixture of beta-human chorionic gonadotropin and alpha-fetoprotein. Overall, nongerminomatous germ cell tumors have a variable prognosis with two-thirds of patients achieving long-term remission.

Pineal parenchymal tumors (PPTs) arise from pineocytes or their precursors. They are less common than intracranial germ cell tumors, accounting for approximately 15% of pineal neoplasms. Whereas pineal germinomas most often occur in male patients, PPTs occur with equal frequency in males and females. Pineocytomas (WHO grade 1) account for 14% to 60% of PPTs and arise from relatively mature, slowly growing cells, whereas pineoblastomas (WHO grade 4) account for 40% of PPTs and arise from undifferentiated, rapidly dividing cells. The remainder of PPTs are usually of intermediate differentiation (Pineal parenchymal tumor of intermediate differentiation (PPTID), WHO grade 2 or 3), and, as their name implies, have histological features between those of pineocytoma and pineoblastoma. Papillary tumor of the pineal region (PTPR, WHO grade 2 or 3) is a relatively newly described, rare tumor, with origins thought to arise from specialized ependymocytes from the sub-commissural organ located in the posterior commissure. PPTs can arise at any age, but their peaks of onset are inversely correlated to their WHO grade; lower grade PPTs, such as pineocytomas, peak later during the third and fourth decades of life; PPTIDs occur in young adults, while higher grade PPTs, such as pineoblastomas, occur earlier in the first decade of life. On imaging, PPTs classically demonstrate a rim of "exploded" calcification that can be helpful in distinguishing them from germ cell tumors. Being composed of more slowly growing cells, pineocytomas rarely disseminate throughout the CSF and subsequently have a favorable prognosis with a 5-year survival of 85% to 100%. Pineoblastomas, on the other hand, tend to be more aggressive with a propensity for CSF dissemination and despite chemoradiation, have a corresponding 5-year survival of 58%.

Congenital lesions, such as epidermoids and arachnoid cysts, are discussed separately in Chapter 31. Vascular lesions of the pineal region, such as aneurysms and vein of Galen malformations, can be distinguished by tracing their contiguity with the adjacent arterial and venous vessels, respectively.

Spectrum of Disease

Germinomas typically are homogeneously enhancing pineal region masses that are hyperdense on CT, engulf calcification, parallel gray matter in signal intensity on MRI, and demonstrate restricted diffusion due to dense cell packing. However, germinomas can demonstrate peripheral calcification, and when they are large, may exhibit heterogeneity resulting from internal necrosis. They also may be seen in the suprasellar region, invading the pituitary stalk and lead to diabetes insipidus, or they may reside intraaxially within the basal ganglia, thalamus, or corpus callosum. Be aware of synchronous germinomas involving the pineal and suprasellar region (case C)!

PPTs are typically isodense or hyperdense to brain parenchyma on noncontrast CT and usually show avid enhancement after contrast administration. Pineoblastomas are typically larger (>3 cm) than pineocytomas on presentation; they frequently demonstrate an irregular morphology and extend beyond the pineal region into the posterior fossa or third ventricle. Pineocytomas tend to be smaller (commonly < 3cm) and show more uniform enhancement. Additionally, not all PPTs show peripheral calcification on CT.

It is important to note that while classic examples of these tumors do exist, the imaging appearance of germ cell tumors and PPTs may overlap and therefore may be indistinguishable.

Differential Diagnosis

1. **Pineal cysts**
2. **Tumors**
   Germ cell tumors (65% of all pineal tumors)
   - Germinoma (40% of all pineal tumors)
   - Nongerminomatous germ cell tumors
   - Teratoma (15% of all pineal tumors)
   - Choriocarcinoma (5% of all pineal tumors)
   - Endodermal sinus tumor

   - Embryonal cell carcinoma
   Pineal parenchymal tumors (15% of all pineal tumors)
   - Pineocytomas
   - Pineal parenchymal tumors of intermediate differentiation
   - Papillary tumors of the pineal region
   - Pineoblastomas
   Tumors of supporting elements or adjacent tissue
   - Meningioma, Astrocytoma, Ependymoma, Lymphoma, Metastases
3. **Congenital lesions**
   Lipoma, epidermoid, dermoid, arachnoid cysts
4. **Vascular lesions**
   Aneurysms of the basilar artery and posterior cerebral artery, vein of Galen malformation, cavernous malformations

Pearls

- Pineal cysts are by far the most common pineal region mass, seen in 20% to 40% of autopsy specimens.
- Pineal region masses displace the internal cerebral veins superiorly, whereas corpus callosum masses displace the internal cerebral veins inferiorly.
- Rule of two-thirds: Two-thirds of pineal region neoplasms are germ cell tumors, two-thirds of intracranial germ cell tumors are germinomas, and two-thirds of germinomas reside in the pineal region.

  Germinomas occur most frequently in Asians within their second and third decades of life, with a male-to-female ratio of 10:1. They are classically homogeneous and hyperdense masses that are isointense to gray matter, enhance avidly after the administration of contrast material, and demonstrate restricted diffusion because of their dense cellular nature.
- Pineal germ cell tumors will classically "engulf" calcification, while PPTs demonstrate peripheral "exploded" calcification.
- Teratomas are heterogeneous with regions of fat and calcium density on CT. On MRI, there is T1 hyperintensity due to fat and/or calcium and T2 and gradient echo hypointensity from calcium.
- Germ cell tumors and PPTs may have overlapping imaging characteristics and visual differentiation may not be possible, although serum and CSF markers can help to differentiate them, as germ cell tumors tend to be hormonally active. Regardless, MRI of the entire spinal neural axis should be imaged to evaluate for drop metastases.

Signs and Complications

Because of the close confines of the pineal region, masses within this location can compress the aqueduct of Sylvius and present with hydrocephalus, or they can abut the tectum and cause Parinaud syndrome (an inability to look upward). Notice in Case A how the temporal horns are dilated out of proportion to the sulcal spaces, indicating obstructive hydrocephalus.

Germinomas, pineoblastomas, and PTPR have the propensity to disseminate throughout the CSF, and imaging of the entire neural axis is necessary to exclude metastases.

Suggested Readings

Barkovich AJ, editor: *Pediatric neuroimaging*, ed 4, Philadelphia, 2005, Lippincott Williams & Wilkins.

Deiana G, Mottolese C, Hermier M, et al: Imagery of pineal tumors. *Neurochirurgie* 61(2-3):113–122, 2015.

Gaillard F, Jones J. Masses of the pineal region: clinical presentation and radiographic features. *Postgrad Med J* 86(1020):597–607, 2010.

Smirniotopoulos JG, Rushing EJ, Mena H: Pineal region masses: differential diagnosis. *Radiographics* 12:577–596, 1992.

Smith AB, Rushing EJ, Smirniotopoulos JG. From the archives of the AFIP: lesions of the pineal region: radiologic-pathologic correlation. *Radiographics* 30(7):2001–2020, 2010.

Solomou AG. Magnetic resonance imaging of pineal tumors and drop metastases: a review approach. *Rare Tumors* 9(3):6715, 2017.

Ueno T, Tanaka YO, Nagata M, et al: Spectrum of germ cell tumors: from head to toe, *Radiographics* 24:387–404, 2004.

24

Cranial Nerve Lesions

HENRY SU, MD, PHD

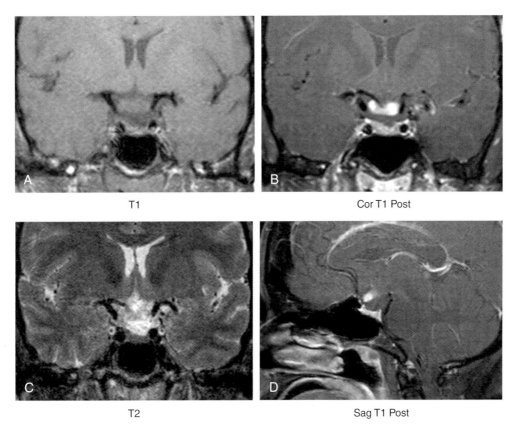

T1   Cor T1 Post

T2   Sag T1 Post

CASE A: A 48-year-old with a history of lupus with severe vision loss. *Cor,* Coronal; *Sag,* sagittal.

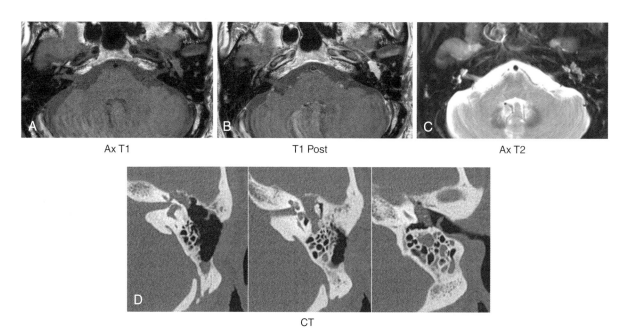

Ax T1   T1 Post   Ax T2

CT

CASE B: A 55-year-old with long-standing left-sided facial weakness. *Ax,* Axial; *CT,* Computed tomography.

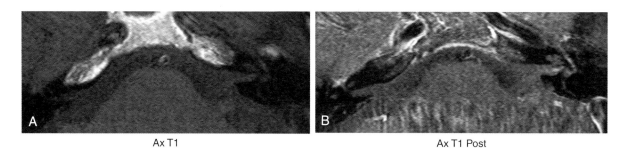

Ax T1   Ax T1 Post

CASE C: A 56-year-old presenting with a 10-day history of left-sided facial weakness. *Ax,* Axial.

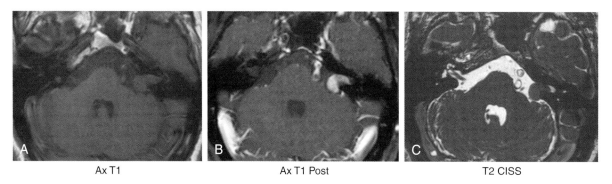

Ax T1   Ax T1 Post   T2 CISS

CASE D: A 63-year-old presenting with left-sided hearing loss. *Ax,* axial; *CISS,* constructive interference in steady state.

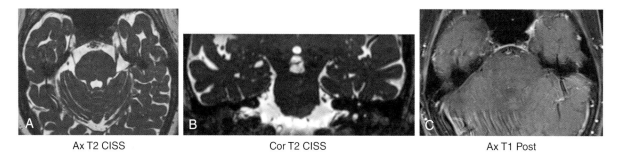

Ax T2 CISS   Cor T2 CISS   Ax T1 Post

CASE E: A 68-year-old presenting with right nasal ala ulceration and associated pruritus. *Ax,* Axial; *CISS,* constructive interference in steady state; *Cor,* coronal.

DESCRIPTION OF FINDINGS

- Case A: Enhancement and diffuse T2 hyperintense signal are seen within the markedly enlarged prechiasmatic optic nerves and optic chiasm.
- Case B: A densely enhancing, T2 hyperintense lesion is seen in the left temporal bone in the expected location of the geniculate ganglion. On the serial axial CT images, correlative soft tissue density is seen along the facial nerve course (geniculate, tympanic, and mastoid segments), with widening of the bony facial nerve canal.
- Case C: Contrast enhancement is seen within the distal intracanalicular portion of the left seventh cranial nerve, with sparing of the cochlear nerve. Additional enhancement is seen in the labyrinthine and tympanic segments of the left facial nerve. The right facial nerve is normal.
- Case D: An expansile, densely enhancing mass is centered in the left CPA and internal auditory canal (IAC). Widening of the porus acusticus and IAC is observed.
- Case E: High-resolution T2 constructive interference in steady-state images demonstrates marked atrophy of the right trigeminal nerve compared with the left trigeminal nerve. No abnormal enhancement is noted.

Diagnosis

Case A: Optic neuritis and chiasmitis
Case B: Left facial nerve schwannoma
Case C: Left-sided Bell palsy (clinical history and negative laboratory values)
Case D: Left vestibular schwannoma
Case E: Trigeminal atrophy and trigeminal trophic syndrome

Summary

Isolated cranial nerve findings can be seen in a number of diseases. Cranial nerves II, V, VII, and VIII are most commonly imaged when specifically looking for pathology.

The most common cause of optic neuritis is multiple sclerosis (MS). T2 hyperintense signal is present in the afflicted optic nerve, and the presence of enhancement and enlargement suggests active disease. The intraorbital optic nerve is most commonly involved. Other differential considerations include neuromyelitis spectrum disorder (bilateral with optic chiasm involvement), myelin oligodendrocyte glycoprotein antibody–associated disease (proximal optic nerves with perineural enhancement), inflammatory (e.g., idiopathic optic neuritis and pseudotumor), infectious, and neoplastic etiologies. In Case A, not only are the diffusely enlarged optic nerves involved in the prechiasmatic segment, but the chiasm itself demonstrates marked T2 hyperintense signal and enhancement. This patient had been diagnosed with systemic lupus erythematosus. In young patients whose optic nerves show nodular mass-like characteristics, the diagnosis of optic glioma should be considered even when the lesion is nonenhancing.

The facial nerve (cranial nerve VII) is another common site of pathology. Postcontrast sequences through this region are performed routinely, but interpretation can be challenging at times because not all enhancement is considered abnormal. Mild enhancement often is seen in the geniculate, tympanic, and mastoid portions because of the rich perineural venous plexus in these locations. However, the presence of enhancement is abnormal in the cisternal, canalicular, or proximal extracranial facial nerve portions.

Linear enhancement with minimal expansion can be seen in persons with Bell palsy, as shown in Case C. The classic intracanalicular facial nerve fundal "tuft" of enhancement is considered the best diagnostic sign. The typical clinical presentation of Bell palsy requires no imaging follow-up because the symptoms typically resolve. Atypical clinical history necessitates a search for an underlying etiology. Other infectious etiologies also can result in facial nerve enhancement, such as Lyme disease (which can involve the root entry zone) or herpes zoster (which can also include enhancement of cranial nerve VIII). If the enhancement along the facial nerve course is masslike or expanded, then additional etiologies would include neoplastic processes, as seen in Case B.

A T2 hyperintense lesion demonstrating intense gadolinium enhancement is typical of a schwannoma. When these lesions become large enough, however, enhancement and T2 signal characteristics may become heterogeneous if associated internal necrosis is present. These peripheral nerve sheath tumors can arise from any of the peripheral cranial nerves, but they are seen most often along the facial, trigeminal, and vestibulocochlear nerves. Bony anatomy and detailed soft tissue evaluation is often better achieved with CT examination because bony expansion of the entire facial canal is readily evident on CT. Although the signal characteristics in this case are typical for a facial schwannoma, the parotid gland should be scrutinized to ensure that this enhancement does not represent perineural spread of tumor. Treatment of facial nerve schwannomas revolves around the degree of facial nerve compromise. The major differential consideration for a facial nerve schwannoma is a hemangioma.

Schwannomas of the vestibulocochlear complex also are known as *vestibular schwannomas* because they usually arise from the vestibular nerve. Mass effect on the cochlear nerve yields the clinical symptoms of hearing loss. The signal characteristics are similar to those previously described for facial schwannomas. High-resolution T2 imaging (constructive interference in steady state or fast imaging employing steady-state acquisition) sequences are very helpful because they yield high-resolution anatomic detail. The differential diagnosis of enhancing lesions in the cerebellopontine angle (CPA)/IAC location includes facial schwannomas and other neoplasms such as meningiomas (indicated by the presence of a dural tail, T2 isointense to brain parenchyma, dense enhancement, no IAC expansion, eccentricity) and metastases (associated leptomeningeal disease, no IAC expansion). Statistically, vestibular schwannomas are the most common tumor in this location, and differentiation from facial nerve schwannomas can be difficult if a labyrinthine tail is not present to suggest cranial nerve VII etiology. The presence of bilateral IAC lesions and multiple peripheral nerve sheath tumors should raise the suspicion for neurofibromatosis type 2.

What may appear as an enlarged nerve on one side may represent a diminutive cranial nerve on the contralateral side. Nerve atrophy is a nonspecific finding indicating axon loss and demyelination of a chronic nature. For instance, optic nerve atrophy can be seen after enucleation. Trigeminal nerve atrophy, as seen in Case E, has been described following surgery, herpetic infection, and cerebrovascular accident. In this case, the patient also presented with superficial skin ulcers involving the right side of the face, including the nasal ala; these dermatologic manifestations are referred to as *trigeminal trophic syndrome* and occur with peripheral or central trigeminal nerve damage. Studies of trigeminal neuralgia show that the trigeminal nerve is approximately 20% smaller on the affected side compared with the normal side.

Differential Diagnosis

1. **Location-dependent**
   Inflammation (MS)
   Infection (postviral such as herpetic, Lyme disease)
   Neoplastic (glioma [cranial nerve II], peripheral nerve sheath tumor—schwannomas [cranial nerves III–XII], meningiomas, metastases, other)
   Granulomatous (often affects multiple cranial nerves; e.g., sarcoid, tuberculosis)

Pearls

- Facial nerve enhancement can be normal in the geniculate, tympanic, and mastoid segments. Always inspect the ipsilateral parotid gland for a potential source of abnormal facial nerve enhancement. If the clinical presentation of Bell palsy is atypical, it is necessary to look for the source.
- Vestibular schwannomas are the most common lesion involving the IAC. They should be differentiated from facial nerve schwannomas (which have labyrinthine enlargement) and meningiomas (which show the presence of a dural tail, are T2 hypointense, are eccentric, and less often enter the porus acusticus).
- Asymmetry of cranial nerves may be due to atrophy.

Signs and Complications

Signs include the facial nerve "tuft" sign, as seen in Bell palsy.

Suggested Readings

Devor M, Govrin-Lippmann R, Rappaport ZH: Mechanism of trigeminal neuralgia: an ultrastructural analysis of trigeminal root specimens obtained during microvascular decompression surgery, *J Neurosurg* 96(3):532–543, 2002.

Erbay SH, Bhadelia RA, O'Callaghan M, et al: Nerve atrophy in severe trigeminal neuralgia: noninvasive confirmation at MR imaging—initial experience, *Radiology* 238(2):689–692, 2006.

Frohman LP, Frieman BJ, Wolansky L: Reversible blindness resulting from optic chiasmitis secondary to systemic lupus erythematosus, *J Neuroophthalmol* 21(1):18–21, 2001.

Gebarski SS, Telian SA, Niparko JK: Enhancement along the normal facial nerve in the facial canal: MR imaging and anatomic correlation, *Radiology* 183(2):391–394, 1992.

Lin YC, Wang AG, Yen MY: Systemic lupus erythematosus-associated optic neuritis: clinical experience and literature review, *Acta Ophthalmol* 87(2):204–210, 2009.

McMonagle B, Al-Sanosi A, Croxson G, et al: Facial schwannoma: results of a large case series and review, *J Laryngol Otol* 122(11):1139–1150, 2008.

Mulkens TH, Parizel PM, Martin JJ, et al: Acoustic schwannoma: MR findings in 84 tumors, *AJR Am J Roentgenol* 160(2):395–398, 1993.

Neoh CY, Tan AW: Trigeminal trophic syndrome: an unusual cause of a non-healing cheek ulcer, *Singapore Med J* 48(1):e22–e24, 2007.

Saremi F, Helmy M, Farzin S, et al: MRI of cranial nerve enhancement, *AJR Am J Roentgenol* 185(6):1487–1497, 2005.

Veillon F, Taboada LR, Eid MA, et al: Pathology of the facial nerve, *Neuroimaging Clin N Am* 18(2):309–320, 2008.

25
Lytic Skull Lesions

JUAN E. SMALL, MD, MSC

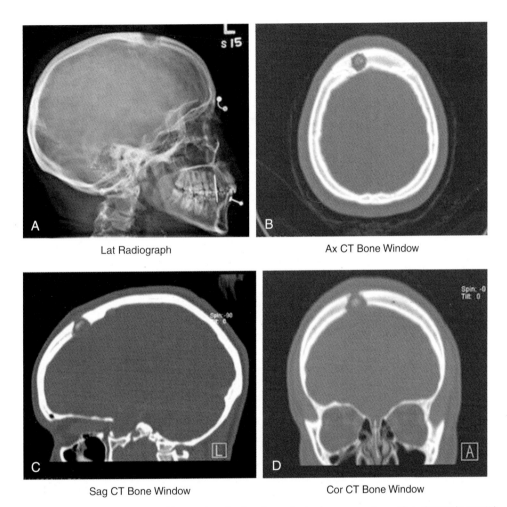

Lat Radiograph

Ax CT Bone Window

Sag CT Bone Window

Cor CT Bone Window

CASE A: A 15-year-old with a history of panic disorder and migraines presenting with a change in mental status. *Ax*, Axial; *Cor*, coronal; *CT*, Computed tomography; *Lat*, lateral; *Sag*, sagittal.

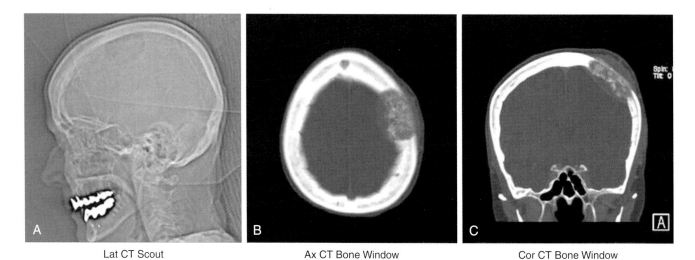

Lat CT Scout   Ax CT Bone Window   Cor CT Bone Window

CASE B: A 69-year-old with a history of multiple paragangliomas and squamous cell and basal cell skin cancer presenting with a palpable left parietal calvarial lesion. *Ax*, Axial; *Cor*, coronal; *CT*, Computed tomography; *Lat*, lateral.

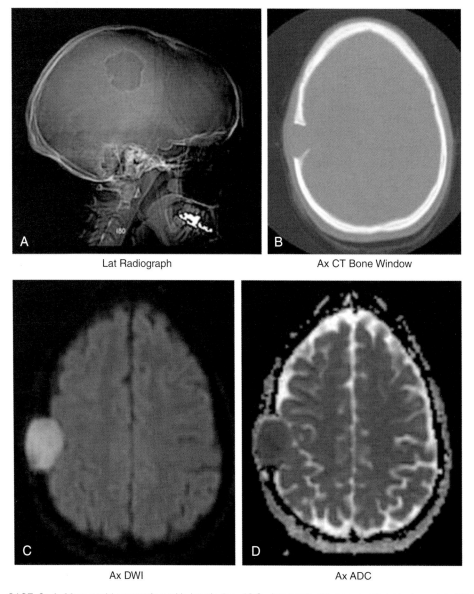

Lat Radiograph   Ax CT Bone Window

Ax DWI   Ax ADC

CASE C: A 30-year-old presenting with headache. *ADC,* Apparent diffusion coefficient; *Ax*, axial; *CT*, Computed tomography; *DWI,* diffusion-weighted imaging; *Lat*, lateral.

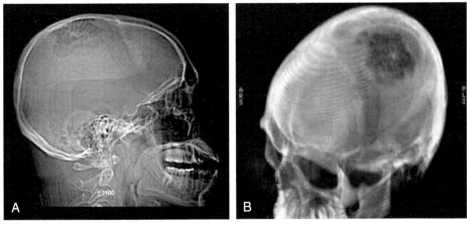

Lat Radiograph   3D CT Recon

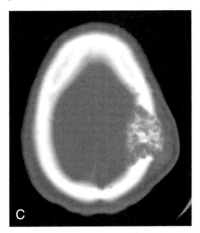

Ax CT Bone Window

CASE D: A 38-year-old presenting with a palpable left-sided calvarial lesion. *Ax*, Axial; *CT*, Computed tomography; *Lat*, lateral; *Recon*, reconstruction.

DESCRIPTION OF FINDINGS

- Case A: A well-defined lytic lesion is centered in the paramedian right frontal calvarium, without marginal sclerosis, and demonstrates asymmetric involvement of the inner table to a greater extent than the outer table ("beveled" edge). A central nodule of residual bone density is evident within the lytic lesion ("button sequestrum").
- Case B: A large left frontoparietal lesion with a permeative, aggressive pattern of calvarial destruction with erosion through the inner and outer tables and extension into the soft tissues and another smaller lytic lesion in the midline frontal calvarium.
- Case C: A well-defined right parietal calvarial lesion with dense sclerotic margins involving both the inner and outer tables of the skull, without internal trabeculation, and demonstrating marked hyperintensity on diffusion-weighted imaging (DWI) and isointensity compared with brain parenchyma on apparent diffusion coefficient (ADC) maps.
- Case D: A well-defined lytic lesion centered in the diploic space with a "spoke wheel" or "reticulated" internal structure pattern of coarse trabeculation radiating from the center to the periphery. Extension into the soft tissues is noted.

Diagnosis

Case A: Eosinophilic granuloma
Case B: Metastasis
Case C: Epidermoid cyst
Case D: Hemangioma

Summary

Focal skull/calvarial lesions may arise from bones, or they may arise from adjacent tissues and secondarily invade bone. When evaluating a skull lesion, the first step is to determine whether it is lytic or sclerotic. Once a lesion has been determined to be lytic, the next step is to evaluate it for benign versus aggressive characteristics. Benign lesions tend to have well-defined borders with sclerotic margins, whereas malignant lesions tend to have a permeative, destructive appearance.

In addition to pathologic entities, surgical defects and normal variants such as arachnoid granulations, venous lakes, large emissary veins, and parietal thinning may appear as areas of calvarial lucency. Before discussing the differentiating features of lytic skull lesions, it is helpful to get a sense of how commonly different entities occur. Broadly, metastases are common, especially in adults. Less common lesions include epidermoid cysts, Langerhans cell histiocytosis, lymphoma, plasmacytoma or multiple myeloma, Paget disease, hemangioma, dermoid cyst, fibrous dysplasia, leptomeningeal cyst, and osteomyelitis. Rare lesions include cephalocele, neurosarcoidosis, sinus pericranii, and aneurysmal bone cyst.

The differential diagnosis of a lytic skull lesion is strongly influenced by the age of the patient. In adults and elderly patients, metastases are by far the most common lytic skull lesions, with the most common primary tumors being breast, lung, melanoma, thyroid, and renal cells. Children and young adults, on the other hand, tend to present more frequently with eosinophilic granulomas (Langerhans cell histiocytosis), dermoids, epidermoids, fibrous dysplasia, meningoceles,

leptomeningeal cysts, or hemangiomas. Although children and young adults rarely present with metastases, the histology tends to be neuroblastoma and leukemia.

Close inspection of the margins of a lytic skull lesion is important. Permeative margins suggest an aggressive lesion, such as metastasis or infection. Epidermoids, dermoids, and other slowly growing lesions demonstrate dense sclerotic margins. Histiocytosis often demonstrates beveled edges.

Close inspection of the internal structure of a lytic skull lesion also is important. A button sequestrum (i.e., central residual bone density within the lytic lesion) is a classic sign of eosinophilic granuloma (histiocytosis), but this feature also has been noted in breast cancer metastasis, osteomyelitis, and epidermoid. A spoke wheel or reticulated internal structure is a classic sign of hemangioma.

Spectrum of Disease

The spectrum of disease has been detailed in the previous section.

Differential Diagnosis

1. **Epidermoid cyst:** A well-defined lesion with dense sclerotic margins involving both the inner and outer tables of the skull, without internal trabeculation, and demonstrating marked hyperintensity on DWI.
2. **Dermoid cyst:** A well-defined, cystic-appearing lesion expanding the diploid space. CT demonstrates fat density, and T1-weighted MRI demonstrates hyperintensity due to the fat component.
3. **Langerhans cell histiocytosis/eosinophilic granuloma:** This lesion generally is seen in patients aged 5 to 15 years old. It is a homogeneously enhancing, T1 hypointense and T2 hyperintense, well-defined lytic lesion without marginal sclerosis. It has beveled edges, usually due to greater involvement of the inner table compared with the outer table. The classic sign is a "hole within a hole" or button sequestrum (central residual bone density within the lytic lesion) on CT.
4. **Plasmacytoma/multiple myeloma:** An enhancing lytic lesion demonstrating scalloped and poorly marginated nonsclerotic borders with a "punch hole" appearance.
5. **Paget disease:** This disease appears as a well-defined lucent lesion with cortical thickening and coarse trabeculation during its lytic phase, known as "osteoporosis circumscripta."
6. **Hemangioma:** A well-defined, strongly enhancing lytic lesion centered in the diploic space with a spoke wheel or reticulated internal structure pattern of coarse trabeculation radiating from the center to the periphery. T1 hyperintensity within the lesion is a differentiating feature of this lesion. Extension into the soft tissues is not uncommon.
7. **Leptomeningeal cyst:** A late posttraumatic complication of a skull fracture, generally in patients younger than 3 years who present with an expanding, smoothly marginated skull defect with protruding meningeal elements and gliosis with or without cystic change in the adjacent brain parenchyma.

8. **Metastasis:** The majority of metastases have a permeative, aggressive pattern of calvarial destruction that often is multiple and appears classically in patients with a known primary malignancy. Sclerotic lesions occur predominantly in association with prostate and breast carcinomas.

9. **Osteomyelitis:** A permeative/"moth-eaten" aggressive pattern of calvarial destruction, often adjacent to a source of infection such as the mastoid air cells or the paranasal sinuses.

10. **Cephalocele:** Congenital or acquired herniation of intracranial elements through a skull defect.

11. **Sinus pericranii:** Generally, a midline or paramedian vascular scalp lesion communicating intracranially with a dural venous sinus by way of a transcalvarial vein and expanding with increases in intracranial pressure.

Pearls

- Close inspection of the margins of a lytic skull lesion is important:
  - Permeative margins suggest an aggressive lesion such as metastases or infection (among other lesions).
  - Epidermoids, dermoids, and other slowly growing lesions demonstrate dense sclerotic margins.
  - Histiocytosis often demonstrates beveled edges.
- Close inspection of the internal structure of a lytic skull lesion is important:
  - A button sequestrum (central residual bone density within the lytic lesion) is a classic sign of eosinophilic granuloma (histiocytosis), but this feature also has been noted in persons with breast cancer metastasis, osteomyelitis, and epidermoid.
  - A spoke wheel or reticulated internal structure is classic for hemangioma.
- A helpful mnemonic for lytic or mixed lytic/sclerotic calvarial lesions is HELP ME:
  - **H**emangioma
  - **E**pidermoid/dermoid
  - **L**eptomeningeal cyst/leukemia/lymphoma
  - **P**aget disease, postsurgical
  - **M**etastases, multiple myeloma
  - **E**osinophilic granuloma, **E**ncephalocele

Signs and Complications

Signs and complications generally are related to invasion or mass effect upon adjacent structures.

Suggested Readings

Garfinkle J, Melançon D, Cortes M, et al: Imaging pattern of calvarial lesions in adults, *Skeletal Radiol* 40(10):1261–1273, 2011.

Lloret I, Server A, Taksdal I: Calvarial lesions: a radiological approach to diagnosis, *Acta Radiol* 50(5):531–542, 2009.

Willatt JM, Quaghebeur G: Calvarial masses of infants and children. A radiological approach, *Clin Radiol* 59(6):474–486, 2004.

Yalçin O, Yildirim T, Kizilkiliç O, et al: CT and MRI findings in calvarial non-infectious lesions, *Diagn Interv Radiol* 13(2):68–74, 2007.

26
Skull Fracture Versus Sutures

JALIL AFNAN, MD, MRCS AND JUAN E. SMALL, MD, MSC

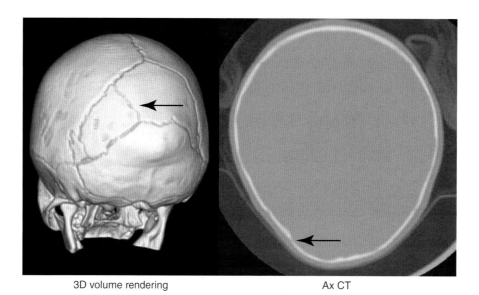

3D volume rendering · Ax CT

CASE A: A 9-month-old infant after a fall. *Ax*, Axial; *CT*, Computed tomography; *3D*, three dimensional.

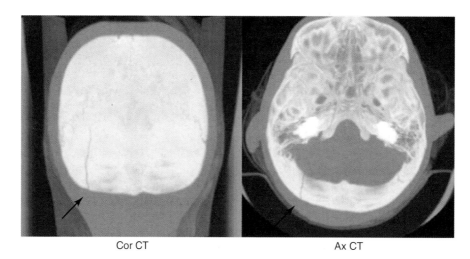

Cor CT · Ax CT

CASE B: A 45-year-old after a fall. *Ax*, Axial; *Cor*, coronal; *CT*, Computed tomography.

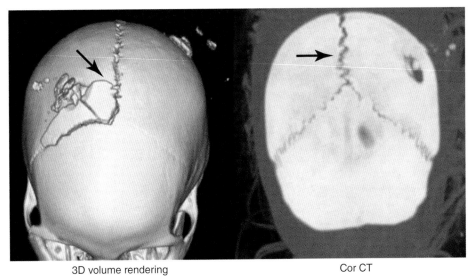

3D volume rendering   Cor CT

CASE C: Head trauma. *Cor*, Coronal; *CT*, Computed tomography; *3D*, three dimensional.

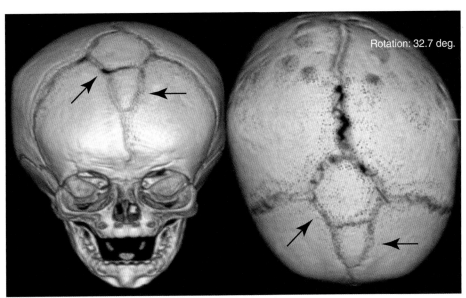

3D volume rendering

CASE D: A 3-month-old infant after a fall. *3D*, three dimensional.

DESCRIPTION OF FINDINGS

- Case A: Well-defined accessory, sutures noted in the posterior skull are contiguous with, but not crossing, the right lambdoid and persistent mendosal sutures and are adjacent to the superior nuchal ridge. No acute fracture is identified.
- Case B: A sharply demarcated linear lucency without associated sclerosis, consistent with an acute fracture, is observed within the right occipital bone.
- Case C: An ill-defined comminuted fracture of the anterior right parietal bone that extends to the adjacent right coronal and sagittal sutures that appear mildly diastase.
- Case D: There are accessory bones between metopic, sagittal, and coronal sutures. The margins are sclerotic, and no evidence of suture diastasis is found.

Diagnosis

Case A: Accessory suture
Case B: Acute, nondisplaced right occipital fracture
Case C: Comminuted parietal fracture and suture diastasis
Case D: Accessory bones

Summary

At times, differentiating between a linear skull fracture, an accessory cranial suture, and suture diastasis poses a diagnostic dilemma. Important rules of thumb to remember are that an acute linear fracture is often a unilateral finding with a sharp, nonsclerotic border; it is frequently associated with suture diastasis and often crosses suture lines. Accessory sutures, on the other hand, have a zigzag or sinusoid pattern with sclerotic borders. These sutures, which often are bilateral, merge with an adjacent suture and are not associated with suture diastasis.

Evaluation must include an accurate clinical history and a physical examination. Absence of a subgaleal hematoma, overlying contusion, or soft tissue injury markedly reduces the likelihood of a nondisplaced fracture. The utility of computed tomography with three-dimensional reformatting is evident in clinically challenging cases. Other than sutures and accessory sutures, vascular channels and venous sinus grooves may have similar imaging characteristics.

Accessory cranial sutures are rare and are thought to arise from incomplete union of normal ossification centers. Examples include the six ossification centers of the occipital bone and two ossification centers of the parietal bone. Four ossification centers—the bilateral lateral exoccipital, ventral basioccipital, and dorsal supraoccipital ossification centers—are found around the foramen magnum.

Fusion of cranial sutures begins in childhood as the dense connective tissue is sequentially replaced by an osseous synchondrosis. Incomplete fusion or the presence of accessory sutures may mistakenly result in false-positive fracture identification, particularly in the pediatric population.

A final entity to consider is wormian bones. Wormian bones are accessory bones occurring along the length of a suture, most commonly the lambdoid suture (os incae) or between the parietal bone and greater wing of the sphenoid (pterion ossicle). Although they result in additional sutures and/or sutures that appear unusual, these bones should not be confused with fractures.

Spectrum of Disease

The spectrum of disease is detailed in the preceding section.

Pearls

- Features of an acute fracture:
  - Sharp, nonsclerotic borders
  - Often unilateral
  - Associated with suture diastasis
  - Often crosses a suture line
- Features of an accessory suture:
  - A zigzag pattern with sclerotic borders
  - Often bilateral
  - Often merges with an adjacent suture
  - Is not associated with suture diastasis

Signs and Complications

A "growing fracture," or craniocerebral erosion results from interposition of dura and arachnoid with development of a leptomeningeal cyst that may widen a preexisting fracture line. A fulminant infectious process may cause increased intracranial pressure and suture diastasis in a pediatric patient; this process can be confused with a fracture.

Suggested Readings

Allen WE III, Kier EL, Rothman SL: Pitfalls in the evaluation of skull trauma. A review, *Radiol Clin North Am* 11(3):479–503, 1973.

Choudhary AK, Jha B, Boal DK, et al: Occipital sutures and its variations: the value of 3D-CT and how to differentiate it from fractures using 3D-CT?, *Surg Radiol Anat* 32(9):807–816, 2010.

Connor SE, Tan G, Fernando R, et al: Computed tomography pseudo-fractures of the mid face and skull base, *Clin Radiol* 60(12):1268–1279, 2005.

Franken EA Jr.: The midline occipital fissure: diagnosis of fracture versus anatomic variants, *Radiology* 93(5):1043–1046, 1969.

Idriz S, Patel JH, Ameli Renani S, et al: CT of normal developmental and variant anatomy of the pediatric skull: distinguishing trauma from normality, *Radiographics* 35(5):1585–1601, 2015.

Lustrin ES, Robertson RL, Tilak S: Normal anatomy of the skull base, *Neuroimaging Clin N Am* 4(3):465–478, 1994.

Miller AJ, Kim U, Carrasco E: Differentiating a mendosal suture from a skull fracture, *J Pediatr* 157(4):691, 2010.

Nakahara K, Miyasaka Y, Takagi H, et al: Unusual accessory cranial sutures in pediatric head trauma—case report, *Neurol Med Chir (Tokyo)* 43(2):80–81, 2003.

Sanchez T, Stewart D, Walvick M, et al: Skull fracture vs. accessory sutures: how can we tell the difference?, *Emerg Radiol* 17(5):413–418, 2010.

Tharp AM, Jason DR: Anomalous parietal suture mimicking skull fracture, *Am J Forensic Med Pathol* 30(1):49–51, 2009.

27

Clivus Lesions

MICHAEL T. PREECE, MD AND PAUL M. BUNCH, MD

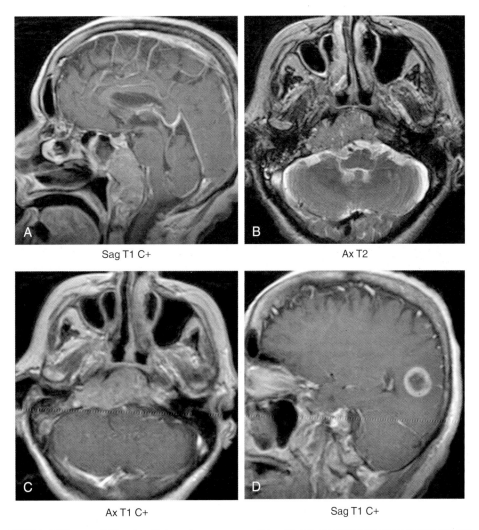

A	B
Sag T1 C+	Ax T2

C	D
Ax T1 C+	Sag T1 C+

CASE A: A 68-year-old female with breast cancer presenting with a 3-month history of worsening cervical spine pain. *Ax,* Axial; *Sag,* sagittal.

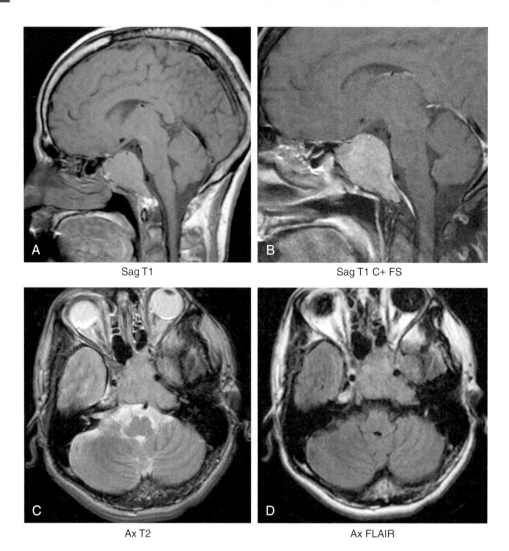

Sag T1

Sag T1 C+ FS

Ax T2

Ax FLAIR

CASE B: A 47-year-old male presenting with worsening headaches and double vision. *Ax*, Axial; *FLAIR*, fluid attenuated inversion recovery; *FS*, fat saturated; *Sag*, sagittal.

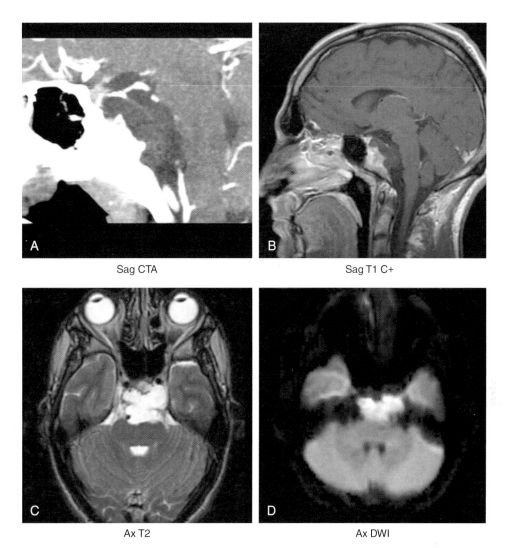

Sag CTA

Sag T1 C+

Ax T2

Ax DWI

CASE C: A 31-year-old male presenting with a 1-week history of progressive headaches and a new blurry vision in the left eye. *Ax,* Axial; *CTA,* computed tomography angiography; *DWI,* diffusion-weighted imaging; *Sag,* sagittal.

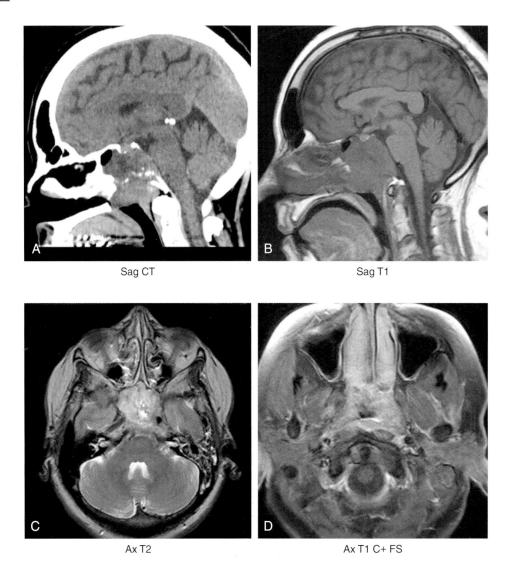

Sag CT

Sag T1

Ax T2

Ax T1 C+ FS

CASE D: A 57-year-old female presenting with intermittent foul-tasting epistaxis and new-onset headache and diplopia. *Ax,* Axial; *CT,* Computed tomography; *FS,* fat saturated; *Sag,* sagittal.

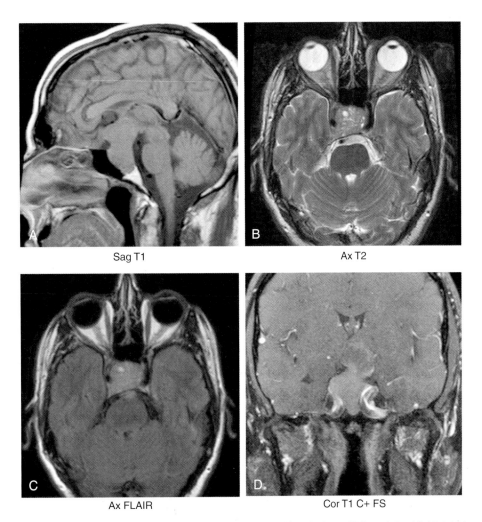

Sag T1   Ax T2

Ax FLAIR   Cor T1 C+ FS

CASE E: A 48-year-old male presenting with a 3-day history of headache and bilateral visual field defects. *Ax*, Axial; *Cor*, coronal; *FLAIR*, fluid attenuated inversion recovery; *FS*, fat saturated; *Sag*, sagittal.

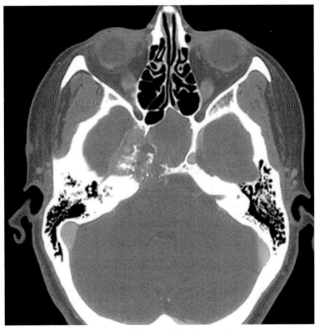

Ax CT Bone Window

CASE F: A 39-year-old female presenting with right-sided headaches and a right cranial nerve VI palsy. *Ax*, Axial; *CT*, Computed tomography.

DESCRIPTION OF FINDINGS

CT and MR images from six patients with lesions affecting the clivus:

- Case A: A heterogeneous, T2 isointense to hypointense, avidly enhancing soft tissue mass is centered within the clivus and also involves the right petrous apex. An additional ring-enhancing lesion is seen in the left parieto-occipital region. Note the normal appearance of the pituitary gland and preservation of the nasopharyngeal mucosa on the sagittal midline image.
- Case B: A homogenous expansile clival mass exhibits slight intrinsic T1 hyperintense signal and intermediate T2 signal. The tumor abuts the internal carotid artery flow voids. Involvement of the sellar floor is noted with upward displacement of the pituitary gland. There is homogeneous enhancement.
- Case C: A destructive mass arises from the posterior clivus with effacement of the prepontine cistern and associated scalloping of the pons. The soft tissue component of the mass is low in attenuation on CT with restricted diffusion, T1 hypointensity, and marked T2 hyperintensity noted on MRI. There is minimal associated enhancement. The mass partially encases the basilar artery.
- Case D: A large destructive soft tissue mass involves the clivus, sphenoid sinus, and nasopharynx. The axial postcontrast image best demonstrates involvement of the nasopharynx and longus colli musculature. T2 signal is intermediate and heterogeneous. Note the normal appearance of the pituitary gland on the sagittal T1-weighted image.
- Case E: A large mass remodels the superior clivus. The mass is centered in the sella with marked upward displacement of the optic chiasm (accounting for the patient's visual disturbance). Small cystic spaces are seen on the T2-weighted image. There is mild enhancement.
- Case F: A destructive expansile lesion is centered in the right petroclival synchondrosis with ring and arc mineralization suggestive of chondroid matrix.

Diagnosis

Case A: Metastatic disease
Case B: Plasmacytoma
Case C: Chordoma
Case D: Nasopharyngeal carcinoma
Case E: Pituitary macroadenoma
Case F: Chondrosarcoma

Summary

A wide spectrum of diseases affects the clivus and paraclival structures, including primary neoplasms, metastatic tumors, inflammatory processes, and hematopoietic disorders. Although these conditions often provide a diagnostic challenge for the radiologist, CT and MRI characteristics of these lesions can help establish an appropriately weighted differential diagnosis.

Chordomas are rare, locally aggressive tumors that arise from embryonic remnants of the primitive notochord. Lesions may occur throughout the axial skeleton, with approximately 30% to 50% involving the sacrum, 30% to 35% occurring at the skull base, and 15% to 30% involving the spine. Masses typically present in the third to fifth decades with headache and/or a variety of cranial neuropathies. The CT appearance is that of a centrally located expansile soft tissue mass with associated extensive lytic bone destruction. Internal calcifications within the mass usually represent fragments of residual clival bone rather than tumor matrix. Lesions often are characterized on MRI by marked T2 hyperintensity, likely reflecting the high fluid content of vacuolated components. Solid enhancement is typically seen.

Metastases to the skull base particularly affect patients with carcinoma of the breast and prostate. Metastases occur late in the course of the disease, with an overall median survival of approximately 2.5 years. Although imaging characteristics are nonspecific, lesions often are distinguished by a history of primary malignancy and by the multiplicity of lesions.

Plasmacytomas are tumors of monoclonal proliferation of immunoglobulin-secreting plasma cells. These tumors more commonly involve the bone (70%) but may less commonly be entirely extramedullary. Patients with solitary plasmacytoma are at risk for progression to multiple myeloma. Lesions typically present during the fifth to ninth decades as an osteolytic soft tissue mass with mild-to-moderate homogenous enhancement. As opposed to the typical T2 hyperintense appearance of chordoma, plasmacytomas are isointense to gray matter on T2-weighted images as a result of a high nuclear to cytoplasmic ratio.

Nasopharyngeal carcinoma is an epithelial neoplasm with a strong Epstein-Barr virus association. Although relatively uncommon in the United States, nasopharyngeal carcinoma is endemic in areas of southern China. Once lesions have invaded bony structures and/or the paranasal sinuses, they are classified as T3 lesions. T4 lesions have intracranial extension or involvement of the cranial nerves, hypopharynx, parotid gland, or orbit. A nasopharyngeal carcinoma with clival involvement typically extends more anteriorly than does a chordoma with involvement of the nasopharynx. Nasopharyngeal carcinoma has associated nodal metastases in up to 90% of cases.

Pituitary macroadenomas can extend inferiorly to involve the clivus. Consider a pituitary macroadenoma as the cause of a clival lesion when the normal pituitary gland is either not identifiable or is inseparable from the mass.

Although chondrosarcomas and chordomas often have similar MRI signal characteristics (e.g., marked T2 hyperintensity), these lesions often can be distinguished by location. Chondrosarcomas typically occur off midline at the petroclival synchondrosis, whereas chordomas most often occur in the midline. Additionally, chordomas typically exhibit relatively low apparent diffusion coefficient (ADC) values on diffusion-weighted imaging, whereas chondrosarcomas exhibit relatively high ADC values.

Spectrum of Disease

Although chordomas typically are characterized as T2 hyperintense, heterogeneous T2 signal may result from intratumoral calcification, hemorrhage, or proteinaceous contents (Fig. 27.1). For differentiating chordoma and ecchordosis physaliphora, refer to Chapter 33, Ecchordosis Physaliphora Versus Chordoma.

Differential Diagnosis

1. Metastasis
2. Plasmacytoma
3. Fibrous dysplasia
4. Chordoma
5. Ecchordosis physaliphora
6. Chondrosarcoma

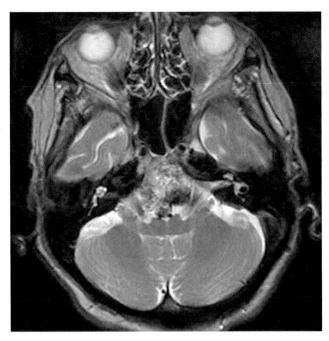

• **Fig. 27.1** A clival chordoma demonstrating T2 heterogeneity as a result of intralesional hemorrhage.

7. Nasopharyngeal carcinoma
8. Sphenoid mucocele
9. Pituitary macroadenoma
10. Clival meningioma
11. Lymphoma

Pearls

- Chordomas are characterized by marked T2 hyperintensity and a midline location.
- Intermediate T2 signal, low diffusivity, and homogeneous enhancement can be seen with plasmacytoma and lymphoma.

- A known primary malignancy and the presence of multiple lesions suggest metastatic disease.
- Nasopharyngeal carcinoma involves the mucosa of the nasopharynx and is associated with nodal metastases in up to 90% of cases.
- A large skull base mass with no identifiable pituitary tissue suggests pituitary macroadenoma.
- Although chordoma and chondrosarcoma are both markedly T2 hyperintense, an off midline location, chondroid matrix, and relatively high ADC all favor chondrosarcoma over chordoma.

Signs and Complications

Destructive clival lesions often present with headache and/or cranial neuropathies. The abducens nerve (cranial nerve VI) is most often affected because of the location of a segment of the nerve at the petroclival venous confluence (Dorello canal).

Suggested Readings

Abunimer A, Aiken A, Baugnon K, et al: Central skull base anatomy and pathology: a review, *Semin Ultrasound CT MR* 42:266–280, 2021.

Bhatoe HS, Kotwal N, Badwal S: Clival pituitary adenoma with acromegaly: case report and review of the literature, *Skull Base* 17:265–268, 2007.

Caers J, Paiva B, Zamagni E, et al: Diagnosis, treatment, and response assessment in solitary plasmacytoma: updated recommendations from a European expert panel, *J Hematol Oncol* 11:10, 2018.

Chan AT, Teo PM, Johnson PJ: Nasopharyngeal carcinoma, *Ann Oncol* 13:1007–1015, 2002.

Erdem E, Angtuaco EC, Van Hemert R, et al: Comprehensive review of intracranial chordoma, *Radiographics* 23:995–1009, 2003.

Goel A, Phalke U, Cacciola F, et al: Giant pituitary adenoma invading the clivus, *Neurol India* 53:105–107, 2005.

Neelakantan A, Rana AK: Benign and malignant diseases of the clivus, *Clin Radiol* 69:1295–1303, 2014.

Yeom KW, Lober RM, Mobley BC, et al: Diffusion-weighted MRI: distinction of skull base chordoma from chondrosarcoma, *AJNR Am J Neuroradiol* 34:1056–1061, 2013.

28

Hyperdense Cerebellum

JUAN E. SMALL, MD, MSC

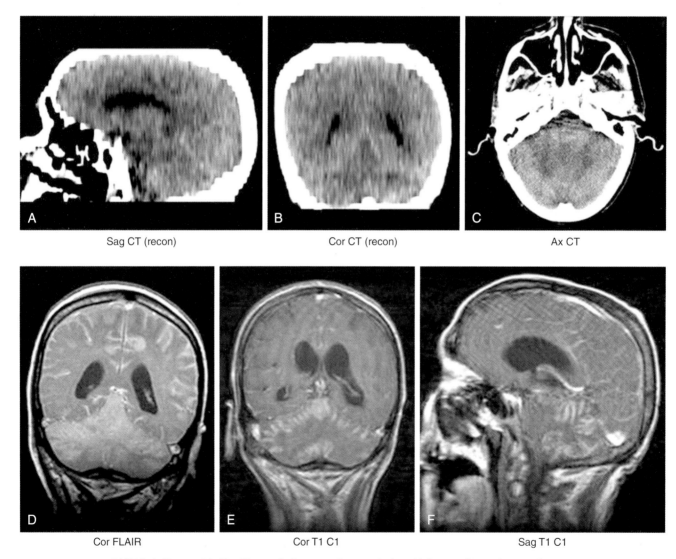

Sag CT (recon)

Cor CT (recon)

Ax CT

Cor FLAIR

Cor T1 C1

Sag T1 C1

CASE A: A 45-year-old with a history of a liver transplant presenting with fever and mental status changes. *Ax,* Axial; *Cor,* coronal; *CT,* Computed tomography; *FLAIR,* fluid attenuated inversion recovery; *recon,* reconstruction; *Sag,* sagittal.

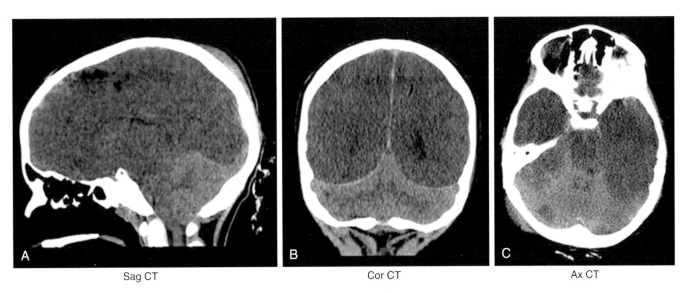

Sag CT   Cor CT   Ax CT

CASE B: An 11-year-old who was struck by a car. *Ax,* Axial; *Cor,* coronal; *CT,* Computed tomography; *Sag,* sagittal.

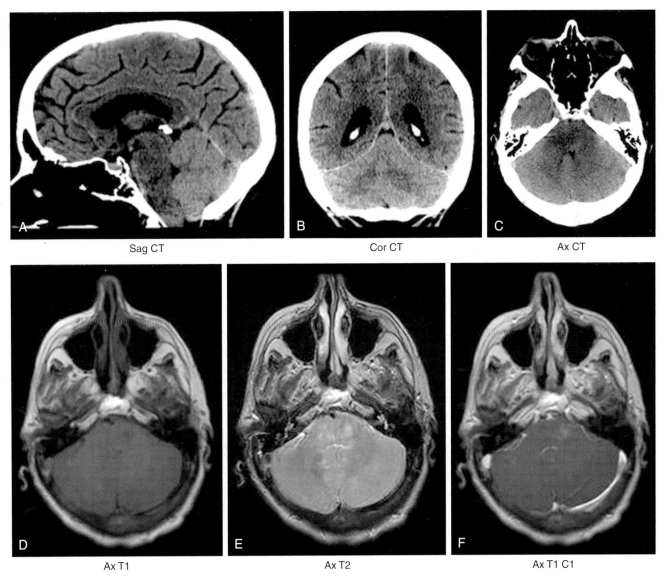

Sag CT   Cor CT   Ax CT

Ax T1   Ax T2   Ax T1 C1

CASE C: A 67-year-old presenting with a 2-month history of increasing headaches, dizziness, and nausea. *Ax,* Axial; *Cor,* coronal; *CT,* Computed tomography; *Sag,* sagittal.

DESCRIPTION OF FINDINGS

- Case A: Prominent heterogeneous cerebellar hyperdensity is noted on sagittal, coronal, and axial CT images. Additional occipital lobe hyperdensity is evident on the sagittal reconstruction, indicating that the pathology is not limited to the posterior fossa. A coronal fluid-attenuated inversion recovery (FLAIR) image demonstrates cerebellar folia edema and diffuse sulcal hyperintensity involving the posterior fossa and supratentorial sulci. Leptomeningeal enhancement is evident on postcontrast coronal and sagittal images. In conjunction, the patient's history of liver transplantation (suggesting immunocompromised), fever, and leptomeningeal enhancement most prominently involving the posterior fossa point toward the correct diagnosis of meningitis with cerebellar involvement.
- Case B: The cerebellum is markedly hyperdense when compared with the abnormally diffuse hypodense appearance of the supratentorial brain. Sulcal effacement also is present in the supratentorial compartment. The findings are consistent with a diffuse, cerebral anoxic insult resulting from respiratory arrest after the patient sustained trauma. A right parieto-occipital subgaleal hematoma is noted on sagittal and axial images, providing further evidence of trauma.
- Case C: Mass-like enlargement of a mildly heterogeneously hyperdense cerebellum is noted on sagittal, coronal, and axial CT images. In addition, mass-like enlargement of a heterogeneously hypodense pons is noted on sagittal CT. Of note, the supratentorial compartment, including the sulci, is normal in appearance. MRI demonstrates heterogeneous T2 hyperintensity and patchy enhancement associated with mass-like enlargement of the pons, cerebellar peduncles, and cerebellum consistent with neoplastic infiltration.

Diagnosis

Case A: Meningitis with cerebellar involvement
Case B: Diffuse cerebral anoxia with sparing of the cerebellum
Case C: Infiltrative neoplasm (presumed glioma)

Summary

Differences in the density of the cerebellum compared with that of the supratentorial brain parenchyma can present a diagnostic dilemma. The first step for the imaging interpreter is to attempt to identify whether the difference in density is a result of supratentorial versus infratentorial pathology. More commonly, cerebellar hyperdensity is a result of the "normal" cerebellum visually standing out as it contrasts with abnormal diffuse supratentorial hypodensity. A distinctive CT appearance has been termed the "reversal sign." It is seen on noncontrast CT images when diffuse supratentorial edema is present and the gray matter appears hypodense in relation to the adjacent white matter (normally, the gray matter appears hyperdense compared to white matter). In contrast, the normal cerebellum and brainstem have much higher attenuation, and these structures appear prominently hyperdense compared with the predominant supratentorial hypodensity. The mass effect with effacement of sulci in the supratentorial compartment points to the supratentorial compartment as the predominant site of injury.

The reversal sign may result from a variety of insults that eventually lead to diffuse cerebral anoxic insult. Etiologies include accidental and nonaccidental trauma, hypoxia, asphyxia, drowning, status epilepticus, and any other causes of global ischemia. The sign indicates irreversible brain damage.

Quite rarely, abnormal diffuse cerebellar hyperdensity may be a result of bacterial or fungal meningitis with cerebellar involvement or posterior fossa leptomeningeal carcinomatosis with cerebellar invasion, or it may be a result of a diffusely infiltrative neoplasm with dense cell packing such as a lymphoma, a high-grade glioma, or an embryonal tumor with multilayered rosettes. The abnormal expanded appearance of the cerebellar folia points to the posterior fossa as the true site of pathology.

Spectrum of Disease

The cause of a diffusely hyperdense cerebellum seen on CT scans can be further discerned with MRI. In patients with anoxia, the cerebellum appears normal, and diffuse FLAIR hyperintensity and restricted diffusion are noted to involve the cerebral cortex and deep gray nuclei. Patients with meningitis or leptomeningeal carcinomatosis with cerebellar involvement have leptomeningeal and parenchymal enhancement and FLAIR hyperintensity in the subarachnoid space and parenchyma. Usually, cerebellar expansion also is present. Patients with an intraaxial high-grade neoplasm have patchy enhancement, patchy restricted diffusion, and marked cerebellar enlargement. MRI scans also are useful for the detection of brainstem compression and hydrocephalus.

Differential Diagnosis

The differential diagnosis is delineated in Figs. 28.1 and 28.2.

Pearls

- The first step in the diagnosis of apparent cerebellar hyperdensity is to attempt to identify whether the difference in density is a result of supratentorial or infratentorial pathology.
- The most common cause of a diffusely hyperdense cerebellum is diffuse hypodensity in the supratentorial brain as a result of anoxia and edema.
- Quite rarely, abnormal diffuse cerebellar hyperdensity may be a result of meningitis with cerebellar involvement, posterior fossa leptomeningeal carcinomatosis with brain invasion, or a primary high-grade infiltrative neoplasm.
- Hemosiderosis can cause diffuse cerebellar hyperdensity; the hyperdensity is usually subtle, and no mass effect is present.
- The most common cause of more focal cerebellar hyperdensity is hemorrhage.

Signs and Complications

The "reversal sign" is seen on noncontrast CT images as the opposite of the normal attenuation of supratentorial gray and white matter, with the gray matter appearing hypodense in relation to the adjacent white matter. In contrast, the normal attenuation of the cerebellum and brainstem is much higher, appearing prominently hyperdense compared with the predominant supratentorial hypodensity. The sign indicates irreversible brain damage.

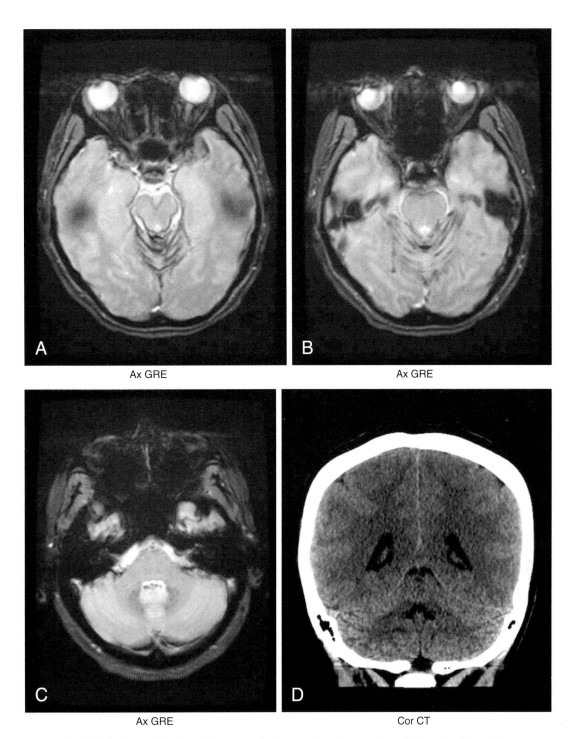

• **Fig. 28.1** A 41-year-old with a history of cervical cord astrocytoma and superficial cerebral hemosiderosis. Axial gradient refocused echo images through the cerebellum (**A, B,** and **C**) demonstrate susceptibility blooming involving the cerebellar folia, consistent with the patient's known history of hemosiderosis. Note, on the coronal computed tomography image (**D**), that only minimal folia hyperdensity is seen, which is quite different and much more subtle in appearance than the differential diagnostic considerations previously presented. *Ax,* Axial; *Cor,* coronal; *CT,* Computed tomography; *GRE,* gradient refocused echo.

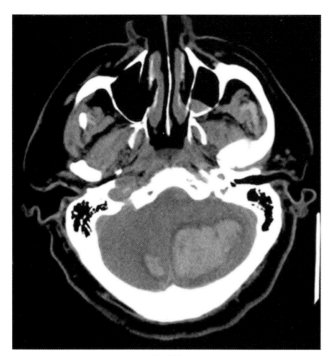

Ax CT

• **Fig. 28.2** A 70-year-old with a severe headache the previous night was found unresponsive the next morning. An axial *(Ax)* computed tomography *(CT)* image through the cerebellum demonstrates hypertensive cerebellar hemorrhages, which are easily distinguished from the differential diagnostic considerations previously presented because of their focality and surrounding rim of hypodense edema.

Suggested Readings

De Bruecker Y, Claus F, Demaerel P, et al: MRI findings in acute cerebellitis, *Eur Radiol* 14(8):1478–1483, 2004.

Han BK, Towbin RB, De Courten-Myers G, et al: Reversal sign on CT: effect of anoxic/ischemic cerebral injury in children, *AJNR Am J Neuroradiol* 10(6):1191–1198, 1989.

Kavanagh EC: The reversal sign, *Radiology* 245(3):914–915, 2007.

Sawaishi Y, Takada G: Acute cerebellitis, *Cerebellum* 1(3):223–228, 2002.

29

Low-Lying Cerebellar Tonsils

FARAHNAZ GOLRIZ, MD

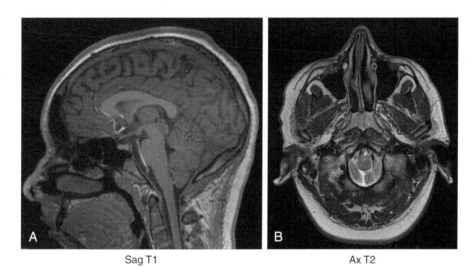

Sag T1   Ax T2

CASE A: A 16-year-old male with headache. *Ax,* Axial; *Sag,* sagittal.

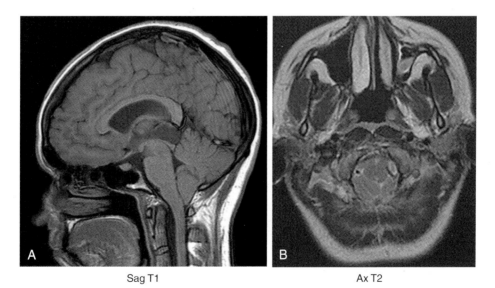

Sag T1   Ax T2

CASE B: A 27-year-old female with new-onset headache. *Ax,* Axial; *Sag,* sagittal.

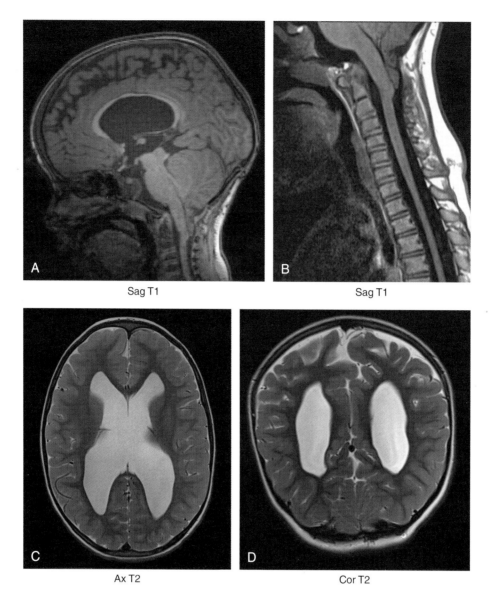

Sag T1

Sag T1

Ax T2

Cor T2

CASE C: A 5-year-old male with history of myelomeningocele status post closure, and ventriculomegaly status post endoscopic third ventriculostomy during first year of life presented for follow-up. *Ax,* Axial; *Cor,* coronal; *Sag,* sagittal.

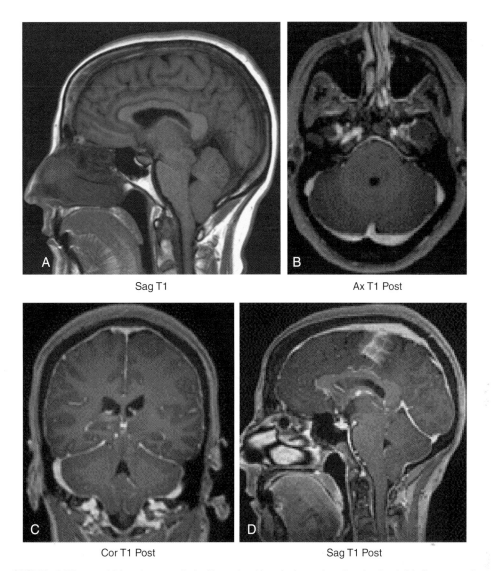

Sag T1   Ax T1 Post

Cor T1 Post   Sag T1 Post

CASE D: A 50-year-old female presented with postural headache and neck pain. *Ax,* Axial; *Cor,* coronal; *Sag,* sagittal.

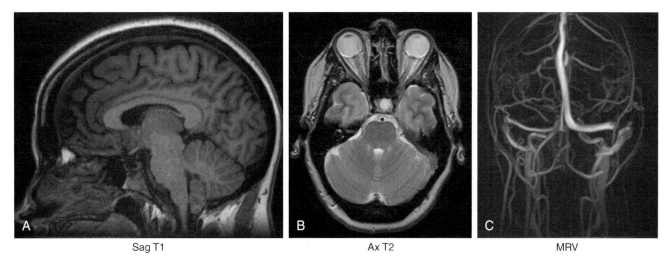

Sag T1   Ax T2   MRV

CASE E: A 36-year-old female with history of rheumatoid arthritis, and Hashimoto thyroiditis on predni-sone presented with new-onset headache and blurry vision. She has bilateral papilledema on exam. *Ax,* Axial; *MRV,* magnetic resonance venography; *Sag,* sagittal.

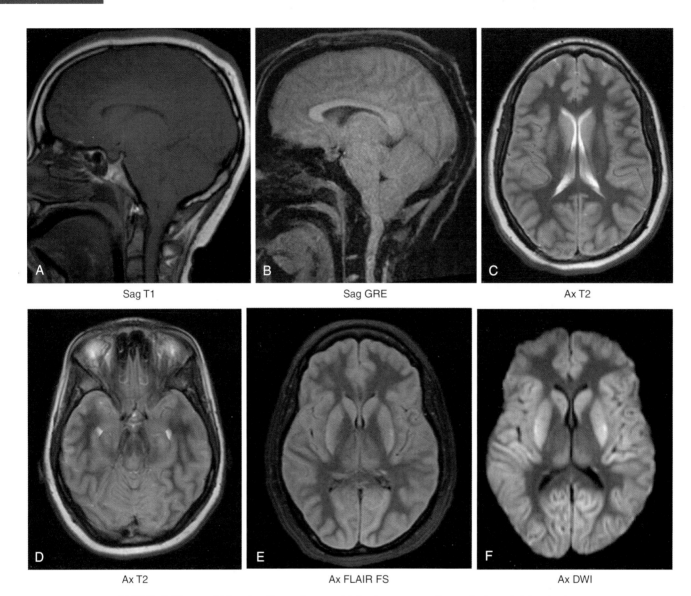

Sag T1   Sag GRE   Ax T2

Ax T2   Ax FLAIR FS   Ax DWI

CASE F: A 32-year-old female with cardiac arrest following severe asthma attack and delayed return of spontaneous circulation (ROSC). *Ax,* Axial; *DWI,* diffusion-weighted imaging; *FLAIR,* fluid attenuated inversion recovery; *GRE,* Gradient refocused echo; *Sag,* sagittal.

DESCRIPTION OF FINDINGS

- Case A: The cerebellar tonsils are 4 mm below the foramen magnum with a normal rounded configuration and preserved cerebrospinal fluid (CSF) space dorsal to the cerebellar tonsils.
- Case B: There are pointed "peg-like" cerebellar tonsils > 5 mm below the foramen magnum with crowding at the foramen magnum, partial effacement of the foramen of Luschka, and effacement of the CSF space dorsal to the cerebellar tonsils.
- Case C: There is a small posterior fossa with descent of the cerebellar tonsils into the upper cervical canal, mild tectal beaking, and interdigitating gyri. The fourth ventricle is inferiorly displaced and effaced. Moderate dilatation of the third and lateral ventricles with a fenestrated septum pellucidum, as well as a defect along the inferior aspect of the third ventricle consistent with prior endoscopic third ventriculostomy are also noted.
- Case D: There is caudal displacement of the cerebellar tonsils with sagging brain configuration and associated decreased pontomammillary distance, closed pons-midbrain angle, and flattening of the pons against the clivus. On postcontrast T1-weighted images, there is smooth, diffuse dural thickening and enhancement, as well as engorgement of the dural sinuses.
- Case E: Mild downward displacement of cerebellar tonsils with a partially empty sella, mild flattening of the posterior aspects of both globes with slight protrusion of the optic nerve heads into the orbits, and mild distension of the optic nerve sheaths are noted. MR venography shows severe narrowing of the distal transverse and proximal sigmoid sinuses bilaterally. Subsequent lumbar puncture showed opening pressure of 35 cmH2O.
- Case F: There is diffuse cerebral swelling, resulting in diffuse sulcal, ventricular, and cisternal effacement with associated downward tonsillar herniation resulting in mass effect on the brainstem. There is also diffuse FLAIR hyperintensity and restricted diffusion throughout the cerebral cortex and deep gray nuclei consistent with global hypoxic-ischemic injury in the setting of cardiac arrest.

Diagnosis

Case A: Low-lying cerebellar tonsils
Case B: Chiari I malformation
Case C: Chiari II malformation
Case D: Spontaneous intracranial hypotension
Case E: Idiopathic intracranial hypertension
Case F: Brain swelling and tonsillar descent secondary to intracranial hypertension due to global hypoxic-ischemic injury

Summary

The cerebellar tonsils may normally lie up to 5 mm below the foramen magnum, and normal cerebellar tonsils show normal rounded configuration.

Chiari I malformation refers to caudal displacement of at least one of the cerebellar tonsils below the foramen magnum by more than 5 mm, resulting in crowding of the foramen magnum and compression of the cerebellar tonsils. The inferiorly displaced cerebellar tonsils are typically peg-shaped/pointed due to compression at the foramen magnum. The posterior fossa may be small and flat, and associated skull base anomalies and spinal cord syrinx could be present. Possible associated skull base anomalies include platybasia, basilar impression, assimilation of C1 to the occiput, and segmentation anomalies. Patients with Chiari I typically do not have additional intracranial anomalies.

Chiari II malformation, which also presents with a small posterior fossa and caudal protrusion of pointed cerebellar tonsils below the foramen magnum by >5 mm is, however, a very distinct entity from Chiari I malformation. Chiari II malformation is associated with a spinal dysraphism resulting in an underdeveloped small posterior fossa and multiple intracranial anomalies. The degree of tonsillar ectopia and crowding at the craniocervical junction is typically greater in Chiari II compared to Chiari I malformations. Intracranial findings in Chiari II malformations include a compressed and elongated fourth ventricle, a beaked tectum, cervicomedullary kinking, enlarged massa intermedia, low-lying torcula, dysgenesis of the corpus callosum (90% of cases), and hydrocephalus in nearly all cases. Additional intracranial findings include interdigitation of gyri in the setting of an incomplete falx, absent septum pellucidum, polymicrogyria, and stenogyria.

Reduced intracranial pressure in patients with spontaneous intracranial hypotension (SIH) results in downward herniation of the cerebellar tonsils in 25% to 75% of cases, which may lead to misdiagnosis of Chiari I malformation. Additional intracranial findings of intracranial hypotension can help to make the correct diagnosis. These findings include sagging brainstem with associated decreased pontomammillary distance (< 5.5 mm) and reduced pons-midbrain angle (<50 degrees), and elongated "fat" appearance of the midbrain and pons, smooth diffuse dural thickening and enhancement in up to 83% of cases, distended dural sinuses in 75% of cases, and subdural collections in 15% to 50% of cases. The optic chiasm and hypothalamus are also often draped over the sella, effacing the suprasellar cistern. The pituitary gland appears prominent in at least 50% of cases. Imaging of the spine can show enlarged venous plexus, subdural collections, and pachymeningeal enhancement. The misinterpretation of intracranial hypotension as Chiari I may lead to decompressive surgery that worsens the patient's symptoms due to worsening CSF hypovolemia, which in rare cases can be fatal.

Low cerebellar tonsils may be seen in 10% to 20% of patients with idiopathic intracranial hypertension (IIH), which could also be misinterpreted as Chiari I malformation, leading to incorrect surgery. Ancillary imaging signs of IIH in the orbits and brain could help to make the correct diagnosis. Typical imaging signs of IIH in the orbits include flattened posterior globes, intraocular protrusion of the optic nerve heads, and distention of optic nerve sheaths with or without increased tortuosity. A partially empty sella is seen in 70% to 80% of patients with IIH. Transverse sinus narrowing has been reported in 65% to 90% of patients with IIH, identified on MR or CT venography. Narrowing is usually located within the distal transverse sinuses bilaterally. Slit-like ventricles are a rare sign of IIH.

Spectrum of Disease

Any primary or secondary posterior fossa mass, inflammatory process, infectious process, subacute ischemic process, or hemorrhagic process may cause tonsillar herniation secondary to local mass effect. Secondary causes of intracranial hypertension can also lead to tonsillar herniation.

Differential Diagnosis

1. Isolated low-lying cerebellar tonsils
2. Chiari 1 malformation
3. Chiari 2 malformation
4. Spontaneous intracranial hypotension
5. Idiopathic intracranial hypertension
6. Intracranial hypertension secondary to ischemia, inflammation, infection, neoplasm, or hemorrhage

Pearls

- In cases with low cerebellar tonsils below the foramen magnum, look for tonsillar shape. In Chiari malformations, the inferiorly displaced tonsils demonstrate a pointed appearance rather than the normal rounded configuration. On the other hand, the low cerebellar tonsils in patients with SIH and IIH typically demonstrate normal rounded shape.
- The presence of tonsillar herniation can lead to misdiagnosis of SIH and IIH as Chiari I and lead to decompressive surgery, which exacerbates the symptoms of patients with SIH, and rarely can be fatal. It is important to look for ancillary findings of intracranial hypotension and hypertension in patients with low-lying cerebellar tonsils.

Signs and Complications

- Patients with Chiari malformations and intracranial hypertension secondary to inflammatory, infectious, ischemic, and neoplastic processes may develop obstructive hydrocephalus.
- Patients with SIH can be misdiagnosed as having a Chiari malformation, leading to decompressive surgery, which can worsen their symptoms.

Suggested Readings

Aiken AH, Hoots JA, Saindane AM, et al: Incidence of cerebellar tonsillar ectopia in idiopathic intracranial hypertension: a mimic of the Chiari I malformation, *AJNR Am J Neuroradiol* 33(10):1901–1906, 2012.

Amrhein TJ, Kranz PG: Spontaneous intracranial hypotension: imaging in diagnosis and treatment, *Radiol Clin North Am* 57(2):439–451, 2019.

El gammal T, Mark EK, Brooks BS. MR imaging of Chiari II malformation, *AJR Am J Roentgenol* 150(1):163–170, 1988.

Kranz PG, Gray L, Malinzak MD, et al: Spontaneous intracranial hypotension: pathogenesis, diagnosis, and treatment, *Neuroimaging Clin N Am* 29(4):581–94, 2019.

Osborn AG, Hedlund GL, Salzman KL: *Osborn's brain e-book,* ed 2, 2017, Elsevier Health Sciences.

30
T2 Hyperintense Pontine Lesions

SCOTT EDWARD HUNTER, MD, MBA

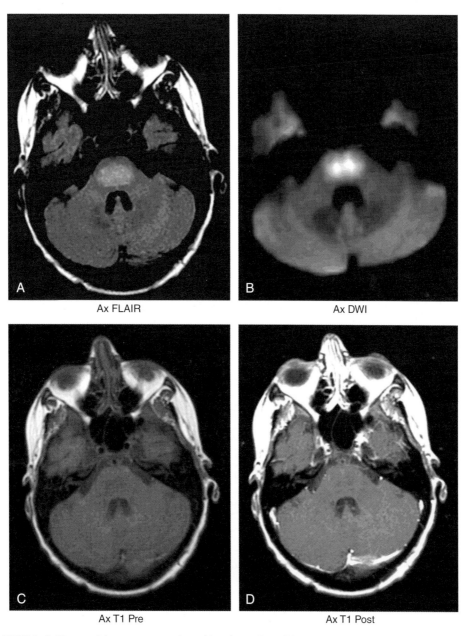

Ax FLAIR

Ax DWI

Ax T1 Pre

Ax T1 Post

CASE A: A 42-year-old woman presenting with orthostasis and hyponatremia. *Ax,* Axial; *DWI,* diffusion-weighted imaging; *FLAIR,* fluid attenuated inversion recovery.

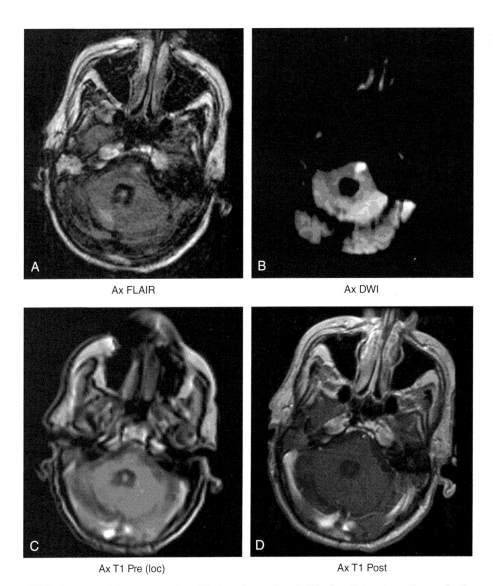

A   Ax FLAIR

B   Ax DWI

C   Ax T1 Pre (loc)

D   Ax T1 Post

CASE B: A 71-year-old man presenting with slurred speech and difficulty with hand-mouth coordination. *Ax,* Axial; *DWI,* diffusion-weighted imaging; *FLAIR,* fluid attenuated inversion recovery.

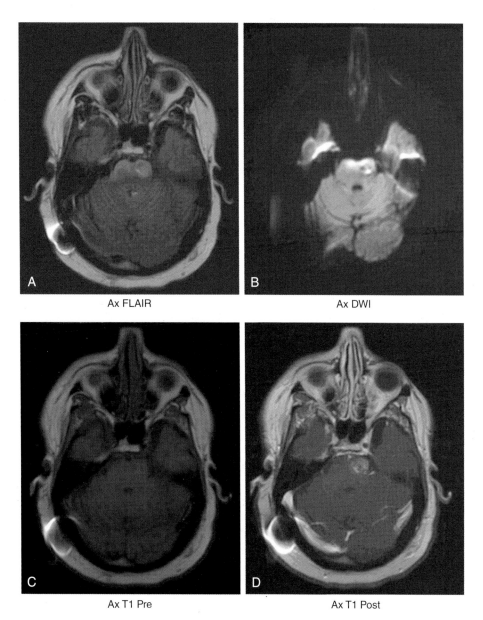

Ax FLAIR

Ax DWI

Ax T1 Pre

Ax T1 Post

CASE C: A 34-year-old man presenting with choking episodes, right-sided weakness, and urinary incontinence. *Ax,* Axial; *DWI,* diffusion-weighted imaging; *FLAIR,* fluid attenuated inversion recovery.

DESCRIPTION OF FINDINGS

- Case A: An axial fluid-attenuated inversion recovery (FLAIR) image demonstrates central hyperintensity of the pons with sparing of the peripheral fibers. Diffusion-weighted MRI shows corresponding restricted diffusion (confirmed by apparent diffusion coefficient (ADC), not shown). T1-weighted pre- contrast and postcontrast MRI discloses no corresponding enhancement.
- Case B: An axial FLAIR image illustrates a left-sided paramedian focus of signal hyperintensity. DWI demonstrates a corresponding wedge-shaped area of restricted diffusion that does not traverse the midline (confirmed by ADC; not shown). T1-weighted precontrast and postcontrast MR images show no enhancement. There is a small chronic infarct in the right superior cerebellum.
- Case C: An axial FLAIR image reveals an expansile region of ventral signal hyperintensity traversing the midline. Diffusion-weighted MRI shows a matching area of restricted diffusion (confirmed by ADC; not shown). T1-weighted precontrast and postcontrast MRI discloses heterogeneous enhancement of the FLAIR hyperintense lesion.

Diagnosis

Case A: Osmotic demyelination
Case B: Basilar perforating artery infarction
Case C: Pontine glioma

Summary

FLAIR/T2 hyperintense pontine lesions may result from multiple different pathologic processes. These etiologies may include ischemic, infectious, inflammatory, autoimmune, neoplastic, or demyelinative processes. Because MRI is the most sensitive and specific technique for characterizing brainstem lesions, this chapter focuses exclusively on this modality.

Osmotic demyelination syndrome (ODS) is a form of acute demyelination caused by rapid shifts in serum osmolality. Approximately half of all lesions related to the syndrome occur in the pons, while the other half occur in extrapontine sites such as the basal ganglia and cerebral white matter. Pontine and extrapontine lesions may often coexist in the same patient. In the pons, ODS lesions are diffuse, grossly symmetric, and invariably affect central pontine fibers while sparing the periphery and the descending corticospinal tracts. A variant of this pattern results in a triangular or "trident" configuration of the affected region, which strongly supports a diagnosis of ODS (Fig. 30.1). On MRI, ODS is characterized by elevated T2/FLAIR signal and intermediate to low T1 signal intensity. DWI and ADC sequences show restricted diffusion in the acute stages of the process, often preceding signal abnormalities on other sequences, which can lag behind clinical findings. Enhancement is not characteristic of ODS, although moderate diffuse enhancement can rarely be seen in the first few weeks, likely because of a disrupted blood-brain barrier. For many patients, imaging abnormalities begin to resolve in the subacute stage.

Pontine infarctions typically result from basilar artery thrombosis or pontine perforator occlusion. Whereas basilar artery thrombosis results in infarction throughout the pons, pontine perforator occlusions, such as the one shown, result in

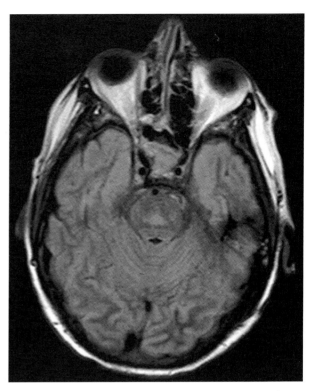

• **Fig. 30.1** Variant appearance of osmotic demyelination syndrome with triangular or "trident" appearance of central pontine T2/fluid attenuated inversion recovery signal abnormality.

unilateral infarctions that do not traverse the midline. The distribution depends on the particular perforating branch that is occluded. Medial and paramedian perforating branches supply the medial and paramedian pons, whereas lateral circumferential perforating branches supply the periphery of the pons. On MRI, infarctions demonstrate restricted diffusion in the acute stage. Within hours, T2/FLAIR hyperintensity accompanies the DWI abnormality in a similar distribution. Accompanying T1 signal in the infarction bed may be isointense to hypointense.

Pontine glioma is a term applied to infiltrative tumors of the brainstem. Because of their location, these tumors generally are not amenable to biopsy and therefore often are diagnosed on the basis of their imaging appearance and clinical presentation. Pathologically, these lesions most often represent low-grade infiltrative fibrillary tumors. MRI typically demonstrates ill-defined expansile T2 signal abnormality of the pons, often with corresponding T1 hypointensity. Expansion can be significant enough to engulf the basilar artery as it courses along the ventral aspect of the pons. Diffusion restriction is characteristically absent, as is enhancement. The presence of these findings, however, may indicate the presence of high-grade tumor.

Spectrum of Disease

T2 hyperintense pontine lesions constitute a heterogeneous group of pathologies with an extensive differential diagnosis.

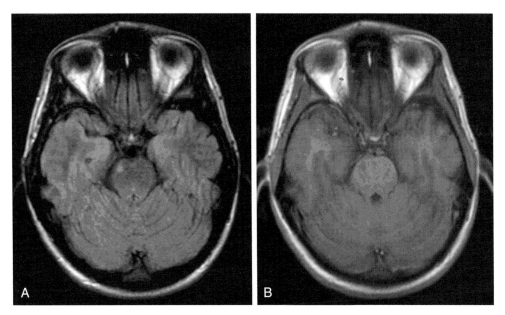

• **Fig. 30.2** Multiple sclerosis. (A) An axial fluid attenuated inversion recovery image demonstrates a focal hyperintense lesion in the right anterior pons. (B) An axial T1-weighted image in the same patient discloses corresponding T1 hypointensity.

Acute disseminated encephalomyelitis, myelin oligodendrocyte glycoprotein antibody–associated disease (MOGAD), neuromyelitis optica spectrum disorder (NMOSD), and multiple sclerosis (Fig. 30.2) are autoimmune-mediated demyelinating processes that may present with pontine involvement and are usually accompanied by supratentorial involvement and frequently accompanied by optic neuritis. Focal pontine lesions accompanied by unilateral optic neuritis, periaqueductal gray matter lesions, and middle cerebellar peduncle lesions as well as by suptratentorial lesions oriented perpendicularly to the lateral ventricles, on the under surface of the corpus callosum, and in a juxtacortical location suggest the diagnosis of multiple sclerosis. Periependymal lesions in the dorsal brainstem, midbrain, and adjacent to the lateral ventricles as well as long corticospinal tract lesions, hemispheric cerebral white matter lesions, long cervical spinal cord lesions, and bilateral optic neuritis extending posteriorly to the chiasm are typical of NMOSD. Diffuse involvement of the pons or middle cerebellar peduncles in conjunction with large asymmetric supratentorial lesions and involvement of the bilateral anterior optic nerves are more common findings in MOGAD. Patchy pontine or middle cerebellar peduncle lesions in conjunction with ill-defined patchy supratentorial white matter lesions and at times basal ganglia lesions suggest the diagnosis of acute disseminated encephalomyelitis (ADEM). MOGAD and ADEM tend to occur in children and young adults and lesions frequently resolve, while MS and NMOSD occur in young and middle-aged women and lesions are more likely to persist and accumulate with time. In all of these demyelinative processes, enhancement and restricted diffusion may be present in the setting of active demyelination. Tissue loss and cavitation are typical of chronic lesions. Pontine perforator occlusion usually results in unilateral focal lesions, corresponding to vascular territories, as previously described. Basilar artery occlusion results in confluent bilateral pontine involvement.

Pontine leukoaraiosis, a disorder characterized by chronic hypoperfusion, often is seen in elderly patients with cardiovascular risk factors. This entity appears as diffuse, central T2/FLAIR hyperintensity without mass effect, corresponding T1 or DWI signal abnormalities or enhancement. The entity frequently occurs in the setting of similar supratentorial white matter changes.

Infectious rhombencephalitis can produce diffuse patchy FLAIR/T2 hyperintensity (Fig. 30.3) and has a variable appearance due to the large number of potential infectious agents. Typically, mild mass effect is present, as concurrent involvement of the cerebellum and remaining brainstem is common. Lesions may show patchy or rim enhancement. A common organism is listeria monocytogenes, frequently seen in infants and older adults as well as immunocompromised patients. Eastern equine encephalitis has a predilection for the brainstem and deep gray nuclei.

Neoplastic processes, such as low-grade gliomas, can yield diffuse expansile FLAIR/T2 hyperintensity without enhancement while high-grade gliomas yield diffuse expansile FLAIR/T2 hyperintensity with patchy enhancement. Gliomas frequently engulf the basilar artery. Primary central nervous system lymphoma is distinguished by its uniform enhancement with restricted diffusion and associated edema. Lymphomatous lesions are more likely to be multiple compared to gliomas.

On rare occasions, posterior reversible encephalopathy syndrome may involve the pons (Fig. 30.4); typically the entire pons is hyperintense on FLAIR and T2-weighted images, has elevated diffusion, and is expanded. Multisystem atrophy is characterized by atrophy of the pons with T2 hyperintense crossing lines, the "hot cross bun" sign in association with tissue loss, and signal abnormality in the middle cerebellar peduncles (Fig. 30.5). Patients with neuro-Behçet syndrome (Fig. 30.6) typically have oral and genital ulcers as well as

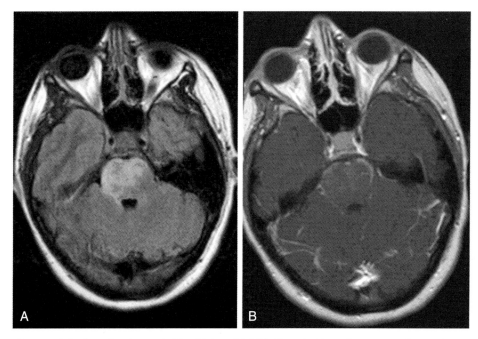

• **Fig. 30.3** Infectious rhombencephalitis. (A) An axial fluid attenuated inversion recovery image demonstrates diffuse pontine T2 hyperintensity. (B) Axial T1 postgadolinium images reveal patchy pontine enhancement.

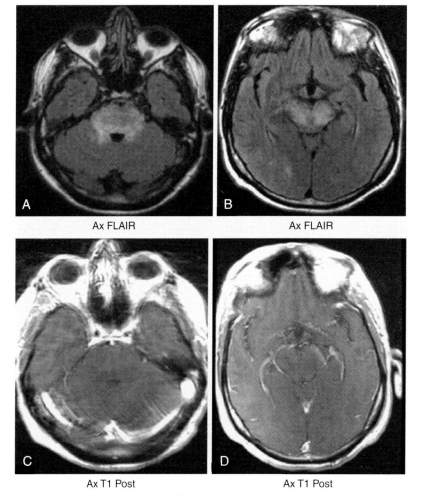

Ax FLAIR   Ax FLAIR

Ax T1 Post   Ax T1 Post

• **Fig. 30.4** Posterior reversible encephalopathy syndrome involving the brainstem. Middle-aged male with hypertension, headache, and confusion. There is mildly expansile FLAIR hyperintensity in the pons and midbrain without associated contrast enhancement. *Ax,* Axial; *FLAIR,* fluid-attenuated inversion recovery.

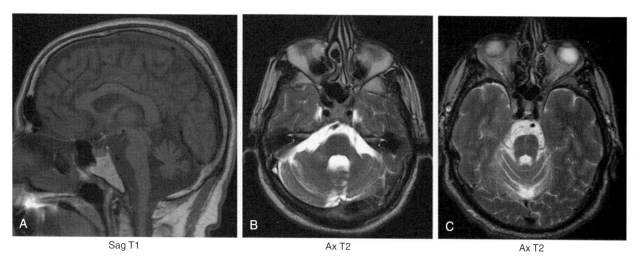

• **Fig. 30.5** Multisystem atrophy—cerebellar type—62-year-old with ataxia. Sagittal T1- and axial T2-weighted images show pontine atrophy. There are also T2 hyperintense lesions in the middle cerebellar peduncles and there are T2 hyperintense crossing lines in the pons, termed the "hot cross bun sign." *Ax,* Axial; *Sag,* sagittal.

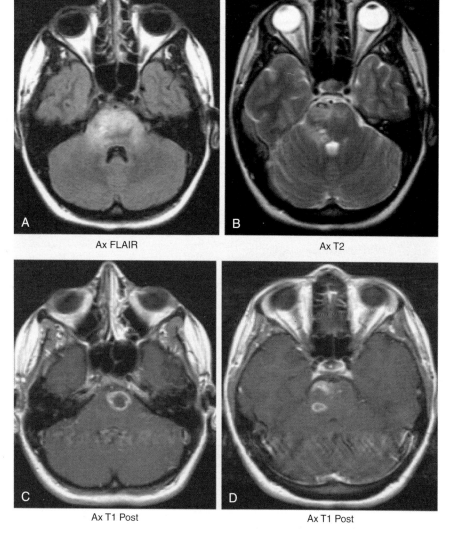

• **Fig. 30.6** Neuro-Behçet. 23-year-old female with oral ulcers, uveitis, and left facial droop. There is expansile, FLAIR/T2 hyperintensity in the pons with associated patchy and ring-enhancing lesions. *Ax,* Axial; *FLAIR,* fluid-attenuated inversion recovery.

expansile FLAIR/T2 hyperintense lesions in the brainstem and basal ganglia with patchy enhancement. They may also have venous sinus thrombosis.

Differential Diagnosis

1. Infarction
2. ODS
3. Pontine glioma
4. Lymphoma
5. Leukoaraiosis
6. Multiple sclerosis
7. Acute demyelinating encephalomyelitis
8. MOGAD
9. NMOSD
10. Infectious rhombencephalitis
11. Posterior reversible encephalopathy syndrome
12. Multisystem atrophy
13. Neuro-Behçet Syndrome

Pearls

- Morphology/location: Osmotic demyelination typically involves the central pons and spares the periphery. A trident configuration is characteristic. Pontine perforating artery infarctions usually are unilateral and rarely traverse the midline. Pontine gliomas often are large, expansile lesions with poorly defined borders.
- Enhancement: Contrast enhancement in ODS is variable but occurs early in the first few weeks of the process when it is present. Pontine perforating artery infarctions may enhance during the subacute phase of infarction. Enhancement of pontine gliomas is atypical and may indicate degeneration to a higher-grade tumor.
- Demographics: Osmotic demyelination may occur in patients of any age, although it is most common in middle-aged patients and is uncommon in children. Pontine infarctions, as with all cerebral infarctions, occur more frequently in patients who are older than 55 years with cardiovascular risk factors such as hyperlipidemia and hypertension. Pontine gliomas, by contrast, occur most frequently in 5- to 10-year-old children and in 20- to 30-year-old adults.

Signs and Complications

Because the imaging features of T2 hyperintense pontine lesions can overlap, clinical history is useful in differentiating potential etiologies. Acute presentations are more typical of ischemic, demyelinative, autoimmune, and infectious lesions, whereas infiltrative gliomas and myelopathies tend to present more insidiously.

ODS invariably presents in the setting of rapid shifts in serum sodium concentration. Although profound chronic hyponatremia is common, ODS may occur in normonatremic patients. Symptoms usually develop 2 to 4 days after rapid correction of hyponatremia and include seizures and mental status changes. Treatment of ODS, once the diagnosis is established, is primarily supportive; no consensus treatment has been determined. The range of outcomes, however, is markedly variable, ranging from complete recovery to spastic quadriparesis, coma, and death.

Basilar perforating artery infarctions may result in pure motor hemiparesis, dysarthria, horizontal gaze palsy, ataxia, and hand clumsiness with abrupt onset. Treatment depends on the condition of the basilar artery. Some patients with severe stenosis may be candidates for stenting and/or angioplasty.

Pontine gliomas occur most frequently in 5- to 10-year-old children. These tumors follow a more indolent course in adults than in children. Pontine gliomas are associated with high morbidity, often because of compression of surrounding structures. Headache, ataxia, dysphagia, and nausea/vomiting are common presentations, and hydrocephalus is a common complication due to compression of the fourth ventricle. Median survival with conventional radiotherapy, with or without chemotherapy, is less than 1 year for children. Pontine gliomas carry a worse prognosis than those of the midbrain or medulla.

Suggested Readings

Banks SA, Morris PP, Chen JJ, et al: Brainstem and cerebellar involvement in MOG-IgG-associated disorder versus aquaporin-4-IgG and MS, *J Neurol Neurosurg Psychiatry* jnnp-2020–325121, 2020.

Guzmán-De-Villoria JA, Fernández-García P, Ferreiro-Argüelles C: Differential diagnosis of T2 hyperintense brainstem lesions: part 1. Focal lesions, *Semin Ultrasound CT MR* 31(3):246–259, 2010.

Guzmán-De-Villoria JA, Ferreiro-Argüelles C, Fernández-García P: Differential diagnosis of T2 hyperintense brainstem lesions: part 2. Diffuse lesions, *Semin Ultrasound CT MR* 31:260–274, 2010.

Kumral E, Bayülkem G, Evyapan D: Clinical spectrum of pontine infarction. Clinical-MRI correlations, *J Neurol* 249(12):1659–1670, 2002.

Purohit B, Kamli AA, Kollias SS: Imaging of adult brainstem gliomas, *Eur J Radiol* 84(4):709–720, 2015.

Singh TD, Fugate JE, Rabinstein AA: Central pontine and extrapontine myelinolysis: a systematic review, *Eur J Neurol* 21(12):1443–1450, 2014.

Tisnado J, Young R, Peck KK, et al: Conventional and advanced imaging of diffuse intrinsic pontine glioma, *J Child Neurol* 31(12):1386–1393, 2016.

Verbalis JG, Goldsmith SR, Greenberg A, et al: Diagnosis, evaluation, and treatment of hyponatremia: expert panel recommendations, *Am J Med* 126(10 Suppl 1):S1–S42, 2013.

Wang KY, Chetta J, Bains P, et al: Spectrum of MRI brain lesion patterns in neuromyelitis optica spectrum disorder: a pictorial review, *Br J Radiol* 91(1086):20170690, 2018.

31

Epidermoid Versus Arachnoid Cyst

JUAN E. SMALL, MD, MSC

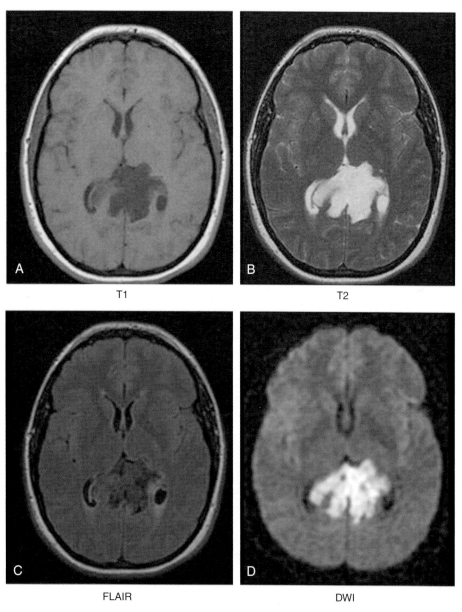

T1   T2

FLAIR   DWI

CASE A: A 33-year-old with a history of chronic headaches. *DWI,* Diffusion-weighted imaging; *FLAIR,* fluid attenuated inversion recovery.

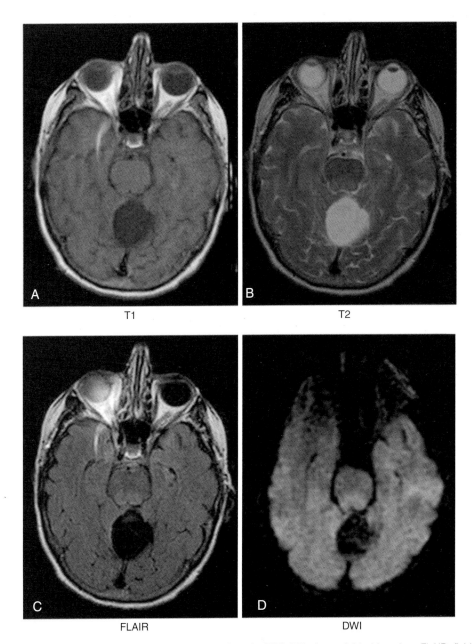

CASE B: A 74-year-old with a history of unsteady gait. *DWI,* Diffusion-weighted imaging; *FLAIR,* fluid attenuated inversion recovery.

DESCRIPTION OF FINDINGS

- Scans demonstrate two different pineal region extraaxial masses roughly following cerebrospinal fluid (CSF) intensity: hypointense on T1-weighted images and hyperintense on T2-weighted images.
- Closer inspection demonstrates that the lesion in Case A has crenulated, irregular margins compared with the smoothly marginated contours of the lesion in Case B.
- In addition, in Case A, the lesion is hyperintense compared with CSF on fluid-attenuated inversion recovery (FLAIR) and diffusion-weighted imaging (DWI). In contrast, the internal signal characteristics of the lesion in Case B are isointense compared with CSF on all sequences, including the FLAIR and DWI sequences.

Diagnosis

Case A: Epidermoid cyst (bright on DWI)
Case B: Arachnoid cyst (dark on DWI)

Summary

A diagnostic dilemma often arises when an extraaxial cystic lesion exhibits signal characteristics that approximate CSF.

As their name implies, arachnoid cysts are space-occupying cystic lesions within the arachnoid space. Their imaging characteristics reflect their internal CSF content. On imaging, they generally appear as unilocular, smoothly contoured cystic lesions that follow CSF on all sequences. Their complications generally relate to mass effect and their location. Scalloping of the adjacent calvarium reflects their long-standing presence.

Epidermoids are benign congenital lesions of ectodermal origin. They are slowly growing lesions that tend to insinuate themselves into the subarachnoid cisterns and sulci and therefore have lobulated, crenulated, and irregular margins. Epidermoid cysts may appear anywhere in the neural axis; however, the most common intracranial sites include the cerebellopontine angle and the sellar region.

On CT, epidermoids appear as lobulated extraaxial masses that generally approximate the density of CSF. However, slight hyperdensity compared with CSF can be seen. Rarely, an epidermoid may present as a hyperdense lesion. By contrast, arachnoid cysts are always isodense to CSF on CT. Enhancement is not seen with either lesion.

Magnetic resonance imaging can readily distinguish epidermoid cysts from arachnoid cysts. The key to differentiating them is DWI: an epidermoid is markedly hyperintense on DWI because of the relatively restricted diffusion of its proteinaceous components compared with CSF and its marked T2 hyperintensity. Epidermoid cysts also are hyperintense compared with CSF on FLAIR images. On the other hand, the fluid within arachnoid cysts is similar to CSF and therefore is markedly hypointense on DWI and FLAIR images. In addition, arachnoid cysts displace vessels and nerves, whereas these structures can travel through epidermoid cysts.

Spectrum of Disease

These lesions may occur in various intracranial compartments (Fig. 31.1).

Differential Diagnosis

1. Epidermoid cyst
2. Arachnoid cyst
3. Neurocysticercosis
4. Dermoid cyst

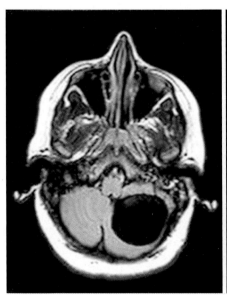 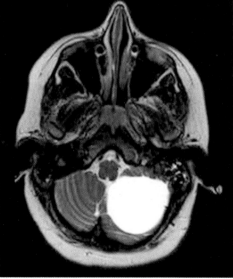 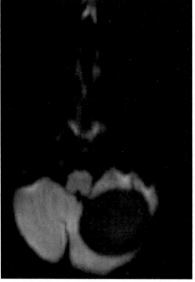

FLAIR   T2   DWI

• **Fig. 31.1** Posterior fossa arachnoid cyst. *DWI,* Diffusion-weighted imaging; *FLAIR,* fluid attenuated inversion recovery.

Pearls

- Diffusion: Both can look like CSF on T1- and T2-weighted sequences, but an epidermoid is markedly hyperintense on DWI, whereas an arachnoid cyst, like CSF, is markedly hypointense.
- FLAIR: An epidermoid cyst is hyperintense compared with CSF, whereas an arachnoid cyst is isointense compared with CSF.

- Morphology: Epidermoid cysts tend to have irregular, crenulated walls, whereas arachnoid cysts tend to have smooth walls.
- Vessels and nerves: Arachnoid cysts displace these structures, whereas vessels can travel through epidermoid cysts.

Signs and Complications

For signs and complications, see Figs. 31.2 and 31.3.

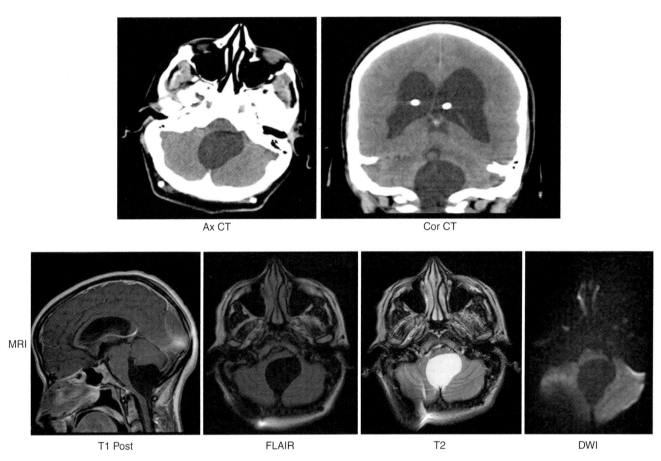

Ax CT   Cor CT

MRI

T1 Post   FLAIR   T2   DWI

- **Fig. 31.2** Complications are generally due to mass effect. This case demonstrates a smoothly marginated, posterior fossa arachnoid cyst. The arachnoid cyst compresses the fourth ventricle, resulting in severe hydrocephalus and necessitating ventriculoperitoneal shunts. *Ax,* Axial; *Cor,* coronal; *CT,* Computed tomography; *DWI,* diffusion-weighted imaging; *FLAIR,* fluid attenuated inversion recovery; *MRI,* magnetic resonance imaging.

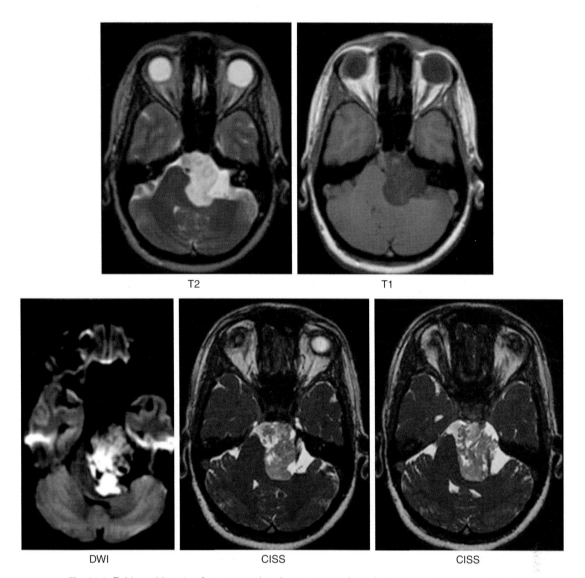

• Fig. 31.3 Epidermoid cysts often surround and encase vessels and nerves as opposed to arachnoid cysts, which displace them. Encased vessels and nerves often make surgical dissection difficult or impossible. This case demonstrates an irregularly marginated left cerebellopontine angle epidermoid cyst exhibiting restricted diffusion. Heavily T2-weighted constructive interference in steady state *(CISS)* images demonstrates that the epidermoid cyst encases the left trigeminal nerve as it exits the effaced brainstem and throughout its course toward Meckel's cave. *DWI,* Diffusion-weighted imaging.

Suggested Readings

Chen S, Ikawa F, Kurisu K, et al: Quantitative MR evaluation of intracranial epidermoid tumors by fast fluid attenuated inversion recovery imaging and echo-planar DWI, *AJNR Am J Neuroradiol* 22: 1089–1096, 2001.

Dutt SN, Mirza S, Chavda SV, et al: Radiologic differentiation of intracranial epidermoids from arachnoid cysts, *Otol Neurotol* 23(1):84–92, 2002.

Gosalakkal JA: Intracranial arachnoid cysts in children: a review of pathogenesis, clinical features, and management, *Pediatr Neurol* 26(2): 93–98, 2002.

Kallmes DF, Provenzale JM, Cloft HJ, et al: Typical and atypical MR imaging features of intracranial epidermoid tumors, *AJR Am J Roentgenol* 169:883–887, 1997.

MacKay CI, Baeesa SS, Ventureyra EC: Epidermoid cysts of the pineal region, *Childs Nerv Syst* 15(4):170–178, 1999.

Osborn AG, Preece MT: Intracranial cysts: radiologic-pathologic correlation and imaging approach, *Radiology* 239(3):651–664, 2006.

Park SH, Chang KH, Song IC, et al: Diffusion-weighted MRI in cystic or necrotic intracranial lesions, *Neuroradiology* 42(10):716–721, 2000.

32

Cyst With a Mural Nodule

JUAN E. SMALL, MD, MSC

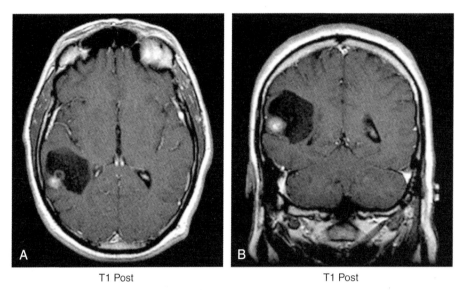

T1 Post · T1 Post

CASE A: A 51-year-old with a history of headaches for 6 weeks now presenting with dizziness and nausea.

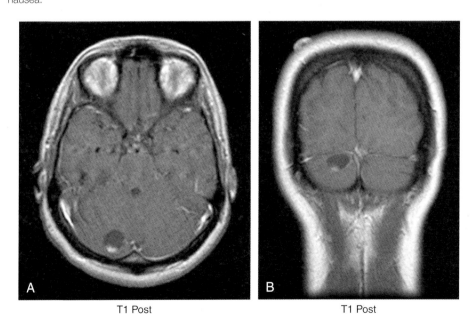

T1 Post · T1 Post

CASE B: A 36-year-old presenting with a 5-day history of progressive confusion, paranoid delusions, and magical thinking.

DESCRIPTION OF FINDINGS

- Case A: A supratentorial right temporal cyst with an enhancing mural nodule. No edema or other lesions are noted.
- Case B: An infratentorial right cerebellar cyst with an enhancing mural nodule. No edema or other lesions are noted.

Diagnosis

Case A: Ganglioglioma
Case B: Hemangioblastoma

Summary

A number of lesions may present with the imaging appearance of a cyst with an enhancing mural nodule, including hemangioblastoma, pilocytic astrocytoma, pleomorphic xanthoastrocytoma, ganglioglioma, neurocysticercosis, and metastases. How, then, can this differential diagnosis be tailored in a useful way? The location of the lesion, coupled with the age of the patient, can help narrow the differential diagnosis (Tables 32.1 and 32.2).

The supratentorial or infratentorial position of the lesion statistically limits the considerations. Because the most common lesion in the posterior fossa in an adult patient is a metastasis, an atypical appearance of a metastasis (as a cyst with an enhancing mural nodule) is an important consideration. In addition, the most common primary posterior fossa mass in an adult patient is a hemangioblastoma, which is associated with von Hippel–Lindau disease. The presence of flow voids within the mural nodule suggests a highly vascular lesion such as a hemangioblastoma, although highly vascular metastasis also may appear in this manner. In adults, it also is important to note that glioblastoma multiforme can at times have a prominent cystic component and can have extensive necrosis with enhancing mural components.

In the pediatric population, on the other hand, the most important consideration when confronted with a posterior fossa mass appearing as a cyst with a mural nodule is a pilocytic astrocytoma. In pediatric patients, adolescents, and young adults, a supratentorial mass appearing as a cyst with a mural nodule raises concern for a ganglioglioma, pleomorphic xanthoastrocytoma, or supratentorial pilocytic astrocytoma. Case A was somewhat atypical considering adult age.

If multiple lesions are present, metastases are the primary consideration. However, if the clinical presentation suggests an infectious etiology, neurocysticercosis, with its scolex as the mural nodule, is the primary diagnostic consideration.

Spectrum of Disease

Hemangioblastoma: Approximately 33% to 60% are a cyst with an enhancing mural nodule; 26% to 35% are predominantly solid; and approximately 5% are nearly purely cystic. It is noteworthy that posterior fossa lesions are more often cystic (70%) and the uncommon supratentorial lesions are more rarely cystic (20%). Approximately 76% appear in the posterior fossa; 9% are supratentorial; 7% appear in the spinal cord; and 5% appear in the brainstem.

Pleomorphic xanthoastrocytoma (Fig. 32.1): Fewer than 48% are a cyst with an enhancing mural nodule; 52% are solid; less than 2% appear in the posterior fossa; and 98% are supratentorial. Only two case reports of spinal cord pleomorphic xanthoastrocytoma exist in the literature.

Pilocytic astrocytoma (Fig. 32.2): 67% percent are a cyst with an enhancing mural nodule (21% have a nonenhancing cyst wall with an enhancing mural nodule and 46% have an enhancing cyst wall with an enhancing mural nodule); 17% are predominantly solid; and 16% are a nonenhancing necrotic mass. The most common location is the cerebellum, but when the lesion is supratentorial, it most commonly occurs in the optic nerve or diencephalon (chiasm/hypothalamus, floor of the third ventricle), thalamus, and rarely occurs in the spinal cord.

Ganglioglioma: Approximately 40% are a cyst with an enhancing mural nodule; 60% are solid, and the most common location is supratentorial, with the temporal lobe as the most common site. This lesion is quite uncommon in the cerebellum, brainstem, and spinal cord.

Differential Diagnosis

1. **Pilocytic astrocytoma:** This lesion is one of the most benign forms of glial neoplasm and the most common astrocytoma in childhood, peaking at approximately 10 years of age. On CT, it often appears as a low-density nodule and may demonstrate calcification in 5% to 25% of patients. The association of optic pathway pilocytic astrocytomas with neurofibromatosis type 1 is well documented.
2. **Hemangioblastoma:** This highly vascular lesion with a subpial nodule demonstrates associated flow voids. On CT, the often high-density nodule does not demonstrate calcification. Approximately 75% are sporadic, and 25% are associated with von Hippel–Lindau disease. Hemangioblastomas are the only brain tumors associated with polycythemia.
3. **Ganglioglioma:** This slow-growth lesion often is associated with a history of chronic seizures and most frequently is

TABLE 32.1	Location	
Posterior Fossa	**Temporal Lobe**	
Pilocytic astrocytoma	Ganglioglioma	
Hemangioblastoma	Pleomorphic xanthoastrocytoma	
Metastasis		

TABLE 32.2	Patient Age	
Child and Adolescent	**Adult**	
Pilocytic astrocytoma	Hemangioblastoma	
Ganglioglioma	Glioblastoma multiforme	
Pleomorphic xanthoastrocytoma	Metastasis	

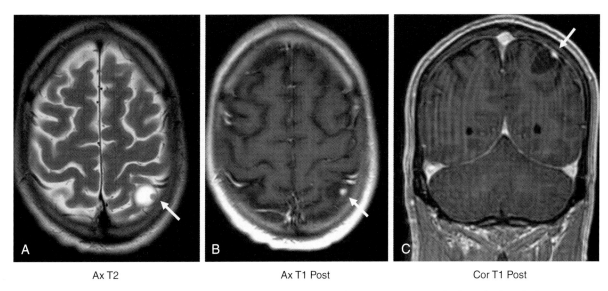

Ax T2   Ax T1 Post   Cor T1 Post

• **Fig. 32.1** Pleomorphic xanthoastrocytoma. Left parietal, T2 hyperintense superficial cerebral cortical cystic lesion with an intensely enhancing nodule abutting the dura with mild dural enhancement *(arrow)*. *Ax,* Axial; *Cor,* coronal.

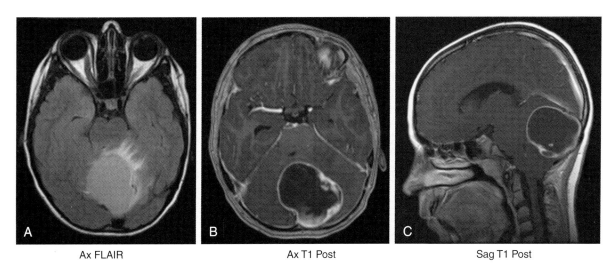

Ax FLAIR   Ax T1 Post   Sag T1 Post

• **Fig. 32.2** Juvenile pilocytic astrocytoma. A young patient with a large predominantly cystic cerebellar mass with peripheral enhancement including avidly enhancing irregular nodular components. *Ax,* Axial; *FLAIR,* fluid attenuated inversion recovery; *Sag,* sagittal.

located in the temporal lobe, although it may occur throughout the cerebrum. One-third of lesions demonstrate calcification. Enhancement is variable. These lesions may remodel adjacent bone.

4. **Pleomorphic xanthoastrocytoma:** This lesion is a rare astrocytoma variant affecting the superficial cerebral cortex and meninges. It often demonstrates a superficial cortical location of a cystic component with an intensely enhancing nodule abutting the leptomeninges. Leptomeningeal involvement is seen in up to 71% of cases.

5. **Glioblastoma multiforme:** This lesion is more commonly a heterogeneous, hemorrhagic, and necrotic mass with thick and irregular avidly enhancing components. It rarely presents with the appearance of a cyst with a mural nodule when it has a prominent cystic component or when there is extensive necrosis with enhancing nodular mural components.

6. **Neurocysticercosis (Fig. 32.3):** In the initial vesicular stage of central nervous system infection, lesions manifest as cystic parenchymal lesions with an internal nodule (the scolex), with little to no perilesional edema and minimal to no enhancement. In the colloidal vesicular stage, the parasite dies, the cyst enhances, and there is surrounding edema. In the granular nodular stage, the edema begins to resolve while enhancement persists. In the nodular calcified stage, there is a calcified cyst remnant with no edema or enhancement.

7. **Metastasis:** Metastasis can be cystic or quite heterogeneous as a result of necrosis, hemorrhage, and liquefaction. Important clues to diagnosis include multiplicity and marked

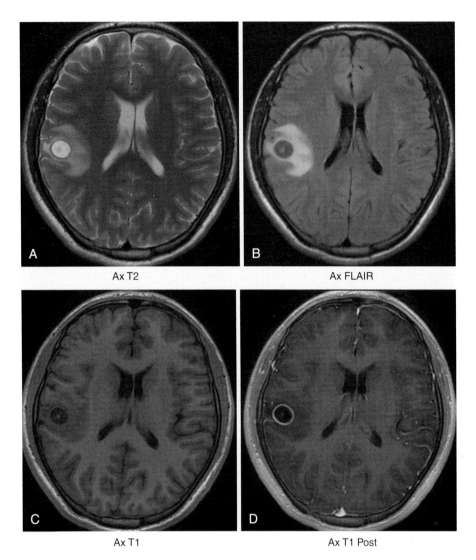

• **Fig. 32.3** Neurocysticercosis. A peripherally enhancing cystic parenchymal lesion with an internal nodule (the scolex) and perilesional edema is consistent with the colloidal vesicular stage of neurocysticercosis. *Ax,* Axial; *FLAIR,* fluid attenuated inversion recovery.

surrounding edema. More common patterns of enhancement include solid, nodular, and ring-like enhancement.

Pearls

- Pilocytic astrocytoma: On CT, it often appears as a low-density nodule that may demonstrate calcification.
- Hemangioblastoma: On CT, it often appears as a high-density nodule that does not demonstrate calcification. It may demonstrate associated flow voids.
- Ganglioglioma: One-third of lesions demonstrate calcification. Gangliogliomas may remodel the inner table of the calvarium.
- Pleomorphic xanthoastrocytoma: This lesion is almost exclusively a supratentorial lesion with a superficial cortical location abutting the meninges and characteristic adjacent meningeal enhancement.
- Neurocysticercosis: The imaging appearance of the scolex within a vesicular cyst is considered pathognomonic.

Signs and Complications

With all of these lesions, always look for complications related to mass effect.

Suggested Readings

Coyle CM, Tanowitz HB: Diagnosis and treatment of neurocysticercosis, *Interdiscip Perspect Infect Dis* 2009:180742, 2009.

Hussein MR: Central nervous system capillary haemangioblastoma: the pathologist's viewpoint, *Int J Exp Pathol* 88(5):311–324, 2007.

Koeller KK, Henry JM: Armed Forces Institute of Pathology: from the archives of the AFIP: superficial gliomas: radiologic-pathologic correlation, *Radiographics* 21(6):1533–1556, 2001.

Koeller KK, Rushing EJ: Armed Forces Institute of Pathology: from the archives of the AFIP: pilocytic astrocytoma: radiologic-pathologic correlation, *Radiographics* 24(6):1693–1708, 2004.

Leung RS, Biswas SV, Duncan M, et al: Imaging features of von Hippel–Lindau disease, *Radiographics* 28(1):65–79, quiz 323, 2008.

Provenzale JM, Ali U, Barboriak DP, et al: Comparison of patient age with MR imaging features of gangliogliomas, *AJR Am J Roentgenol* 174(3):859–862, 2000.

Safavi-Abbasi S, Di Rocco F, Chantra K, et al: Posterior cranial fossa gangliogliomas, *Skull Base* 17(4):253–264, 2007.

Shin JH, Lee HK, Khang SK, et al: Neuronal tumors of the central nervous system: radiologic findings and pathologic correlation, *Radiographics* 22(5):1177–1189, 2002.

Slater A, Moore NR, Huson SM: The natural history of cerebellar hemangioblastomas in von Hippel–Lindau disease, *AJNR Am J Neuroradiol* 24(8):1570–1574, 2003.

33

Ecchordosis Physaliphora Versus Chordoma

JUAN E. SMALL, MD, MSC

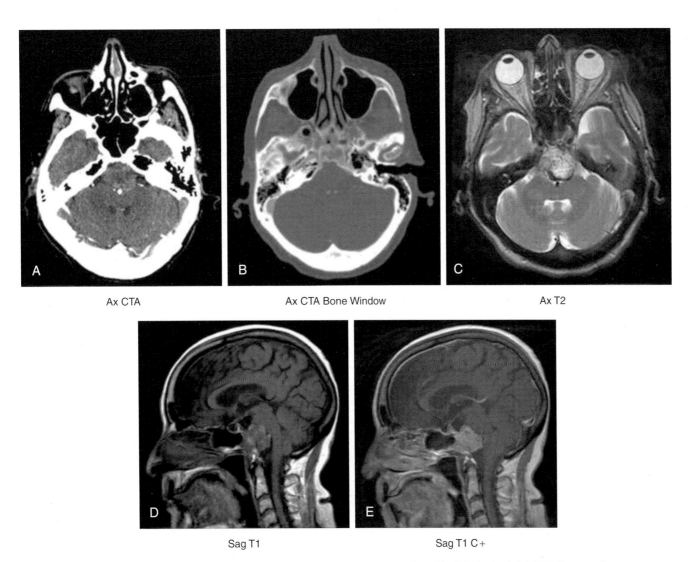

Ax CTA

Ax CTA Bone Window

Ax T2

Sag T1

Sag T1 C+

CASE A: A 70-year-old with a history of breast cancer presenting with diplopia. *Ax*, Axial; *CTA*, Computed tomographic angiography; *Sag*, sagittal.

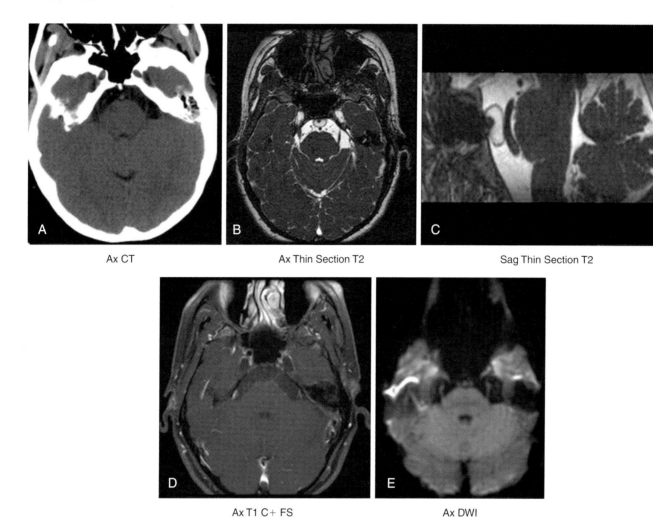

Ax CT

Ax Thin Section T2

Sag Thin Section T2

Ax T1 C+ FS

Ax DWI

CASE B: A 44-year-old presenting with headache and dizziness. *Ax,* Axial; *CT,* Computed tomography; *DWI,* diffusion-weighted imaging; *FS,* fat saturated; *Sag,* sagittal.

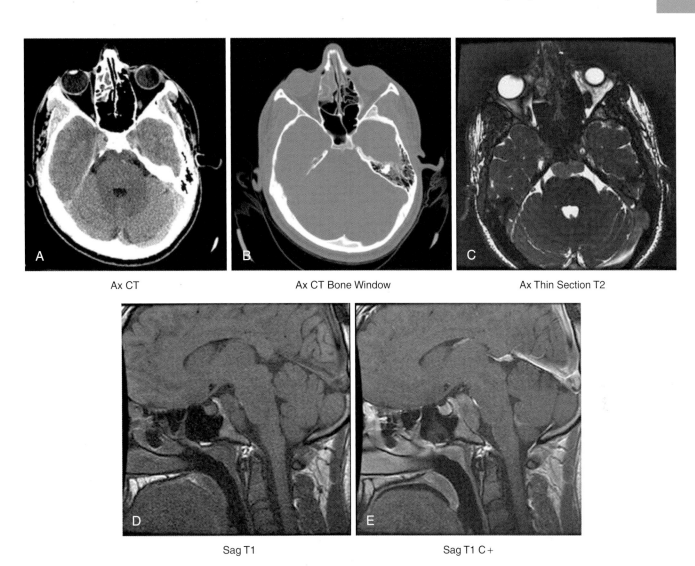

Ax CT   Ax CT Bone Window   Ax Thin Section T2

Sag T1   Sag T1 C+

CASE C: A 19-year-old who sustained trauma. *Ax,* Axial; *CT,* computed tomography; *Sag,* sagittal.

DESCRIPTION OF FINDINGS

- Case A: A clival/retroclival mass associated with bone destruction is evident on CT angiography images (Fig. 33.1A). Prominent high signal intensity is noted on an axial T2 image. Heterogeneous signal and diffuse enhancement are noted on precontrast and postcontrast sagittal T1-weighted images, respectively. Bone destruction, high T2 signal, and enhancement suggest the diagnosis of chordoma.
- Case B: An osseous retroclival stalk/pedicle is evident on an axial CT image (Fig. 33.1B). Axial and sagittal thin-section T2 images demonstrate an intradural, prepontine, cystic retroclival lesion attached to the dorsal clivus by the osseous stalk/pedicle without evidence of bony destruction. No enhancement is noted on the postcontrast fat-saturated T1-weighted axial image. A nonenhancing, cystic prepontine lesion attached to the clivus by an osseous stalk is the hallmark appearance of ecchordosis physaliphora (EP). The lack of diffusion-weighted imaging hyperintensity rules out an epidermoid cyst as a diagnostic consideration.
- Case C: An osseous retroclival stalk/pedicle is evident on an axial CT image (Fig. 33.1C). An axial thin-section T2 image demonstrates an intradural, prepontine, solid-appearing retroclival lesion attached to the dorsal clivus by the osseous stalk/pedicle without evidence of clival bony destruction. Mild diffuse contrast enhancement is present. The presence of enhancement excludes EP as a diagnostic consideration. The lack of bone destruction suggests the diagnosis of intradural/benign chordoma.

Diagnosis

Case A: Chordoma
Case B: EP
Case C: Intradural/benign chordoma

Summary

The differential diagnosis of retroclival lesions includes lesions derived from ectopic notochordal remnants, such as chordoma or EP; metastasis; meningioma, epidermoid, dermoid, and arachnoid cysts.

Clival chordomas generally are symptomatic, T2-hyperintense, enhancing, extradural, locally invasive lesions demonstrating bone destruction and foci of calcification. Although chordomas usually are extradural and osteolytic, rare extraosseous intradural chordomas have been reported, making their imaging differentiation from EP more difficult. Intradural chordomas appear to have a more favorable prognosis than do extradural clival chordomas.

EP has been found in approximately 2% of autopsy specimens and most often appears as an intradural, prepontine, cystic/gelatinous retroclival nodule attached to the dorsal clivus by an osseous stalk/pedicle with lack of clival bony destruction. EP can be particularly difficult to identify because of its general isointense appearance to the surrounding cerebrospinal fluid (CSF) on most MRI sequences. Despite its inconspicuous appearance on most sequences, it is clearly delineated on thin-section heavily weighted T2 sequences (constructive interference in steady-state/fast imaging employing steady-state acquisition [CISS/FIESTA]). Key features for the diagnosis of clival EP include the absence of related symptoms, the lack of contrast enhancement, and the presence of an osseous stalk arising from the basisphenoid portion of the clivus. The lack of symptoms is particularly important, although rare case reports have described symptomatic cases of EP.

The distinction between chordoma and ecchordosis is particularly important because chordoma is considered a malignant neoplasm to be treated by resection and radiation, and ecchordosis is considered a benign congenital malformation that is treated conservatively because of its expected lack of progression/growth. In addition, the imaging interpretation between these two entities is vital because they are pathologically indistinguishable—their microscopic, immunohistochemical, and ultrastructural features are, for all intents and purposes, identical (differentiation is still a matter of debate). The margins of chordoma may demonstrate infiltrative growth, a finding that is not seen with ecchordosis. Some researchers have proposed that proliferation indices may be a helpful differentiating feature, but this proposal is not widely accepted. Although both entities are part of the spectrum of

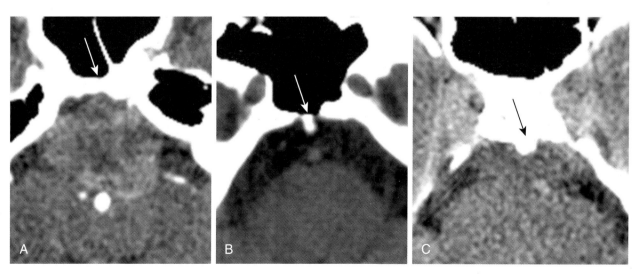

- **Fig. 33.1** Expanded axial computed tomography images on all three unknown cases demonstrate (A) bone destruction in a case of chordoma, (B) a clival bony stalk/pedicle in a case of ecchordosis physaliphora, and a (C) short bony stalk/pedicle as well as the absence of bone destruction in a case of intradural/benign chordoma.

notochordal-related lesions, it is unclear whether ecchordosis can be a precursor to chordoma.

Attempting to distinguish between intradural chordoma and EP can be quite challenging. Particularly confusing is the gray area between the rare case reports of large or symptomatic EP and extraosseous intradural chordomas with a benign course. The issue of whether intradural chordoma and large or symptomatic EP constitute different entities or can be grouped together is still debated. This problem is particularly vexing considering the lack of a widely accepted gold standard for pathologic differentiation. This situation has led some researchers to propose the terms "intradural/benign chordoma" or "giant/symptomatic ecchordosis physaliphora" to encompass all symptomatic intradural extraosseous physaliphorous lesions.

Spectrum of Disease

As previously noted, the terms intradural/benign chordoma or giant/symptomatic EP have been proposed to encompass all symptomatic intradural extraosseous physaliphorous lesions.

Differential Diagnosis

1. **Chordoma:** Hyperintense on T2-weighted images, bone destruction, enhancing
2. **EP:** Osseous stalk/pedicle, nonenhancing, no bone destruction, similar to CSF on most sequences
3. **Metastasis (Fig. 33.2):** Aggressive, relatively T2 hypointense, known primary, enhancing
4. **Lymphoma:** Relatively hypointense on T2-weighted images, invasive, enhancing
5. **Plasmacytoma:** Relatively hypointense on T2-weighted images, invasive, enhancing
6. **Meningioma (Fig. 33.3):** Relatively hypointense on T2-weighted images, densely homogeneously enhancing, dural tail, hyperostosis, may be intraosseous

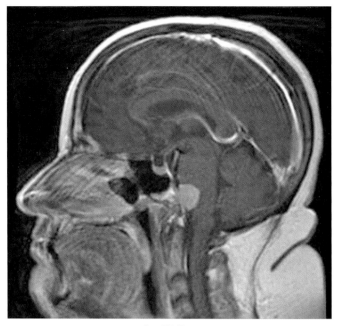

Sag T1 Post

• **Fig. 33.3** A 52-year-old female presenting with headaches. A sagittal T1 postcontrast image demonstrates a dural-based, avidly enhancing retroclival lesion with a dural tail consistent with a meningioma. Calcification and associated hyperostosis were evident on computed tomography images (not shown). *Sag,* sagittal.

7. **Thrombosed basilar aneurysm** lamellated appearance, blood products, contiguous with basilar artery
8. **Epidermoid cyst:** Hyperintense on DWI, nonenhancing
9. **Dermoid cyst:** Hyperintense on T1 and hypointense on T2-weighted images due to fat, nonenhancing
10. **Arachnoid cyst:** Isointense to CSF on all sequences, nonenhancing
11. **Neurenteric cyst:** Associated bone anomalies, variable signal depending on protein content, nonenhancing

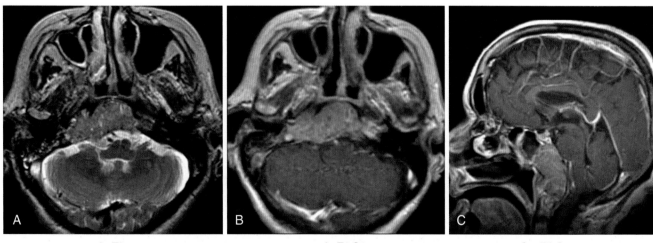

Ax T2   Ax T1 C+   Sag T1 C+

• **Fig. 33.2** Breast carcinoma metastasis. An axial T2-weighted image shows an aggressive, expansile relatively hypointense mass center in the clivus. Axial *(Ax)* and sagittal *(Sag)* contrast-enhanced *(C+)* T1-weighted images show that the lesion avidly enhances, infiltrates adjacent bone, and extends into the prepontine cistern.

Pearls

- Clival chordomas are generally:
  - Symptomatic
  - Locally invasive lesions demonstrating bone destruction
  - Enhancing
  - Hyperintense on T2-weighted images
- Intradural chordomas generally show:
  - Variable enhancement
  - General lack of osseous involvement
  - More favorable prognosis than extradural clival chordomas
- EP is generally:
  - Asymptomatic
  - Nonenhancing
  - Marked by an osseous stalk/pedicle from the basisphenoid portion of the clivus
  - Without clival bony destruction
  - Isointense in appearance to the surrounding CSF on most MRI sequences
  - Clearly delineated on thin-section, heavily weighted T2 sequences (constructive interference in steady-state/fast imaging employing steady-state acquisition).

Signs and Complications

Complications related to retroclival lesions generally are related to invasion of adjacent structures, including the cranial nerves, and mass effect on adjacent structures, such as the brainstem or the basilar artery.

Suggested Readings

Alkan O, Yildirim T, Kizilkiliç O, et al: A case of ecchordosis physaliphora presenting with an intratumoral hemorrhage, *Turk Neurosurg* 19(3):293–296, 2009.

Alli A, Clark M, Mansell NJ: Cerebrospinal fluid rhinorrhea secondary to ecchordosis physaliphora, *Skull Base* 18(6):395–399, 2008.

Bhat DI, Yasha M, Rojin A, et al: Intradural clival chordoma: a rare pathological entity, *J Neurooncol* 96(2):287–290, 2009.

Ciarpaglini R, Pasquini E, Mazzatenta D, et al: Intradural clival chordoma and ecchordosis physaliphora: a challenging differential diagnosis: case report, *Neurosurgery* 64(2):E387–E388, 2009.

Erdem E, Angtuaco EC, Van Hemert R, et al: Comprehensive review of intracranial chordoma, *Radiographics* 23(4):995–1009, 2003.

Ling SS, Sader C, Robbins P, et al: A case of giant ecchordosis physaliphora: a case report and literature review, *Otol Neurotol* 28(7):931–933, 2007.

Mehnert F, Beschorner R, Küker W, et al: Retroclival ecchordosis physaliphora: MR imaging and review of the literature, *AJNR Am J Neuroradiol* 25(10):1851–1855, 2004.

Wolfe JT III, Scheithauer BW: "Intradural chordoma" or "giant ecchordosis physaliphora"? Report of two cases, *Clin Neuropathol* 6(3):98–103, 1987.

Rodrigues JF, da Silva FM, Mangussi-Gomes J, et al: Differential diagnosis of clival lesions – literature review of the clinical and radiological features, *Ann Otolaryngol Rhinol* 4(9):1200, 2017.

34

Atlantooccipital and Atlantoaxial Separation

DANIEL THOMAS GINAT, MD

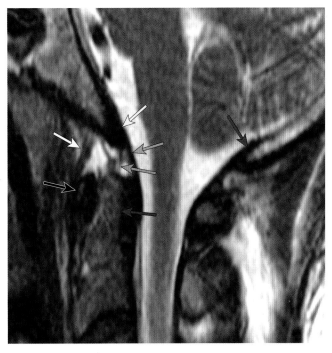

CASE A: Sagittal T2 magnetic resonance imaging shows the anterior atlantooccipital ligament *(white arrow)*, anterior arch of C1 *(black arrow)*, dens *(magenta arrow)*, apical ligament *(blue arrow)*, tectorial membrane *(green arrow)*, basion *(yellow arrow)*, and opisthion *(red arrow)*.

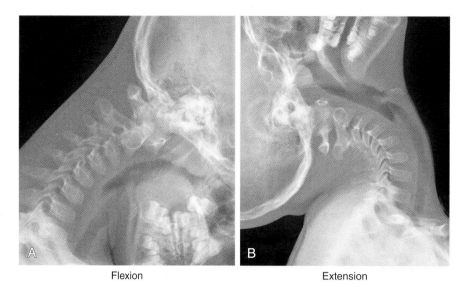

Flexion   Extension

CASE B: Flexion and extension lateral radiographs show normal alignment on the extension view but significant anterior translation of the atlas with respect to the dens on the flexion view.

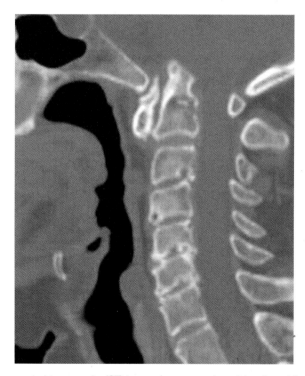

CASE C: Sagittal computed tomography (CT) image shows superior subluxation of the dens through the foramen magnum. Erosive changes also are affecting the dens.

Diagnosis

Case A: Normal anatomy
Case B: Atlantoaxial instability
Case C: Rheumatoid arthritis with cranial settling

Background Summary

Several ligamentous structures secure the atlantoaxial and atlantooccipital (medial and lateral) joints, including the anterior and posterior atlantooccipital ligaments, apical ligament, tectorial membrane, cruciate ligament, and odontoid ligaments (apical and transverse).

Atlantooccipital separation (dissociation or subluxation) results from disruption or laxity of the ligaments between the occiput and atlas. This condition is recognized by widening of the C1-C2 interspinous space, which should measure less than 10 mm, a basion-dens interval of 12 mm or less, and a Power's ratio greater than 1.15. In addition, the occipital condyles should articulate with the lateral masses of C1.

Atlantoaxial separation can result from disruption of the transverse ligament, alar ligament, or tectorial membrane or from fractures of C1 and C2. Atlantoaxial subluxation is defined as an anterior shift of C1 with respect to the dens. The degree of atlantoaxial subluxation can be recognized by a decreased spinal canal diameter and an increased atlantodens interval. On the other hand, atlantoaxial rotatory subluxation and fixation may not necessarily demonstrate an increased atlantodens interval, depending on the subtype. Differentiating between rotatory subluxation and fixation can be accomplished by performing dynamic CT with voluntary head movement. Cranial settling can be considered another form of atlantoaxial subluxation in which there is downward telescoping of the atlas onto the axis body, anterior displacement of the C1 posterior arch, and subsequent ventral and dorsal cervicomedullary compression. In the case of basilar invagination/impression, the C1 arch maintains a relatively normal relationship with C2. In the case of cranial settling, the C1 arch maintains a normal relationship with the occiput, and together the occiput and C1 translate inferiorly upon the remainder of the cervical spine.

As for basilar invagination and platybasia, craniometric parameters are available for quantifying atlantooccipital and atlantoaxial separation. Some of the more common measures are listed and illustrated in Table 34.1. Note that the craniometric references were originally devised for radiographs and CT but can be adapted readily to MRI.

TABLE 34.1	**Craniometric Parameters and Measures**	
Parameter	Description	Schematics on Sagittal MRI
Basion-dens interval	Distance between the inferior tip of the basion to the superior edge of the dens; normally measures <12.5 mm in adults and 8.5 mm in children.	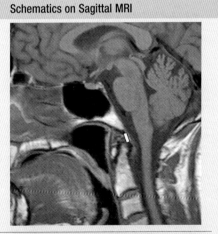
Atlantodens interval	Measured from the posterior margin of the anterior ring of the atlas to the anterior margin of the dens; normally, the atlantodens interval measures <3 mm in adults and 5 mm in children; in turn, a shift of >5 mm suggests the presence of atlantoaxial instability.	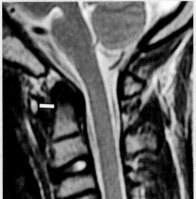

Continued

TABLE 34.1	Craniometric Parameters and Measures—cont'd		
Parameter	**Description**	**Schematics on Sagittal MRI**
Power's ratio	Obtained by dividing the distance between the basion and posterior arch of the atlas *(black line)* by the distance between the opisthion and anterior arch of the atlas *(white line)*; normally, the ratio is <1.0.	
Redlund-Johnell line	Distance between Chamberlain's line and the base of the dens; cranial settling is suggested by <34 mm in male patients and <29 mm in female patients.	

Differential Diagnosis

The patient's history often allows a straightforward diagnosis to be made. Trauma is responsible for the vast majority of cases of atlantooccipital and atlantoaxial separation. Conditions other than trauma to consider are listed in Table 34.2.

Spectrum of Disease

Examples of congenital and acquired manifestations of atlantooccipital and atlantoaxial separation are described and depicted in Table 34.3.

Complications and Treatment

Halo fixation and traction is a relatively well-tolerated option for conservative management of atlantoaxial and atlantooccipital instability. Patients with continued pain or other symptoms may warrant dynamic imaging. Alternatively, craniocervical fusion can be performed, which may consist of atlantoaxial fusion for isolated atlantoaxial instability versus occiput to C2 fusion for atlantoocciput instability or for combined atlantoaxial and atlantoocciput instability. The presence of myelopathy may necessitate decompression, usually via a posterior fossa craniectomy and upper cervical laminectomy. If the patient has associated cervical

TABLE 34.2	Differential Diagnosis of Atlantooccipital Separation and Atlantoaxial Separation	
Finding	**Differential Diagnosis/Etiology**
Atlantooccipital separation	Trauma, Down syndrome, rheumatoid arthritis
Atlantoaxial separation	Trauma, Down syndrome, rheumatoid arthritis, psoriatic arthritis, ankylosing spondylitis, spasmodic torticollis, tumor (chordoma, plasmacytoma), crystal deposition disease (calcium pyrophosphate dihydrate deposition, gout), infection (tonsillitis, pharyngitis)

TABLE 34.3	Spectrum of Disease	
Condition	**Findings**	**Images**
Down syndrome Clues: Diagnosis is typically already evident; radiographic cervical spine evaluation may be performed to screen for nontraumatic atlantooccipital and atlantoaxial instability and to prevent neurologic injury during athletic competitions.	Sagittal T1 MRI shows mild atlantooccipital and atlantoaxial separation, which results in narrowing of the foramen magnum.	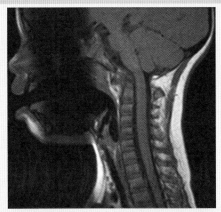
	3D CT surface rendering shows fusion anomaly of the anterior arch of C1 *(arrows)*.	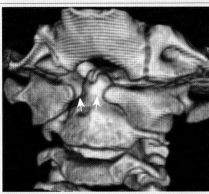
Spontaneous atlantoaxial rotatory fixation clues: Imaging is pathognomonic; 3D CT renderings are most helpful for delineating the relationship of C1 with C2; dynamic imaging helps differentiate subluxation, which is reversible, from fixation, which does not change significantly.	3D CT surface renderings show rotation of the atlas with respect to C2 in the transverse plane, such that the superior articular facets of C2 *(arrows)* do not articulate with the inferior articular facets of C1 *(arrowheads)*.	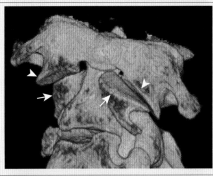
	3D CT surface rendering shows the angle formed between the line that traverses the lateral masses of C1 *(green)* and the line that traverses the lateral masses of C2 *(blue)*.	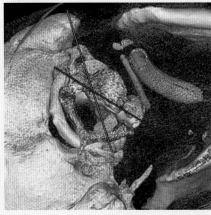

Continued

TABLE 34.3 Spectrum of Disease—cont'd

Condition	Findings	Images
Traumatic atlantooccipital separation Clues: The craniometric aberrations and history are specific; associated severe spinal cord, brainstem, and ligamentous injuries are almost always present; MRI is recommended for evaluating the extent of these injuries.	Sagittal CT image shows widening of the basion-dens interval *(arrows)* and the C1-C2 interspinous space; the patient is intubated.	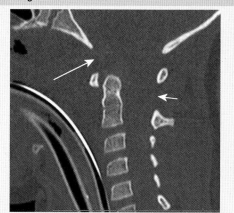
	Sagittal T2 MRI shows extensive high signal in the brainstem and cervical spinal cord *(arrowheads)*; edema is also present in the paraspinal soft tissues.	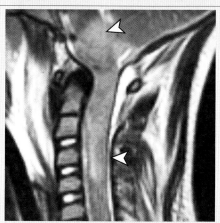
Chordoma Clues: The finding of a midline high T2 signal-enhancing mass with lobulated margins and surrounding bone destruction; there is a predilection for the clivus and upper cervical spine; the mass can disrupt the atlantoaxial ligaments and result in cord compression.	Sagittal T1 MRI with contrast shows a heterogeneously enhancing mass in the dens *(arrow)* with associated mild widening of the anterior atlantodens interval and severe spinal canal narrowing with compression of the spinal cord.	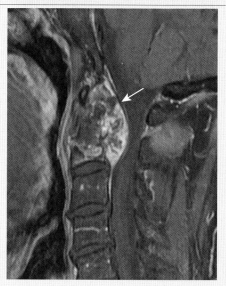

TABLE 34.3   Spectrum of Disease—cont'd

Condition	Findings	Images
	Axial T2 MRI shows that the lesion is lobulated and has a high signal, which is characteristic of a chordoma.	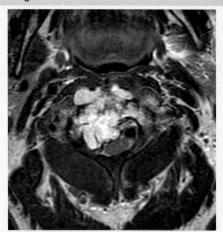
Achondroplasia Clues: • Frontal bossing • Hypoplastic dens and clivus with narrow foramen magnum • Squared contours of the iliac wings have a "tombstone" appearance • Progressive decrease in the lumbar spine interpedicular distance from superior to inferior with spinal stenosis • Posterior scalloping of the vertebral bodies • Short limbs	Sagittal T1 MRI of the head shows frontal bossing *(arrow)*, a short, vertical clivus *(white arrowhead)*, and a hypoplastic dens *(black arrowhead)*, resulting in apparent atlantooccipital separation; in addition, foramen magnum stenosis is present.	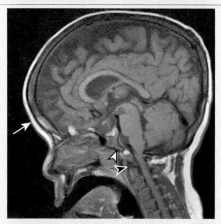
	Sagittal T2 MRI of the lumbar spine shows multilevel scalloping of the posterior vertebral bodies and severe spinal stenosis.	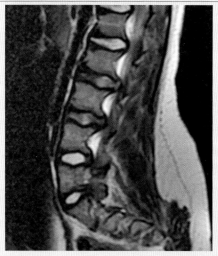

CT, Computed tomography; *MRI,* magnetic resonance imaging.

spine fractures in the setting of traumatic instability, these fractures may be treated via open reduction and internal fixation.

Pearls

- The role of imaging in cases of atlantooccipital and atlantoaxial separation is geared mainly toward evaluating the severity of associated lesions rather than making a diagnosis, which is usually evident at presentation.
- MRI is the modality of choice for evaluating spinal cord and ligamentous involvement, while CT is well suited for identifying associated fractures.
- Atlantooccipital and atlantoaxial separation are processes that occur in three or even four dimensions, and thus three-dimensional, maximum intensity projection, and dynamic imaging are useful for comprehensive assessment.
- As always, flexion/extension views and other forms of dynamic imaging should be performed voluntarily and cautiously.

Suggested Readings

Bertozzi JC, Rojas CA, Martinez CR: Evaluation of the pediatric craniocervical junction on MDCT, *AJR Am J Roentgenol* 192(1):26–31, 2009.

Chang W, Alexander MT, Mirvis SE: Diagnostic determinants of craniocervical distraction injury in adults, *AJR Am J Roentgenol* 192(1): 52–58, 2009.

Hankinson TC, Anderson RC: Craniovertebral junction abnormalities in Down syndrome, *Neurosurgery* 66(suppl 3):32–38, 2010.

Pang D: Atlantoaxial rotatory fixation, *Neurosurgery* 66(suppl 3): 161–183, 2010.

Stiskal MA, Neuhold A, Szolar DB, et al: Rheumatoid arthritis of the craniocervical region by MR imaging: detection and characterization, *AJR Am J Roentgenol* 165:585–592, 1995.

35

Basilar Invagination and Platybasia

DANIEL THOMAS GINAT, MD

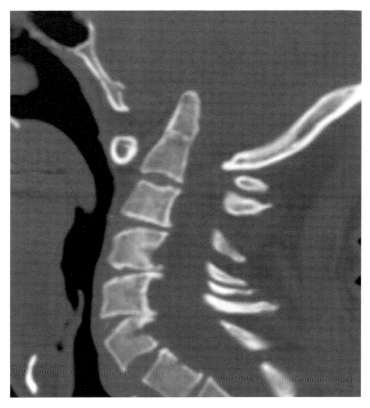

CASE A: Sagittal computed tomography image shows severe superior migration of the dens across the foramen magnum. There is also exaggerated cervical spine lordosis.

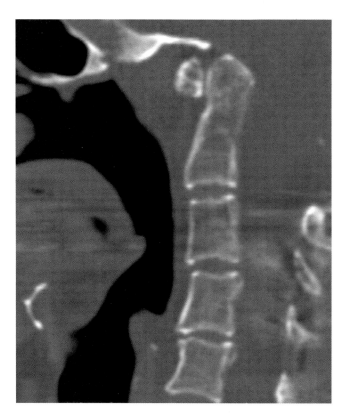

CASE B: Sagittal computed tomography image shows a nearly horizontal configuration of the clivus. In addition, the dens and atlas are positioned far superior to the level of Chamberlain's line. There is also diffuse osteopenia.

Diagnosis

Case A: Basilar invagination
Case B: Platybasia

Background Summary

Basilar invagination is a condition in which the margin of the foramen magnum and upper cervical spine is translated superiorly into the skull base. Primary basilar invagination is a congenital condition. Secondary basilar invagination, or basilar impression, is acquired and often is associated with conditions that result in softening of the skull base.

Platybasia refers to flattening of the skull base, whereby there is an increased basal angle. The clivus assumes a more horizontal orientation than normal. Although platybasia can occur in isolation, it often coexists with basilar invagination.

Several craniometric parameters have been devised to help characterize craniovertebral junction anatomy. Some of the more commonly used measurements are listed and depicted in Table 35.1. Nevertheless, a qualitative assessment is often adequate for characterizing the abnormality.

Because basilar invagination and platybasia are findings, not diagnoses, it is important to search for associated abnormalities to establish a diagnosis (Table 35.2). Familiarity with the embryology and subsequent normal development of the craniovertebral junction can help in the understanding of the imaging appearance of congenital anomalies in this region. For example, the basiocciput, which is separated from the basisphenoid by the sphenooccipital synchondrosis, is derived from fusion of the first four sclerotomes. Failure of the last sclerotome to fuse leads to condylus tertius, whereas underdevelopment of the sclerotomes leads to condylar or basiocciput hypoplasia.

Spectrum of Disease

A wide variety of unrelated conditions can present with basilar invagination and/or platybasia. However, additional findings on the imaging study itself often are present and can

TABLE 35.1	Craniometric Parameters/Measures for Craniovertebral Junction Anatomy	
Parameter	**Description**	**Schematics With Sagittal T1-Weighted MRI**
McRae's line	Extends from the basion to the opisthion, essentially demarcating the foramen magnum, the diameter of which should measure ≥35 mm.	
Chamberlain's line	Extends from the posterior margin of the hard palate to the opisthion; the maximum distance that the odontoid should project above this line ranges from 1 mm ± 3.6–6.6 mm.	

Continued

TABLE 35.1	**Craniometric Parameters/Measures for Craniovertebral Junction Anatomy—cont'd**	
Parameter	**Description**	**Schematics With Sagittal T1-Weighted MRI**
McGregor's line	Line drawn from the posterior margin of the hard palate to the most inferior surface of the occipital bone; the tip of the odontoid should not project more than 4.5 mm above this line.	
Wackenheim's line	Line drawn along the posterior surface of the clivus and extrapolated inferiorly to the upper cervical spine level; normally the line runs tangential to the posterior aspect of the tip of the dens.	
Welcher basal angle	Formed by the intersection of lines drawn from the nasion to the tuberculum sella and from the tuberculum sella to the basion; normally <140 degrees.	

TABLE 35.1	Craniometric Parameters/Measures for Craniovertebral Junction Anatomy—cont'd	
Parameter	**Description**	**Schematics With Sagittal T1-Weighted MRI**
Clivus canal angle	Formed by the intersection of Wackenheim's line and a line prescribed along the posterior aspect of the dens and axis body; normal measurements range between 150 and 180 degrees.	

TABLE 35.2	Differential Diagnosis for Basilar Invagination, Basilar Impression, and Platybasia
Finding	**Differential Diagnosis/Etiology**
Basilar invagination	Congenital occiput anomalies (condylus tertius, condylar hypoplasia, basiocciput hypoplasia, and atlantooccipital assimilation), Arnold–Chiari malformation, craniocleidodysostosis
Basilar impression	Hyperparathyroidism, osteogenesis imperfecta, Hurler syndrome, rickets
Platybasia	Congenital craniofacial anomalies, condylus tertius, osteogenesis imperfecta, craniocleidodysostosis, Down syndrome, Arnold–Chiari malformation, Paget disease, osteomalacia, rickets, trauma

suggest a diagnosis or can at least help narrow the differential diagnosis. In addition, imaging studies of other parts of the body may provide helpful clues. Selected examples of how secondary findings can be useful are described and depicted in Table 35.3.

Complications and Treatment

Basilar invagination and platybasia can result in serious complications, such as canal stenosis and cord compression, which can manifest as motor and sensory deficits, brainstem and lower cranial nerve dysfunction, and vascular compromise. Imaging plays an important role in evaluating patients who present with these complications. In particular, MRI is the study of choice for evaluating the status of the spinal cord. This modality also is well suited for delineating the bony anatomy. CT can be complementary to MRI in indeterminate cases. When patients present with neurologic compromise, intervention is warranted, and imaging should not be delayed. Treatment ranges from application of traction devices to surgical occipitocervical decompression (odontoidectomy and laminectomy) and fusion.

Pearls

- Radiographs, CT, and MRI all have roles in evaluating the craniovertebral junction. MRI is particularly useful for assessing cord compression, which is a surgical emergency.
- The first step in the interpretation of abnormal craniometry of the craniovertebral junction region is to decide whether it is congenital or acquired because this differentiation helps focus the differential diagnosis and course of treatment.
- Identifying associated findings can help narrow the differential imaging diagnosis further or even establish the diagnosis, if it is not already known. Clinical parameters such as the patient's age, history, physical examination findings, and laboratory test results often are helpful as well.
- Conditions that produce softening of the bone predispose to basilar impression and platybasia, whereas conditions that produce ligamentous laxity predispose to atlantoaxial and atlantooccipital separation.
- Although atlas and axis anomalies usually are not associated with basilar invagination, these lesions can result in instability and can be clinically significant, especially if they are a component of a syndrome.

TABLE 35.3 **Spectrum of Disease**

Arnold–Chiari malformation type I
Clues:

- Low-lying/ectopic cerebellar tonsils (>5 mm below the foramen magnum)
- Syringohydromyelia (usually in the cervical spinal cord); often has a "string of sausage" appearance
- Vertebral fusion anomalies such as atlantooccipital assimilation

Sagittal CT image shows atlantooccipital assimilation and considerable basilar invagination; evidence of posterior fossa decompression is seen, including resection of the posterior arch of C1.

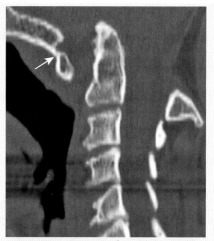

Sagittal T2 MRI also shows basilar invagination but reveals severe indentation of the cervicomedullary junction and syringohydromyelia *(arrows)*; assimilation of the anterior arch of C1 with the basiocciput and sequelae of decompression surgery are again noted.

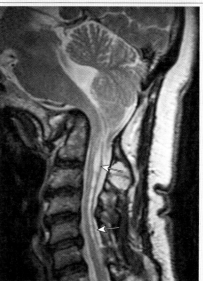

Mucopolysaccharidosis
Clues:

- Findings differ based on the specific type of mucopolysac-charidosis
- The constellation of imaging findings throughout the body in conjunction with clinical param-eters establish the diagnosis

Sagittal CT image shows platybasia; macrocephaly also is present.

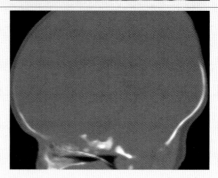

TABLE 35.3 Spectrum of Disease—cont'd

Axial FLAIR MRI shows extensive confluent bilateral white matter signal abnormality, as well as prominent Virchow-Robin spaces; ventricular dilation also is present.

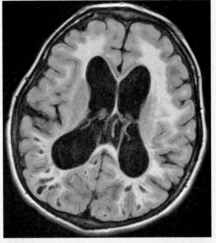

Lateral radiograph of the spine shows a hypoplastic L1 vertebra with inferior beaking *(arrow)* and associated gibbus deformity (focal kyphosis).

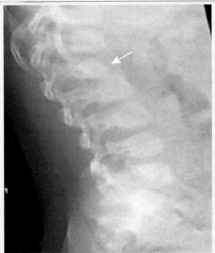

Klippel–Feil syndrome
Clues: Fusion of one or more cervical spine vertebral segments; sometimes the thoracic and lumbar spine also are involved; an omovertebral bone is variably present that extends from the scapula to the posterior elements of a cervical vertebra; patients may have a low hairline and Sprengel deformity

Sagittal T2 MRI shows C4–C5 fusion with "wasp waist" configuration *(arrow)* and at least partial atlantooccipital assimilation and mild basilar invagination.

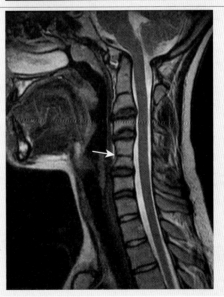

Continued

<table>
<tr><td>TABLE
35.3</td><td>**Spectrum of Disease—cont'd**</td></tr>
</table>

Axial CT image in a different patient shows Sprengel deformity on the left side with a high-riding scapula; an omovertebral bone also is noted *(arrow)*.

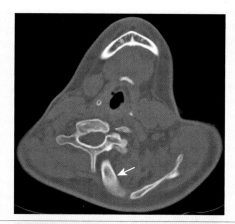

Paget disease
Clues:
- Elderly patient
- May have lucent lesions, such as "blade of grass" appearance in long bones or osteoporosis circumscripta in the skull, mixed sclerotic and lytic areas, such as "cotton wool" appearance in the skull, or sclerotic areas
- Although appearance is variable, the presence of an expanded medullary space and a thickened cortex is highly suggestive

Sagittal T1 MRI shows basilar impression and platybasia; thickening of the calvarium and heterogeneous bone marrow also is apparent.

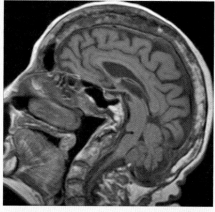

Axial CT image shows circumferential expansion of the calvarium with numerous lucent and sclerotic areas, which produces a characteristic "cotton wool" appearance.

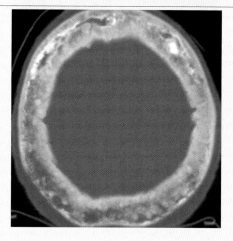

CT, computed tomography; *MRI,* magnetic resonance imaging.

Suggested Readings

Klimo P Jr., Rao G, Brockmeyer D: Congenital anomalies of the cervical spine, *Neurosurg Clin N Am* 18(3):463–478, 2007.

Koenigsberg RA, Vakil N, Hong TA, et al: Evaluation of platybasia with MR imaging, *AJNR Am J Neuroradiol* 26(1):89–92, 2005.

Rojas CA, Bertozzi JC, Martinez CR, et al: Reassessment of the craniocervical junction: normal values on CT, *AJNR Am J Neuroradiol* 28(9):1819–1823, 2007.

Smith JS, Shaffrey CI, Abel MF, et al: Basilar invagination, *Neurosurgery* 66(3 suppl):39–47, 2010.

Smoker WR: Craniovertebral junction: normal anatomy, craniometry, and congenital anomalies, *Radiographics* 14(2):255–277, 1994.

Smoker WR: MR imaging of the craniovertebral junction, *Magn Reson Imaging Clin N Am* 8(3):635–650, 2000.

Siddiqui A, Connor SEJ: Imaging of developmental skull base abnormalities, *Neuroimaging Clin N Am* 31(4):621–647, 2021.

36

Focal Cord Deformities

DANIEL HILL, MD

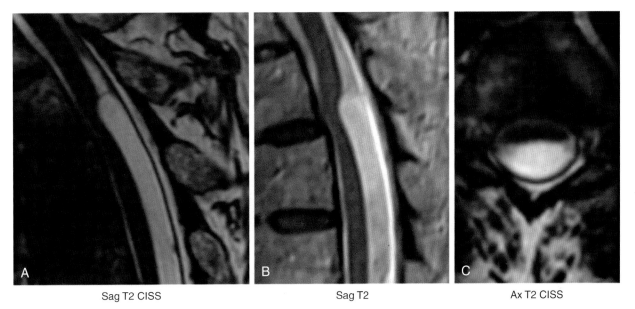

| Sag T2 CISS | Sag T2 | Ax T2 CISS |

CASE A: An 82-year-old who presents with back pain. *Ax*, Axial; *CISS*, constructive interference in steady state; *Sag*, sagittal.

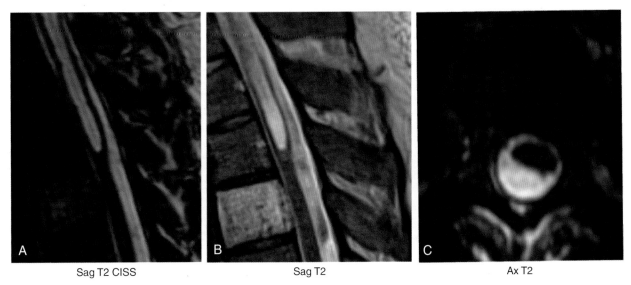

| Sag T2 CISS | Sag T2 | Ax T2 |

CASE B: A 24-year-old who presents with right upper extremity numbness. *Ax*, Axial; *CISS*, constructive interference in steady state; *Sag*, sagittal.

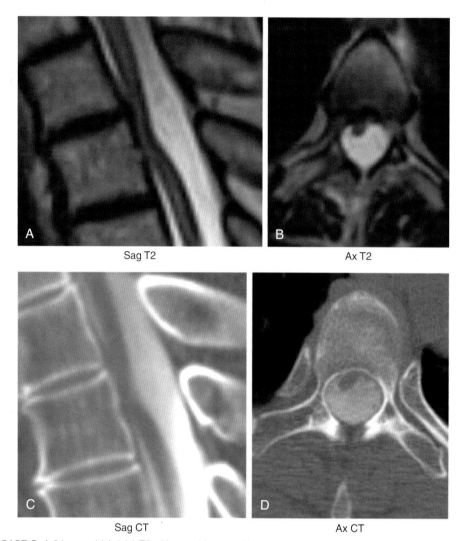

A Sag T2

B Ax T2

C Sag CT

D Ax CT

CASE C: A 64-year-old Axial A T2 with several years of bilateral lower extremity numbness and progressive left lower extremity weakness. *Ax*, Axial; *CT*, Computed tomography; *Sag*, sagittal.

DESCRIPTION OF FINDINGS

CT and MR images from three patients with focal cord deformity.
- Case A: There is dorsal thoracic cord scalloping at the T2–T3 level. The cord is deviated ventrally with homogenous signal widening of the dorsal subarachnoid space. A high-resolution thin-section MR sequence reveals a membrane in the dorsal cerebrospinal fluid (CSF) space most apparent along the superior margin at the site of cord deformity, less well seen on the conventional T2-weighted sequence.
- Case B: There is dorsal thoracic cord flattening at the T3 level, most apparent on the axial images, where the cord is deviated ventrally and to the left. CSF pulsation artifact within the dorsal subarachnoid space is present. A proximal syrinx is partially visualized. An incidental intraosseous hemangioma is present at T4.
- Case C: There is dorsal cord deformity at the upper T4 level with complete effacement of the ventral CSF space. At the apex of the cord deformity, there is suggestion of cord tissue extending beyond the dura into the ventral epidural space.

Diagnosis

Case A: Spinal arachnoid cyst
Case B: Spinal arachnoid web
Case C: Ventral cord herniation

Summary

Focal cord deformity describes the spinal cord morphology resulting from spinal arachnoid cyst, spinal arachnoid web, or cord herniation. These entities most commonly result in short-segment dorsal cord deformity at the mid-thoracic level, with widening of the dorsal subarachnoid space.

A spinal arachnoid cyst represents an extramedullary (intradural or extradural) CSF-filled collection that scallops the spinal cord. These cysts are usually circumscribed, although a cyst membrane is not always visualized on conventional MR sequences. These cysts replace the subarachnoid space with attenuated CSF pulsation artifact on MR. On CT myelogram, there is often differential, slower contrast filling of the arachnoid cyst, although in the setting of wide cyst to subarachnoid space communication there may be near identical filling. Osseous remodeling may also be present.

Arachnoid webs are comprised of thickened arachnoid tissue, possibly due to a remnant cyst. Typically, these webs are not directly visualized on imaging, and secondary imaging features should be recognized. The "scalpel sign" describes a characteristic spinal cord morphology in the sagittal plane. The dorsal cord contour resembles the edge of a surgical scalpel with widening of the dorsal subarachnoid space and relative presentation ventrally.

Spinal cord herniation is a transdural protrusion of the spinal cord into the epidural space, usually posttraumatic, postsurgical, or idiopathic. This is sometimes directly visualized as extradural cord tissue, best seen on high-resolution thin-section MR sequence or CT myelogram. In all cases, there is complete interruption of the CSF space at the site of herniation. The cord contour has been described as "C-shaped". The "nuclear trail sign" has been associated with this entity. This describes linear osseous high-density representing

calcification from prior disk herniation, thought to represent the precursor to a dural defect.

As there is substantial imaging overlap of these entities, misdiagnosis is common. This is further compounded as these diagnoses are often not directly visualized and diagnosis may rely on secondary findings. As such, the imaging approach should be focused on identifying differentiating features.

In nearly all scenarios, acquisition of a high-resolution thin-section MR sequence may enhance direct visualization of the underlying pathology. Similarly, CT myelogram may confirm a space-occupying lesion and provide further detail on the subarachnoid space. An intact ventral subarachnoid space can reliably exclude cord herniation. Alternatively, when cord mass effect is great enough with arachnoid cyst or web, the ventral subarachnoid space may be completely effaced, mimicking cord herniation. Attenuated dorsal CSF pulsation artifact would favor arachnoid cyst, while accentuated CSF pulsation can be seen with arachnoid web. Phase contrast/CSF flow sequence may show disrupted dynamics ventrally or dorsally in the setting of cord herniation or arachnoid web, respectively.

Spectrum of Disease

Associated cord signal abnormality has been documented with arachnoid web and cord herniation, usually not observed with arachnoid cysts. Spinal cord syrinx is most often associated with arachnoid web.

Differential Diagnosis

1. Spinal arachnoid cyst
2. Spinal arachnoid web
3. Cord herniation
4. Dural ectasia
5. Spinal epidermoid cyst

Pearls

- Focal cord deformities are usually at the dorsal mid-thoracic level from spinal arachnoid cyst, spinal arachnoid web, and cord herniation.
- High-resolution thin-section MR sequence and CT myelogram may enhance visualization of a cyst membrane, web, or herniated cord.
- Characteristics of the subarachnoid space and shape of cord deformity may provide diagnostic information.
- Arachnoid cyst replaces the subarachnoid space with attenuated CSF pulsation artifact.
- "Scalpel Sign" is associated with arachnoid web.
- Cord herniation completely interrupts the ventral subarachnoid space.

Signs and Complications

There are no specific clinical features that can distinguish these pathologies. Frequent presenting symptoms include sensory or motor abnormalities and pain, although patients may be asymptomatic as well. Brown–Séquard Syndrome is most closely associated with cord herniation, present in over 50% of cases. Severity of symptoms dictates treatment, which is most typically surgical.

Suggested Readings

Brugières P, Malapert D, Adle-Biassette H, et al: Idiopathic spinal cord herniation value of MR phase contrast imaging, *AJNR Am J Neuroradiol* 20(5): 935–939, 1999.

Haber MD, Nguyen DD, Li S: Differentiation of idiopathic spinal cord herniation from CSF-isointense intraspinal extramedullary lesions displacing the cord, *Radiographics* 34(2):313–329, 2014.

Nada A, Mahdi E, Mahmoud E, et al. Multi-modality imaging evaluation of the dorsal arachnoid web, *Neuroradiol J* 33(6):508–516, 2020.

Parmar H, Park P, Brahma B, et al: Imaging of idiopathic spinal cord herniation. *Radiographics* 28(2):511–518, 2008.

Patel DM, Weinberg BD, Hoch MJ: CT myelography: clinical indications and imaging findings, *Radiographics* 40(2):470–484, 2020.

Schultz R Jr., Steven A, Wessell A, et al. Differentiation of idiopathic spinal cord herniation from dorsal arachnoid webs on MRI and CT myelography, *J Neurosurg Spine* 26(6):754–759, 2017.

37

Spinal Cord Metabolic/Demyelinating Processes

NATHAN M. COLEMAN, MD

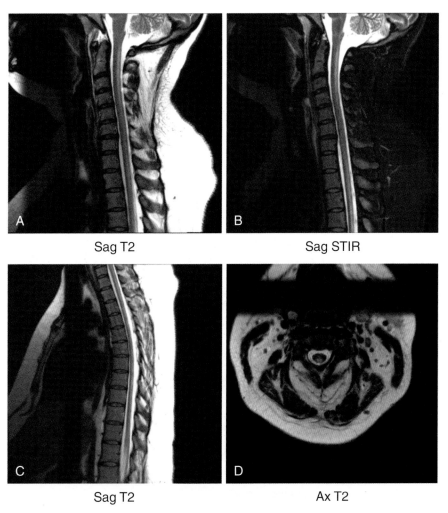

Sag T2

Sag STIR

Sag T2

Ax T2

CASE A: A 30-year-old with several months of numbness and altered temperature sensation in her face and extremities. *Ax,* Axial; *Sag,* sagittal; *STIR,* short tau inversion recovery.

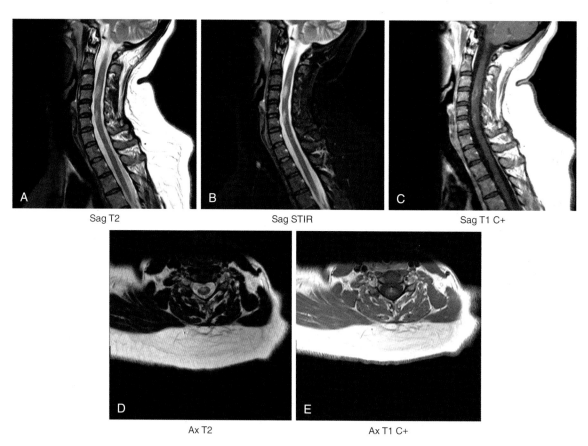

Sag T2   Sag STIR   Sag T1 C+

Ax T2   Ax T1 C+

CASE B: A 37-year-old who presents with multiple waxing and waning neurologic deficits. *Ax,* Axial; *Sag,* sagittal; *STIR,* short tau inversion recovery.

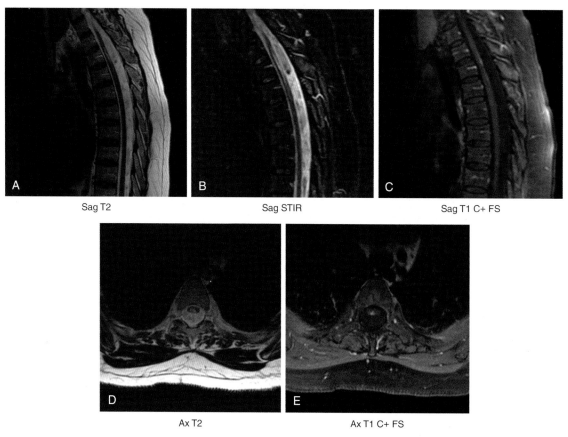

Sag T2   Sag STIR   Sag T1 C+ FS

Ax T2   Ax T1 C+ FS

CASE C: A 55-year-old with subacute onset of lower extremity myelopathic pain, paresthesias, and weakness. Also with subjective intermittent visual changes. *Ax,* Axial; *Sag,* sagittal; *STIR,* short tau inversion recovery.

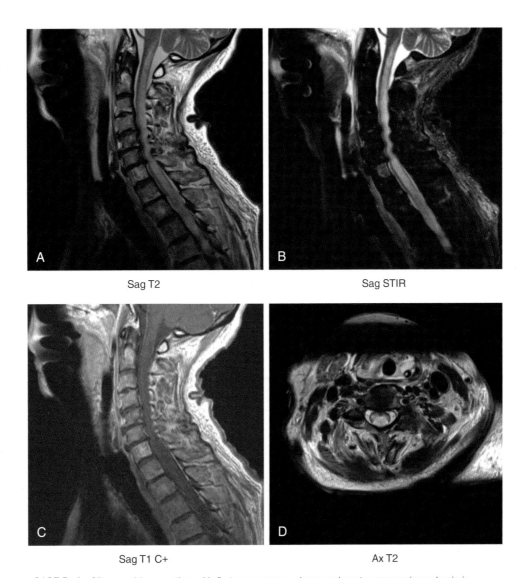

Sag T2

Sag STIR

Sag T1 C+

Ax T2

CASE D: An 80-year-old presenting with first occurrence seizure and acute progressive aphasia in setting of more subacute migrating extremity paresthesias and unintentional weight loss/B symptoms. *Ax,* Axial; *Sag,* sagittal; *STIR,* short tau inversion recovery.

DESCRIPTION OF FINDINGS

MR images from four patients with lesions affecting the spinal cord.
- Case A: There is smooth, longitudinally extensive, nonenhancing T2 and short T1 inversion recovery (STIR) signal hyperintensity of the dorsal columns. Note the lack of expansion or mass effect. This extends nearly the entire length of the cord and appears symmetric on axial images.
- Case B: There are patchy, short-segment T2/STIR hyperintense intramedullary lesions, which appear mildly expansile. While they appear relatively central in location, there is no clear pattern of distribution, and they may be eccentric, unilateral, or symmetric. Several demonstrate at least some degree of enhancement.
- Case C: There is smooth, intermediate length, T2/STIR hyperintensity within the dorsal thoracic cord. There are scattered foci of enhancement within the greater area of signal abnormality.
- Case D: There is markedly expansile, longitudinally extensive T2/STIR hyperintensity and patchy enhancement involving the majority of the cross-sectional area of the cord on axial images.

Diagnosis

Case A: Subacute combined degeneration (SCD)
Case B: Multiple sclerosis (MS) with active demyelination
Case C: Neuromyelitis optica spectrum disorder (NMO/NMOSD)
Case D: Longitudinally extensive transverse myelitis (LETM), potentially idiopathic acute transverse myelitis

Summary

When demyelinating or metabolic diseases of the spinal cord are suspected, an early and important imaging distinction is whether the lesion(s) is/are longitudinally extensive. Some disease processes, particularly MS, characteristically demonstrate "short-segment" involvement of the spinal cord, commonly estimated at less than three contiguous vertebral bodies in length for a single lesion. This contrasts with other processes such as NMO/NMOSD, acute disseminated encephalomyelitis (ADEM), myelin oligodendrocyte glycoprotein antibody—associated disease (MOGAD or anti-MOG), SCD, or other causes of transverse myelitis. While there are clinical similarities among these entities, they are pathologically distinct.

SCD is a chronic sequela of cobalamin (B12) deficiency resulting in demyelination. The primary imaging finding is long-segment T2/STIR signal hyperintensity, most commonly involving the dorsal and sometimes lateral columns of the spinal cord. There is generally little to no enhancement. Cerebral white matter changes may also be present. Clinically it manifests as loss of proprioception and vibratory sensation in the extremities. This may eventually progress to extremity weakness, ataxia, and gait difficulty. Importantly, any etiology of B12 deficiency can lead to SCD. This includes pernicious anemia, Crohn disease or other terminal ileitis (the terminal ileum is the primary site of absorption), proton pump inhibitor use, gastric surgery, celiac disease, nitrous oxide abuse, and methotrexate use. Other metabolic derangements, including copper deficiency or vitamin E deficiency, can have an identical imaging and clinical presentation. HIV-related myelopathy

and other atypical infectious process such as neurosyphilis should also be considered.

MS is an acquired demyelinating disease involving the central nervous system, characteristically disseminated in both space (multiple lesions) and time (different lesions manifest at different times). This is mediated by an autoimmune response to myelin components, with resultant oligodendrocyte loss and, eventually, gliosis/axonal degeneration. On spine magnetic resonance imaging (MRI), typical acute demyelinating presents with T2/STIR hyperintensity, which is often somewhat expansile. Some degree of enhancement is typically present, although it may be patchy or incomplete. Occasionally, reduced diffusivity may be present within the lesion. Chronic lesions generally retain the hyperintense T2/STIR signal but may demonstrate local volume loss. Enhancement should not be evident in chronic demyelination. Lesions are often characterized as either acute/active stage (active demyelination typically with enhancement on imaging), subacute stage (abundant macrophages), and chronic stage (gliosis and parenchymal volume loss). When involvement of the spinal cord is present, patients may present with extremity sensory loss, paresthesias, upper motor neuron signs, and urinary incontinence. CSF testing for oligoclonal bands can be helpful in confirming the diagnosis, particularly in the instance of clinically isolated syndrome.

NMO, or more appropriately NMOSD, was at one time considered to be a variant of MS, but has since been reclassified as its own entity. Specifically, NMOSD is an autoimmune process mediated by antibodies to the aquaporin-4 transporter (AQP4). The classic triad of NMOSD includes optic neuritis, LETM, and positive anti-AQP4 antibody. However, patients may not present with all of these manifestations, or may have additional clinical and imaging findings. MRI findings of the spine commonly include LETM and some degree of cord edema; however, short-segment myelitis may be present in a minority of cases. Lesions are T2/STIR hyperintense, in some cases with superimposed "bright spotty lesions" of hyperintense signal. There are varying degrees of enhancement, including ring enhancement in some instances, and depending on the acuity of imaging. Similar to MS, chronic demyelinating foci are nonenhancing and may exhibit some degree of volume loss. Patients generally present at slightly older age compared to MS and are more predominantly female. If there is a question of NMO in a young, male patient, MOGAD or anti-MOG should be considered as an alternative diagnosis.

LETM is not so much a diagnosis as it is a manifestation of any number of underlying etiologies. Cases without a clearly identifiable cause are sometimes referred to as idiopathic acute transverse myelitis. Generally, an intramedullary lesion is considered "longitudinally extensive" when the craniocaudal extent is greater than three contiguous vertebral bodies. MRI findings generally include expansive T2/STIR hyperintense lesions, which may demonstrate variable enhancement. Hemorrhage is not typically seen and should raise concern for other underlying processes, such as a vascular lesion, neoplasm, or trauma. As mentioned, LETM can be an imaging finding related to NMOSD. Other autoimmune demyelinating and inflammatory processes, such as acute disseminated encephalomyelitis (ADEM), MOGAD or anti-MOG, neurosarcoid, and systemic lupus erythematosus (SLE) are included in this differential. However, acute atypical infection (viral or fungal), cord infarct, paraneoplastic syndrome, or intramedullary neoplasm all may demonstrate a similar imaging appearance. Hence, the role of the imaging interpreter in this instance is to synthesize the imaging findings with available clinical information to propose potential etiologies for the imaging findings.

Spectrum of Disease

There is a great degree of overlap in the imaging presentation of the various demyelinating and metabolic derangements that can afflict the spinal cord. Constructing a differential diagnosis based on characterizing features or patterns is key for the interpreting clinician, and in many cases, a definitive diagnosis will only be made in conjunction with other clinical testing. Particularly, these processes may be challenging to differentiate from other inflammatory (neurosarcoid), infectious (HIV-related myelopathy, neurosyphilis), or even neoplastic disease of the cord. Mass effect is an insufficient finding to suggest underlying neoplasm, as acute demyelinating lesions are often somewhat expansile in appearance due to local cord edema.

Differential Diagnosis

1. MS
2. NMOSD
3. SCD
4. Anti-MOG–related disease
5. ADEM
6. Idiopathic acute transverse myelitis
7. Neurosarcoid
8. Neuro-Behçet
9. Cord infarct
10. Atypical infection
11. Methotrexate toxicity
12. Paraneoplastic syndrome

Pearls

- Use all the available clinical information to help formulate a differential diagnosis. Imaging findings for demyelinating disease of the spine are often nonspecific.

- Longitudinally extensive cord signal abnormality confined to the dorsal columns is highly suggestive of SCD and should prompt assessment for underlying metabolic derangements.
- Short-segment lesions help to differentiate MS from other demyelinating diseases of the spine.
- Enhancement suggests active demyelination.
- Lack of enhancement and volume loss suggests a chronic lesion.
- NMO has a slightly older average age of presentation compared to MS, and even greater female predilection. There may also be preferential involvement of the central rather than peripheral cord.
- Idiopathic acute transverse myelitis is exceedingly rare; however, LETM is a more commonly seen fulminant manifestation of a wide variety of demyelinating, inflammatory, and even infectious conditions.

Suggested Readings

Chee CG, Park KS, Lee JW, et al: MRI features of aquaporin-4 antibody-positive longitudinally extensive transverse myelitis: insights into the diagnosis of neuromyelitis optica spectrum disorders, *AJNR Am J Neuroradiol* 39(4):782–787, 2018.

Goodman BP, Chong BW, Patel AC, et al: Copper deficiency myeloneuropathy resembling B12 deficiency: partial resolution of MR imaging findings with copper supplementation, *AJNR Am J Neuroradiol* 27(10):2112–2114, 2006.

Jain RS, Kumar S, Mathur T, et al: Longitudinally extensive transverse myelitis: a retrospective analysis of sixty-four patients at tertiary care center of North-West India, *Clin Neurol Neurosurg* 148:5–12, 2016.

Kitley J, Waters P, Woodhall M, et al: Neuromyelitis optica spectrum disorders with aquaporin-4 and myelin-oligodendrocyte glycoprotein antibodies: a comparative study, *JAMA Neurol* 71(3):276–283, 2014.

Lee MJ, Aronberg R, Manganaro MS, et al: Diagnostic approach to intrinsic abnormality of spinal cord signal intensity, *Radiographics* 39(6):1824–1839, 2019.

Ravina B, Loevner LA, Bank W: MR findings in subacute combined degeneration of the spinal cord: a case of reversible cervical myelopathy, *AJR Am J Roentgenol* 174(3):863–865, 2000.

Thompson AJ, Banwell BL, Barkhof F, et al: Diagnosis of multiple sclerosis: 2017 revisions of the McDonald criteria, *Lancet Neurol* 17(2):162–173, 2018.

38

Enhancing Intramedullary Spinal Cord Lesions

JUAN E. SMALL, MD, MSC AND HENRY SU, MD, PHD

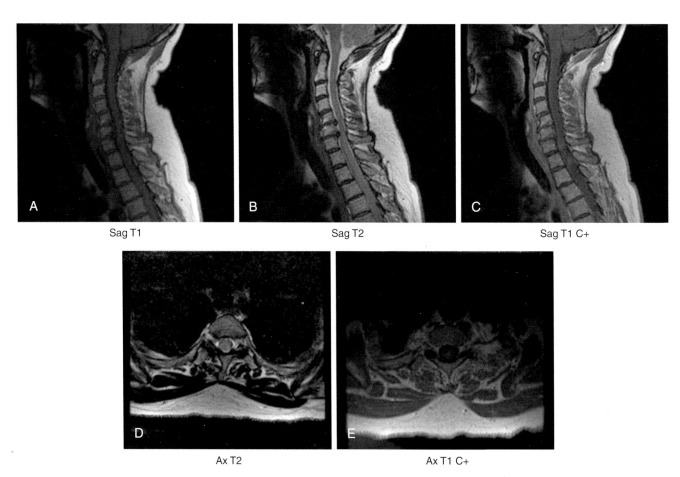

Sag T1   Sag T2   Sag T1 C+

Ax T2   Ax T1 C+

CASE A: A 60-year-old presenting with progressive lower extremity numbness. *Ax,* Axial; *Sag,* sagittal.

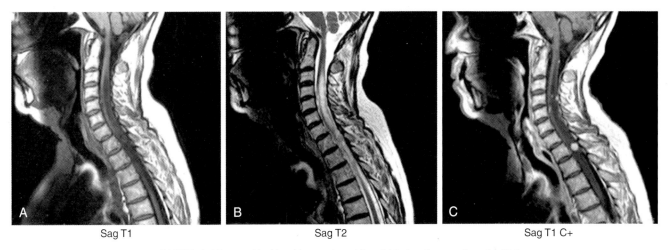

Sag T1   Sag T2   Sag T1 C+

CASE B: A 64-year-old with a history of von Hippel–Lindau disease. *Sag,* Sagittal.

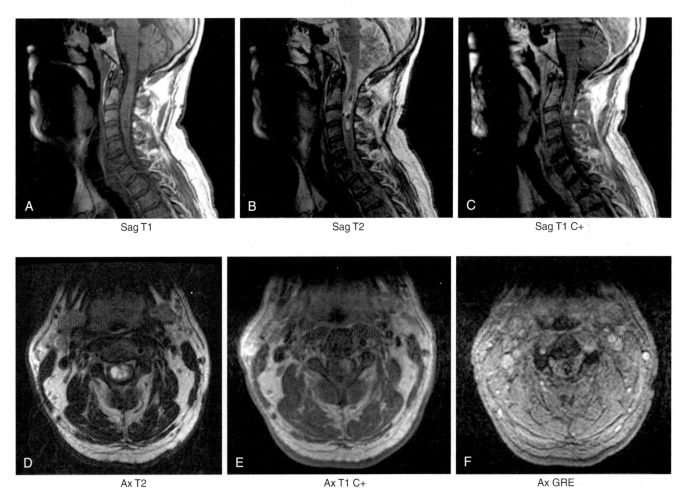

Sag T1   Sag T2   Sag T1 C+

Ax T2   Ax T1 C+   Ax GRE

CASE C: A 47-year-old with a 1-year history of gradually progressive neck and hand pain and pain radiating into his arms. *Ax,* Axial; *GRE,* gradient refocused echo; *Sag,* sagittal.

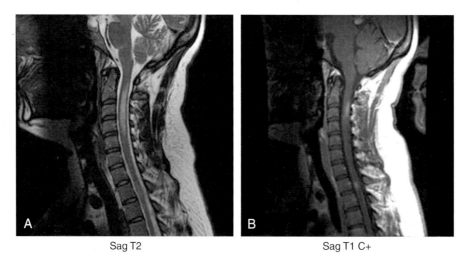

A — Sag T1

B — Sag T2

C — Sag T1 FS C+

D — Brain Ax T1 C+

CASE D: A 46-year-old with metastatic cervical cancer. *Ax,* Axial; *FS,* frequency shifted; *Sag,* sagittal.

A — Sag T2

B — Sag T1 C+

CASE E: A 29-year-old with systemic lupus erythematosus presenting with left arm pain. *Sag,* Sagittal.

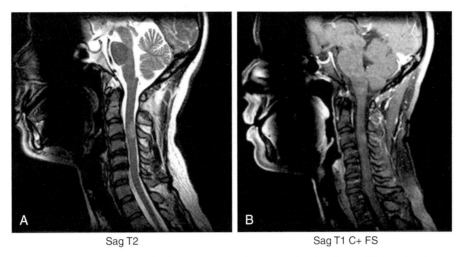

| Sag T2 | Sag T1 C+ FS |

CASE F: A 39-year-old presenting with numbness, weakness, and unsteadiness. *FS,* fat saturated; *Sag,* sagittal.

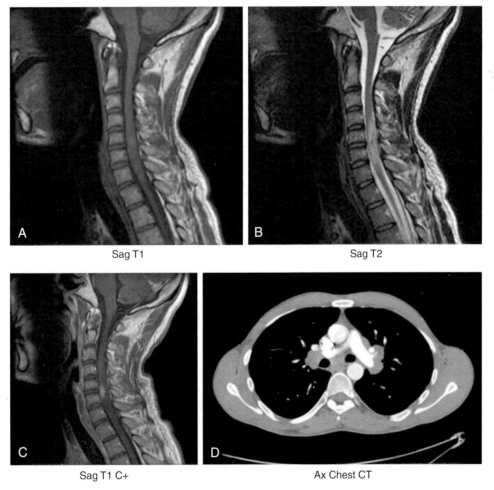

| Sag T1 | Sag T2 |

| Sag T1 C+ | Ax Chest CT |

CASE G: A 32-year-old presenting with upper extremity pain and Lhermitte sign. *Ax,* Axial; *CT,* Computed tomography; *Sag,* sagittal.

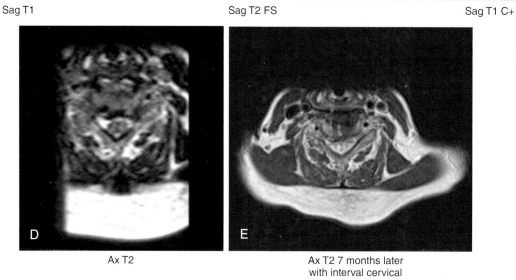

A Sag T1

B Sag T2 FS

C Sag T1 C+

D Ax T2

E Ax T2 7 months later with interval cervical spinal cord decompression surgery

CASE H: A 66-year-old presenting with right-sided weakness, numbness, and severe headaches. *Ax,* Axial; *FS,* fat saturated; *Sag,* sagittal.

DESCRIPTION OF FINDINGS

- Case A: Marked lower cervical and upper thoracic spinal cord expansion is noted with mild associated enhancement. No cystic or hemorrhagic features were identified.
- Case B: Multiple, predominantly small, enhancing intramedullary nodules are noted with a disproportionately large associated syrinx, resulting in marked cord expansion in a patient with a known history of von Hippel–Lindau disease.
- Case C: Focal, prominent spinal cord expansion is present and is associated with a well-marginated, heterogeneous, solid, and cystic enhancing intramedullary mass with hemorrhagic components identified on a gradient refocused echo image.
- Case D: Several enhancing cervical and thoracic intramedullary lesions with marked edema are present. Additional cerebral intraparenchymal lesions also are noted in a patient with a known metastatic cervical carcinoma.
- Case E: Two cervical T2 hyperintense intramedullary lesions with associated enhancement are noted in a patient with a known history of systemic lupus erythematosus (SLE). Note that the upper cervical lesion spans more than three vertebral body segments and that cord expansion is mild.
- Case F: An enhancing T2 hyperintense lesion with minimal cord expansion is noted in a patient with a known history of multiple sclerosis (MS). Note that the lesion spans less than one to two vertebral body segments.
- Case G: An irregularly marginated enhancing lesion associated with more extensive T2 hyperintense spinal cord signal abnormality and mild cord in a patient with a known history of sarcoidosis and bilateral hilar adenopathy is evident on a chest CT scan.
- Case H: Disk-osteophyte complexes that are present at the C4–C5 and C5–C6 disk levels in association with ligamentum flavum thickening result in severe central spinal canal stenosis and ventral and dorsal cord compression. An abnormal central spinal cord T2 hyperintense signal extends from the C4–C7 levels, with focal central intramedullary enhancement at the level of maximal compression at the C5–C6 level, consistent with compressive cervical myelopathy. A follow-up study after surgical decompression demonstrates central cord myelomalacia consistent with chronic spinal cord infarction.

Diagnosis

Case A: Astrocytoma
Case B: Hemangioblastomas
Case C: Ependymoma
Case D: Intramedullary metastases
Case E: Transverse myelitis
Case F: MS with active demyelination
Case G: Intramedullary neurosarcoidosis
Case H: Compressive myelopathy

Summary

For practical purposes, enhancing spinal cord lesions can be divided into neoplastic and nonneoplastic etiologies. Differentiating between these etiologic categories can be challenging, but imaging characteristics may help narrow the differential diagnosis, and the clinical history may further tailor the diagnostic considerations.

The foremost consideration is whether spinal cord enlargement, which is a hallmark for neoplastic etiologies, is present. When an enhancing intramedullary lesion with marked fusiform enlargement of the spinal cord is encountered, a spinal cord neoplasm should be given serious consideration. Caution is necessary when only minimal or mild spinal cord enlargement is evident because nonneoplastic entities in the acute setting can produce inflammatory edema and cord expansion. Follow-up imaging may help reveal whether the expansion is due to an increase in the number of cells, as seen in tumors, or a transient increase related to inflammation.

Differential considerations for enhancing intramedullary spinal cord neoplasms include ependymoma, astrocytoma, hemangioblastoma, lymphoma, and metastasis. Ependymomas and astrocytomas, which are the most common lesions in adults, always should be given serious consideration when one is confronted with a heterogeneously enhancing intramedullary mass that is expanding the cord. Although a tissue diagnosis can be suggested on the basis of imaging, a biopsy is required to make a definitive distinction.

Ependymomas are the most common intramedullary tumor in adults (particularly in the lower spinal cord) and the second most common intramedullary tumor in children. Although ependymomas most commonly occur intracranially, up to one-third may be seen in the spinal cord, with the lower spinal cord/conus involved more often than the remainder of the cord. Ependymomas arise from the ependymal cells surrounding the central spinal cord canal and thus typically demonstrate a more central location compared with astrocytomas, particularly when they are still small. However, they usually present as larger, heterogeneously enhancing hemorrhagic masses with well-defined margins. A "cap sign" may be evident with a T2 hypointense rim at the tumor poles as a result of hemorrhage and cord edema. Although findings such as central location, a heterogeneous signal including hemorrhagic components, and a well-defined lesion with a "cap sign" are not pathognomonic, they favor the diagnosis of ependymoma rather than astrocytoma.

Astrocytomas are the most common intramedullary tumor in children and the second most common intramedullary tumor in adults. Astrocytomas tend to involve the mid-to-upper spinal cord more often than the lower spinal cord. Astrocytomas virtually always present with fusiform expansion of the spinal cord. They usually appear as a heterogeneously enhancing, necrotic, ill-defined mass lesion without a well-demarcated margin, reflecting their infiltrative nature. Cystic changes are seen in one-fourth to one-third of these lesions, and hemorrhage is less common than in ependymomas. When astrocytomas are small, an eccentric location within the spinal cord is seen, in contrast with the central location of a small ependymoma.

Intramedullary hemangioblastoma also should be considered in the differential diagnosis of an enhancing intramedullary neoplasm. Spinal cord hemangioblastomas may be sporadic or associated with von Hippel–Lindau syndrome. Intramedullary hemangioblastomas most often present as a small, avidly enhancing nodule or as a cyst with an enhancing mural nodule. A suggestive feature is their association with a disproportionately large syrinx in contrast to the small size of the enhancing lesion. The presence of surrounding serpiginous flow voids may be a diagnostic clue, reflecting the highly vascular nature of hemangioblastomas.

Other much less common neoplastic entities to consider in the appropriate clinical setting are lymphomas and metastases. Lymphomas most commonly involve the vertebral bodies or the epidural space rather than the cord (Fig. 38.1). Although cord involvement is quite rare, when it is present, it most commonly appears as a solitary intramedullary cord lesion. Cervical spinal cord involvement is most common, with thoracic and lumbar involvement seen less commonly. Surrounding edema and avid enhancement are typical, although lymphomas may present with homogeneous, irregular, or heterogeneous enhancement. Metastatic involvement of the spinal cord is exceedingly rare, with lung, breast, melanoma, renal, and colorectal cancer being the most common primary tumors of origin. Known metastatic dissemination and the presence of multiple soft tissue and vertebral body lesions may provide diagnostic clues.

When enlargement of the spinal cord is absent or only minimal in association with an enhancing intramedullary cord lesion, nonneoplastic lesions such as demyelinating, vascular, granulomatous, inflammatory, and infectious pathologies should be considered. The diagnostic considerations within this category include MS, transverse myelitis, cavernous malformation, subacute infarct, arteriovenous malformation (AVM), neurosarcoidosis, and abscess.

Acute demyelination in the setting of MS is associated with plaque enhancement, and lesions typically are smaller than two vertebral segments in length. Chronic lesions can persist as nonenhancing T2 hyperintense foci and may demonstrate focal cord atrophy. MS plaques in the cord usually are peripheral and dorsally positioned in the cord and involve both gray and white matter. In a patient suspected of a demyelinating disease such as MS or transverse myelitis, a concomitant MRI of the brain may be quite helpful. The presence of intracranial lesions of differing ages ("disseminated in space and time") and spinal cord lesions spanning less than two vertebral body segments suggests MS. On the other hand, acute transverse myelitis typically extends three to four vertebral segments in length, and enhancement may be variable. Transverse myelitis may be associated with viral infections, vaccination, SLE, and paraneoplastic syndromes.

Vascular lesions presenting as an enhancing intramedullary lesion include cavernous malformations, AVMs, and subacute cord infarction. The spinal cord is a relatively uncommon site for cavernous malformations, with only approximately 3% to 5% occurring at this site. The characteristic MRI features of the chronic lesion include multilobular T1 or T2 hyperintensity in a "popcorn-like" configuration with a complete T2 hypointense peripheral rim reflecting the susceptibility of chronic blood products (Fig. 38.2).

This hemosiderin ring typically "blooms" on susceptibility imaging. In the setting of acute hemorrhage, hematoma, associated edema, and cord expansion can obscure these more characteristic findings.

An intramedullary AVM nidus may be seen as a variably enhancing tangle of vessels with feeding serpentine flow voids and draining perimedullary veins (Fig. 38.3). As with arteriovenous fistulas, venous hypertension may lead to cord edema.

Intramedullary enhancement also can be seen, with spinal cord infarction typically appearing as diffuse enhancement 10 to 21 days after the infarction occurs. Infarction occurs most commonly in the thoracic and thoracolumbar spine and often is related to aortic disease. T2 hyperintense signal abnormality usually extends more than one vertebral body segment, and slight cord expansion may be seen. Intramedullary enhancement can be confused with a neoplastic process.

Spinal cord injury from subacute and chronic compressive myelopathy also can present with intramedullary enhancement. Venous hypertension and neovascularization in areas of gliosis may explain the presence of enhancement, which may decrease or resolve after surgical decompression. However, intramedullary enhancement on preoperative MRI can be a poor prognostic factor.

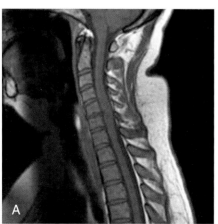
Sag T1

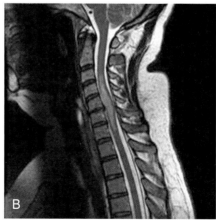
Sag T2

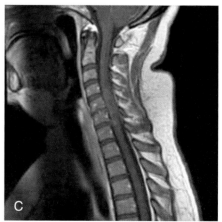
Sag T1 C+

• **Fig. 38.1** Lymphoma. A 56-year-old presented with extremity weakness and hyperreflexia. (A) Sagittal *(Sag)* T1, (B) sagittal T2, and (C) sagittal T2 postcontrast images of the cervical spine demonstrate an ill-defined mildly and predominantly peripherally enhancing intramedullary lesion associated with mild cord expansion. Findings of a spinal cord biopsy were consistent with lymphoma.

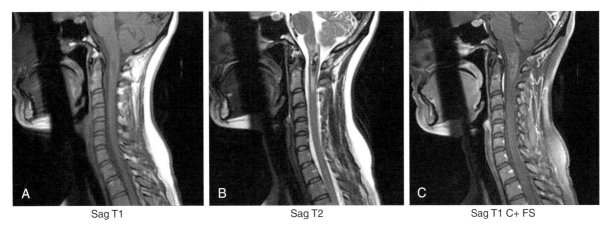

Sag T1 Sag T2 Sag T1 C+ FS

• **Fig. 38.2** Cavernous malformation. A 33-year-old had a 3-day history of right facial numbness that extended into the right neck and arm. (A) Sagittal *(Sag)* T1, (B) sagittal T2, and (C) sagittal T1 fat-saturated *(FS)* postcontrast images of the cervical spine demonstrate a mildly enhancing, heterogeneous, intramedullary lesion with a prominent peripheral rim of T2 hypointensity. Mild surrounding edema is noted as a result of acute hemorrhage. A cavernous malformation was diagnosed pathologically.

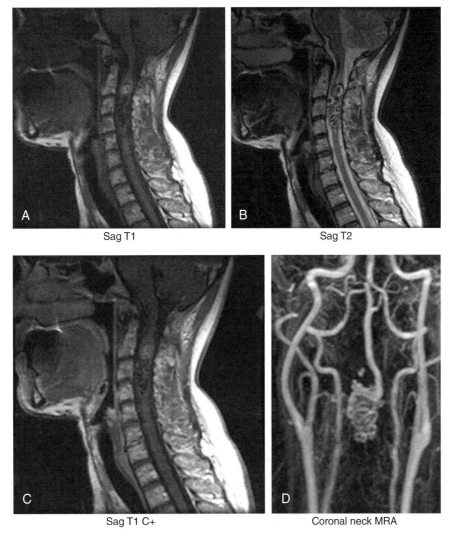

Sag T1 Sag T2

Sag T1 C+ Coronal neck MRA

• **Fig. 38.3** Intramedullary arteriovenous malformation. (A) Sagittal *(Sag)* T1, (B) sagittal T2, and (C) sagittal T1 fat-saturated postcontrast images of the cervical spine demonstrate intramedullary serpiginous flow voids expanding the upper cervical spinal cord. (D) Coronal neck magnetic resonance angiography *(MRA)* demonstrates a dilated anterior spinal artery supplying an enhancing tangle of vessels correlating with the magnetic resonance images and consistent with an intramedullary arteriovenous malformation.

Granulomatous, inflammatory, and infectious processes are less common etiologies of a nonexpansile or mildly edematous enhancing spinal cord lesion, but should be considered in the appropriate clinical setting. Thoracic lymphadenopathy (hilar and paratracheal adenopathy) is the most common imaging finding in persons with sarcoidosis. Intracranial neurosarcoidosis typically presents as nodular basilar-predominant intracranial leptomeningeal enhancement. Spinal cord involvement is exceedingly rare. The imaging features of intramedullary sarcoid with enhancement and mild spinal cord enlargement are nonspecific, but correlation with thoracic and clinical findings can help make the diagnosis.

Although they are rare, spinal cord abscesses typically present as a peripherally enhancing intramedullary lesion with surrounding edema and cord expansion (Fig. 38.4). Restricted diffusion can be a helpful finding. A detailed clinical history and the presence of systemic infectious symptoms are of critical assistance in making the diagnosis.

Spectrum of Disease

The spectrum of disease is delineated in Figs. 38.5 to 38.7.

Differential Diagnosis

1. Neoplastic
2. Astrocytoma
3. Ependymoma
4. Hemangioblastoma
5. Lymphoma
6. Metastases
7. Demyelinative
8. MS
9. Transverse myelitis
10. Vascular
11. Cavernous malformation
12. Subacute infarct

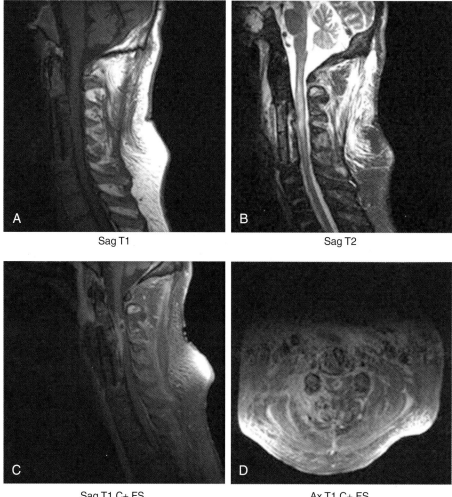

Sag T1	Sag T2
Sag T1 C+ FS	Ax T1 C+ FS

• **Fig. 38.4** Intramedullary abscess. (A) Sagittal *(Sag)* T1, (B) sagittal T2, and (C) sagittal T1 fat-saturated *(FS)* postcontrast images of the cervical spine in a patient with a history of upper cervical spine corpectomies demonstrate marked perivertebral soft tissue swelling and phlegmonous change. An intramedullary T2 hyperintense signal is noted surrounding a peripherally enhancing intramedullary lesion that is best evident on (D) the axial *(Ax)* T1 fat-saturated postcontrast image, consistent with a spinal cord abscess.

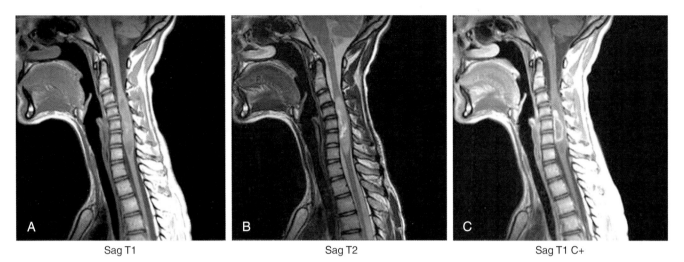

Sag T1   Sag T2   Sag T1 C+

• **Fig. 38.5** An astrocytoma with well-defined borders. A 14-year-old presented with right-handed weakness. (A) Sagittal *(Sag)* T1, (B) sagittal T2 fat-saturated, and (C) sagittal T1 postcontrast images of the cervical spine demonstrate prominent mid cervical spinal cord expansion associated with a peripherally enhancing, pathologically proven astrocytoma. Note the well-defined borders of the lesion on the sagittal T2 image, which is a more typical finding of ependymoma, underscoring the reality that astrocytomas and ependymomas cannot always be reliably differentiated by imaging.

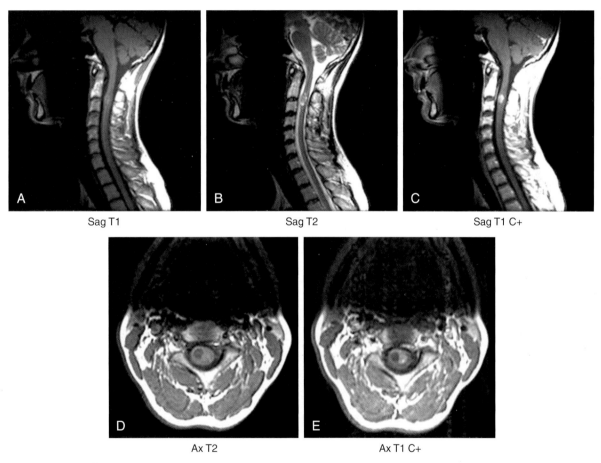

Sag T1   Sag T2   Sag T1 C+

Ax T2   Ax T1 C+

• **Fig. 38.6** These images provide an example of how a small, central versus peripheral location of an intramedullary neoplasm may be helpful in making a diagnosis. A 38-year-old female presented with burning neck pain. (A) Sagittal *(Sag)* T1, (B) sagittal T2, and (C) sagittal T1 postcontrast images of the cervical spine demonstrate a heterogeneous, solid, and cystic enhancing intramedullary lesion focally expanding the cord. (D) Axial *(Ax)* T1 and (E) axial T2 postcontrast images through the solid and cystic enhancing lesion demonstrate a central location, typical of a small ependymoma. Ependymoma was diagnosed pathologically.

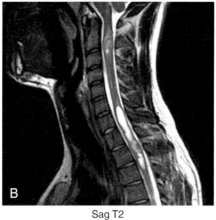
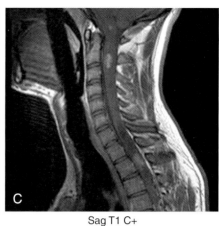

Sag T1   Sag T2   Sag T1 C+

• **Fig. 38.7** Ependymomas are associated with neurofibromatosis type 2 (NF2). (A) Sagittal *(Sag)* T1, (B) sagittal T2, and (C) sagittal T1 postcontrast images of the cervical spine demonstrate cord expansion associated with multiple heterogeneously enhancing solid and cystic intramedullary ependymomas in a 22-year-old male with NF2.

13. AVM
14. Granulomatous/inflammatory/infectious
15. Neurosarcoid
16. Abscess

Pearls

- The foremost consideration is whether significant spinal cord enlargement is present, which is a hallmark for neoplastic etiologies. When the imaging characteristics of a lesion are an enhancing intramedullary lesion with marked fusiform enlargement of the spinal cord, a spinal cord neoplasm should be the top differential consideration.
- A well-defined enhancing lesion with a central location, a heterogenous signal including hemorrhagic components, and a "cap sign" favor the diagnosis of ependymoma rather than astrocytoma.
- Astrocytomas virtually always present with fusiform expansion of the spinal cord and present as a heterogeneously enhancing, necrotic, ill-defined, infiltrative lesion without a well-demarcated margin. Hemorrhage is less common than in ependymomas and, when the lesion is small, an eccentric location within the cord contrasts with the typical central location of an ependymoma.
- A history of von Hippel–Lindau disease or a disproportionately large syrinx in association with a small enhancing lesion suggests a hemangioblastoma. Prominent associated serpiginous flow voids may be evident.
- Spinal cord lymphoma and metastases are relatively uncommon differential considerations.
- The presence of intracranial lesions of differing ages and spinal cord lesions spanning less than two vertebral body segments suggests MS.
- Acute transverse myelitis typically extends three to four vertebral segments in length and may be associated with viral infections, vaccination, SLE, and paraneoplastic syndromes.

- Consider a subacute infarct or compressive myelopathy as a differential consideration to neoplasm when an enhancing intramedullary lesion is encountered.
- When compressive myelopathy is noted, intramedullary enhancement on preoperative MRI may be a poor prognostic factor.
- Cavernous malformations have a characteristic imaging appearance, including "popcorn-like" T1 or T2 hyperintensity with a prominent T2 hypointense peripheral rim with blooming on susceptibility imaging. In the setting of acute hemorrhage, hematoma, associated edema, and cord expansion can obscure these more characteristic findings.
- An intramedullary tangle of enhancing vessels with a feeding artery and draining veins is suggestive of an intramedullary spinal cord AVM.
- A clinical history of sarcoidosis or the presence of bilateral hilar and paratracheal lymphadenopathy aid in the rare diagnosis of intramedullary neurosarcoidosis.
- A detailed clinical history and the presence of systemic infectious symptoms can be of critical assistance in the diagnosis of spinal cord abscess.

Signs and Complications

Complications are related to the specific intramedullary location and level of the lesion.

Suggested Readings

Choi KH, Lee KS, Chung SO, et al: Idiopathic transverse myelitis: MR characteristics, *AJNR Am J Neuroradiol* 17(6):1151–1160, 1996.

Christoforidis GA, Spickler EM, Recio MV, et al: MR of CNS sarcoidosis: correlation of imaging features to clinical symptoms and response to treatment, *AJNR Am J Neuroradiol* 20(4):655–669, 1999.

Do-Dai DD, Brooks MK, Goldkamp A, et al: Magnetic resonance imaging of intramedullary spinal cord lesions: a pictorial review, *Curr Probl Diagn Radiol* 39(4):160–185, 2010.

Houten JK, Cooper PR: Spinal cord astrocytomas: presentation, management and outcome, *J Neurooncol* 47(3):219–224, 2000.

Hynson JL, Kornberg AJ, Coleman LT, et al: Clinical and neuroradiologic features of acute disseminated encephalomyelitis in children, *Neurology* 56:1308–1312, 2001.

Krings T, Lasjaunias PL, Hans FJ, et al: Imaging in spinal vascular disease, *Neuroimaging Clin N Am* 17(1):57–72, 2007.

Ozawa H, Sato T, Hyodo H, et al: Clinical significance of intramedullary Gd-DTPA enhancement in cervical myelopathy, *Spinal Cord* 48:415–422, 2010.

Pretorius PM, Quaghebeur G: The role of MRI in the diagnosis of MS, *Clin Radiol* 58(6):434–448, 2003.

Scotti G, Gerevini S: Diagnosis and differential diagnosis of acute transverse myelopathy. The role of neuroradiological investigations and review of the literature, *Neurol Sci* 22(Suppl 2):S69–S73, 2001.

Tartaglino LM, Croul SE, Flanders AE, et al: Idiopathic acute transverse myelitis: MR imaging findings, *Radiology* 201(3):661–669, 1996.

Tartaglino LM, Friedman DP, Flanders AE, et al: Multiple sclerosis in the spinal cord: MR appearance and correlation with clinical parameters, *Radiology* 195(3):725–732, 1995.

39

Enhancing Intramedullary Conus Lesions

JUAN E. SMALL, MD, MSC

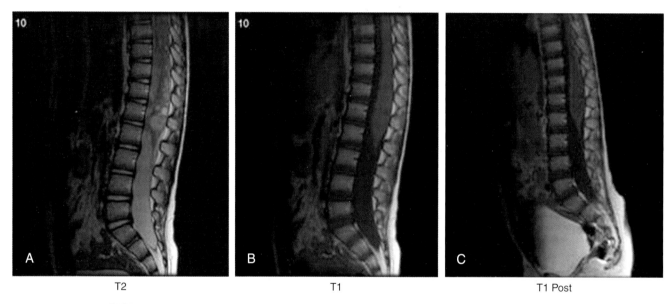

| T2 | T1 | T1 Post |

CASE A: A 3-year-old who has been limping and favoring the left lower extremity for approximately 1 month.

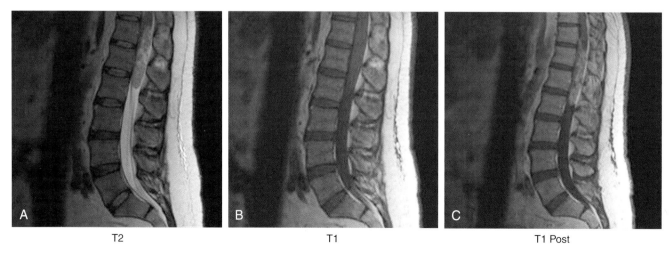

| T2 | T1 | T1 Post |

CASE B: A 46-year-old presenting with progressive bilateral lower extremity weakness and gait difficulty.

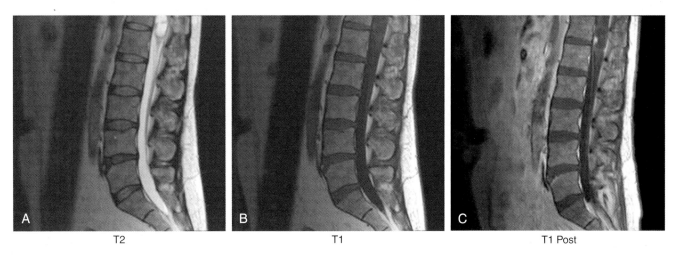

| T2 | T1 | T1 Post |

CASE C: A 38-year-old with von Hippel–Lindau (VHL) disease presenting with bowel and bladder dysfunction.

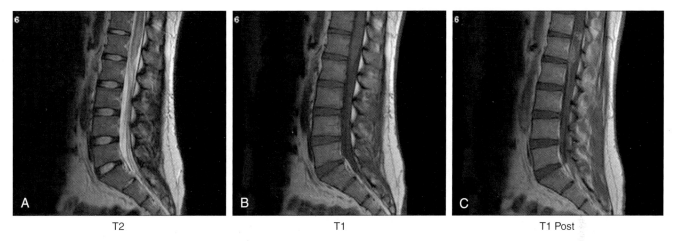

| T2 | T1 | T1 Post |

CASE D: A 29-year-old Brazilian with numbness in both legs, difficulty walking, and urinary retention.

DESCRIPTION OF FINDINGS

- Case A: A heterogeneous, solid and cystic, T2 hyperintense, T1 hypointense, nonenhancing mass in a child that is expanding the conus.
- Case B: A heterogeneous, T2 hyperintense, avidly enhancing conus mass with a distinct plane between the tumor and the conus noted on T2 images.
- Case C: A T2 hyperintense, solid and cystic conus mass with a cyst and enhancing mural nodule configuration.
- Case D: Nodular, irregular enhancement of the peripheral conus with marked associated edema.

Diagnosis

Case A: Astrocytoma
Case B: Myxopapillary ependymoma
Case C: Hemangioblastoma
Case D: Schistosomiasis

Summary

In adults, the most common intramedullary neoplastic lesion of the conus and filum terminale is an ependymoma.

Although astrocytomas are more common in the cervical and upper thoracic cord, they represent the second most common conus tumor in adults. In children, however, astrocytomas of the conus are more common than ependymomas.

Unfortunately, ependymomas and astrocytomas of the conus can have a similar appearance. Both generally appear as T2 hyperintense, expansile heterogeneous enhancing lesions. Imaging signs that favor ependymoma are a central location, well-demarcated edges, hemorrhagic components, cysts, marked surrounding edema, an associated syrinx, and intense homogeneous enhancement. Astrocytomas, on the other hand, are weakly favored by their usually eccentric intramedullary location, ill-defined borders, and patchy enhancement, with lack of enhancement in up to 30%. They are less likely to have hemorrhage, cysts, significant associated edema, or syrinx formation.

Hemangioblastomas rarely affect the conus, although their association with von Hippel–Lindau (VHL) disease or their characteristic appearance as a cyst and mural nodule can be particularly suggestive of this diagnosis. Most hemangioblastomas, however, are sporadic, and they frequently present as a well-circumscribed, solid, densely enhancing lesion with flow voids, surrounding edema, and a disproportionately large associated syrinx. Dilated tortuous associated vessels may be evident.

Nonneoplastic conditions also may involve the conus and mimic tumors on MRI. These include cavernous malformations, inflammatory lesions (such as sarcoid and demyelinating lesions), and infectious etiologies (such as tuberculosis, schistosomiasis, and cysticercosis). Laboratory analysis of cerebrospinal fluid may help differentiate neoplastic from nonneoplastic etiologies.

Rarely, other neoplastic conditions, such as lymphoma and intramedullary metastasis, affect the conus (Fig. 39.1). Multiplicity of lesions and clinical history are important aids to diagnosis.

Spectrum of Disease

The spectrum of disease is detailed in the preceding section.

Differential Diagnosis

1. Myxopapillary ependymoma
2. Astrocytoma
3. Hemangioblastoma
4. Infection (schistosomiasis, tuberculosis, cysticercosis)
5. Granulomatous lesions
6. Metastasis
7. Demyelinating lesions

Pearls

- Myxopapillary ependymomas of the conus:
  - The most common neoplastic conus lesion in adults

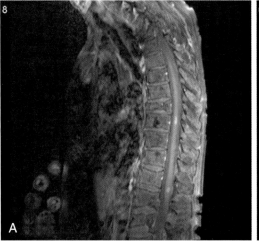

T1 Post

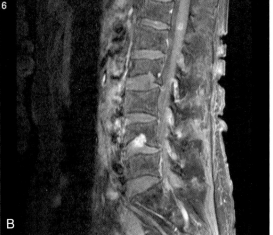

T1 Post

• **Fig. 39.1** A 71-year-old with a history of breast cancer who presented with progressive weakness. Multiple metastatic enhancing lesions are noted, including bony metastases and intramedullary enhancing lesions involving the lower thoracic cord and the conus.

- The second most common neoplastic conus lesion in children
- Imaging signs that weakly favor ependymoma are a central location, well-demarcated edges, hemorrhagic components, cysts, marked associated edema, associated syrinx, and intense homogeneous enhancement
- Astrocytomas of the conus:
  - The most common neoplastic conus lesion in children
  - The second most common neoplastic conus lesion in adults
  - Imaging signs that weakly favor astrocytoma are eccentric intramedullary location, ill-defined borders, and patchy enhancement, with lack of enhancement in up to 30%
- Hemangioblastoma of the cord:
  - Variable imaging appearance as a highly vascular enhancing nodule or a cyst with a mural nodule
  - Dilated tortuous-associated vessels may be evident
  - May present with an associated, disproportionately large syrinx

- Association with VHL disease
- Other lesions that may mimic intramedullary tumors are demyelinating lesions and sarcoid and infections, such as schistosomiasis, tuberculosis, and cysticercosis

Signs and Complications

Signs and complications generally are related to location, mass effect, and edema.

Suggested Readings

Ebner FH, Roser F, Acioly MA, et al: Intramedullary lesions of the conus medullaris: differential diagnosis and surgical management, *Neurosurg Rev* 32(3):287–300, 2009.

Gebauer GP, Farjoodi P, Sciubba DM, et al: Magnetic resonance imaging of spine tumors: classification, differential diagnosis, and spectrum of disease, *J Bone Joint Surg Am* 90A(suppl 4):146–162, 2008.

Koeller KK, Rosenblum RS, Morrison AL: Neoplasms of the spinal cord and filum terminale: radiologic-pathologic correlation, *Radiographics* 20(6):1721–1749, 2000.

40

Hemorrhagic Intramedullary Lesion

JASON LAUER, MD

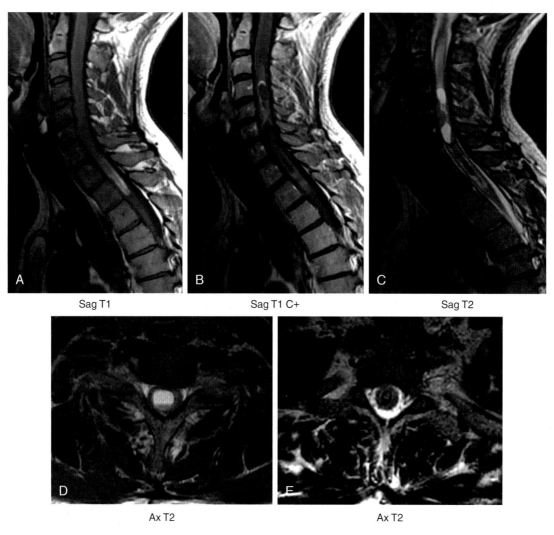

Sag T1   Sag T1 C+   Sag T2

Ax T2   Ax T2

CASE A: A 42-year-old with neck pain. *Ax,* Axial; *Sag,* sagittal.

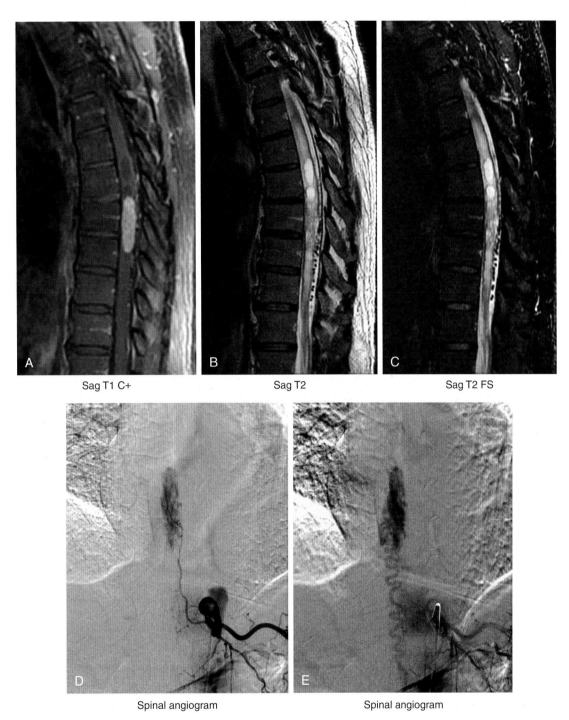

Sag T1 C+   Sag T2   Sag T2 FS

Spinal angiogram   Spinal angiogram

CASE B: A 30-year-old with upper extremity sensory changes and weakness. *Ax*, Axial; *FS*, fat saturated.

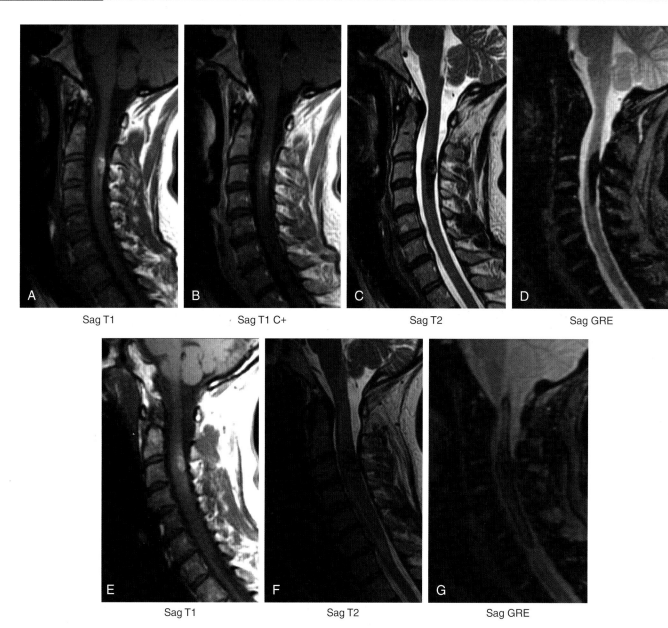

A   Sag T1   B   Sag T1 C+   C   Sag T2   D   Sag GRE

E   Sag T1   F   Sag T2   G   Sag GRE

CASE C: A 35-year-old with episodic upper extremity sensorimotor deficit. Initial and follow-up images 8 years later after an episode of sudden paraplegia are provided. *GRE*, Gradient refocused echo; *Sag*, sagittal.

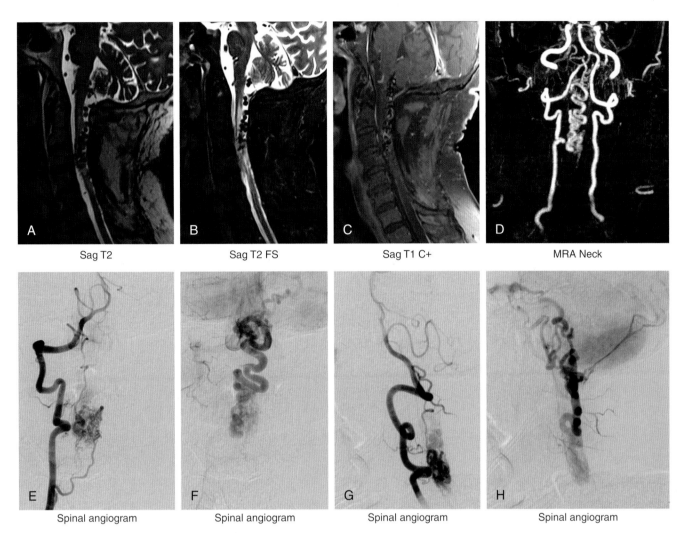

Sag T2   Sag T2 FS   Sag T1 C+   MRA Neck

Spinal angiogram   Spinal angiogram   Spinal angiogram   Spinal angiogram

CASE D: A 50-year-old with sudden onset right upper and lower extremity paresthesia. *FS*, fat saturated; *MRA*, Magnetic resonance angiography; Axial; *Sag*, sagittal.

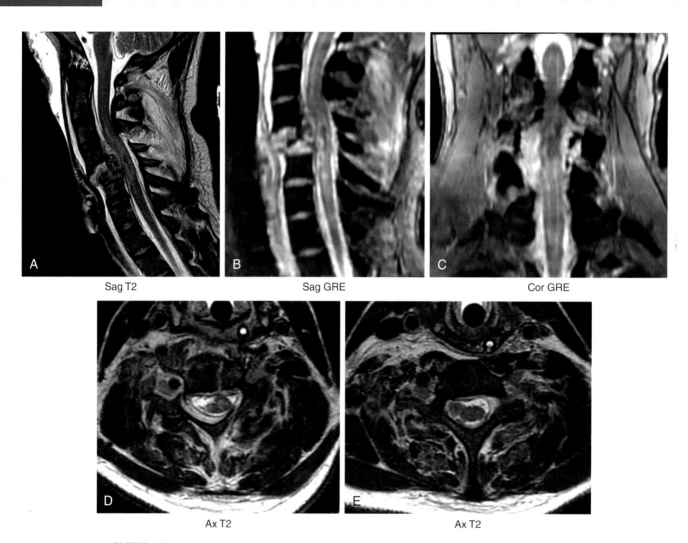

Sag T2

Sag GRE

Cor GRE

Ax T2

Ax T2

CASE E: A 30-year-old presents after high-speed motor vehicle accident. *Ax*, Axial; *Cor*, coronal; *GRE*, Gradient refocused echo; *Sag*, sagittal.

- Case A: An intramedullary lesion centered in the cervical spinal cord demonstrates intrinsic T1 hyperintensity caudally with peripheral and solid enhancement cephalad. Axial and sagittal T2 images demonstrate a complex syrinx associated with the lesion. There is T2 hyperintense fluid—T2 isointense hemorrhage level layering within a component of the syrinx and a T2 hypointense hemosiderin cap within the inferior margin. Lesion appears centered within the cord on axial images. These findings are consistent with pathologically proven ependymoma.
- Case B: An avidly and solidly enhancing mass involves the thoracic spinal cord at T8–T9 levels. T2-weighted and T2/short TI inversion recovery (STIR) images demonstrate heterogenous signal associated with the enhancing component as well as perilesional cyst and/or syrinx formation along the cephalad aspect. There is T2/STIR hyperintensity within the surrounding spinal cord consistent with vasogenic edema. Also note the prominent tortuous flow voids along the dorsal aspect of the lesion. Axial images were not helpful in confirming a peripheral location of the lesion due to its size. Digital subtraction angiography (DSA) following a left T10 intercostal artery injection demonstrates marked opacification of the lesion from the feeding posterior spinal artery followed by prompt venous shunting via corkscrew-like vessels from the caudal aspect of the lesion. Overall findings of an avidly enhancing mass with mark arteriovenous shunting are consistent with pathologically proven hemangioblastoma.
- Case C: An intramedullary lesion at the C3 level demonstrates "popcorn-like" intrinsic T1 hyperintensity with no discrete enhancing components. T2-weighted sagittal image shows marked T2 hypointensity within and surrounding the lesion. Blooming of the lesion extending to C4 level is seen on gradient echo image. After 8 years of observation, acute symptoms prompted repeat imaging, which showed similar size of the lesion on T1- and T2-weighted images; nevertheless, marked hemosiderin deposition spanning six levels is revealed on gradient echo imaging, suggesting chronic hemorrhage. Imaging findings are consistent with pathologically proven cavernous malformation.
- Case D: Conglomerate of flow voids involving the intramedullary cervical cord with extramedullary feeder and drainage vessels. Associated T2 hyperintense signal is seen in the cord, with mild enhancement surrounding some of the vessels. DSA demonstrates a feeding vessel off the right vertebral artery, opacification of the vessel conglomerate, and a serpentine draining vessel flowing to the cavernous sinus. Findings are consistent with an intramedullary arteriovenous malformation.
- Case E: Burst fracture-dislocation with retropulsion of C5 fragments into the spinal canal compressing the cord, resulting in marked T2 hyperintense signal within the cord consistent with contusion-related edema. Centrally within the contused spinal cord, there is superimposed lobulated T2 hypointense signal, accentuated on multiplanar reformatted gradient recall echo images, consistent with intramedullary hemorrhage. Axial T2-weighted images demonstrate evidence of spinal cord laceration as well, with one slice inferior showing associated and distinct extramedullary hematoma anterolateral to the spinal cord.

Diagnosis

Case A: Ependymoma

Case B: Hemangioblastoma

Case C: Cavernous malformation

Case D: Intramedullary arteriovenous malformation

Case E: Traumatic intramedullary hemorrhage

Summary

The appearance of hemorrhage within an intramedullary lesion will vary based on the age of hemoglobin products, noting that hemorrhagic lesions often will contain blood products of different ages. Signature MR features of hemorrhage include intrinsic T1 hyperintensity for early and late subacute hemorrhage due to presence of intra- and extracellular methemoglobin and pan-hypointense signal for chronic hemorrhages secondary to hemosiderin. The presence of a hemorrhagic intramedullary lesion, particularly within the cervical spine, should raise suspicion for an ependymoma, as it is the most common intramedullary tumor among adults (occurring both sporadically and as a feature of neurofibromatosis type II [NF-2]/multiple inherited schwannomas, meningiomas, and ependymoma [MISME]) and demonstrates a particular propensity for intralesional hemorrhage. Ependymomas are often identified by their central location (originating from ependymal cells of the central canal) and slow, noninfiltrative growth pattern, which explains secondary findings such as spinal canal widening and remodeling. Peritumoral cysts and syrinx formation are common but not specific. The "hemosiderin cap," characterized by T2 hypointensity at the upper or lower margins of a lesion, is most associated with ependymomas but can also be seen with any hypervascular lesion with a propensity for hemorrhage.

Lesional hypervascularity, and thus its propensity for hemorrhage, can be inferred by the presence of avid enhancement and/or visualization of perilesional feeding vessels, both of which are common features of the hemangioblastoma, the third commonest intramedullary lesion in adults. As capillary-rich neoplasms, hemangioblastomas will demonstrate intense peripheral or solid enhancement, although this feature in isolation is not sufficient to distinguish hemangioblastoma from ependymoma. In contradistinction to the centrally located ependymomas arising from the central canal, hemangioblastomas arise from the pial surface of the cerebellum or spinal cord, and thus smaller hemangioblastomas can be readily identified by their peripheral, often dorsal distribution along the spinal cord pial surface. Larger hemangioblastomas may be difficult to confine to the pial surface, and in fact due to its meningeal origin, the hemangioblastoma may present as a pure intramedullary lesion, a mixed intramedullary-extramedullary lesion, or even a pure extramedullary lesion. Larger hemangioblastomas can likewise demonstrate extensive syrinx formation and evidence of prior hemorrhage, including a "hemosiderin cap," making distinction from other hemorrhagic lesions difficult. A clue that the lesion represents a hemangioblastoma over an ependymoma is the presence of multiple enlarged feeding arteries and draining veins associated with the lesion, which will appear as flow voids on spin echo or gradient echo sequences. Dedicated vascular imaging, such as magnetic resonance angiography (MRA) or DSA, may show prolonged contrast stain of the primary tumor and delineate the complex vascular nature of its feeding artery(ies) and draining venous structure(s). Multiplicity of lesions can further suggest a diagnosis of hemangioblastoma as a feature of von Hippel–Lindau (VHL) syndrome if history is consistent; however, sporadic, solitary hemangioblastomas account for two-thirds of all cases, which highlights the importance of imaging features to make the diagnosis.

If an intramedullary lesion fails to demonstrate discrete enhancement, this can shift the differential away from neoplastic lesions, allowing for consideration of vascular malformations, such as cavernous malformations. Cavernous malformations are commonly encountered in the supratentorial brain (often incidentally) but can uncommonly appear as intramedullary lesions in the spinal cord where they are frequently symptomatic. Considered to be slow flow venous malformations, cavernous malformations of the spine can remain indolent or even regress, allowing for observation of asymptomatic lesions. This highlights the importance of accurate imaging diagnosis of cavernous malformations to avoid unnecessary biopsies and resections. Key MR imaging features of the cavernous malformation include a speckled "popcorn" pattern of intrinsic T1 signal representing blood products of various ages, circumscribed by a rim of T2 hypointense hemosiderin staining, which will be accentuated on susceptibility sensitive sequences. Enhancement is characteristically absent or minimal, and perilesional spinal cord signal is likewise normal unless recent hemorrhage, which may produce T2 hyperintense vasogenic edema within the surrounding spinal cord. Notably absent within cavernous malformations is an abnormal network of perilesional feeding and draining vessels, which would indicate the presence of a spinal cord arteriovenous malformation (AVM). Analogous to intracranial AVMs, the type II spinal AVM involves an intramedullary nidus typically fed by branches of the anterior and/or posterior spinal artery and drained by the coronal venous plexus on the cord surface. The network of abnormal feeding and draining vessels around the nidus manifests as serpentine flow voids that cluster around the nidus within the spinal cord giving a "bag of worms" appearance on imaging, classically described as "glomus type." The AVM vessel conglomerate can extend into the dorsal subarachnoid space and be superimposed on secondary extramedullary flow voids, which represent venous shunts as a result of venous hypertension from the high-flow type II AVM nidus. The spinal cord surrounding the AVM may demonstrate findings consistent with prior hemorrhage including heterogenous signal on T1- and T2-weighted images, with areas of T2 hypointense hemosiderin staining from chronic hemorrhage (accentuated on susceptibility sensitive sequences) and T2 hyperintense signal within the surrounding cord from vasogenic edema, particularly following recent hemorrhage. Enhancement of either the nidus or the spinal cord may be present but is nonspecific, presenting somewhat of a diagnostic dilemma if one considers that large hemangioblastomas also enhance and have prominent flow voids corresponding to feeding and draining pial vessels. Subtle differences between the enhancement of the two lesions may be helpful, as enhancement of the AVM nidus would be expected to be irregular and less robust compared to hemangioblastoma. Likewise, careful discrimination of intramedullary T2 hypointense flow voids from nonspecific background T2 hypointense hemosiderin staining, along with the absence of other features such as syringes and perilesional cysts, also may be helpful in teasing out a diagnosis of type II spinal AVM. The constellation of MR findings allows one to suggest the diagnosis of spinal AVM; however, DSA is often required to delineate the complex angioarchitecture of these lesions and identify perinidal aneurysms, which are commonly found. Type II spinal cord AVMs are congenital and present in younger adults with acute neurological symptoms from subarachnoid hemorrhage or progressive myelopathy. Sporadic cases as well as syndromic cases occur, notably as features of Klippel-Trenaunay-Weber and Rendu-Osler-Weber syndromes.

The final hemorrhagic intramedullary lesion to consider is the traumatic intramedullary hemorrhage. As the name suggests, a differential diagnosis for this lesion is often not necessary as patient history along with secondary imaging findings of trauma allow for the diagnosis to be made with high confidence. Commonly associated with spinal column fractures or subluxation following high-velocity trauma or even short falls in the elderly, acute spinal cord injury may take the form of an isolated acute cord contusion characterized by T2 hyperintense edema within the cord at the level of injury, which portends a better prognosis if hemorrhage is absent. However, if cord hematoma is seen, usually as hypointense intramedullary signal on T2-weighted or susceptibility sensitive sequences, the prognosis for the patient is far worse. It is important to report the presence and extent of intramedullary hemorrhage if present as well as additional traumatic findings not apparent on CT such as ligamentous injuries, occult fractures, disk herniations, and extraaxial hemorrhages.

Differential Diagnosis

1. Hypervascular neoplastic lesions
2. Vascular malformations
3. Trauma
4. Hemorrhagic intramedullary metastasis (rare)

Pearls

- Although there is some imaging overlap among hemorrhagic intramedullary lesions, certain imaging features can help lead one to the proper diagnosis.
- Ependymomas and hemangioblastomas can sometimes be distinguished from their axial location within the spinal cord. Look for additional findings that may indicate syndromic causes (NF-2 or VHL).
- Susceptibility sensitive sequence may be helpful for detecting subtle areas of chronic hemorrhage within the lesion.
- In addition to hemosiderin deposition, other causes for T2 hypointensity or susceptibility include calcification, which should be considered as a possibility.
- Flow voids should be distinguished from hemosiderin, as their presence suggests the presence of a vascular malformation or possibly hemangioblastoma.

Suggested Readings

Kim LJ, Spetzler RF: Classification and surgical management of spinal arteriovenous lesions: arteriovenous fistulae and arteriovenous malformations, *Neurosurgery* 59(5 suppl 3):S3-195–S13-201, 2006.

Miyanji F, Furlan JC, Aarabi B, et al: Acute cervical traumatic spinal cord injury: MR imaging findings correlated with neurologic outcome—prospective study with 100 consecutive patients, *Radiology* 243(3): 820–827, 2007.

Otten M, Mccormick P: Natural history of spinal cavernous malformations. In *Handbook of Clinical Neurology*, 143:233–239, 2017, Elsevier.

Tobin MK, Geraghty JR, Engelhard HH, et al: Intramedullary spinal cord tumors: a review of current and future treatment strategies, *Neurosurgeon Focus* 39(2):E14, 2015.

41

Solitary Enhancing Intradural, Extramedullary Lesions

JUAN E. SMALL, MD, MSC

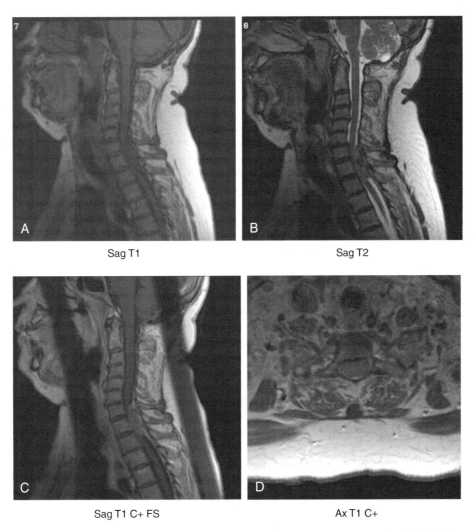

Sag T1

Sag T2

Sag T1 C+ FS

Ax T1 C+

CASE A: A 56-year-old with a history of chronic lower back pain and leg weakness who had fallen in the shower. *Ax*, Axial; *FS*, fat saturated; *Sag*, sagittal.

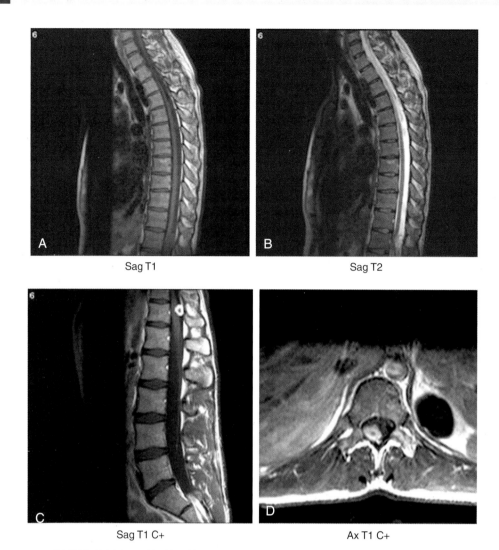

Sag T1

Sag T2

Sag T1 C+

Ax T1 C+

CASE B: A 28-year-old with a history of neurofibromatosis type 2. *Ax,* Axial; *Sag,* sagittal.

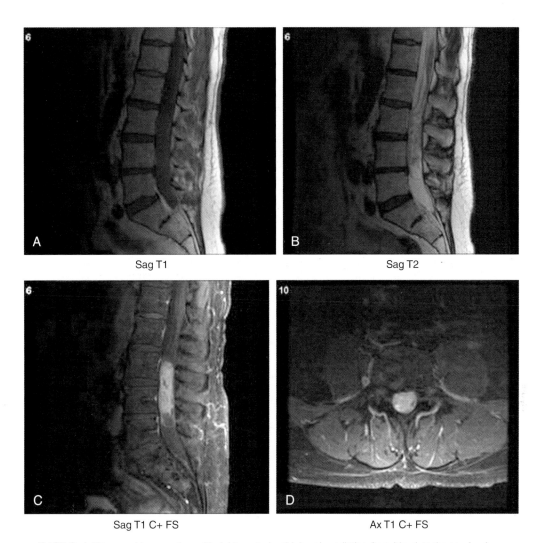

Sag T1

Sag T2

Sag T1 C+ FS

Ax T1 C+ FS

CASE C: A 78-year-old presenting with right posterior thigh pain radiating from his gluteal area. *Ax,* Axial; *FS,* fat saturated; *Sag,* sagittal.

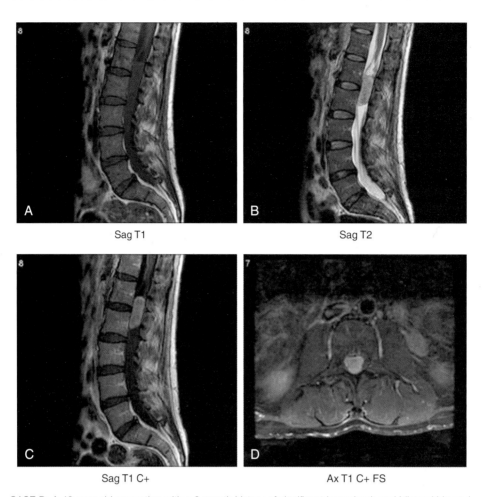

Sag T1

Sag T2

Sag T1 C+

Ax T1 C+ FS

CASE D: A 40-year-old presenting with a 2-month history of significant lower back and bilateral hip and leg pain. *Ax,* Axial; *FS,* fat saturated; *Sag,* sagittal.

DESCRIPTION OF FINDINGS

- Case A: An intradural, extramedullary, avidly enhancing, T2 hypointense, posterior dural-based mass with dural enhancement centered at the level of the cervicothoracic junction. The mass fills the central canal and markedly compresses the cord. Important clues to the diagnosis of meningioma are central calcification, which is evident as hypointensity on T2-weighted imaging along the dural enhancement associated with the lesion.

- Case B: An intradural, extramedullary, peripherally enhancing, T2 hyperintense mass at the level of T12. The effect of the mass on the adjacent cord is noted. The prominent T2 hyperintensity of the lesion and the rim enhancement are important clues to the diagnosis of nerve sheath tumor (schwannoma).

- Case C: An intradural, extramedullary, heterogenous, avidly enhancing mass, demonstrating heterogenous T2 hyperintensity, is centered below the conus medullaris. Although lesions of the cauda equina or filum terminale are nearly impossible to distinguish from each other on imaging, pathology findings proved that this lesion was a schwannoma.

- Case D: An intradural, extramedullary, T2 mildly hyperintense, avidly enhancing, smoothly marginated mass that is displacing cauda equina nerve roots and filling the thecal sac at the level of L1/L2. The conus terminates above the level of this lesion. Although lesions of the cauda equina or filum terminale are nearly impossible to distinguish from each other on imaging, pathology findings proved that this lesion was a myxopapillary ependymoma of the filum terminale.

Diagnosis

Case A: Meningioma
Case B: Nerve sheath tumor—schwannoma
Case C: Schwannoma
Case D: Myxopapillary ependymoma

Summary

The most common (30% to 35%) intradural extramedullary spinal cord lesions are nerve sheath tumors (e.g., schwannomas and neurofibromas) and meningiomas (25%). However, several other less common differential considerations are ependymoma of the filum terminale, drop metastases, lipoma, dermoid, arachnoid cyst, neurenteric cyst, hemangioblastoma, and paraganglioma.

When first evaluating an enhancing intradural extramedullary lesion, the pattern of enhancement (whether solid or ring/peripheral) helps narrow the differential considerations. Common solidly enhancing lesions include schwannomas, neurofibromas, meningiomas, drop metastases, and ependymomas. Lesions typically exhibiting ring/peripheral enhancement include cystic schwannomas and cystic or calcified meningiomas.

Nerve sheath tumors generally are T2 hyperintense because they have a high water content. However, they often exhibit a central T2 hypointense area. Two types of benign nerve sheath tumors can be distinguished: schwannomas and neurofibromas. Schwannomas are generally solitary, well-demarcated, encapsulated lesions that may have hemorrhage, cysts or fatty degeneration and are associated with neurofibromatosis type 2. Neurofibromas are well circumscribed but not encapsulated and usually associated with neurofibromatosis type 1. Neurofibromas generally are not associated with hemorrhage, cysts, and fatty degeneration. Malignant degeneration of nerve sheath tumors is uncommon, and calcification is rare compared with meningiomas. Nerve sheath tumors can be purely

intradural, partially intradural and partially extradural with a dumbbell shape, or purely extradural.

Meningiomas generally present in the fifth and sixth decades and are seen more often in female patients. Meningiomas of the spine tend to be well-circumscribed lesions that are isointense to the spinal cord on T2-weighted sequences. Calcification is present in approximately 75% of cases, and intense homogenous enhancement of noncalcified portions is generally seen. Meningiomas typically are posterolateral in location when in the thoracic or lumbar spine, but in the cervical region they tend to be anterior. Approximately 80% are thoracic, 16% are cervical, and 3% are lumbar. Metastases usually are multiple or demonstrate diffuse nodular or linear enhancement. They may be seen in the setting of neurofibromatosis type 2.

Although, as previously detailed, a long list of other entities should be considered when evaluating a solidly enhancing intradural extramedullary lesion, it is important to remember that ependymomas (particularly the myxopapillary type) can occur anywhere along the filum terminale. Ependymomas typically demonstrate marked enhancement with variable areas of necrosis, hemorrhage, or cyst formation.

An important secondary intradural extramedullary solitary lesion consideration is metastatic disease (leptomeningeal carcinomatosis/drop metastases). However, metastases usually are multiple or demonstrate diffuse nodular or linear enhancement. Leptomeningeal metastatic disease is seen 75% of the time in the lumbar region, likely as a result of gravity. In the pediatric population, primary intracranial neoplasms tend to be a more common cause than systemic malignancies. In adults, breast cancer is the most common cause, followed by lung cancer and melanoma.

Spectrum of Disease

Figs. 41.1 to 41.5 illustrate the spectrum of disease.

Pearls

Table 41.1 provides criteria that are helpful in differentiating nerve sheath tumors from meningiomas.

Signs and Complications

Signs and complications generally are related to mass effect.

Differential Diagnosis

1. Nerve sheath tumor (schwannoma, neurofibroma), 30% to 35%
2. Meningioma, 25%
3. Ependymoma of the filum terminale
4. Drop metastases/leptomeningeal carcinomatosis
5. Lipoma
6. Dermoid (commonly in the region of the conus/cauda equina and often associated with spinal dysraphism)
7. Arachnoid cyst
8. Neurenteric cyst
9. Hemangioblastoma
10. Paraganglioma

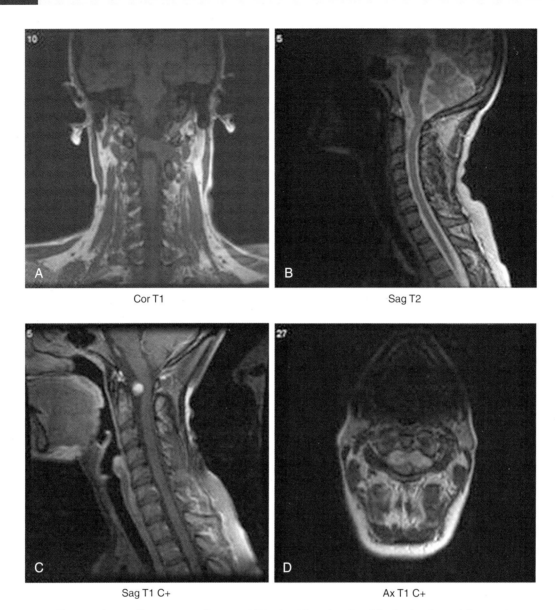

Cor T1

Sag T2

Sag T1 C+

Ax T1 C+

• **Fig. 41.1** A neurofibroma presenting as a bilobed, avidly enhancing, intradural, extramedullary mass anterior to the cervical cord at the level of the dens. *Ax,* Axial; *Cor,* coronal; *Sag,* sagittal.

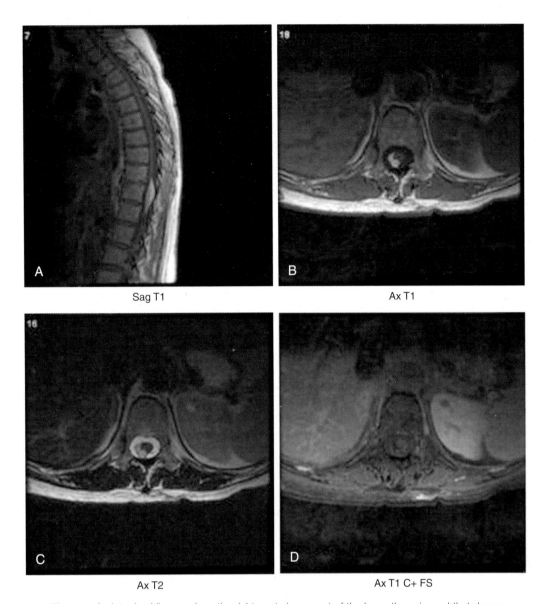

• **Fig. 41.2** An intradural lipoma along the right posterior aspect of the lower thoracic cord that demonstrates isointense signal characteristics to fat, including intrinsic T1 and T2 hyperintensity and signal saturation on postcontrast fat-saturated images. *Ax,* Axial; *FS,* fat saturated; *Sag,* sagittal.

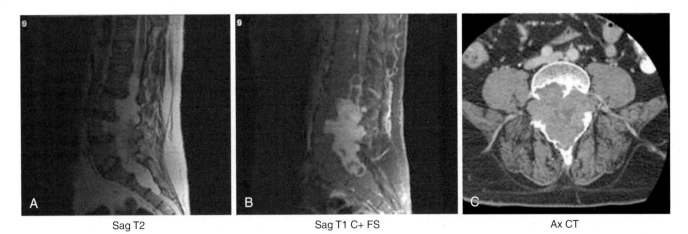

• **Fig. 41.3** A malignant schwannoma presenting as a large, aggressive, heterogenous T2 hyperintense avidly enhancing mass that is eroding and invading adjacent bony structures. This case is presented to remind the reader that these lesions may show quite aggressive features on presentation. *Ax,* Axial; *CT,* Computed tomography; *FS,* fat saturated; *Sag,* sagittal.

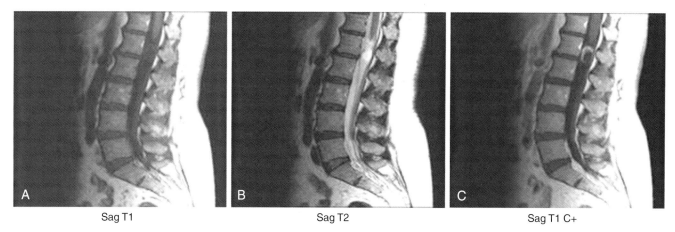

• **Fig. 41.4** A schwannoma with cystic changes presenting as a solid and cystic lesion inferior to the conus. Solid areas of enhancement are noted superiorly, with a cystic component inferiorly. *Sag,* Sagittal.

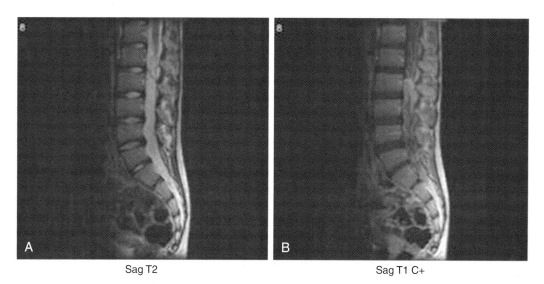

• **Fig. 41.5** A heterogenous myxopapillary ependymoma of the filum terminale. *Sag,* Sagittal.

TABLE 41.1	Nerve Sheath Tumors vs. Meningiomas	
	Nerve Sheath Tumors	**Meningiomas**
MR signal characteristics	"Target" sign: central area of T2 hypointense signal not representing calcification; peripheral, heterogeneous, or homogeneous enhancement; no dural enhancement	Calcification, dural attachment T2 isointense to cord, dense enhancement, dural enhancement
Number	Neurofibromas are generally multiple because they usually are associated with NF1; schwannomas generally are solitary, except in the setting of NF2 or schwannomatosis	Generally solitary except in the setting of meningiomatosis and NF2
Mobility	Mobile because of a lack of dural attachment	Nonmobile because of dural attachment
Location	Generally more anteriorly located; can be purely intradermal, partially intradermal and partially extradural, or purely extradural	Generally posterolateral in location, except in the cervical region, where the location is usually anterior; intradural

NF1, 2, Neurofibromatosis type 1, 2.

Suggested Readings

Abul-Kasim K, Thurnher MM, McKeever P, et al: Intradural spinal tumors: current classification and MRI features, *Neuroradiology* 50(4): 301–314, 2008.

Beall DP, Googe DJ, Emery RL, et al: Extramedullary intradural spinal tumors: a pictorial review, *Curr Probl Diagn Radiol* 36(5):185–198, 2007.

42

Multiple Enhancing Intradural, Extramedullary Lesions

JUAN E. SMALL, MD, MSC

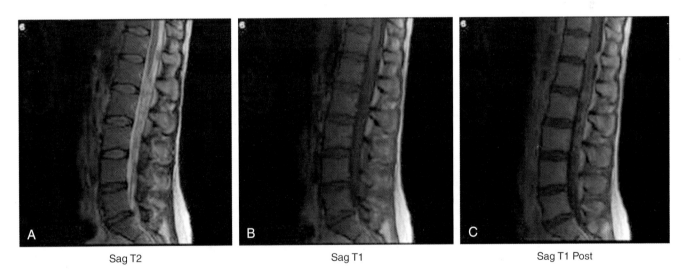

Sag T2

Sag T1

Sag T1 Post

CASE A: A 40-year-old presenting with a 1-week history of worsening ascending numbness/tingling, urinary retention, saddle anesthesia, and decreased rectal tone. *Sag*, Sagittal.

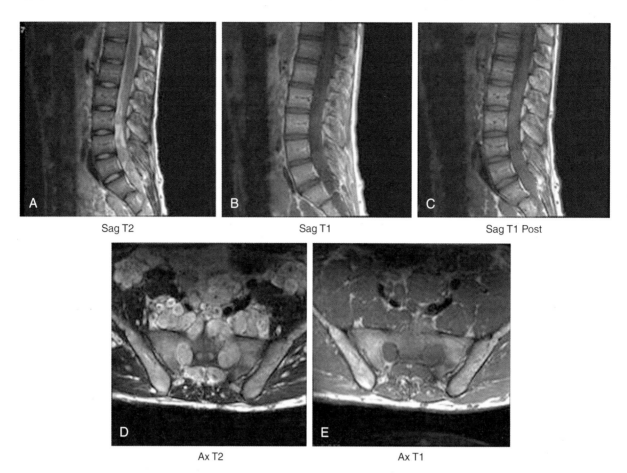

CASE B: A 22-year-old with a history of a known disorder. *Ax,* Axial; *Sag,* sagittal.

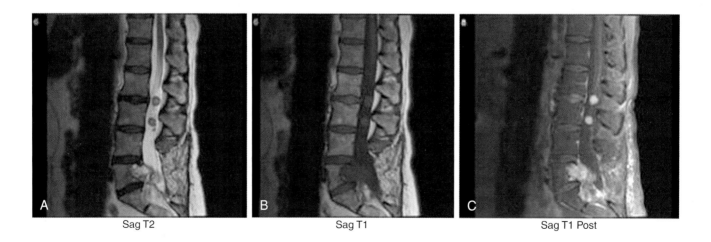

CASE C: A 42-year-old presenting with recurrent schwannoma proven by pathology and a brain magnetic resonance imaging scan negative for vestibular schwannoma. *Sag,* Sagittal.

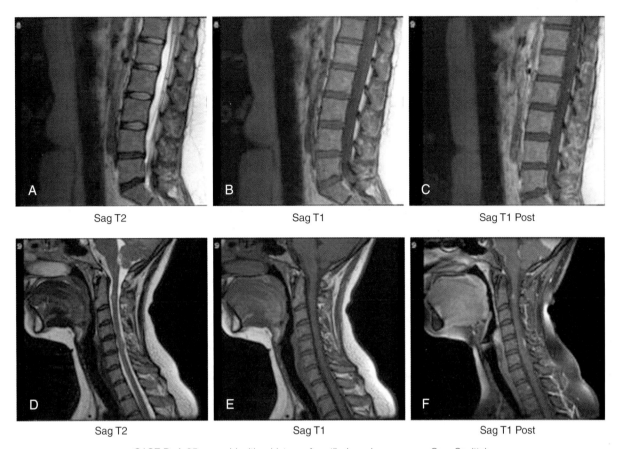

Sag T2   Sag T1   Sag T1 Post

Sag T2   Sag T1   Sag T1 Post

CASE D: A 25-year-old with a history of vestibular schwannomas. *Sag*, Sagittal.

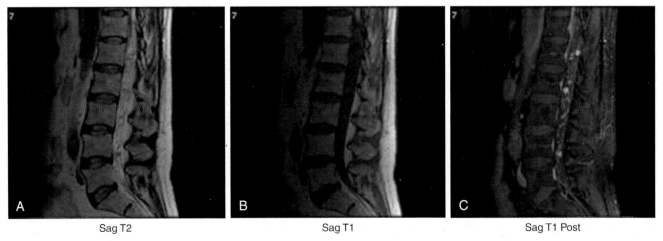

Sag T2   Sag T1   Sag T1 Post

CASE E: A 57-year-old with a history of von Hippel–Lindau disease. *Sag*, Sagittal.

DESCRIPTION OF FINDINGS

- Case A: Abnormal nodular enhancement is noted surrounding the conus and extending along the cauda equina.
- Case B: Fusiform, mildly enhancing masses involving the cauda equina nerve roots and extending through widened sacral neural foramina into the region of the lumbar plexus. There are additional pelvic and soft tissue lesions. Multiple lesions demonstrate "target signs" with central low signal intensity and peripheral high signal intensity on T2-weighted images.
- Case C: Two intradural, extramedullary, avidly enhancing nodular lesions are noted inferior to the conus in a patient with a history of an aggressive-appearing recurrent schwannoma located at the level of L5/S1 in the absence of vestibular schwannomas.
- Case D: Multiple lumbar, intradural, extramedullary, avidly enhancing, rounded lesions are noted along the nerve roots. In addition, cervical images demonstrate enhancing intramedullary lesions (ependymomas) and a partially imaged, dural-based, extraaxial mass superior to the cerebellum (tentorial meningioma).
- Case E: Multiple intradural, extramedullary enhancing spinal lesions are noted along with multiple prominent serpiginous vessels, suggesting highly vascular lesions in a patient with a known history of von Hippel–Lindau (VHL) disease.

Diagnosis

Case A: Leptomeningeal carcinomatosis (pathology: diffuse large B-cell lymphoma)

Case B: Neurofibromatosis type 1 (NF1), plexiform neurofibroma

Case C: Schwannomatosis

Case D: Neurofibromatosis type 2 (NF 2), schwannomas

Case E: von Hippel–Lindau disease (VHL), hemangioblastomas

Summary

When assessing multiple intradural, extramedullary lesions, it is helpful to order the differential diagnoses with respect to their likelihood based on incidence. The most commonly encountered entities are metastases/leptomeningeal carcinomatosis and neoplastic lesions related to NF1 or NF2. Less commonly, multiple schwannomas, neurofibromas, and meningiomas may occur in the nonsyndromic patient. Furthermore, multiple intradural, extramedullary hemangioblastomas occur either sporadically or in patients with VHL disease. In addition, granulomatous diseases such as sarcoidosis, tuberculosis, and fungal infections also can present as multiple, enhancing, intradural, extramedullary lesions.

NF1 is associated with neurofibromas that can be discrete or plexiform in nature. Plexiform neurofibromas present as a network-like fusiform enlargement of multiple enhancing nerve roots. Target signs may be evident within neurofibromas with central low signal intensity and peripheral high signal intensity on T2-weighted images. Neurofibromas occasionally can undergo malignant degeneration.

NF2 is associated with multiple schwannomas, meningiomas, and ependymomas. When multiple intradural, extramedullary enhancing spinal lesions are noted in the setting of NF2, they are schwannomas, and/or meningiomas. These lesions generally are distinguished by their growth along nerve roots (schwannomas) versus a dural attachment (meningiomas), T2 characteristics (schwannomas are T2 hyperintense, meningiomas

are isointense), enhancement characteristics (meningiomas classically homogeneously enhance, schwannomas may have heterogeneous enhancement or rim enhancement), and the presence of calcification (meningiomas frequently calcify whereas schwannomas typically do not).

It is important to note that not all patients with multiple schwannomas have NF2. In persons with schwannomatosis (a neurocutaneous disorder), multiple schwannomas occur in the absence of vestibular schwannomas and other lesions associated with NF2.

Metastatic disease/leptomeningeal carcinomatosis of the spine may represent drop metastases from a central nervous system primary lesion such as a medulloblastoma, ependymoma, or glioblastoma, or it may represent metastatic disease from a systemic primary source such as lung cancer, breast cancer, melanoma, lymphoma, or leukemia. Abnormal enhancement may be seen in various patterns, including linear enhancement; diffuse, sheet-like coating of the cord and/or nerve roots ("sugar coating"); or multifocal discrete nodules along the cord and nerve roots. In approximately 75% of cases, leptomeningeal enhancement is seen in the lumbar region, likely as a result of the effects of gravity.

Hemangioblastomas are most commonly intramedullary lesions that arise near the surface of the cerebellum and spinal cord. These tumors usually present sporadically as single lesions or in the setting of VHL disease. Rarely, hemangioblastomas occur in a disseminated leptomeningeal pattern (hemangioblastomatosis) or as multiple extradural lesions extending along the cauda equina and filum terminale. The typical imaging pattern is multiple avidly enhancing nodules with prominent associated vessels.

Spectrum of Disease

The spectrum of disease is detailed in the preceding section.

Differential Diagnosis

1. Plexiform neurofibroma or multiple neurofibromas (usually associated with NF1)
2. Multiple schwannomas and/or meningiomas associated with NF2
3. Schwannomatosis
4. Metastases/leptomeningeal carcinomatosis
5. Hemangioblastomas/hemangioblastomatosis
6. Sarcoidosis
7. Tuberculosis
8. Fungal infections

Pearls

- The most commonly encountered entities are neoplastic lesions related either to metastases/leptomeningeal carcinomatosis or NF1 and NF2.
- Plexiform neurofibromas have a distinctive imaging characteristics: a network-like, fusiform enlargement of multiple enhancing nerve roots. They also may have target signs with central low signal intensity and peripheral high signal intensity on T2-weighted images.

- Schwannomas and meningiomas occur in NF2. Schwannomas tend to be well-defined, rounded, or oval lesions that grow along nerve roots, are T2 hyperintense, do not calcify, and have variable enhancement patterns. Meningiomas have a dural attachment, are T2 isointense, frequently calcify, and often homogeneously enhance.
- Not all patients with multiple schwannomas have NF2. In persons with schwannomatosis (a neurocutaneous disorder), multiple schwannomas occur in the absence of vestibular schwannomas and other stigmata of NF2.
- Metastatic disease/leptomeningeal carcinomatosis may be seen in various patterns, including linear enhancement; diffuse, sheet-like coating of the cord and/or nerve roots (sugar coating); or multifocal discrete nodules along the cord and nerve roots.
- Leptomeningeal dissemination of hemangioblastomas is rare. These lesions densely enhance and may be associated with prominent vessels.
- Granulomatous diseases such as sarcoidosis, tuberculosis, and fungal infections present with multiple leptomeningeal nodules.

Signs and Complications

Neurofibromas occasionally can degenerate into malignant peripheral nerve sheath tumors.

Suggested Readings

Abul-Kasim K, Thurnher MM, McKeever P, et al: Intradural spinal tumors: current classification and MRI features, *Neuroradiology* 50(4):301–314, 2008.

Beall DP, Googe DJ, Emery RL, et al: Extramedullary intradural spinal tumors: a pictorial review, *Curr Probl Diagn Radiol* 36(5):185–198, 2007.

Ferner RE: Neurofibromatosis 1 and neurofibromatosis 2: a twenty first century perspective, *Lancet Neurol* 6(4):340–351, 2007.

Lim R, Jaramillo D, Poussaint TY, et al: Superficial neurofibroma: a lesion with unique MRI characteristics in patients with neurofibromatosis type 1, *AJR Am J Roentgenol* 184(3):962–968, 2005.

Westhout FD, Mathews M, Paré LS, et al: Recognizing schwannomatosis and distinguishing it from neurofibromatosis type 1 or 2, *J Spinal Disord Tech* 20(4):329–332, 2007.

43

Cystic Intradural Extramedullary Lesions

HUI J. JENNY CHEN, MD

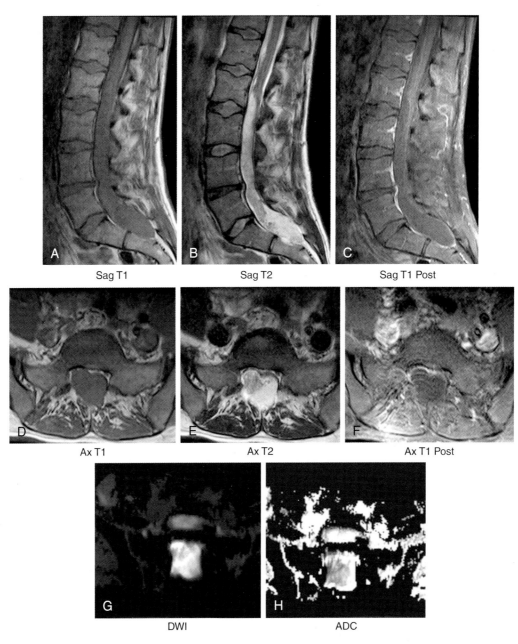

Sag T1	Sag T2	Sag T1 Post
Ax T1	Ax T2	Ax T1 Post
DWI	ADC	

CASE A: A 42-year-old presenting with worsening lower extremity discomfort. *ADC,* Apparent diffusion coefficient; *Ax,* axial; *DWI,* diffusion-weighted imaging; *Sag,* sagittal.

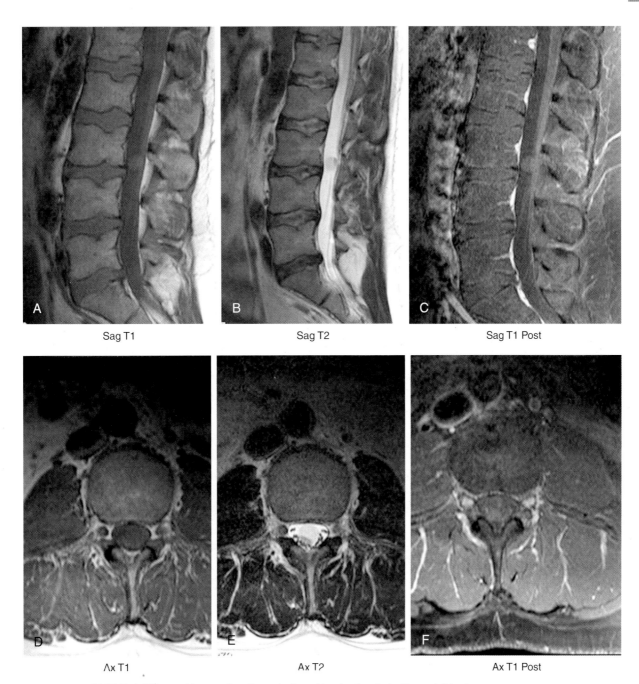

Sag T1

Sag T2

Sag T1 Post

Ax T1

Ax T2

Ax T1 Post

CASE B: A 37-year-old presenting for evaluation of low back pain for the past 3 to 4 years.
Ax, Axial; *Sag*, sagittal.

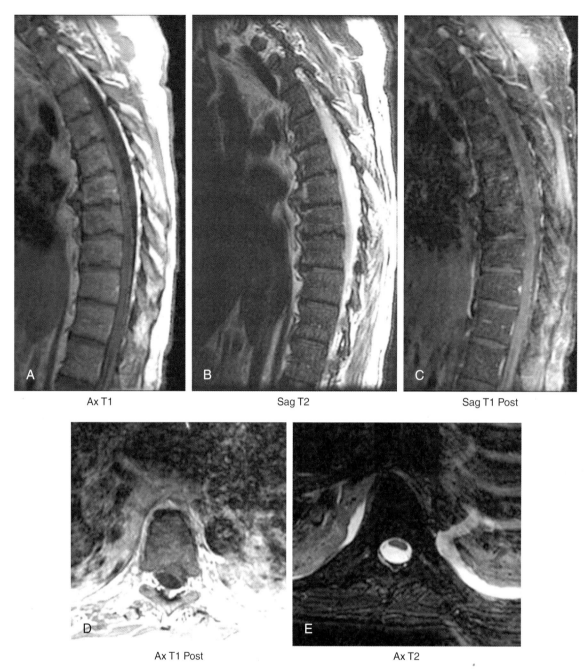

A   Ax T1

B   Sag T2

C   Sag T1 Post

D   Ax T1 Post

E   Ax T2

CASE C: A 35-year-old presenting with back pain. *Ax,* Axial; *Sag,* sagittal.

DESCRIPTION OF FINDINGS

MRI demonstrates three cases of intradural extramedullary (IDEM) cystic-appearing masses of the spine.
- Case A: The images show a T1 hypointense, T2 hyperintense, nearly isointense to cerebrospinal fluid (CSF), nonenhancing IDEM, cystic-appearing mass in the lower spinal canal scalloping the posterior vertebral bodies. Diffusion-weighted images demonstrate relative diffusion restriction.
- Case B: The images show a T1 mildly hyperintense compared with CSF, T2 mildly hypointense compared with CSF, nonenhancing cystic IDEM mass inferior to the conus that is displacing adjacent cauda equina nerve roots posteriorly.
- Case C: A T1 and T2 isointense to CSF, nonenhancing IDEM lesion displaces the cord anteriorly. On an axial T2 image, a subtle thin cystic wall is noted.

Diagnosis

Case A: Epidermoid cyst
Case B: Neurenteric cyst
Case C: Dorsal intradural arachnoid cyst

Summary

The spinal meninges include the dura, arachnoid, and pia mater. A reasonable differential diagnosis for spinal cystic masses can be generated based on the location of the mass relative to these meningeal layers. These can be classified into intramedullary or extramedullary lesions, and within the latter, it can be divided into intradural (IDEM) or extradural lesions. There are several clues one can use to figure out where a lesion is relative to the dura and spinal cord:
- Intramedullary lesions typically expand the cord, while extramedullary lesions compress the cord to a smaller caliber.
- An IDEM lesion compresses the spinal cord and forms an acute angle with the cord with a "marble above the carpet"

appearance. The "marble" is the lesion, and the "carpet" is the dura.
- An extradural lesion compresses on both the spinal cord and the dura, often effacing the CSF space and forming an obtuse angle with the CSF on sagittal T2 images. This is also known as "marble under the carpet" appearance (Fig. 43.1).
- An additional useful tip to identify extradural space even when the dura is not well seen is a lack of CSF pulsation artifact.

The major differential diagnoses with their characteristic MRI findings are listed in Table 43.1.

Arachnoid Cyst

An arachnoid cyst is defined as a space that contains CSF and is limited by arachnoid matter. Arachnoid cysts are identical in signal intensity to CSF on all sequences. An arachnoid cyst can be congenital or acquired (resulting from infection or trauma).

The Nabors' classification of arachnoid cysts includes the following types:
Type I: Extradural cyst without neural element
Type II: Extradural cyst with neural element (e.g., Tarlov and perineural cysts)
Type III: Intradural cyst

This discussion focuses on type III arachnoid cysts. The size of arachnoid cysts is variable. Posttraumatic cysts often are larger than congenital ones.

With the exception of cysts with neoplastic and infectious etiologies, most patients can be treated conservatively. Surgical intervention is reserved for patients with significant neurologic symptoms generally resulting from mass effect. Fenestration and partial resection often are the options if the cysts are large or ventrally located. The surgical outcome is usually favorable.

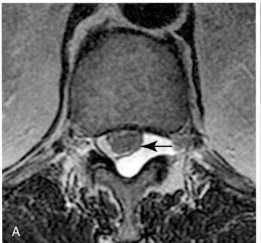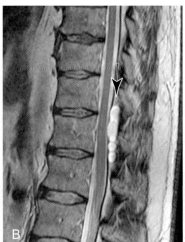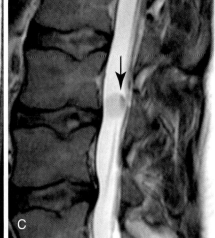

• **Fig. 43.1** Extradural versus intradural extramedullary (IDEM) cysts. (A) Axial T2 image of an extradural arachnoid cyst with clear displacement of the dura *(arrow)*. (B) The same arachnoid cyst on a sagittal T2 image compressing the dorsal thecal sac and effacing the dorsal cerebrospinal fluid space *(arrow)*. (C) A sagittal short T1 inversion recovery image of an IDEM cyst that displaces the nerve roots and forms a meniscus with the cerebrospinal fluid *(arrow)*.

TABLE 43.1 Cystic Intradural Extramedullary Lesions

Pathology	Craniocaudal	Axial	T1/T2[a]	DWI	Enhancement
Neurenteric cyst	Cervicothoracic junction; conus	Ventral or ventrolateral	Isointense to hyperintense/ hyperintense	Hypointense	None
Arachnoid cyst[b]	Thoracic spine (young); lumbosacral spine (adult)	Posterior or posterolateral	Isointense/isointense	Hypointense	None
Epidermoid cyst	Evenly throughout spine	No predilection	Isointense/isointense	Hyperintense	None unless infected
Dermoid cyst	Lumbosacral and cauda equina	No predilection	Heterogeneous; markedly hyperintense		None unless infected
Neurocysticercosis	Lumbosacral	Dorsal thoracic	Isointense to slightly hyper-intense/isointense to slightly hyperintense	Hypointense	No enhancement or ring enhancement

[a]Relative to cerebrospinal fluid signal intensity.
[b]Nabors type III arachnoid cyst.

Dermoid and Epidermoid Cysts

Dermoid and epidermoid cysts can be either congenital or acquired. Congenital lesions arise from the inclusion of ectodermal elements during neural tube development. Acquired lesions often are the result of iatrogenic implantation during lumbar puncture. They can be both unilocular and multilocular.

On T1- and T2-weighted images, most epidermoid cysts are similar in signal (but not completely isointense) to CSF. There is significant diffusion restriction in epidermoid cysts compared with CSF. Dermoid cysts frequently have T1 hyperintense foci due to fat components and usually are heterogeneous on T1- and T2-weighted images.

Both dermoid and epidermoid cysts can have associated dermal sinus tracts.

Neurenteric Cysts

Neurenteric cysts result from failed separation of the endoderm from the ectoderm during the third week of embryogenesis. They are lined by alimentary tract mucosa and have a definitive connection with the spinal canal. Therefore, they can be seen in communication with an extraspinal cystic component in the mesentery, the mediastinum, and the gut.

Neurenteric cysts frequently are associated with spinal segmentation abnormalities, which can be an important clue to diagnosis. These lesions have a predilection for the cervical spine, but they can be seen anywhere along the spinal canal. Because of variable proteinaceous content, the neurenteric cyst may appear hyperintense to CSF on T1 imaging.

Beyond these more common entities, infections such as neurocysticercosis could be considered for patients in the appropriate clinical setting. Cystic degeneration of peripheral nerve sheath tumor or meningioma is known to occur, but this is extremely rare.

Spectrum of Disease

Synovial cysts, which are extradural extramedullary cystic lesions of the spine, sometimes are confused with intradural lesions. Synovial cysts are associated with degenerative and posttraumatic changes in the spine. They communicate with the facet joint and are lined by the synovium. The cyst often is isointense to slightly hyperintense to CSF on T1 imaging and slightly hyperintense or hypointense to CSF on T2 imaging, but signal characteristics may be variable (Fig. 43.2). A T2 hypointense peripheral rim often is seen, likely from calcification or hemorrhage in the margin of the cyst (Fig. 43.3). Hemorrhage within the cyst also is possible. Synovial cysts may result in severe cord, nerve root, and thecal sac compression.

Differential Diagnosis

1. Arachnoid cyst (type III)
2. Dermoid/epidermoid cyst
3. Neurenteric cyst
4. Tumor with cystic/necrotic component
   Cystic schwannoma spine
   Metastasis
5. Parasitic infection
   Hydatid cyst
   Neurocysticercosis

See Table 43.1 for a brief outline of the diagnostic approach to cystic IDEM lesions based on conventional MRI features.

Pearls

- Arachnoid cysts generally are isointense to CSF. When the arachnoid cystic wall is not well visualized, the lack of CSF pulsation artifact within the cyst can be useful in distinguishing the arachnoid cyst from surrounding CSF. In addition, due to its indolent nature, surrounding bony

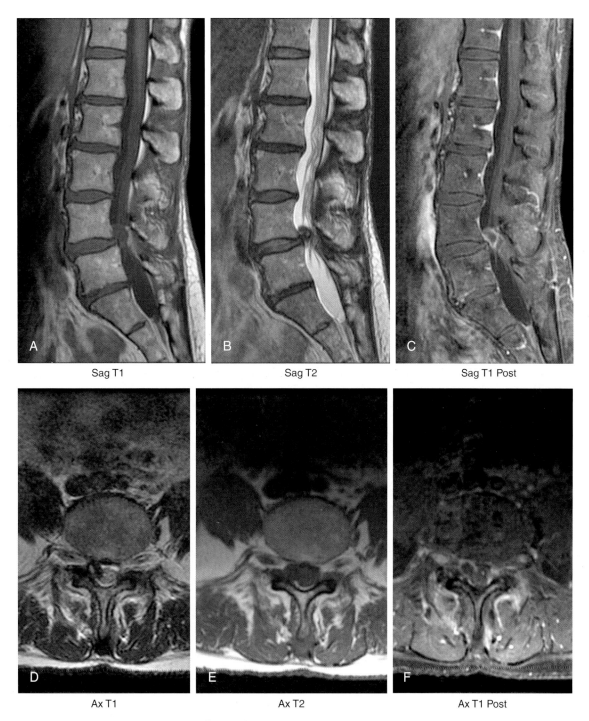

Sag T1   Sag T2   Sag T1 Post

Ax T1   Ax T2   Ax T1 Post

• **Fig. 43.2** A synovial cyst. (A–C) An epidural T1 and T2 hypointense mass with small T2 focal hyperintensity centered in the right lateral recess of the spinal canal is exerting mass effect on the adjacent caudal nerve roots. (D–E) A thin peripheral rim of enhancement is evident on postcontrast T1 images. *Ax,* Axial; *Sag,* sagittal.

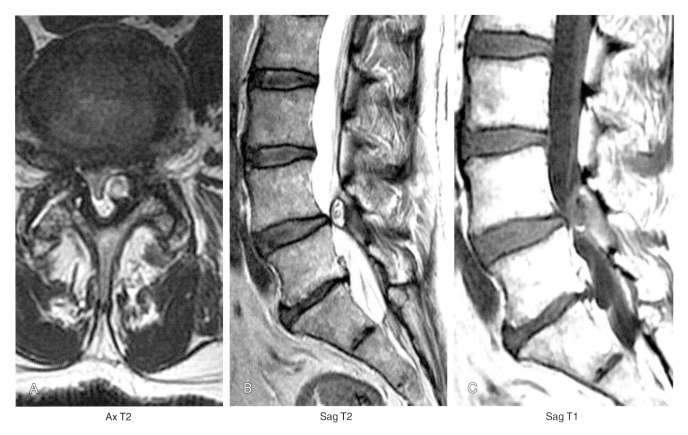

Ax T2   Sag T2   Sag T1

• **Fig. 43.3** A synovial cyst similar to that in Fig. 43.2 with deformity of the thecal sac and nerve root compression. A prominent T2 hypointense peripheral rim is evident. *Ax,* Axial; *Sag,* sagittal.

remodeling with associated widening of the spinal canal or neural foramina usually is seen.

• It is important to consider parasitic diseases in the differential diagnosis for small cystic IDEM lesions. These diseases include hydatid and neurocysticercosis cysts. They typically are in dependent locations, such as the lumbosacral and dorsal thoracic regions (Fig. 43.4).

• Dermoid cysts often are more heterogeneous than CSF and epidermoids. They have T1 hyperintense, fatty components. Both dermoid and epidermoid cysts can be associated with nearby dermal sinus tracts. Epidermoid cysts have restricted diffusion.

• Spine segmentation anomalies are frequently seen in conjunction with neurenteric cysts.

• An important differential diagnosis for a dorsal arachnoid cyst is a ventral dural defect. Features that would favor a ventral dural defect over an arachnoid cyst (Case C) include acute angular ventral cord deviation, cord deviation less than two thoracic segments or 3 cm, absence of CSF ventral or ventrolateral to the cord, absence of CSF loculation dorsal to the cord, absence of delayed myelographic CSF opacification dorsal to the cord, and the presence of a ventral extradural cyst containing CSF.

Signs and Complications

Cystic IDEM lesions often result in chronic nonspecific clinical findings, including chronic back pain, neuropathy, paresthesia, paraparesis, and/or gait ataxia.

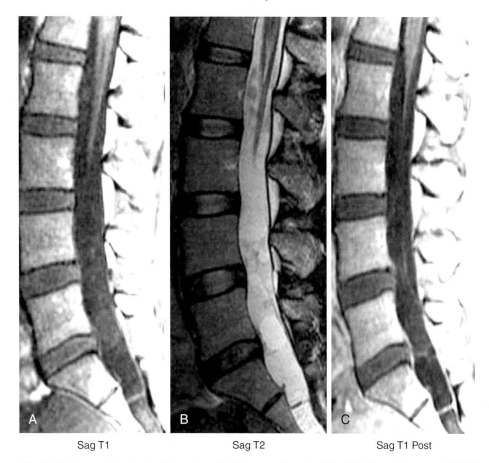

Sag T1   Sag T2   Sag T1 Post

• **Fig. 43.4** Neurocysticercosis of the spine. Multiple nonenhancing, T1 slightly hyperintense to CSF, T2 slightly hyperintense to CSF, intradural, extramedullary cysts are seen in the dependent portion of the thecal sac. *Sag,* Sagittal.

Suggested Readings

Beall DP, Googe DJ, Emery RL, et al: Extramedullary intradural spinal tumors: a pictorial review, *Curr Probl Diagn Radiol* 36(5):185–198, 2007.

da Conceição Araújo Filho S, da Silva HB, de Albuquerque LAF, et al: Giant intradural extramedullary arachnoid cyst of the thoracic spine, *J Clin Neurosci* 16(10):1369–1371, 2009.

Evans A, Stoodley N, Halpin S: Magnetic resonance imaging of intraspinal cystic lesions: a pictorial review, *Curr Probl Diagn Radiol* 31(3): 79–94, 2002.

Güneçs M, Akdemir H, Tuqcu B, et al: Multiple intradural spinal hydatid disease: a case report and review of literature, *Spine* 34(9):E346–E350, 2009.

Kasliwal MK, Kale SS, Sharma BS, et al: Totally cystic intradural extramedullary schwannoma, *Turk Neurosurg* 18(4):404–406, 2008.

Khosla A, Wippold FJ II: CT Myelography and MR imaging of extramedullary cysts of the spinal canal in adult and pediatric patients, *AJR Am J Roentgenol* 178(1):201–207, 2002.

Menezes AH, Traynelis VC: Spinal neurenteric cysts in the magnetic resonance imaging era, *Neurosurgery* 58(1):97–105, 2006.

Morley S, Naidoo P, Robertson A, et al: Thoracic ventral dural defect: idiopathic spinal cord herniation, *Australas Radiol* 50(2):168–170, 2006.

Secer HI, Anik I, Celik E, et al: Spinal hydatid cyst mimicking arachnoid cyst on magnetic resonance imaging, *J Spinal Cord Med* 31(1):106–108, 2008.

Silbergleit R, Brunberg JA, Patel SC, et al: Imaging of spinal intradural arachnoid cysts: MRI, myelography and CT, *Neuroradiology* 40(10): 664–668, 1998.

Wu S, Sharma KK, Ho CL: Lumbar spinal epidural capillary hemangioma: a case report and literature review, *Am J Case Rep* 23:e936181, 2022.

44

Nerve Root Enlargement

FARGOL BOOYA, MD

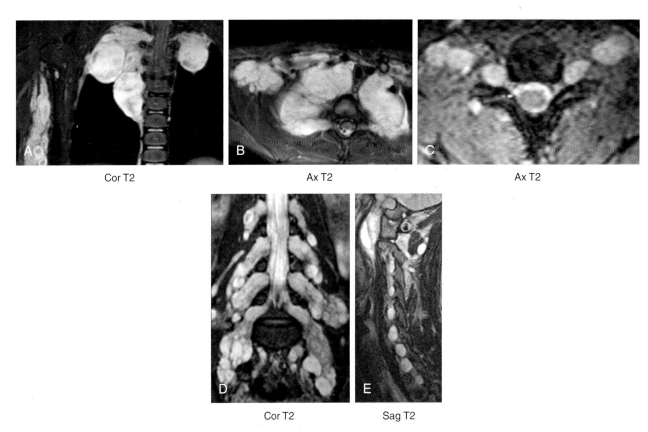

Cor T2   Ax T2   Ax T2

Cor T2   Sag T2

CASE A: A 24-year-old with a history of neurofibromatosis type 1 presenting with a 3-month history of weakness and tremors in right hand. *Ax*, Axial; *Cor*, coronal; *Sag*, sagittal.

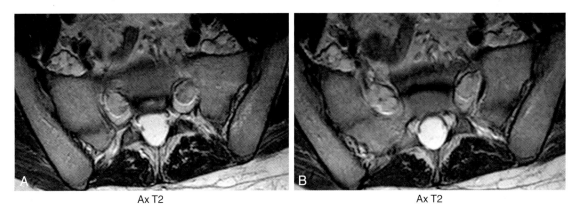

Ax T2   Ax T2

CASE B: A 17-year-old with foot deformity and scoliosis. *Ax*, Axial.

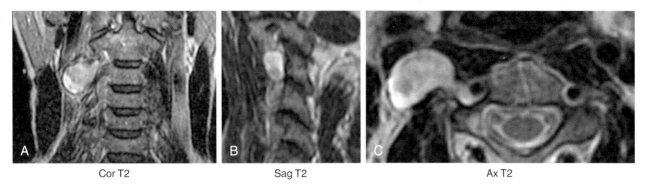

Cor T2   Sag T2   Ax T2

CASE C: A 59-year-old presenting with pain and sensation of a mass in the right side of the neck. *Ax,* Axial; *Cor,* coronal; *Sag,* sagittal.

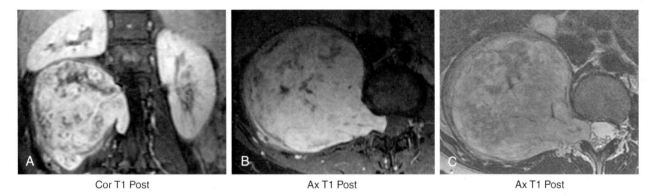

Cor T1 Post   Ax T1 Post   Ax T1 Post

CASE D: A 35-year-old presenting with 2 weeks of increasing dull pain in the right upper quadrant. *Ax,* Axial; *Cor,* coronal.

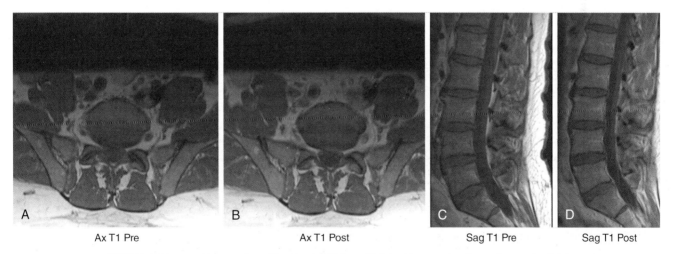

Ax T1 Pre   Ax T1 Post   Sag T1 Pre   Sag T1 Post

CASE E: A 24-year-old presenting with a 2-week history of bilateral lower extremity weakness. *Ax,* Axial; *Sag,* sagittal.

DESCRIPTION OF FINDINGS

- Case A: Bilateral, enhancing, plexiform, mass-like enlargement of the cervical nerve roots extending into the extraforaminal paraspinal region.
- Case B: Enhancement and diffuse enlargement of the sacral foraminal nerve roots and extraforaminal sacral nerves bilaterally.
- Case C: An extramedullary mass expanding the right C2–C3 neural foramen. The mass has a target appearance with central hypointensity on T2-weighted images.
- Case D: A heterogeneously enhancing large right upper quadrant mass extends out of the spinal canal through a right upper lumbar neural foramen.
- Case E: Diffuse enhancement of the cauda equina nerve roots and pia of the conus medullaris.

Diagnosis

Case A: Plexiform neurofibromas in the setting of neurofibromatosis type 1 (NF1)

Case B: Charcot–Marie–Tooth (CMT) disease

Case C: Solitary benign peripheral nerve sheath tumor confirmed by biopsy

Case D: Malignant peripheral nerve sheath tumor confirmed by excisional biopsy

Case E: Abnormal enhancement of the peripheral nerves in the setting of Guillain–Barré disease (GBD) (diagnosis was confirmed by electromyography and nerve conduction velocity testing)

Summary

Differential considerations for abnormal enlargement or abnormal enhancement of the peripheral nerve roots can be distinguished partly on the basis of the dominant imaging finding. The predominant feature can be abnormal morphology, an unusual pattern of enhancement, or the presence of a tumoral mass.

Abnormal morphology of the peripheral nerves may be seen with the chronic neuropathies—for example, chronic sensory motor peripheral neuropathies such as CMT disease or chronic immune demyelinating polyneuropathy (CIDP). In these entities, sequential episodes of demyelination and remyelination lead to a concentric "onion skin" or "light bulb" appearance.

The presence of a solitary tumor of the peripheral nerve is suggested by an enhancing mass that grows along the nerve, often extending out of the neural foramina. A solitary nerve sheath tumor may represent either a solitary neurofibroma or schwannoma or a malignant peripheral nerve sheath tumor. If it is associated with diffuse enlargement of the peripheral nerve roots, entities such as NF1 and neurofibromatosis type 2 (NF2) should be considered. Patients with NF1 and NF2 have characteristic bilateral peripheral nerve involvement with evidence of chronicity, such as enlargement of the neural foramina from dural ectasia or bony scalloping or remodeling from the nerve root sheath tumors themselves. Neurofibromas may arise sporadically or in association with NF1. A neurofibroma may arise at any point along a peripheral nerve and presents as fusiform enlargement of the nerve. From an imaging point of view, schwannomas cannot definitely be differentiated from neurofibromas. In practice, the major distinction between a

schwannoma and a solitary neurofibroma is that a schwannoma can be resected while sparing the underlying nerve, whereas resection of a neurofibroma requires sacrifice of the underlying nerve. The hallmark lesion of NF1 is the plexiform neurofibroma. This lesion is composed of sheets of neurofibromatous tissue that may infiltrate and encase major nerves, blood vessels, and other vital structures. These lesions look like rope or a branching bag of worms. Malignant peripheral nerve sheath tumors, once called neurofibrosarcomas, can arise de novo or from degeneration of a plexiform neurofibroma; however, this complication is rare. A plexiform neurofibroma has an 8% to 12% lifetime risk of transformation.

Abnormal enhancement of the nerve roots can be seen with neoplastic, infectious, and inflammatory/autoimmune causes, as seen with GBD. The pattern of enhancement, chronicity, and other imaging findings coupled with a thorough history can help pare down this differential diagnosis.

Spectrum of Disease

Neurofibromatosis Type 1

Different types of spinal neurofibromas are recognized in persons with NF1. Localized neurofibroma is seen in 90% of patients with NF1. Plexiform neurofibroma is less common and presents with diffuse enlargement of the nerve roots with a bulky mass or a rope-like appearance.

Neurofibromatosis Type 2

Meningiomas, schwannomas, and ependymomas are the hallmarks of NF2. More than half of patients with this disorder present with extraspinal findings. Approximately half present with extramedullary, intradural tumors, and they may present with cord compression.

Chronic Immune Demyelinizing Polyneuropathy/Congenital Hypertrophic Neuropathy

One cannot distinguish CIDP/congenital hypertrophic neuropathy (hereditary motor sensory neuropathy or CMT disease) from an imaging standpoint. Enlargement and abnormal T2 hyperintensity of the nerve roots, plexi, and peripheral nerves are noted. Nerve size may vary from small to very large. Muscle denervation signals also may be seen. Brain magnetic resonance imaging may demonstrate subclinical demyelination in cases of CIDP.

Abnormal Enhancement of the Nerve Roots

The entities presenting with abnormal enhancement of the peripheral nerves may not necessarily cause thickening or enlargement of the nerve roots. For example, GBD causes avid enhancement of the cauda equina nerve roots with slightly thickened but not nodular enhancement compared with the chronic recurring diseases such as CIDP.

Differential Diagnosis

1. Arachnoiditis (chemical or postsurgical): The absence of discrete nerve roots in the thecal sac (empty thecal sac sign) may be apparent because nerve roots adhere to the dural wall. Irregular distortion and clumping of nerve roots and/or a septated appearance of cerebrospinal fluid (CSF) in the thecal sac may be noted.

2. Lateral meningocele: CSF signal intensity meningeal protrusion may be present through the neural foramen, which is highly associated with NF1, but it may be seen separately. This entity may be confused with nerve sheath tumors but will not enhance on postcontrast imaging.

3. Brachial plexus traction injury resulting in a pseudomeningocele: Brachial plexus traction injury resulting in a pseudomeningocele is a lateral CSF-containing dural outpouching with no neural elements. The patient usually has a history of trauma followed by paralysis.

4. Sarcoidosis: Sarcoidosis may have a varied presentation in the spine. The usual presentation is leptomeningeal and intramedullary mass-like lesions. Sarcoidosis is very unlikely to present as enlargement of the nerve roots.

5. Conjoined nerve roots: Conjoined nerve roots are an asymmetric anomalous origin of an enlarged nerve roots sleeve containing nerve roots from two levels. Because of normal enhancement of the dorsal root ganglia enhancement and neural foraminal remodeling, this entity may be confused with a peripheral nerve sheath tumor.

Pearls

- In the differential of peripheral nerve enlargement, CIDP/congenital hypertrophic neuropathy should be considered.

The hallmark of CIDP is "onion skin" enlargement of the peripheral nerves.

- Multilevel bulky nerve root tumors in a patient with stigmata of NF1 or NF2 suggests multiple neurofibromas and/or schwannomas.
- Enhancement of the cauda equina nerve roots with little or no enlargement and no nodularity suggests GBD.

Signs and Complications

Most common signs/symptoms include sensory and motor symptoms in the affected territory. Pain also may be present. Plexiform neurofibromas and tumors of the nerve roots also may present with myelopathy and complications related to the effect of the mass.

Suggested Readings

Egelhoff JC, Bates DJ, Ross JS, et al: Spinal MR findings in neurofibromatosis types 1 and 2, *AJNR Am J Neuroradiol* 13(4):1071–1077, 1992.

Khong PL, Goh WH, Wong VC, et al: MR imaging of spinal tumors in children with neurofibromatosis 1, *AJR Am J Roentgenol* 180(2):413–417, 2003.

Murphey MD, Smith WS, Smith SE, et al: From the archives of the AFIP. Imaging of musculoskeletal neurogenic tumors: radiologic-pathologic correlation, *Radiographics* 19(5):1253–1280, 1999.

Odaka M, Yuki N, Hirata K: Patients with chronic inflammatory demyelinating polyneuropathy initially diagnosed as Guillain-Barré syndrome, *J Neurol* 250(8):913–916, 2003.

Schady W, Goulding PJ, Lecky BR, et al: Massive nerve root enlargement in chronic inflammatory demyelinating polyneuropathy, *J Neurol Neurosurg Psychiatry* 61(6):636–640, 1996.

Stull MA, Moser RP Jr., Kransdorf MJ, et al: Magnetic resonance appearance of peripheral nerve sheath tumors, *Skeletal Radiol* 20(1):9–14, 1991.

Woodruff JM, et al: Neurofibroma. In Kleihues P, Cavenee WK, editors: *Tumors of the nervous system*, Lyon, France, 2000, IARC Press.

45

Extramedullary Abnormal Vessels

MARIA BRAILEANU, MD

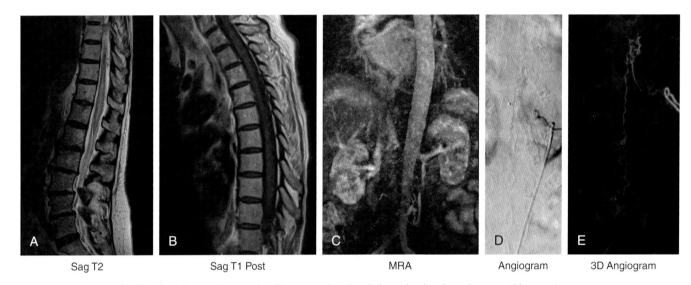

A	B	C	D	E
Sag T2	Sag T1 Post	MRA	Angiogram	3D Angiogram

CASE A: An 85-year-old presents with progressive chronic lower back pain and neuropathic symptoms including bladder function loss and inability to walk. *MRA*, Magnetic resonance angiography; *Sag*, sagittal.

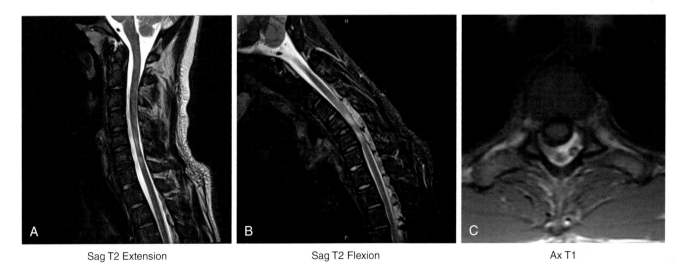

A	B	C
Sag T2 Extension	Sag T2 Flexion	Ax T1

CASE B: A 16-year-old presents with progressive asymmetric right upper extremity weakness and functional loss. *Ax*, Axial; *Sag*, sagittal.

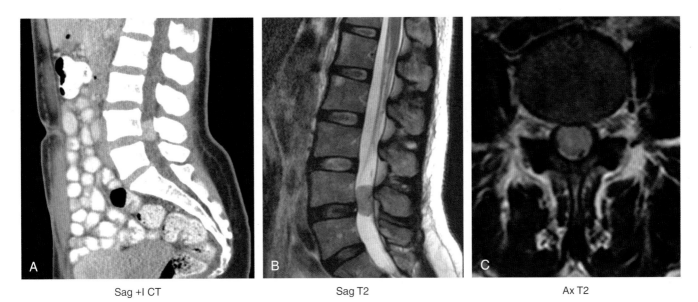

Sag +I CT   Sag T2   Ax T2

CASE C: A 45-year-old presents with lower back and right-sided sciatic pain. *Ax,* Axial; *CT,* Computed tomography; *Sag,* sagittal.

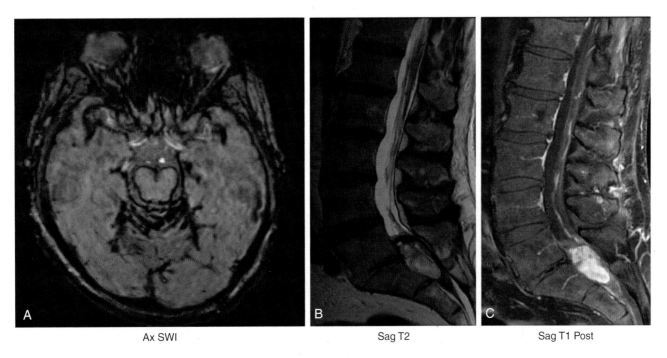

Ax SWI   Sag T2   Sag T1 Post

CASE D: A 65-year-old presents with headache. *Ax,* Axial; *Sag,* sagittal; *SWI,* susceptibility-weighted imaging.

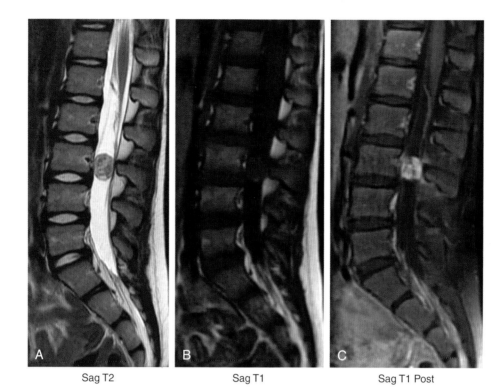

Sag T2   Sag T1   Sag T1 Post

CASE E: An 8-year-old presents with back pain and constipation. *Sag*, Sagittal.

DESCRIPTION OF FINDINGS

CT, magnetic resonance imaging (MRI), MRA, and digital subtraction angiography (DSA) images from four patients with abnormal extramedullary vessels of the spine.

- Case A: There is T2 hyperintense signal and expansion of the spinal cord extending from the levels of T9 to L1 with associated extramedullary dorsal flow voids. On post contrast T1 sequences, the dorsal vessels enhanced. On MRA, irregular vascularity arises from the left infrarenal aorta. On DSA and 3D angiographic reconstructions, arteriovenous shunting is noted from the left T10 segmental artery, with dilated and tortuous venous structures noted within the spinal canal.
- Case B: There is T2 hyperintense signal and volume loss of the cervical spinal cord at the levels of C5 to C7. On flexion sequences, there is enlargement of the posterior epidural space and prominence of the venous plexus involving the cervical spine. The dorsal dura compresses the cervical cord in flexion. There is loss of the dorsal dural attachment to the lamina. Follow-up MRA is negative for a vascular malformation (not shown).
- Case C: A well-circumscribed hyperdense mass is seen in the spinal canal at the level of L4 to L5 on CT. On MRI, the lesion is associated with the nerve roots. Flow voids are noted along the surface of the lesion and extending along the nerve roots to the conus.
- Case D: There is hemosiderin staining of the basal cisterns and posterior fossa on brain MRI. On spinal MRI, an avidly enhancing hemorrhagic mass is seen at the level of L5 to S1. Associated extramedullary vessels extend superiorly adjacent to the nerve roots to the conus.
- Case E: An enhancing highly vascular lesion is seen at the level of L3 arising from the nerve roots. Prominent serpiginous vessels extend superiorly from the mass to the conus.

Diagnosis

Case A: Arteriovenous fistula (AVF)
Case B: Hirayama disease
Case C: Paraganglioma
Case D: Hemangioblastoma
Case E: Hemangioma

Summary

Extramedullary abnormal vessels within the spinal canal include a heterogenous group of pathologies, which can be purely vascular or associated with other lesions. For example, intradural dorsal AVFs are spinal vascular malformations. On the other hand, atypical spinal paragangliomas are vascular lesions that are associated with extramedullary serpiginous vessels. Benign vascular findings, such as anatomical variants, as well as enhancing epidural disease, such as an epidural abscess, may mimic extramedullary vascular lesions. Correlation with clinical symptoms and history is especially important in the diagnosis. Apart from initial CT and MR examinations, follow-up imaging, such as flexion/extension MRI, MRA, and DSA, may be required for further workup and confirmation of diagnosis.

Spinal dural AVFs are a type of spinal arteriovenous malformation (AVM). Intradural dorsal AVFs (type I) make up 80% of all spinal AVMs. Other types of spinal AVFs include extradural (epidural) and ventral intradural (perimedullary, type IV a/b/c; please see companion case Fig. 45.1). Patients are typically males in their late 40s to early 60s presenting with progressive lower extremity weakness and pain. On MRI, the cord may appear enlarged with abnormal signal. On MRA, the fistula may be at a different spinal level. DSA is the gold standard for diagnosis.

Hirayama disease is a cervical flexion myelopathy that causes upper extremity weakness in young male patients.

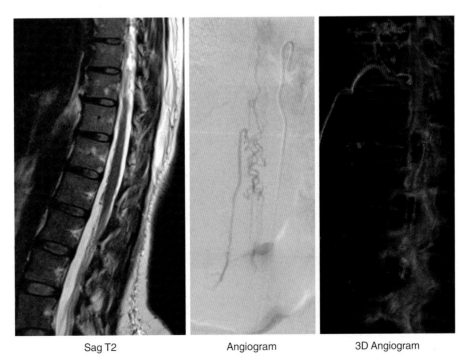

Sag T2   Angiogram   3D Angiogram

• **Fig. 45.1** A 45-year-old with long-standing back pain. Magnetic resonance imaging demonstrates ventral flow voids along the thoracolumbar spine. Digital subtraction angiography with 3D reconstruction demonstrates a type IV spinal arteriovenous fistula of the left T11 segmental artery. *Sag*, Sagittal.

Compression of the cord with flexion causes damage to the lower cervical anterior horns. Imaging features of Hirayama include lower cervical cord volume loss, abnormal cervical cord T2 hyperintensity, detachment of the dura from the lamina, and loss of the cervical lordosis. Follow-up flexion MRI sequences may demonstrate the forward displacement of the dura, causing compression of the cervical cord and increased prominence of the dorsal epidural space and epidural venous plexus. Unlike spinal AVFs, follow-up MRA will be negative for underlying vascular lesion.

Spinal paragangliomas are highly vascular neuroendocrine lesions that are attached to the filum terminale or lumbar nerve roots. Spinal location of paragangliomas is rare and they account for only 3% to 4% of all cauda equina tumors. Both children and older adults are affected with a slight male predilection. Clinical symptoms are usually secondary to lesion mass effect causing back pain, and occasionally cauda equina symptoms; endocrine symptoms and associated subarachnoid hemorrhage are very rare. These lesions are classified as WHO grade I. On MRI, lesions are well-circumscribed masses with serpentine flow voids, which can extend along the surface of the tumor and the spinal cord. On DSA, lesions demonstrate early arterial blushing that persists into the early venous phase.

Hemangioblastomas are typically intramedullary tumors (as described in Chapter 38, Enhancing Intramedullary Spinal Cord Lesions). Rarely, these lesions may be extramedullary in the lumbosacral spine. Hemangioblastomas may be sporadic in adults or be associated with von Hippel–Lindau syndrome in 32% of cases (See companion case Fig. 45.2). Clinical presentation depends on the location of the lesion. Hemangioblastomas are highly vascular with larger lesions demonstrating flow voids and associated abnormal extramedullary vessels. Extramedullary hemangioblastomas are typically associated with the nerve roots.

Unlike vertebral hemangiomas, central and peripheral nervous system hemangiomas are extremely rare. In the spinal cord, the lesion can arise from the blood vessels of the nerve roots, pial surface of the cord, or inner surface of the dura. Patients may present with symptoms secondary to mass effect from the lesion or from associated hemorrhage. On MRI, the lesion will markedly enhance with intertumoral flow voids. The lesion may have both extra- and intramedullary components. Tortuous vessels and arterial feeders may be present (See companion case Fig. 45.3).

Spectrum of Disease

Spectrum of pathological findings is described in the preceding section. Enhancing lesions in the epidural space, such as an epidural abscess or metastatic lesion, may mimic extramedullary vascular pathology. Additional mimics in the epidural space include the benign dilatation of the epidural venous plexus and MRI flow-related artifact.

Differential Diagnosis

1. **Spinal AVM**
   • Spinal AVF (Fig. 45.1)
2. **Hirayama disease**

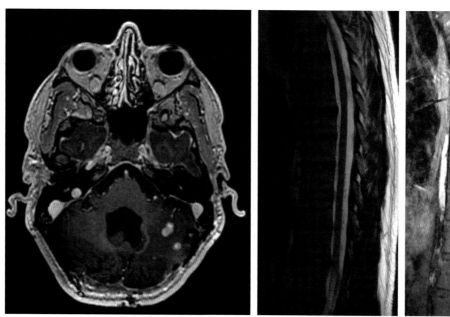
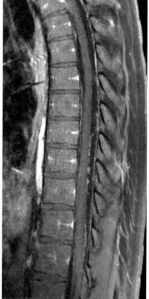

Ax T1 Post   Sag T2   Sag T1 Post

• **Fig. 45.2** A 35-year-old with von Hippel-Lindau and multiple posterior fossa hemangioblastomas. There are no cord lesions, but patient has abnormal extramedullary vessels of the lower thoracic spine which were negative for vascular malformation on prior magnetic resonance angiography (not shown). *Ax,* Axial; *Sag,* sagittal.

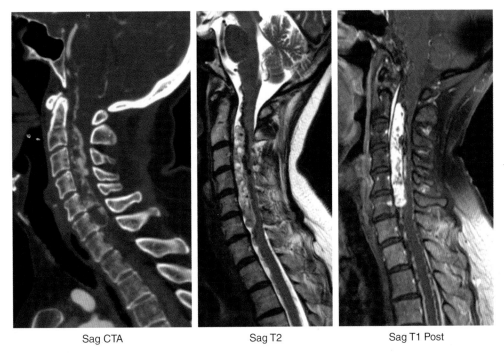

Sag CTA   Sag T2   Sag T1 Post

• **Fig. 45.3** A 60-year-old with an inoperable presumed cervical hemangioma. An enhancing lesion with flow voids spans the levels of C2 to C6. Multiple prominent serpiginous flow voids are noted within the mass. Associated extramedullary vessels extend superiorly along the cervical cord to the craniocervical junction and inferiorly along the thoracic cord. *CTA*, Computed tomography angiography; *Sag*, sagittal.

3. **Epidural enhancing lesions (mimics)**
   • Abscess
   • Hematoma (Fig. 45.4)
   • Metastatic lesion
4. **Cerebrospinal fluid (CSF) flow-related artifact**
5. **Benign dilation of the venous plexus**
   • Epidural venous plexus engorgement (secondary to pelvic venous congestion, for example)
6. **Vascular intramedullary/extramedullary lesions**
   • Hemangioblastoma (Fig. 45.2)
   • Paraganglioma
   • Hemangioma (Fig. 45.3)

Pearls

• Spinal AVFs generally occur in older male patients with lower extremity symptoms. The cord may demonstrate enlargement and abnormal T2 signal. Flow voids will be present along the cord surface. Follow-up MRA and DSA is warranted.
• Hirayama generally occurs in young male patients with upper extremity symptoms. The cord may demonstrate volume loss and abnormal T2 signal. On flexion and extension sequences, there may be prominence of the

dorsal epidural venous plexus with compression of the cervical cord by the dura. Angiographic imaging will be negative for AVF/AVM.
• Paragangliomas are well-circumscribed highly vascular masses along the filum terminale/nerve roots with associated serpentine flow voids. These lesions are very rare in the spine.
• Hemangioblastomas can be associated with von Hippel-Lindau syndrome. Lesions are rarely extramedullary in the spine. Lesions are typically associated with the lumbar nerve roots and serpentine flow voids (Fig. 45.2).
• Hemangiomas are very rare in the central and peripheral nervous system.

Signs and Complications

When AVFs are treated early with endovascular or surgical approach, the patient's lower extremity symptoms may improve. Compressive myelopathy secondary to Hirayama disease in the cervical spine typically causes upper extremity weakness and atrophy; treatment is usually conservative. Paragangliomas may cause symptoms secondary to mass effect on the filum terminale and lumbar nerve roots, similar to hemangioblastomas and hemangiomas. Lesions may require resection if the patient is symptomatic.

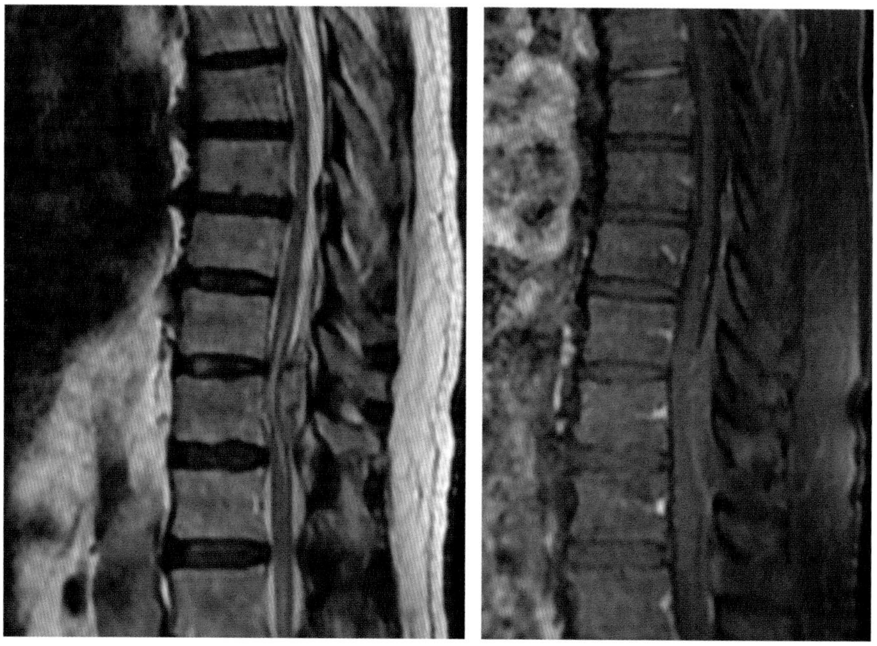

Sag T2   Sag T1 Post

• **Fig. 45.4** An 87-year-old on anticoagulation presents with bilateral lower extremity paralysis. Magnetic resonance imaging demonstrates a nonenhancing epidural hematoma centered at T11 mimicking an extramedullary vascular abnormality. *Sag*, Sagittal.

Suggested Readings

Baker KB, Moran CJ, Wippold FJ II, et al: MR imaging of spinal hemangioblastoma, *AJR Am J Roentgenol* 174(2):377–382, 2000.

Freeman CW, Lazor JW, Loevner LA, et al: Variations of the CNS venous system mimicking pathology: spectrum of imaging findings, *J Neuroimaging* 29(6):673–688, 2019.

Koeller KK, Shih RY: Intradural extramedullary spinal neoplasms: radiologic-pathologic correlation, *Radiographics* 39(2):468–490, 2019.

Lehman VT, Luetmer PH, Sorenson EJ, et al: Cervical spine MR imaging findings of patients with Hirayama disease in North America: a multisite study, *AJNR Am J Neuroradiol* 34(2):451–456, 2013.

McEvoy SH, Farrell M, Brett F, et al: Haemangioma, an uncommon cause of an extradural or intradural extramedullary mass: case series with radiological pathological correlation, *Insights Imaging* 7(1):87–98, 2016.

Morris JM: Imaging of dural arteriovenous fistula, *Radiol Clin North Am* 50(4):823–39, 2012.

Ozpinar A, Weiner GM, Ducruet AF: Epidemiology, clinical presentation, diagnostic evaluation, and prognosis of spinal arteriovenous malformations, *Handb Clin Neurol* 143:145–152, 2017.

Shih RY, Koeller KK: Intramedullary masses of the spinal cord: radiologic-pathologic correlation, *Radiographics* 40(4):1125–1145, 2020.

46

Epidural Rim-Enhancing Lesion

BASHAR KAKO, MD

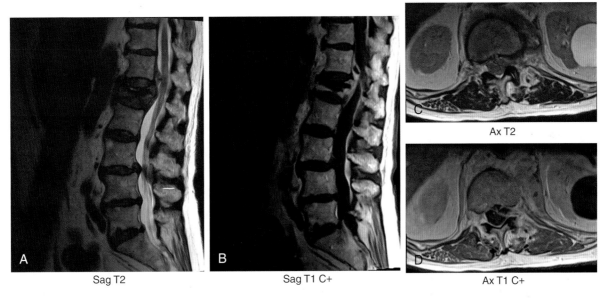

Sag T2   Sag T1 C+   Ax T2   Ax T1 C+

CASE A: A 75-year-old with history of osteoporosis who presents with 2 weeks' history of severe lower back pain that developed after carrying a heavy shopping bag. *Ax*, Axial; *Sag*, sagittal.

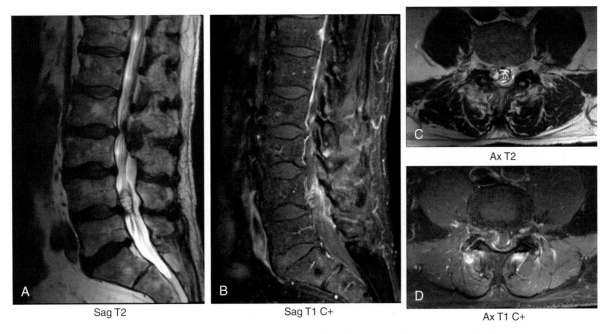

Sag T2   Sag T1 C+   Ax T2   Ax T1 C+

CASE B: A 62-year-old who presents with back pain with radiation to the legs not responsive to conservative measures. *Ax*, Axial; *Sag*, sagittal.

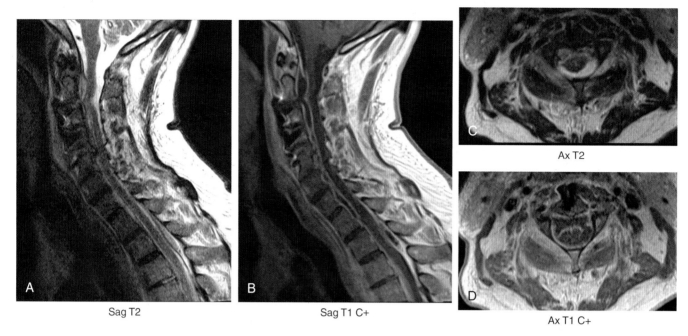

Sag T2

Sag T1 C+

Ax T2

Ax T1 C+

CASE C: A 60-year-old status post recent C2–C4 fusion, anterior cervical discectomy and fusion, presented with neck pain and fever. *Ax*, Axial; *Sag*, sagittal.

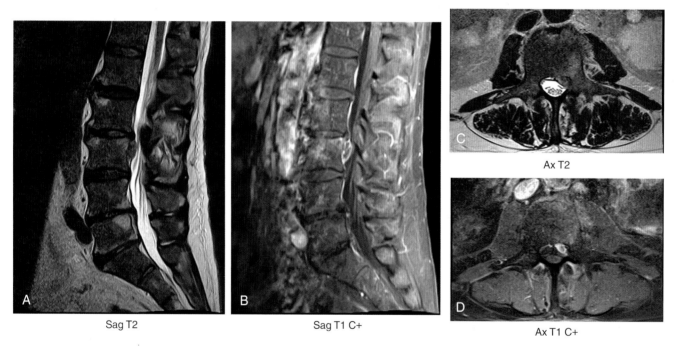

Sag T2

Sag T1 C+

Ax T2

Ax T1 C+

CASE D: A 68-year-old with left lower back pain. *Ax*, Axial; *Sag*, sagittal.

DESCRIPTION OF FINDINGS

Magnetic resonance (MR) images from four patients with epidural rim-enhancing lesions.

- Case A: There is a compression fracture of L1 vertebral body and an associated heterogenous predominantly T2 hypointense ventral epidural collection extending superiorly to the T12 level resulting in moderate narrowing of the spinal canal. There is mild peripheral enhancement associated with the collection. There is also mild paravertebral and psoas muscle edema and enhancement at that level.
- Case B: There is a large predominantly T2 hyperintense extracanalicular lesion along the medial aspect of the right L4–L5 facet joint where there are severe degenerative changes. The lesion demonstrates faint peripheral enhancement and causes substantial narrowing of the right lateral recess and the right lateral spinal canal.
- Case C: There are postoperative changes related to C2–C4 ACDF with a rim-enhancing epidural fluid collection extending from the cervical to the thoracic region. The collection exerts mass effect on the cord. Additionally, there is edema in the paravertebral soft tissues.
- Case D: There is multilevel spondylosis with a ventral epidural T2 hypointense peripherally enhancing lesion at the level of L3. The lesion effaces the left ventral thecal sac as well as the left subarticular zone with mass effect on the descending left L3 nerve root.

Diagnosis

Case A: Late acute to early subacute epidural hematoma secondary to a compression fracture
Case B: Facet synovial cyst
Case C: Postoperative epidural abscess
Case D: Sequestered disc fragment

Summary

There are multiple entities that can present as peripherally enhancing epidural lesions, including facet joint synovial cysts, sequestered disc fragments, and epidural fluid collections such as abscesses and subacute hematomas. Although they can be a diagnostic challenge, MR imaging Characteristics of these lesions as well as the clinical history can aid in establishing a diagnosis.

Facet joint synovial cysts are a result of facet joint degeneration. These, depending on the size and location, can present with back pain with or without radicular symptoms. The lumbar spine is most commonly involved. The intrinsic MR appearance on T1- and T2-weighted sequences is variable depending on the presence or absence of hemorrhagic and/or proteinaceous contents. However, these cysts are most commonly seen in the posterolateral epidural space abutting an arthritic facet joint. A thin rim of enhancement is commonly seen.

Similarly, sequestered disc fragments are related to degenerative changes and can present with back pain with or without radicular symptoms. They represent an extruded disc material without continuity to the intervertebral disc. The lower lumbar spine is the most common location. On MR imaging, sequestered disc fragments are usually seen along the anterior or anterolateral aspect of the thecal sac associated with parent disc height loss, protrusion, and/or degeneration. Sequestered disc fragments are usually of intermediate to low signal intensity on T1-weighted images and intermediate to high signal intensity on T2-weighted images. Thin peripheral enhancement of the sequestered fragment is sometimes seen.

Spinal epidural abscesses are mostly due to bacterial or fungal infections. They usually develop as a result of hematogenous spread in the setting of endocarditis, contiguous extension in the setting of adjacent discitis/vertebral osteomyelitis, or direct inoculation from penetrating trauma or surgical intervention. Intravenous drug abuse, immunocompromised state, and chronic conditions such as diabetes mellitus are predisposing factors. *Staphylococcus aureus* is the most common causative pathogen. Most common locations involved are the lower thoracic and lumbar spine. Epidural abscesses classically span multiple levels and are usually isointense to hypointense on T1-weighted images and hyperintense on T2/short TI inversion recovery (STIR)-weighted sequences. Peripheral enhancement is usually seen surrounding a necrotic abscess. These collections characteristically restrict diffusion on diffusion-weighed imaging. Additional imaging findings, including discitis/osteomyelitis, paravertebral/paraspinal edema and/or collections, and postsurgical changes provide important supportive diagnostic clues.

Spinal epidural/extradural hematomas usually occur in the setting of trauma, recent instrumentation, or anticoagulation therapy. MR signal characteristics vary depending on the age of the hematoma. Hematomas typically extend over multiple levels. Subacute hematomas may demonstrate variable peripheral enhancement due to chemical irritation. The presence of intrinsic T1 hyperintensities within the collection can be seen in subacute hematomas, indicating the presence of methemoglobin. Additionally, T2* gradient refocused echo (GRE) sequence demonstrates susceptibility artifacts due to blood products. Additional findings, such as spine fractures and postsurgical changes, are important supportive clues.

Summary

Lesion	Imaging Features/Location	Supportive Clues
Facet joint synovial cyst	• Posterolateral epidural space lesion abutting an arthritic facet joint • Variable MR imaging signal	Back pain with or without same-sided radicular symptoms
Sequestered disc fragments	• Lesion anterior or anterolateral to the thecal sac with associated parent disc degeneration • Variable MR imaging signal	Back pain with or without same-sided radicular symptoms
Spinal epidural abscess	• Usually span multiple levels • T2WI/STIR hyperintense; DWI: restrict diffusion	Fever Elevated inflammatory markers Spondylodiscitis Recent surgery Adjacent soft tissue involvement
Subacute spinal epidural hematoma	• Usually span multiple levels • Intrinsic T1 hyperintensities can be seen due to presence of methemoglobin. • T2* GRE sequence accentuates susceptibility artifact.	Trauma/fractures Recent surgery Anticoagulation therapy

Differential Diagnosis

Metastasis

Pearls

- Facet joint synovial cysts are usually seen in the posterolateral epidural space abutting an arthritic facet joint.
- Sequestered disc fragments are usually anterior or anterolateral to the thecal sac with associated parent disc degeneration.
- Spinal epidural collections usually extend craniocaudally. Abscesses characteristically restrict diffusion. Fever, spondylodiscitis, recent surgery, and/or adjacent soft tissue involvement can be supportive clues for an abscess. History of spinal fractures/trauma, recent surgery, and intrinsic T1 hyperintensity within the collection raise concern for a hematoma.

Suggested Readings

Gala FB, Aswani Y: Imaging in spinal posterior epidural space lesions: a pictorial essay, *Indian J Radiol Imaging* 26(3):299–315, 2016.

Wolf M, Weber MA: Neuroimaging of the traumatic spine, *Magn Reson Imaging Clin N Am* 24(3):541–561, 2016.

Numaguchi Y, Rigamonti D, Rothman MI, et al: Spinal epidural abscess: evaluation with gadolinium-enhanced MR imaging, *Radiographics* 13(3):545–559, discussion 559–560, 1993.

Eastwood JD, Vollmer RT, Provenzale JM: Diffusion-weighted imaging in a patient with vertebral and epidural abscesses, *AJNR Am J Neuroradiol* 23(3):496–498, 2002.

Fardon DF, Williams AL, Dohring EJ, et al: Lumbar disc nomenclature: version 2.0: recommendations of the combined task forces of the North American Spine Society, the American Society of Spine Radiology and the American Society of Neuroradiology, *Spine J* 14(11):2525–2545, 2014.

Khan AM, Girardi F: Spinal lumbar synovial cysts. Diagnosis and management challenge, *Eur Spine J* 15(8):1176–11782, 2006.

47

Vertebral Anomalies

RILEY BRAZIL, MD, MPH AND SIMONE MONTOYA, MD

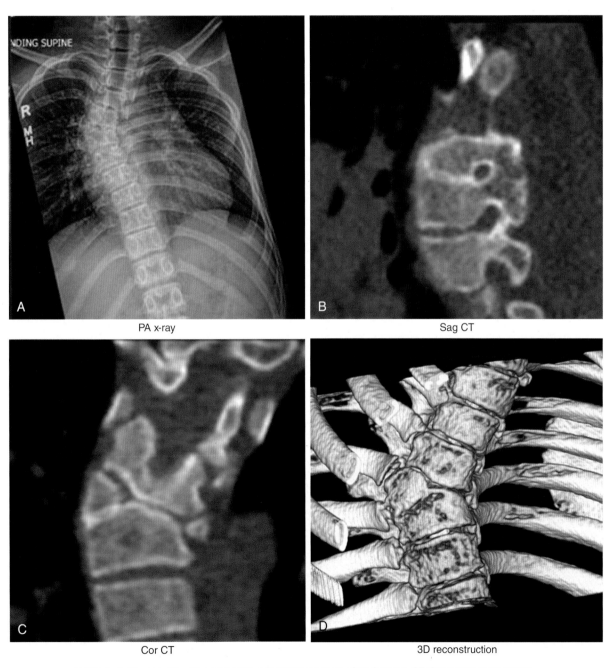

PA x-ray

Sag CT

Cor CT

3D reconstruction

CASE A: A 13-year-old with progressive congenital scoliosis. *Cor,* Coronal; *CT,* Computed tomography; *PA,* posteroanterior; *Sag,* sagittal.

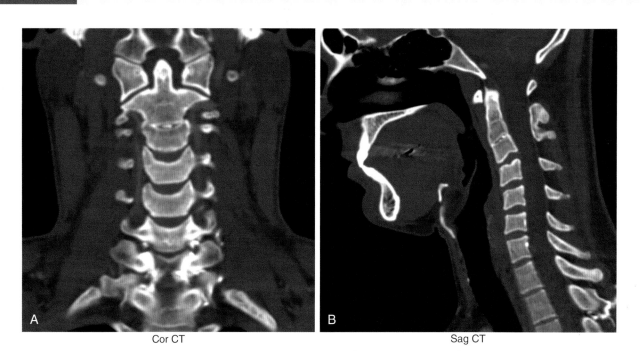

Cor CT

Sag CT

CASE B: A 31-year-old with nontraumatic neck pain and dizziness (incidental finding). *Cor,* Coronal; *CT,* Computed tomography; *Sag,* sagittal.

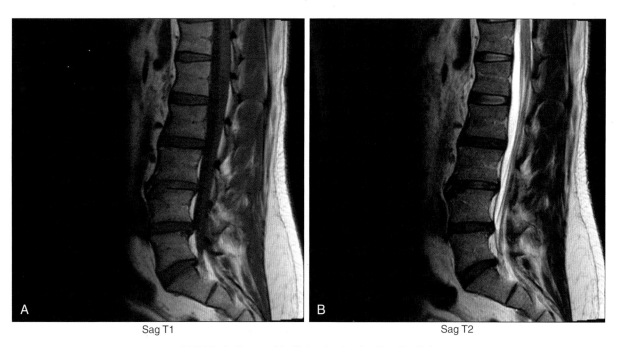

Sag T1

Sag T2

CASE C: A 42-year-old with low back pain. *Sag,* Sagittal.

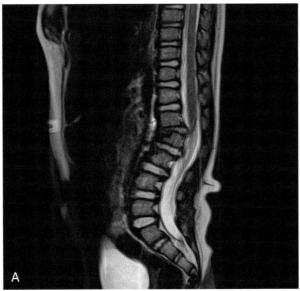

Sag T2

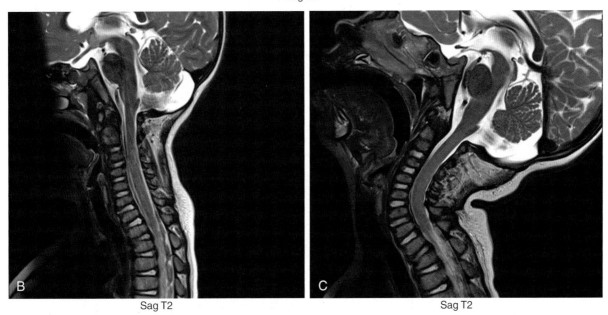

Sag T2

Sag T2

CASE D: A 3-year-old with known genetic disorder. *Sag,* Sagittal.

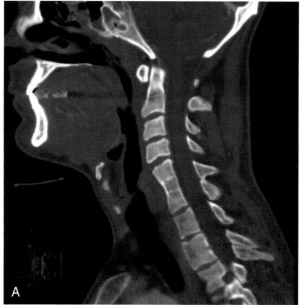

Sag CT

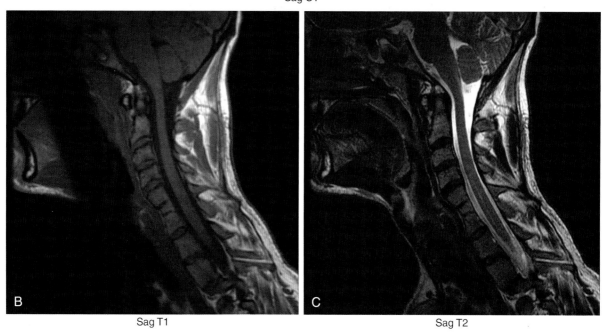

Sag T1   Sag T2

CASE E: A 27-year-old with polytrauma (incidental finding). *CT,* Computed tomography; *Sag,* sagittal.

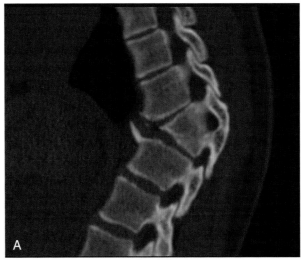

Sag CT

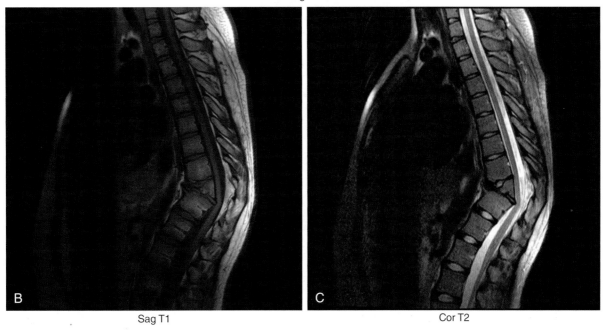

Sag T1   Cor T2

CASE F: A 21-year-old immigrant with longstanding spinal deformity. *Cor,* Coronal; *CT,* Computed tomography; *Sag,* sagittal.

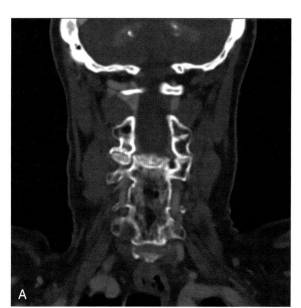

Cor CT

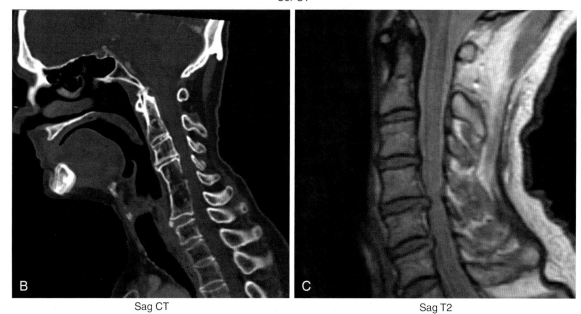

B   C

Sag CT   Sag T2

CASE G: A 77-year-old undergoing surveillance imaging for tongue base squamous cell carcinoma treated with chemoradiation. *Cor,* Coronal; *CT,* Computed tomography; *Sag,* sagittal.

DESCRIPTION OF FINDINGS

CT and MR images from six patients with anomalous vertebral body findings.

- Case A: There is wedged-shaped osseous structure located at the right lateral aspect of the thoracic spinal column, consistent with an incompletely formed T5 vertebral body. There is accompanying focal dextroscoliosis (right-convex curvature).
- Case B: There is incomplete segmentation of the C2 and C3 vertebral bodies, which are slightly diminutive in size relative to the other cervical levels. There are conjoined posterior elements and a rudimentary intervening C2 to C3 discs.
- Case C: There is a well-corticated osseous structure at the anterosuperior margin of the L4 vertebral body, corresponding to an unfused secondary ossification center. Disc material herniates through the superior endplate between this ossific body and the remainder of the vertebral body.
- Case D: There is anterior beaking of the vertebral bodies ("bullet-shaped" vertebrae). The L2 vertebral body is hypoplastic, resulting in focal thoracolumbar kyphosis and gibbous deformity. C1 arch hypoplasia and ligamentous thickening contribute to narrowing at the craniocervical junction, although there is no evident instability or brainstem/spinal cord compression. Flattening of the tuberculum sella results in "J-shaped" sellar configuration.
- Case E: The C5, C6, and C7 vertebral bodies are fused. The C6 vertebra is hypoplastic, resulting in spinal column narrowing with a "wasp waist" configuration.
- Case F: The T9 vertebral body is wedge-shaped, with endplate irregularity involving the T8 to T9 and T9 to T10 disc spaces. There is resultant focal kyphotic deformity, with adjacent extravertebral disease suggesting contiguous spread of a disease process.
- Case G: There is osseous fusion of the C4, C5, and C6 vertebral bodies across the interspaces, without intervening disc material; however, the posterior elements are not fused. Prior MRI demonstrates lack of vertebral body fusion and present intervertebral discs, indicating an iatrogenic rather than congenital/developmental process.

Diagnosis

Case A: Hemivertebra
Case B: Block vertebra
Case C: Limbus vertebra
Case D: Mucopolysaccharidosis, type 1 (Hurler syndrome)
Case E: Klippel–Feil syndrome
Case F: Tuberculous spondylodiscitis (Pott disease)
Case G: Iatrogenic noninstrumented fusion

Summary

Vertebrae are formed during development by the alignment of paired sclerotomes, which then undergo segmentation. As a result, each sclerotome provides a disc space, half of a vertebrae superiorly and half of a vertebrae inferiorly. Failure of either of these two steps, sclerotome pairing and segmentation, will give rise to two groups of congenital malformations. Congenital variants from pairing dysfunction include hemivertebrae and wedge vertebrae, whereas variants from segmentation dysfunction include butterfly vertebrae, block vertebrae, and unilateral bars (Fig. 47.1). Transitional lumbosacral vertebrae, although congenital, are not discussed here.

Hemivertebrae are the result of complete failure of a primary vertebral ossification center. The more typical lateral hemivertebrae result from an unpaired sclerotome and are asymmetric in

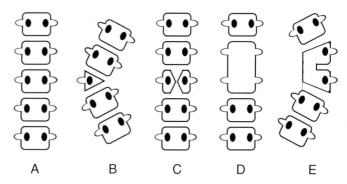

• Fig. 47.1 Congenital variants. A, Normal formation. B, Lateral hemivertebra and C, Butterfly vertebra; failure of somite pairing. D, Block vertebra and E, Unilateral bar; failure of segmentation.

the coronal plane. A rarer form of posterior hemivertebrae exists involving about 10% of cases and results from failure of anterior ossification. Hemivertebrae can impact spine curvature on the basis of orientation, relation to adjacent levels and growth pattern; this is further discussed in the Spectrum of Disease section of this chapter. Posterior subtypes predispose to kyphosis, whereas the more common lateral subtype is associated with scoliosis.

Butterfly vertebrae, also called sagittal cleft vertebrae, are distinct from hemivertebrae morphologically, developmentally, and clinically. They tend not to contribute to scoliosis nor kyphosis and are often incidental findings. Rarely, they may be symptomatic in young adults, in the setting of mid to low back pain. These butterfly vertebrae can be sporadic or can co-occur with other rare congenital conditions, most frequently spondylocostal dysostosis or Alagille syndrome.

Limbus vertebra, not to be mistaken for a limbus fracture, involves incomplete ossification of the vertebral ring apophysis, due to isolation of an ossification center that normally lies along the ring apophysis.

Block vertebra maintain the typical shape of vertebrae but remain unsegmented. This lack of segmentation, which resembles fusion, can occur anteriorly (the vertebral body) or posteriorly (the posterior facets) or both. When involving the cervical spine, it may be considered a variation of Klippel–Feil syndrome, which is discussed further in the Spectrum of Disease section of this chapter.

On occasion, these congenital formations can mimic more common pathology. For example, a butterfly vertebra can resemble a burst or compression fracture, although distinction can be made on the basis of the integrity of the cortex in the former entity. A posterior limbus vertebra can mimic disc herniation both clinically and radiographically, but is a much rarer entity and would be distinguished by the presence of the ossification center. History of trauma or infection, if present, may be useful to identify an acquired rather than congenital etiology, and examination with MRI for edema or effusion may rule out acute fracture. In areas where tuberculosis is prevalent, tuberculous spondylopathy (Pott disease) is a common cause for vertebral deformity and scoliosis.

Vertebral segment ankylosis can occur later in life, as in surgical fusion or in ankylosing spondylitis, and can resemble block vertebrae. Similarly, discal calcification may also occur in various pathologies. Acquired fusion or calcification tends to occur overtime with joint hypertrophy, resulting in a much wider anterior-posterior profile than seen in congenital vertebral fusions like block vertebrae. Correlation with other arthritic change throughout the body may increase the likelihood of acquired as opposed to congenital fusion.

Finally, it is important to distinguish between these congenital vertebral anomalies and congenital scoliosis. While some of these congenital anomalies may induce scoliosis—which could appropriately be categorized as congenital scoliosis—many patients with congenital anomalies may not develop clinical symptoms of scoliosis. Furthermore, an important distinction should be made between congenital scoliosis and the vastly more common idiopathic juvenile scoliosis, which is developmental and for which a cause is not identified, as well as neuromuscular scoliosis and other structural causes of scoliosis, which are often acquired. Features of a congenital anomaly that are hypothesized to induce clinical congenital scoliosis are discussed in the Spectrum of Disease section of this chapter.

Spectrum of Disease

Congenital vertebral anomalies can vary in terms of their impact on spinal alignment ranging from little to no effect on the bend of the spine of anomalies (like most butterfly vertebra, incarcerated or nonsegmented subtypes of hemivertebrae, and the block vertebra of Case B), to severe congenital scoliosis (like unsegmented bars, fully segmented hemivertebrae of Case A, or the wedge vertebra of Case E). When considering the potential effect of a spinal anomaly on spinal bend, consider features such as endplate shape, disc height/thickness, and restriction of joint spaces due to fusion.

This effect is exemplified by the various types of hemivertebrae. Segmented hemivertebrae have full-thickness disc tissue superiorly and inferiorly and no attachment to either adjacent level; as they grow, progressive wedging may result in worsening scoliosis. Semisegmented hemivertebrae are attached to one adjacent level, while nonsegmented hemivertebrae are attached to both adjacent vertebrae and thus are limited in their growth and not usually associated with scoliosis. Incarcerated hemivertebrae are confined within a space formed by the adjacent levels and do not extend to the vertebral margins; these have little effect on spinal curvature, as their growth is compensated by the surrounding vertebrae. The presence of a unilateral bar—from failed segmentation of the posterior processes—can result in a rigid "lock" on one side of the deformity and can contribute to worsening of axial deviation as the patient's contralateral endplates grow.

Klippel–Feil syndrome is a catch-all term referring to a heterogeneous group of presentations with congenital fusion of two or more cervical vertebrae. The classic clinical triad is a short neck with restricted movement and a low hairline, and there are a number of known associations such as Sprengel deformity (congenital elevation of the scapula). Although there is a female predilection, these deformities were thought to be sporadic, hence in the original classification was based on location and extent of fusion and the presence or absence of other vertebral abnormalities; however, familial cohorts with variable penetration have been identified.

For pediatric radiologists, some rare genetic conditions are associated with these vertebral anomalies. Assessment for additional skeletal dysplasias and extraskeletal anomalies can be diagnostic, as can referral to genetic testing. A more comprehensive list of associated syndromes can be referenced in the Differential Diagnosis section of this chapter.

Differential Diagnosis

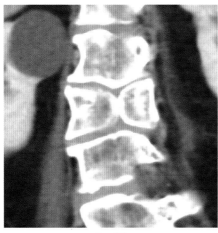
Cor CT

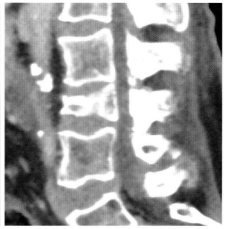
Sag CT

1. L3 butterfly vertebra with superior and inferior midline clefts (coronal CT); the cortices remain intact, and the vertebral body margins remain confined to the borders of the spinal column (sagittal CT).

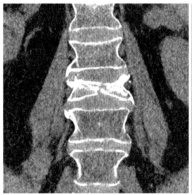

| Cor CT | Sag CT |

2. L3 burst fracture; the fracture line disrupts the superior and inferior endplates (coronal CT) and the vertebral body margins extend beyond the anterior and posterior spinal lines (sagittal CT).

Congenital Entities
- Hemivertebrae
- Butterfly vertebrae
- Block vertebrae
- Bullet vertebrae
  - Mucopolysaccharidoses
  - Achondroplasia
  - Congenital hypothyroidism
- Idiopathic scoliosis
- Congenital scoliosis and kyphosis

Acquired Entities
- Fracture
- Vertebral ankylosis
- Surgical fusion
- Disc herniation
- Calcification of annulus fibrosus

Associated Congenital Syndromes
- Skeletal Dysplasias
  - Scheuermann disease
  - Chondroplasias
  - Dysostoses
  - Goldenhar syndrome
  - Klippel–Feil syndrome
  - Crouzon syndrome
  - Pfeiffer syndrome
- Inborn Errors of Metabolism
  - Mucopolysaccharidoses
  - Lathosterolosis
- Tumor Suppressor Mutations
  - Neurofibromatosis type 1
  - Gorlin syndrome
- Syndromes with Multisystem Involvement
  - Down syndrome
  - VATER/VACTERL syndrome
  - MURCS syndrome
  - Aicardi syndrome
  - Alagille syndrome
  - Fryns syndrome
  - Kabuki syndrome
  - Myhre syndrome

- Behçet disease
- Kallman syndrome

Pearls

- Consider the degree of disc involvement to categorize malformations, noting the contour of the endplates and degree of cortication/sclerosis.
- Consider the presence of edema on MRI to distinguish acute fractures/deformity from variant anatomy in the context of recent trauma or infection.
- Consider the extent of degenerative change to approximate the likelihood of spondylosis.
- Consider local extravertebral findings, which may indicate contiguous disease spread such as tumor, inflammatory, or infectious etiologies that could mimic the appearance of a congenital finding.
- Specific features of the patients' medical record could prove essential in interpretation of an unusual vertebral finding, particularly known congenital conditions, potential disease states that contribute to chronic pathologic fractures and past surgical history.
- Identification of vertebral anomalies in newborns or infants should warrant consideration of additional imaging and potential referral to genetic testing and counselling to rule out genetic syndromes.

Signs and Complications

The "wasp waist" sign is a classic presentation of Klippel–Feil syndrome. It is characterized by a slimmer axial diameter at the level of the block vertebrae than the diameter of superior and inferior vertebrae.

The main complications of these congenital anomalies are scoliosis and kyphosis, although many patients with these malformations experience no such complication. If no anomalous vertebrae are noted in a case of scoliosis, these other etiologies should be considered. Etiologies of scoliosis and kyphosis include idiopathic, congenital (which can be osteogenic or neurogenic), neuromuscular, dysplastic, tumor-induced, and tuberculous. Scoliosis caused by vertebral malformations comprise the osteogenic subtype of congenital scoliosis, as opposed to neuropathic congenital scoliosis, which is associated with abnormal cord findings (i.e., tethered cord, syringomyelia, Chiari malformations, etc.).

In general, two characteristics of the affected vertebrae should be noted when an anomaly is discovered: the vertebral level and the morphology of the adjacent discs. Low thoracic or lumbar anomalies are more likely to be associated with abnormal curvature of the spine. Additionally, the shape of adjacent discs can potentially compensate for a wedge vertebra as in the case of incarcerated hemivertebrae. Scoliosis and kyphosis, when present, can also contribute to altered loading mechanics and therefore the extent of premature degenerative change should be noted.

Additional and more rare complications of congenital anomalies can include cord impingement, especially in cases of posterior limbus vertebrae, and atlantoaxial instability, especially in cases of Down syndrome and Klippel–Feil syndrome.

Suggested Readings

Chaturvedi A, Klionsky NB, Nadarajah U, et al: Malformed vertebrae: a clinical and imaging review, *Insights Imaging* 9(3):343–355, 2018.

Clarke RA, Catalan G, Diwan AD, et al: Heterogeneity in Klippel-Feil syndrome: a new classification, *Pediatr Radiol* 28(12):967–974, 1998.

Huang PY, Yeh LR, Tzeng WS, et al: Imaging features of posterior limbus vertebrae, *Clin Imaging* 36(6):797–802, 2012.

Johal J, Loukas M, Fisahn C, et al: Hemivertebrae: a comprehensive review of embryology, imaging, classification, and management, *Childs Nerv Syst* 32(11):2105–2109, 2016.

Katsuura Y, Kim HJ: Butterfly vertebrae: a systematic review of the literature and analysis, *Global Spine J* 9(6):666–679, 2019.

Laloo F, Herregods N, Jaremko JL, et al: MRI of the axial skeleton in spondyloarthritis: the many faces of new bone formation, *Insights Imaging* 10(1):67, 2019.

Musson RE, Warren DJ, Bickle I, et al: Imaging in childhood scoliosis: a pictorial review, *Postgrad Med J* 86(1017):419–427, 2010.

48

Single Aggressive Vertebral Body Lesion

DANIEL B. CHONDE, MD, PHD

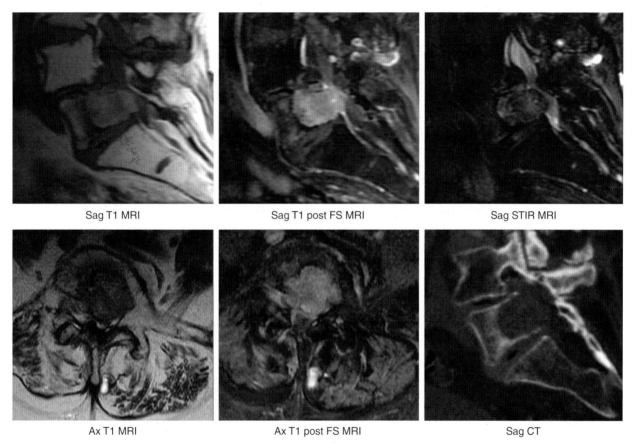

Sag T1 MRI   Sag T1 post FS MRI   Sag STIR MRI

Ax T1 MRI   Ax T1 post FS MRI   Sag CT

CASE A: A 78-year-old who presents with back pain. *Ax*, Axial; *CT*, Computed tomography; *FS*, fat saturated; *MRI*, magnetic resonance imaging; *Sag*, sagittal; *STIR*, short tau inversion recovery.

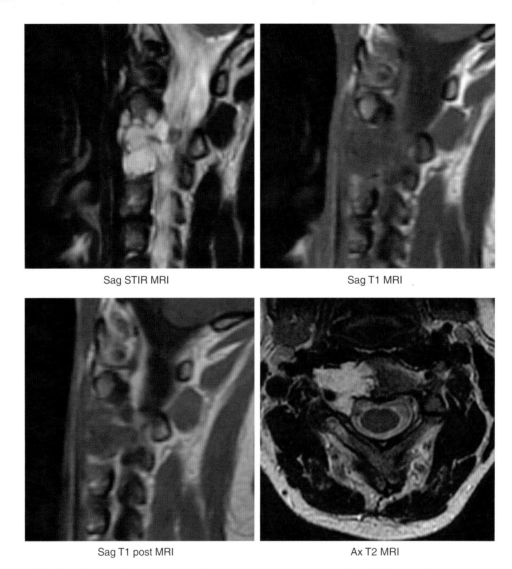

Sag STIR MRI

Sag T1 MRI

Sag T1 post MRI

Ax T2 MRI

CASE B: A 47-year-old who presents with right neck pain after fall. *Ax*, Axial; *MRI*, magnetic resonance imaging; *Sag*, sagittal; *STIR*, short tau inversion recovery.

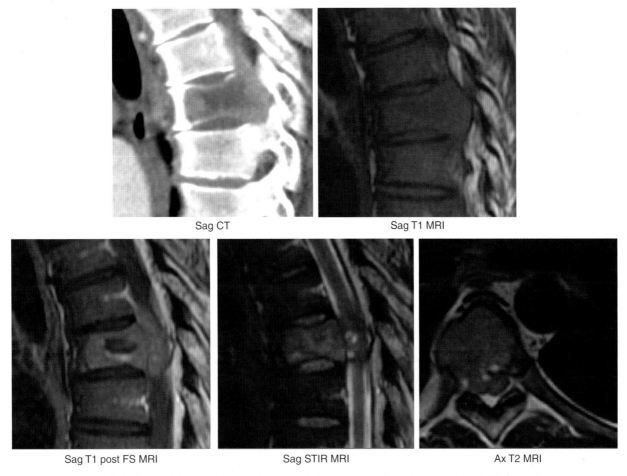

Sag CT   Sag T1 MRI

Sag T1 post FS MRI   Sag STIR MRI   Ax T2 MRI

CASE C: A 32-year-old male who presents with back pain radiating down his legs. *Ax*, Axial; *CT*, Computed tomography; *FS*, fat saturated; *MRI*, magnetic resonance imaging; *Sag*, sagittal; *STIR*, short tau inversion recovery.

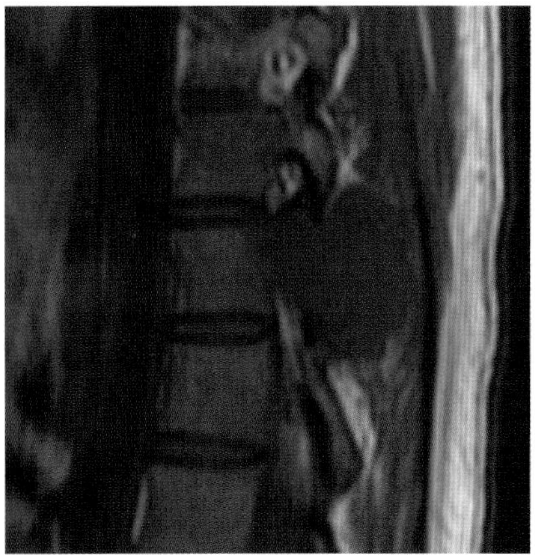

Sag T1 MRI

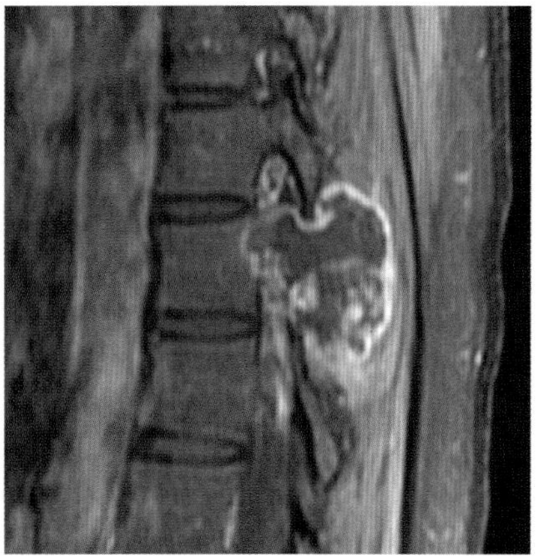

Sag T1 post FS MRI

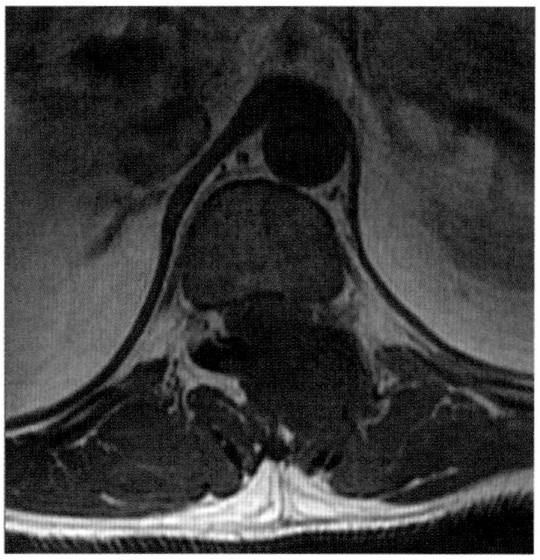

Ax T1 MRI

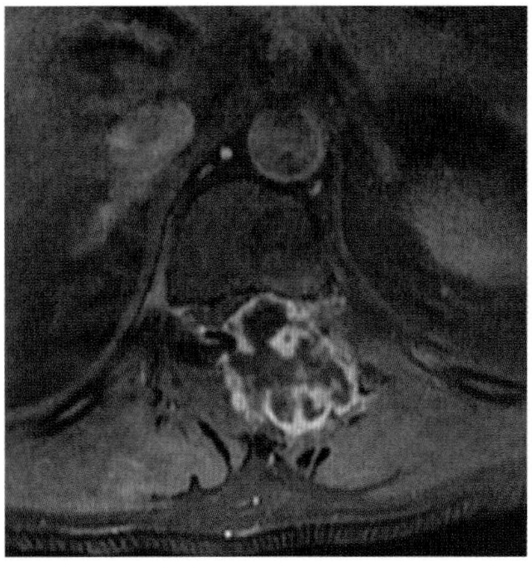

Ax T1 post FS MRI

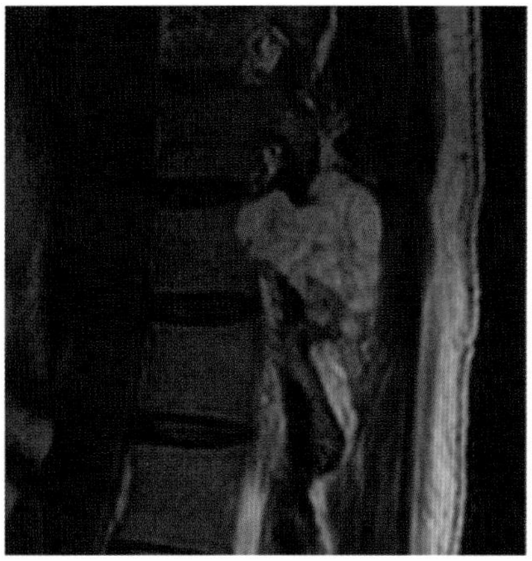

Sag T2 MRI

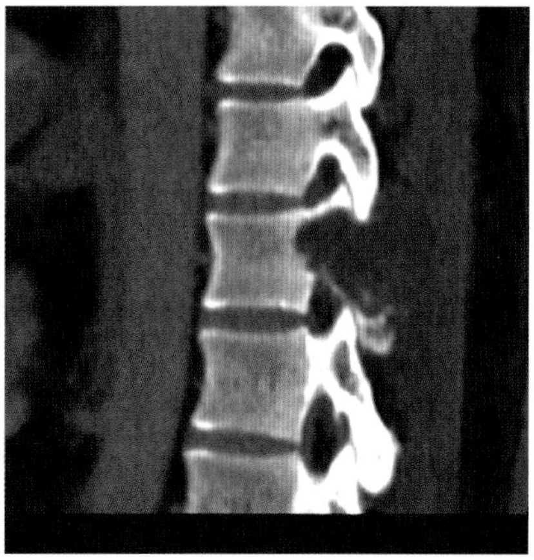

Sag CT

CASE D: A 33-year-old who presents with several months of intermittent back pain, left leg numbness, and urinary retention/constipation. *Ax*, Axial; *CT*, Computed tomography; *FS*, fat saturated; *MRI*, magnetic resonance imaging; *Sag*, sagittal.

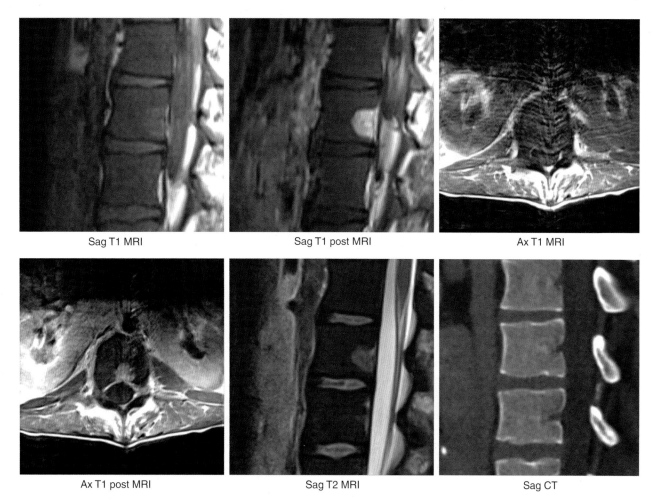

Sag T1 MRI   Sag T1 post MRI   Ax T1 MRI

Ax T1 post MRI   Sag T2 MRI   Sag CT

CASE E: A 25-year-old who presents with back pain, night sweats, vertical diplopia, and deconjugate gaze. *Ax*, Axial; *CT*, Computed tomography; *MRI*, magnetic resonance imaging; *Sag*, sagittal.

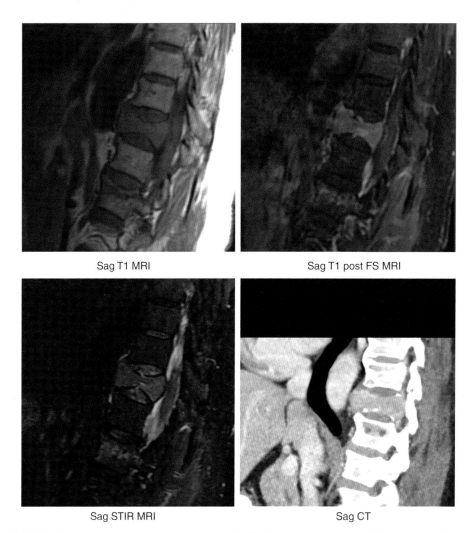

Sag T1 MRI

Sag T1 post FS MRI

Sag STIR MRI

Sag CT

CASE F: A 66-year-old who presents with back pain. *CT*, Computed tomography; *FS*, fat saturated; *MRI*, magnetic resonance imaging; *Sag*, sagittal; *STIR*, short tau inversion recovery.

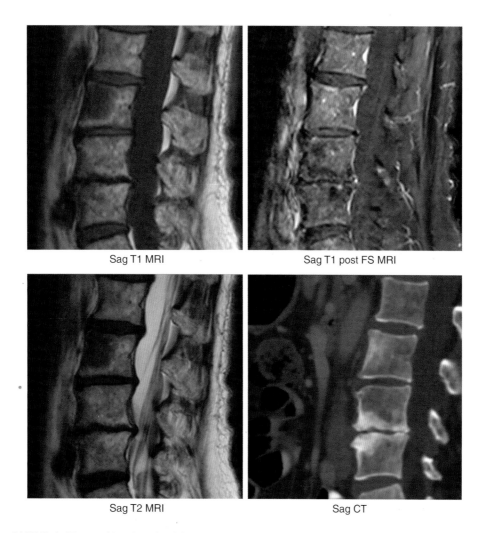

Sag T1 MRI

Sag T1 post FS MRI

Sag T2 MRI

Sag CT

CASE G: A 67-year-old undergoing follow-up of an incidentally noted lumbar spine lesion of prior pelvic MRI. *CT*, Computed tomography; *FS*, fat saturated; *MRI*, magnetic resonance imaging; *Sag*, sagittal.

DESCRIPTION OF FINDINGS

- Case A: A heterogenous lobulated enhancing mass is centered in the posterior aspect of the vertebral body. CT demonstrates a lytic lesion with reactive sclerosis surrounding the lesion.
- Case B: a mildly enhancing, intensely T2 hyperintense lesion is centered in the right aspect of C1. Note the prominent lobulations of the mass which has a signal intensity similar to that of cerebrospinal fluid.
- Case C: There is an enhancing lucent lesion in the posterior aspect of the vertebral body with a pathologic fracture. The lesion, with the accompanying extraosseous component, demonstrates multiple T2 hyperintense cystic elements.
- Case D: There is an intensely T2 hyperintense erosive lesion centered in the left posterior element of the vertebral body with intense peripheral enhancement. T2 imaging demonstrates an internal structure with rings and arcs.
- Case E: There is an intrinsically T2/STIR hyperintense, enhancing lesion along the posterior element of the vertebral body at the location of the basivertebral vein. There is no obviously corresponding lesion on the CT, nor evidence of reactive changes in the bonelike sclerosis.
- Case F: There is a pathologic fracture of the vertebral body which demonstrates homogeneously abnormal signal on all series indicative of a uniform marrow replacing process.
- Case G: There is a solitary T1 hypointense lesion centered in the vertebral body with relative T2 hypointensity and mild enhancement. CT demonstrates a linear patter of sclerosis and rarefaction.

Diagnosis

Case A: Metastasis
Case B: Chordoma
Case C: Giant cell tumor (GCT)
Case D: Chondrosarcoma
Case E: Lymphoma
Case F: Plasmacytoma
Case G: Hemangioma

Summary

The presence of multiple osseous vertebral lesions usually suggests a malignant etiology: metastases, multiple myeloma, or lymphoproliferative disorders—the three of which happen to be the most common malignant spinal tumors. A solitary osseous lesion, on the other hand, can present a diagnostic dilemma in its identification and determining its malignant potential. In many cases, both CT and MR may be helpful in characterizing a lesion as they present complementary information—MR providing the superior soft tissue contrast and allowing detection of fluid-fluid levels, and CT offering superior evaluation of the tumor matrix and characterization of the surrounding mineralization. In some cases, nuclear medicine studies, including positron emission tomography (PET) and bone scans, may provide additional information, e.g., accumulation of Tc-99m–labeled red blood cells in a hemangioma.

The differential for solitary vertebral lesions depends on the location of the abnormality. Mainly, if the lesion is centered in the vertebral body versus posterior elements (including the pedicles). To complicate matters, a subset of vertebral body lesions commonly extends into the posterior elements, just as a subset of posterior element lesions commonly extend into the vertebral body. Consigning ourselves to the aggressive appearing lesions centered in the vertebral body, we consider metastatic disease, chordoma, GCT, lymphoma, plasmacytoma, and hemangioma with one addition, chondrosarcoma, which is typically based in the posterior elements, but commonly extends into the vertebral body. Additional lesions which are not considered include osteosarcoma which rarely involves the spine (only about 4% of cases) and typically are centered in the posterior elements, and Ewing sarcoma, which in its primary vertebral form is rare, typically involves the posterior elements and is a tumor of the young.

A true solitary vertebral body lymphoma, i.e., without any nodal disease, is rare. Termed primary bone lymphoma, solitary lesions are more likely to occur in the long bones of the appendicular skeleton. Multifocal primary bone lymphoma, which is more common to have vertebral involvement, is discussed in the following case. Primary bone lymphoma is typically due to non-Hodgkin lymphoma, with diffuse large B cell-lymphoma as the most common cell type. Primary osseous lymphoma of bone can have a variety of appearances on CT and radiograph with lytic, sclerotic, mixed lytic, and sclerotic lesions or in some cases completely normal with or without extraosseous extension. The most common presentation is a lytic lesion with a permeative appearance resulting in a wide zone of transition, with or without extraosseous soft tissue. When the CT appearance of the bone is subtle or not evident, magnetic resonance imaging (MRI) can provide invaluable information, as the hypercellular lymphoma replaces the typical marrow signal leading to hypointensity on T1. These lesions typically demonstrate T2 signal, which is hyperintense to muscle, although the degree of fibrosis within the tumor may affect the T2 intensity.

A subset of lymphoproliferative disorders, plasmacytomas are an abnormal proliferation of plasma cells, lymphocytes which secrete antibodies. When there are multiple visceral or osseous sites of disease, the term multiple myeloma is used.

Discounting the lymphoproliferative tumors, chordomas are the most common primary malignant neoplasm of the spine in adults. Derived from malignant transformation of remnants of the notochord, the progenitor scaffold of the clivus and spinal cord which are formed around it, chordomas can develop along the entirety of its course. In the skull base, the notochord takes a sigmoid course, reaching the surface of the bone at three locations: dorsum sellae, pharyngeal surface, and dorsal clivus. In the spine its course is much more regular, situated between the anterior two-thirds and posterior one-third of the eventual vertebral bodies and excreted during formation to the interspinous region, eventually forming the nucleus pulposus of the intervertebral disc. Notochord remnants are most common in the skull base and sacrococcygeal region and thus so are chordomas with 50% of cases in the sacrococcygeal region, 35% in the skull base, and the remaining 15% in the vertebral bodies. Chordomas are relatively indolent lesions, typically presenting on CT as well-circumscribed lytic lesions with prominent lobulated soft tissue components, which may include a pseudocapsule and variable degrees of stromal elements, mucin, hemorrhage, and sequestered bone.

On MR imaging, the neoplastic tissues have signal characteristics similar to the nucleus pulposus, and intense T2 signal and T1 signal which is hypointense to isointense in comparison to skeletal muscle. Enhancements in these lesions are variable, but typically at least moderate. Of note, as the expansile soft tissue invades adjacent vertebrae, it typically spares the disc.

The pathognomonic appearance for hemangioma is an irregular exaggeration of the trabeculated pattern on CT, giving it a polka dot appearance on axial imaging and alternating bands of high and low density on sagittal imaging, aptly named the corduroy sign. Atypical and aggressive hemangiomas, defined below and include hemangiomas that erode the cortex, expand the vertebral body, or appear to have prominent soft tissue components on CT or other forms of imaging, will typically continue to have the polka dot or corduroy appearance, and thus, when in doubt, request the CT. The appearance of these lesions on MRI is best understood by their histopathology, mainly that they are composed of an overgrowth of capillary sized blood vessels in a loose edematous cartilaginous matrix surrounding reactive changes: sclerosis of the remaining vertically oriented trabeculated bone, the presence of fibrous scar tissue, and an overgrowth of fat. The overgrowth of fat will lead to hyperintensity on standard T1 and T2 imaging, while fat-suppressed imaging, including short tau inversion recovery (STIR), will show a relative dropout in the signal of these lesions. Similarly, the high water content of these lesions will present as hyperintensity on T2 imaging and explain the residual hyperintense signal on fat-suppressed T2 images. Sclerotic trabecula and overgrown vasculature will appear as vertically oriented hypodensities and flow voids on noncontrast enhanced T1 sequences, which may give it an appearance akin to the polka dot and corduroy signs present on CT. The presence of flow voids remains one of the most important signs on MR to suggest a hemangioma. The relative composition of edematous stroma, fat, and vascular channels can affect the MR appearance of a hemangioma and thus lesions with less prominent fat components are termed *atypical* hemangiomas. Furthermore, when features like erosions of the cortical bone or extension beyond the vertebral body, these lesions are referred to as *aggressive* hemangiomas. Of note, all hemangiomas will have some degree of variable enhancement.

GCTs get their name from the characteristic multinucleated osteoclast-monocyte linage type giant cell, which is a principal component of the lesion. The other components include mononuclear stromal cells, the predominant replicating neoplastic cell in this lesion, and secondarily recruited histiocytes which are recruited by the stromal cells and eventually fuse to form more giant cells. Despite the fact GCTs can demonstrate hematogenous spread with resulting lung nodules and occasionally can undergo malignant transformation to a high-grade sarcoma, these tumors are considered benign.

The recruitment and stimulation of phagocytic cells results in the lytic appearance of these tumors on CT imaging. The continued expansion of the lesion with its osteoclastic activity can result in cortical thinning, expansion of the bone, and in some cases destruction of the cortical bone with an expansile soft tissue component—all of which are considered aggressive features. Given the increased soft tissue contrast of MRI, MRI has a role in delineating soft tissue extension; otherwise the tumor demonstrates relatively nonspecific intermediate to decreased T1 signal, increased T2 signal, and enhancement.

It is not uncommon for GCTs to develop multiseptated cystic blood-filled spaces that lack an epithelial lining which can present as fluid-fluid levels on MRI. These changes have recently been referred to as aneurysmal bone cyst-like changes, as aneurysmal bone cysts are considered a unique neoplastic lesion. However, the presence of aneurysmal bone cyst-like changes is not isolated to GCTs and can also be seen in chondrosarcoma.

In this list of differential diagnoses, chondrosarcoma is the outlier, as it typically is centered in the posterior elements of the vertebrae. Chondrosarcomas develop from chondrocytes, allowing them to develop in cartilaginous joints and within rests of chondrocytes that can occur throughout any bone formed via endochondral ossification. Based on a 1989, single site report of 20 patients, the spatial distribution of chondrosarcoma is 15% in the vertebral body, 40% in the posterior elements, and 45% in both. There are several subtypes of chondrosarcomas, ranging from low grade to high grade; however, there are a number of unifying imaging features. Hallmark to cartilaginous tumors is the ring-and-arc appearance of calcification which occurs throughout the chondroid matrix produced by the tumor. This translates to rings and arcs on CT and generally an intense T2 signal from the high water content chondroid matrix on MRI. Larger and more aggressive tumors may demonstrate a central area void of calcification as it is growing faster than it can calcify. Additionally, cartilaginous tumors have a lobulated appearance. Aggressive lesions will demonstrate increased cortical thinning, breach, and soft tissue components with increasing cellularity. Enhancement of these lesions will be heterogeneous based on degree of stroma and fibrovascular septations.

Metastasis is presented last, as in the setting of a solitary vertebral body lesion, it can resemble many of the other lesions, making it the first and last item on the differential. For example, thyroid and renal cell carcinoma may present with lytic metastases which can mimic a GCT.

Differential Diagnosis

1. Metastasis
2. Chordoma
3. Giant cell tumor
4. Lymphoma
5. Plasmacytoma
6. Hemangioma
7. Chondrosarcoma

Pearls

- CT and MR provide complementary information when characterizing a single aggressive vertebral body lesion.
- Location is key: chordomas, GCTs, lymphomas, plasmacytomas, and hemangiomas tend to present in the vertebral body while chondrosarcomas present in the posterior elements.

- Alternating bands of high and low density on CT can help identify a hemangioma.
- Aneurysmal bone cysts are not unique to GCTs; chondrosarcomas can have them as well.
- Chondrosarcomas and chordomas are intensely T2 bright.

Suggested Readings

Balke M, Schremper L, Gebert C, et al: Giant cell tumor of bone: treatment and outcome of 214 cases, *J Cancer Res Clin Oncol* 134(9): 969–978, 2008.

Chakarun CJ, Forrester DM, Gottsegen CJ, et al: Giant cell tumor of bone: review, mimics, and new developments in treatment, *Radiographics* 33(1):197–211, 2013.

Cross JJ, Antoun NM, Laing RJ, et al: Imaging of compressive vertebral haemangiomas, *Eur Radiol* 10(6):997–1002, 2000.

Gaudino S, Martucci M, Colantonio R, et al: A systematic approach to vertebral hemangioma, *Skeletal radiology* 44(1):25–36, 2015.

Hirsh LF, Thanki A, Spector HB: Primary spinal chondrosarcoma with eighteen-year follow-up: case report and literature review, *Neurosurgery* 14(6):747–749, 1984.

Katonis P, Alpantaki K, Michail K, et al: Spinal chondrosarcoma: a review, *Sarcoma* 2011:378957, 2011.

Kim YS, Han IH, Lee IS, et al: Imaging findings of solitary spinal bony lesions and the differential diagnosis of benign and malignant lesions, *J Korean Neurosurg Soc* 52(2):126–132, 2012.

Krishnan A, Shirkhoda A, Tehranzadeh J, et al: Primary bone lymphoma: radiographic–MR imaging correlation, *Radiographics* 23(6):1371–1383, 2003.

Lim CY, Ong KO: Imaging of musculoskeletal lymphoma, *Cancer imaging* 13(4):448, 2013.

Mechri M, Riahi H, Sboui I, et al: Imaging of malignant primitive tumors of the spine, *Journal of the Belgian Society of Radiology* 102(1): 56, 2018.

Restrepo R, Zahrah D, Pelaez L, et al: Update on aneurysmal bone cyst: pathophysiology, histology, imaging and treatment, *Pediatric Radiology* 52(9):1601–1614, 2022.

Rodallec MH, Feydy A, Larousserie F, et al: Diagnostic imaging of solitary tumors of the spine: what to do and say, *Radiographics* 28(4): 1019–1041, 2008.

Yao ML, Patel VK, Parnes GJ: Know your notochord: a pictorial review of notochord remnants, *Neurographics* 10(1):19–25, 2020.

49
Posterior Element Lesions

KENNETH S. ALLISON, MD

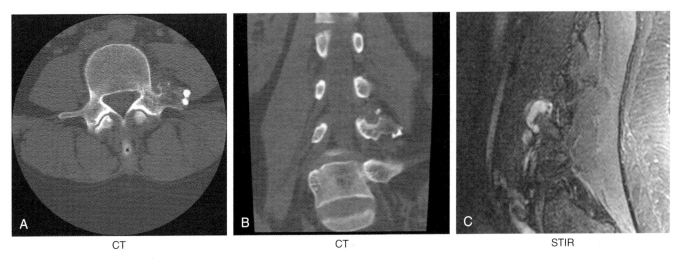

CT   CT   STIR

CASE A: A 54-year-old presenting with back pain and left L3 radiculopathy. *CT*, Computed tomography; *STIR*, short T1 inversion recovery.

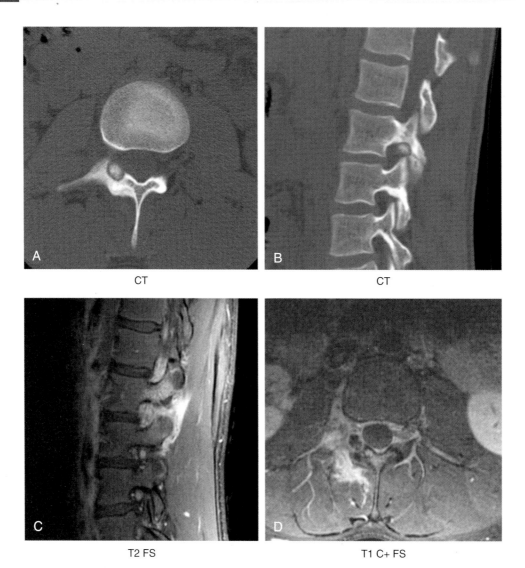

A
CT

B
CT

C
T2 FS

D
T1 C+ FS

CASE B: A 19-year-old presenting with right lower back pain. *CT*, Computed tomography; *FS*, fat saturated.

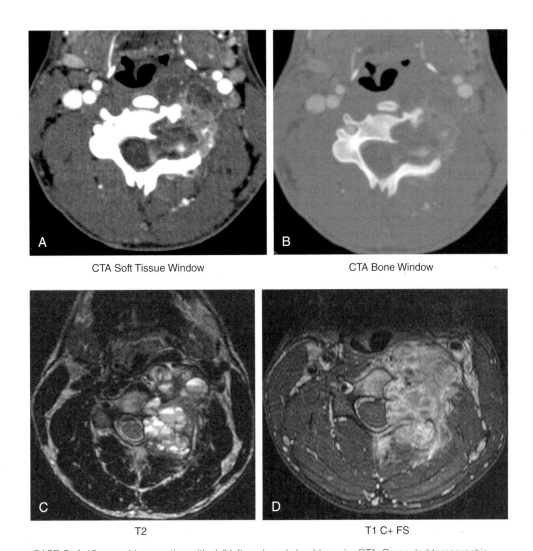

CTA Soft Tissue Window

CTA Bone Window

T2

T1 C+ FS

CASE C: A 19-year-old presenting with dull left neck and shoulder pain. *CTA*, Computed tomographic angiography; *FS*, fat saturated.

CT

CT

T1 C+ FS

Bone Scan

CASE D: A 12-year-old presenting with neck stiffness and pain. *CT,* Computed tomography; *FS,* fat saturated.

DESCRIPTION OF FINDINGS

- Case A: An exophytic bone lesion arises from the left L4 transverse process and demonstrates continuity of its cortex and medullary cavity with those of the transverse process. Short T1 inversion recovery images reveal a cartilaginous cap along the superior-medial aspect of the lesion. A review of all studies and sequences also showed impingement upon the exiting left L3 nerve root, explaining the patient's symptoms.
- Case B: A lesion centered in the right L2 pars interarticularis region is calcified centrally and has a well-circumscribed radiolucent rim with surrounding bony sclerosis. It measures approximately 1.2 cm in maximal diameter. Magnetic resonance imaging (MRI) shows edema within the adjacent bone marrow and inflammatory changes in the adjacent soft tissues.
- Case C: A multilobulated, expansile, heterogeneously enhancing mass is centered in the left C4 pedicle and also involves the left lamina and left posterolateral vertebral body. It encases and narrows the left vertebral artery and extends into the left extradural spinal canal, partially effacing the thecal sac. No matrix is perceptible. T2-weighted MRI demonstrates multiple fluid-fluid levels within the mass.
- Case D: An expansile lytic lesion is centered in the left pedicle of the C5 vertebra, extending laterally into the articular mass and measuring approximately 1.6 cm in maximal diameter. Several small central calcifications are noted, along with adjacent bony sclerosis. T2-weighted images (not shown) and contrast-enhanced MRI demonstrate extensive reactive inflammatory changes in the adjacent bone and soft tissues. There is avid radiotracer uptake on the bone scan.

Diagnosis

Case A: Osteochondroma
Case B: Osteoid osteoma
Case C: Aneurysmal bone cyst (ABC)
Case D: Osteoblastoma

Summary

Lesions of the vertebral column encompass a wide variety of pathologies, most of which may arise in or involve the vertebral body, the posterior elements, or both. This discussion is confined to some lesions that characteristically or predominately affect the posterior elements.

Osteoid osteomas are benign lesions that, when found in the spine (as in approximately 10% of cases), typically are located in the posterior elements. CT is the imaging modality of choice and will reveal a radiolucent nidus measuring less than 1.5 to 2.0 cm in diameter (sometimes with central calcification) with surrounding reactive sclerosis. The MRI appearance is variable depending on the degree of vascularity, calcification, and sclerosis of the lesion, but often edema is prominent within the adjacent bone marrow and soft tissues. If present, the classic clinical history of a young patient (between 10 and 20 years) with intensely painful scoliosis that is worse at night and is relieved by aspirin or other nonsteroidal antiinflammatory drugs may help clinch the diagnosis.

Osteoblastomas are similar pathologically to osteoid osteomas but are larger, measuring more than 1.5 to 2.0 cm, and often present with dull localized pain and/or focal neurologic symptoms. They usually affect the posterior elements,

although progression to involve the vertebral body is common. The imaging appearance of osteoblastomas may be identical to that of large osteoid osteomas, but osteoblastomas are more likely than osteoid osteomas to be expansile and contain multifocal matrix calcification (which may simulate chondroid matrix). Osteoblastomas may also appear to be quite aggressive, with bone destruction and extension into the adjacent soft tissues. The MRI appearance is nonspecific and may be difficult to distinguish from infection or malignancy. MRI therefore is mainly helpful for assessing any extension into the spinal canal or soft tissues and for delineating the associated inflammatory response, which may be considerable. Osteoblastomas also demonstrate marked radiotracer uptake upon bone scintigraphy.

Spinal osteochondromas can arise from any portion of the vertebra but predominately arise from the posterior elements and are most often encountered in the atlantoaxial region of the cervical spine. Their imaging appearance is the same as that of osteochondromas encountered elsewhere in the skeleton: an osseous excrescence with marrow and cortex in continuity with those of the underlying bone and a cartilaginous cap.

ABCs are benign lesions that mainly affect young patients (younger than 20 years) and are composed largely of multiloculated, cystic, blood-filled spaces. They most often are found in the posterior elements but frequently grow to involve the vertebral body. They also may extend into the adjacent soft tissues. CT and MRI of ABCs will confirm their multiloculated, cystic nature (i.e., "soap bubble" appearance) and often will demonstrate their characteristic, multiple fluid-fluid levels related to layering blood products within the cysts. Although most ABCs are considered solitary lesions, up to one-third are seen in association with preexisting lesions such as giant cell tumor, osteoblastoma, chondroblastoma, and osteosarcoma. The presence of solid, enhancing portions of the lesion may indicate a secondary ABC, although rare solid variants of ABCs also exist.

Many other lesions may affect the posterior elements, although without a clear posterior predilection per se. These lesions include metastases, which are the most common spinal tumors overall. Other lesions include lymphomas, myelomas, chondrosarcomas, osteosarcomas, Ewing sarcomas, giant cell tumors, and chondroblastomas.

Differential Diagnosis

1. Metastasis
2. Osteoid osteoma
3. Osteoblastoma
4. Osteochondroma
5. ABC
6. Osteosarcoma
7. Chondrosarcoma
8. Ewing sarcoma
9. Lymphoma
10. Myeloma/plasmacytoma
11. Giant cell tumor

Pearls

- The most common spinal tumors overall are metastases.
- The differential diagnosis for multiple fluid-fluid levels includes ABC, giant cell tumor, and telangiectatic osteosarcoma.
- Because they are similar pathologically and radiographically, osteoid osteomas and osteoblastomas often are distinguished on the basis of size (less than and greater than 1.5 to 2.0 cm, respectively).

Signs and Complications

The signs and complications are detailed in the preceding sections.

Suggested Readings

Murphey MD, Andrews CL, Flemming DJ, et al: From the archives of the AFIP. Primary tumors of the spine: radiologic pathologic correlation, *Radiographics* 16(5):1131–1158, 1996.

Rodallec MH, Feydy A, Larousserie F, et al: Diagnostic imaging of solitary tumors of the spine: what to do and say, *Radiographics* 28(4): 1019–1041, 2008.

Sansur CA, Pouratian N, Dumont AS: Part II: spinal-cord neoplasms—primary tumours of the bony spine and adjacent soft tissues, *Lancet Oncol* 8(2):137–147, 2007.

50

Multiple Lytic Lesions of the Spine

PARTH Y. PATEL, MD AND DANIEL L. NOUJAIM, MD

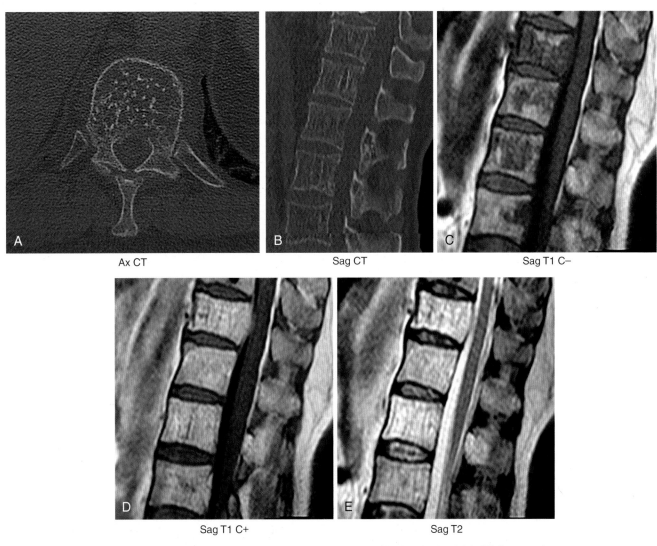

Ax CT   Sag CT   Sag T1 C−

Sag T1 C+   Sag T2

CASE A: A 63-year-old male presenting with a 2-day history of back pain. *Ax*, Axial; *CT*, Computed tomography; *Sag*, sagittal.

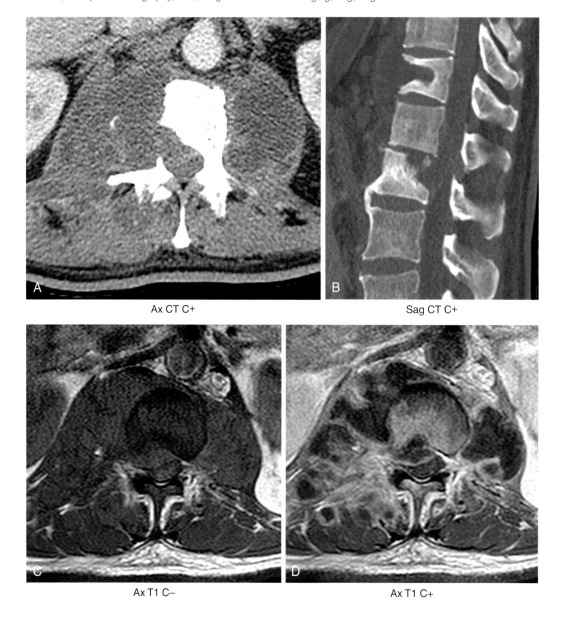

| Sag CT | Sag T1 | Sag T2 |

CASE B: A 61-year-old male presenting with progressive bilateral extremity weakness and pain.
CT, Computed tomography; *MRI*, magnetic resonance imaging; *Sag*, sagittal.

| Ax CT C+ | Sag CT C+ |

| Ax T1 C− | Ax T1 C+ |

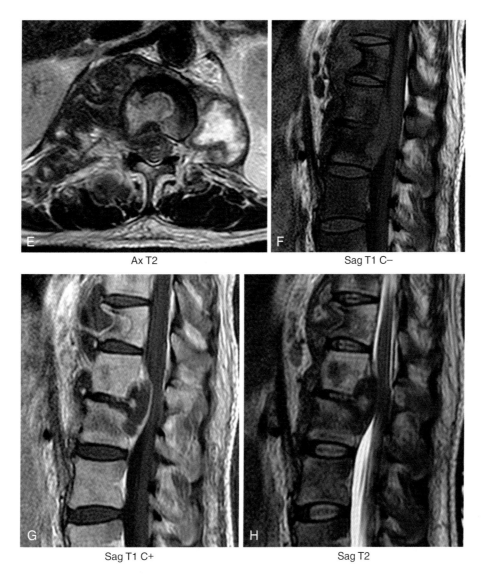

CASE C: A 39-year-old Indonesian male presenting with unintentional weight loss, night sweats, and back pain. *Ax*, Axial; *CT*, Computed tomography; *Sag*, sagittal.

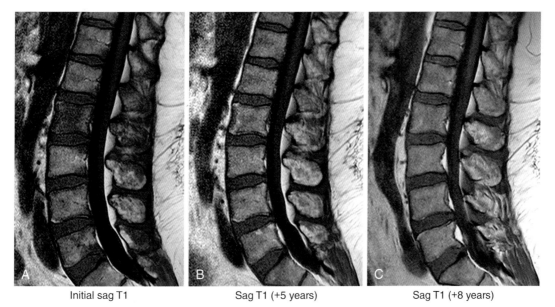

CASE D: A 62-year-old male initially presents with acute low back pain. Images from three separate points in time are shown while on long-term corticosteroid therapy for a systemic illness. *Sag*, Sagittal.

DESCRIPTION OF FINDINGS

- Case A: Axial CT images show punctate sclerotic foci within the vertebral body with relative surrounding lucency, giving a characteristic polka-dotted appearance, with apparent thinning of the posterior cortex of the uppermost vertebral level. Sagittal CT images demonstrate multilevel vertically oriented sclerotic striations throughout the thoracic spine, similar to a corduroy or jail bar pattern. Follow-up magnetic resonance (MR) images show multilevel patchy T1 hypointense and T2 hyperintense signal characteristics with avid enhancement. There is suggestion of ventral epidural extension of this process at the uppermost vertebral level. Notably, the lesions have small foci of intralesional T1 signal compatible with fatty elements, which is most notably seen within the second lowest spinous process on the sagittal MR sequences.
- Case B: Sagittal CT shows multiple rounded, lytic lesions throughout the thoracic spine, with surrounding sclerotic rim. Follow-up MR images demonstrate multiple T1 and T2 hypointense rounded foci of bone marrow replacement throughout the thoracic spine. One of these marrow replacing lesions demonstrates a small central focus of T2 hyperintensity compatible with central necrosis.
- Case C: CT images demonstrate extensive osseous destruction of the anterior T11 and posterior L1 vertebral bodies. There is substantial bilateral paraspinal soft tissue abnormality, which demonstrates peripheral enhancement and central nonenhancement, suggesting fluid collections. There is a punctate calcification within the right paraspinal collection. Follow-up MR images of this region demonstrate vertebral body destruction, multilobulated paraspinal fluid collections, and peripheral enhancement with subligamentous extension over multiple vertebral levels. There is associated involvement of the spinal canal, with ventral effacement of the thecal sac and posterior displacement of the cord. Note sparing of the intervertebral disc spaces relative to the degree of osseous and paraspinal involvement.
- Case D: Initial sagittal MR image of the thoracolumbar spine demonstrates a diffusely T1 hypointense lesion involving a majority of the L2 vertebral body, with significantly less involvement at the L3 and L5 vertebral bodies. There is additional T1 hypointense signal characteristics of the visualized posterior elements. Sagittal images 5 and 8 years later demonstrate gradual normalization of marrow signal abnormalities within these respective vertebral levels.

Diagnosis

Case A: Multiple aggressive vertebral hemangiomas
Case B: Multiple myeloma
Case C: Tuberculous spondylitis (Pott disease)
Case D: Osseous spinal sarcoidosis

Summary/Spectrum of Disease

Most lytic lesions seen within the spinal column in adults and the elderly consist of either osseous metastatic disease or multiple myeloma. Metastasis is the most common vertebral tumor with up to 70% of those with osseous metastatic disease having spinal column involvement. Apart from breast and prostate cancer, most primary tumors cause lytic osseous metastases, most commonly involving the posterior vertebral body, pedicles, and lamina, with irregular margins and destruction of the cortex on CT. When hemorrhage, edema, or necrosis occur within these lesions, T1- and T2-weighted MR images can be variable in appearance, although typically T1 hypointense to normal bone marrow. Multiple myeloma is another common consideration when approached with multiple lytic lesions in the spine, as it is the most common

primary malignant osseous neoplasm. Characteristically having well-defined margins without periosteal reaction, these lesions can also show demineralization. It is critical to assess for any known history of malignancy when identifying new lytic lesions on imaging, as these two differentials tend to be the most common pathologies encountered.

However, not all lytic lesions in the spine fall into these categories, as benign, infectious, and inflammatory conditions can mimic these classic appearances. As the most common benign vertebral lesion, hemangiomas can occasionally have malignant-appearing features. Typically, hemangiomas appear as lytic lesions with internal thickened trabecula within the vertebral body, resulting in a polka dot pattern on axial CT and a corduroy pattern on coronal and sagittal reformats. MR imaging appearance is variable and dependent upon the degree of fatty versus vascular elements, which are T1 and T2 hyperintense, respectively. Atypical hemangiomas can mimic metastases due to low fat content of these lesions limiting T1 hyperintense components that are typically seen in vertebral hemangiomas. Additionally, aggressive vertebral hemangiomas demineralize and extend through the vertebral cortex to involve the paraspinal or epidural spaces, mimicking the appearance of extraosseous extension of bony metastatic disease, as seen on Case A.

Infectious etiologies can be an overlooked diagnoses when presented with multiple lytic osseous lesions. Pyogenic discitis-osteomyelitis typically begins by hematogenous spread to the vertebral endplate with early involvement of the adjacent disc space and opposing level endplate. However, atypical infections, such as tuberculous spondylitis and brucellosis, should be considered when a lytic lesion is centered in the vertebral marrow space with paraspinal and subligamentous spread that spares adjacent disc spaces. Infectious lesions often destroy midline ligamentous attachment to the posterior longitudinal ligament, while neoplastic lesions may respect this attachment in the early stages of the disease.

Additionally, chronic systemic processes, such as Langerhans cell histiocytosis and sarcoidosis, can occasionally have a lytic appearance with spinal involvement. Given that many of these conditions have a nonspecific appearance on CT and MR imaging—typically T1 hypointense and T2 hyperintense with post-contrast enhancement—proper review of a patient's past medical history is critical to avoid an erroneous diagnosis. Occasionally proper therapy and management can result in gradual resolution of these lytic lesions (as seen in Case D) or focal changes within the lesion itself (i.e., central necrosis within partially treated myelomatous lesion in Case B). Furthermore, radiation therapy can cause signal alterations in the bone marrow on MR imaging and may be complicated by geographic areas of osteonecrosis.

Differential Diagnosis

1. Osseous metastatic disease
2. Multiple myeloma
3. Vertebral hemangiomas
4. Tuberculosis
5. Lymphoma

6. Sarcoidosis
7. Radiation necrosis
8. Benign osseous lesions (i.e., Langerhans cell histiocytosis, Brown Tumor)

Signs and Complications

Complications are generally related to associated pathologic fractures of the involved vertebral body. This clinically manifests as acute onset back pain typically. Additionally, myelopathy and radiculopathy related to spinal cord compression are of clinical concerns in these patients, as epidural involvement of these processes are not infrequent.

Pearls

- While metastatic disease and multiple myeloma may be the most common lytic spinal column lesions, it is critical to note any underlying infectious or inflammatory conditions of the patient, as tuberculosis, sarcoidosis, and others can have similar appearances on initial imaging.
- Acute vertebral body fractures should not be underestimated, especially in the absence of trauma, as many may have additional findings to point toward an underlying etiology, such as metastases.

- Epidural extension from the vertebral body may be seen in other settings outside of metastatic disease, as associated findings, such as a thickened trabeculated pattern, may suggest an underlying aggressive hemangioma as the proper etiology.
- Preservation of the posterior longitudinal ligament attachment to the posterior vertebral body with adjacent lytic lesions may imply an underlying, noninfectious etiology, such as multiple myeloma or hemangioma.

Suggested Readings

Dutoit JC, Verstraete KL: MRI in multiple myeloma: a pictorial review of diagnostic and post-treatment findings, *Insights Imaging* 7:553–569, 2016.

Kim DH, Rosenblum JK, Panghaal VS, et al: Differentiating neoplastic from nonneoplastic processes in the anterior extradural space, *Radiology* 260(3):825–830, 2011.

Olubiyi OI, Brown F, Teytelboym OM: Lucent lesions of vertebral body: differential diagnosis, *Contemporary Diagnostic Radiology* 42(11):1–7, 2019.

Rodallec MH, Feydy A, Larousserie F, et al: Diagnostic imaging of solitary tumors of the spine: what to do and say, *Radiographics* 28:1019–1041, 2008.

Silva HS, Zamora C, Castillo M: Multifocal and diffuse spinal lesions that may mimic metastases, *Neurographics* 9(3):163–181, 2019.

Soni N, Bathla G, Maheshwarappa RP: Imaging findings in spinal sarcoidosis: a report of 18 cases and review of the current literature, *Neuroradiol J* 32(1):17–28, 2019.

51

Sacral Masses

SCOTT EDWARD HUNTER, MD, MBA

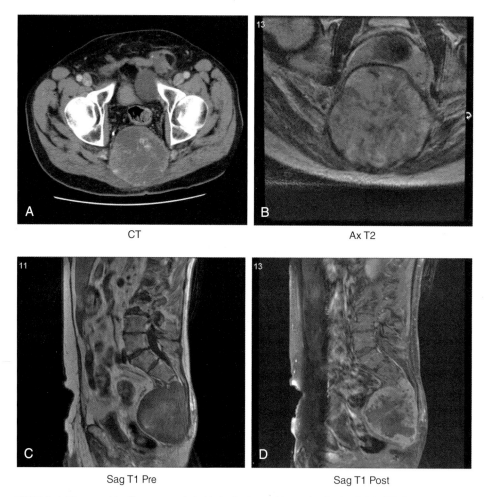

CT

Ax T2

Sag T1 Pre

Sag T1 Post

CASE A: A 71-year-old with severe pain in his buttocks and lower back. *Ax*, Axial; *CT*, Computed tomography; *Sag*, sagittal.

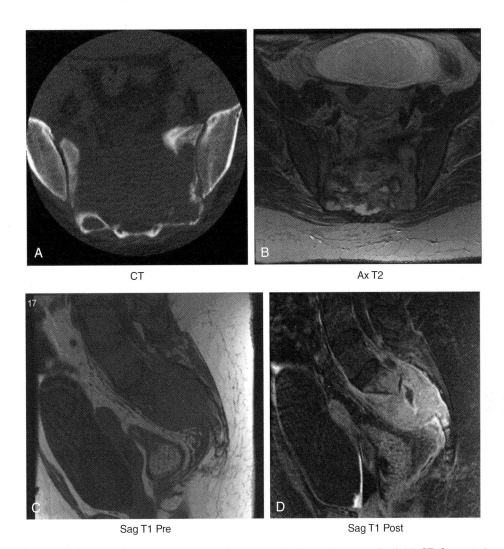

CT

Ax T2

Sag T1 Pre

Sag T1 Post

CASE B: A 20-year-old with progressive pain in her lower back and buttocks. *Ax*, Axial; *CT*, Computed tomography; *Sag*, sagittal.

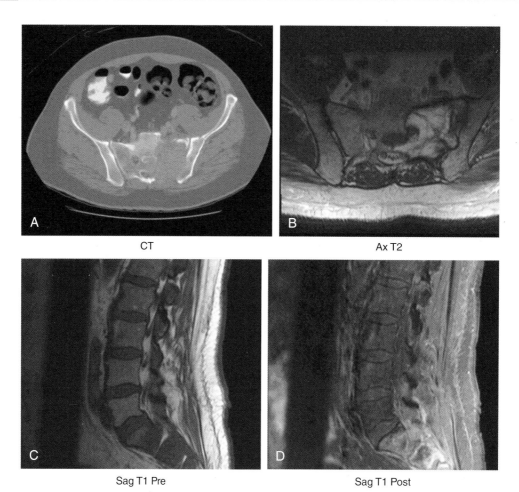

CASE C: A 52-year-old with progressive lower back and left leg pain. *Ax*, Axial; *CT*, Computed tomography; *Sag*, sagittal.

DESCRIPTION OF FINDINGS

- Case A: A CT scan of the sacrum depicts a large, well-delineated, midline sacral mass extending into the presacral region. Scattered amorphous calcifications are present. A T2-weighted MRI scan shows heterogeneous hyperintensity. T1-weighted precontrast and postcontrast MRI scans illustrate avid peripheral enhancement of the predominantly T1 hypointense mass.
- Case B: A CT scan of the sacrum illustrates a large, expansile lytic lesion with a narrow zone of transition extending to the sacroiliac joints bilaterally. No residual bony matrix is present. T2-weighted MRI scan demonstrates corresponding T2 hyperintense soft tissue throughout the visualized sacrum with involvement of the visualized sacral foramina. T1-weighted precontrast and postcontrast images show heterogeneous enhancement of an amorphous T1 hypointense sacral mass with extension into both the presacral and epidural spaces.
- Case C: A CT scan of the sacrum reveals an asymmetric, ill-defined, lytic lesion in the left hemisacrum that traverses the left-sided neural foramina and extends to the left sacroiliac joint. No bony matrix is apparent in the involved regions. T2-weighted MRI shows heterogeneous hyperintensity. T1-weighted precontrast and postcontrast MRI discloses heterogeneous enhancement of the T1 hypointense mass, which abuts the cartilaginous disk spaces.

Diagnosis

Case A: Chordoma
Case B: Giant cell tumor
Case C: Multiple myeloma

Summary

Sacral masses may represent primary or secondary neoplasms. Primary sacral tumors include malignant entities such as chordomas, osteosarcomas, Ewing sarcomas, and plasmacytomas as well as more benign entities such as giant cell tumors, hemangiomas, aneurysmal bone cysts (ABCs), and osteoblastomas. Secondary malignancies may result from hematogenous or direct spread of metastatic disease. Approximately 7% of all sacral neoplasms are primary and 93% are secondary.

Chordomas are the most common primary tumor of the sacrum, constituting 40% of primary sacral neoplasms. Nearly half of all chordomas occur in the sacrum, whereas only 15% occur in the remainder of the spine; 35% occur in the clivus, the second most common site of involvement. Chordomas originate from intraosseous notochordal rests and almost always occupy a midline or paramedian location in the distal sacrum. On CT, chordomas appear as large lytic masses with associated soft tissue components that often extend into the presacral space or spinal canal. Internal calcifications or sequestered bony fragments are evident in 30% to 70% of these lesions. On MRI, these tumors exhibit a low to intermediate T1 signal and very high T2 signal intensity. Superimposed T1 hyperintense foci indicate hemorrhage or proteinaceous components, while superimposed T2 hyperintense foci typically indicate septations or hemorrhage. Although enhancement is characteristic, gadolinium avidity is variable.

Giant cell tumors are the second most frequent primary tumor of the sacrum and occur in this location in 1% to 8% of cases. Most of these lesions arise in long bones, typically the distal femur and proximal tibia. In contrast to chordomas,

sacral giant cell tumors are frequently eccentric and abut or extend across the sacroiliac joint. On CT, these lesions are lytic and expansile, with a narrow zone of transition and a characteristic absence of bony matrix. On MRI, giant cell tumors exhibit low to intermediate T1 signal intensity and intermediate to high T2 signal intensity. Their T2 signal intensity is generally less than that of chordomas. Enhancement is typically heterogeneous due to areas of necrosis.

Multiple myeloma represents a monoclonal proliferation of malignant plasma cells of the bone marrow. Plasmacytoma is the unifocal form of multiple myeloma and usually has a better prognosis than multiple myeloma. CT often discloses a large, expansile lytic lesion. The classic appearance of multiple "punched-out" lesions is an alternative appearance. On MRI, plasmacytomas and myeloma lesions are hypointense to normal marrow on T1-weighted sequences and hyperintense on T2-weighted sequences. Variable enhancement is demonstrated on MRI. These lesions rarely traverse disc spaces.

Spectrum of Disease

Sacral masses constitute a heterogeneous group of lesions with an extensive differential diagnosis. These lesions include primary lesions of bone, including those described in this chapter: primary neural tumors and metastatic lesions.

Primary bone lesions presenting as sacral masses are overwhelmingly lytic in appearance. For example, sacral ABCs, which constitute approximately 20% of spinal ABCs, typically appear as expansile lytic lesions with a predilection for the posterior elements. Their CT and MRI appearance often can be distinguished from that of other osteolytic lesions by the presence of multiloculated, septated, blood-filled cavities with fluid-fluid levels (Fig. 51.1). Sacral ABCs typically occur in the

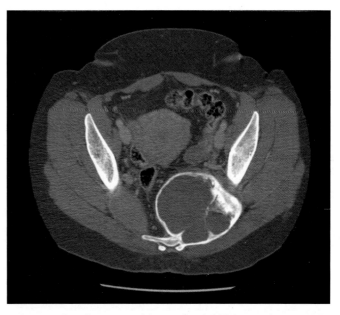

• **Fig. 51.1** Sacral aneurysmal bone cyst. Axial computed tomography image demonstrates a large multiloculated expansile lytic cyst in the left lower sacrum. A dominant loculation demonstrates a fluid-fluid level, a characteristic finding of these lesions.

second decade of life with a slight female predominance and may be suspected on the basis of patient demographics. Another osteolytic mass is the sacral osteoblastoma, which constitutes 17% of all spinal osteoblastomas and often occurs in association with ABCs. Although its CT appearance is variable, the most common pattern is that of an expansile lytic lesion centered in the posterior elements with multiple small calcifications and a peripheral sclerotic rim. An osteoid matrix is often evident on CT. By MRI, these lesions often demonstrate variable T2 signal, depending on the extent of tumor ossification. Enhancing peritumoral edema is often a prominent feature and may mimic malignancy.

Although chondrosarcoma is the most common malignant primary bone neoplasm in adults, sacral involvement is unusual. When a chondrosarcoma is present in the sacrum, it is often eccentric and may traverse the sacroiliac joint (Fig. 51.2). This appearance is distinct from that of chordomas, which tend to occupy a central position. Typically lytic and destructive in appearance, a chondrosarcoma may have a cartilaginous matrix, with a "ring-and-arc" pattern on both CT and T2-weighted MRI, although a matrix is variably present.

Primary neural tumors presenting as sacral masses may include nerve sheath tumors, such as neurofibromas and schwannomas. These tumors originate from lumbar or sacral nerve roots and appear as intradural extramedullary masses, frequently with extradural components that assume a characteristic dumbbell shape and extend through the neural foramina. However, in advanced cases, these lesions may cause sacral destruction and contain large soft tissue components, rendering their appearance nonspecific (Fig. 51.3). Both neurofibromas and schwannomas may exhibit a "target" appearance on T2-weighted sequences, with central low signal surrounded by high signal.

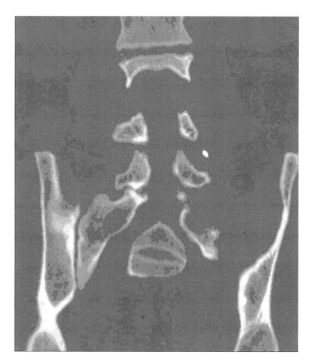

• **Fig. 51.3** A neurofibroma. A coronal reformatted image from a computed tomography scan demonstrates widening of the left L5-S1 neural foramen and destruction of the left hemisacrum by a large neurofibroma in a patient with neurofibromatosis type 1.

Differential Diagnosis

1. Chordoma
2. Giant cell tumor
3. Osteoblastoma
4. ABC
5. Metastasis
6. Multiple myeloma

Pearls

- Morphology: Chordomas are lobulated in contour. Giant cell tumors typically are aggressive, often with cortical breakthrough. Multiple myeloma may appear as a solitary, large, infiltrative lesion with soft tissue components that span the intraosseous and extraosseous compartments. Alternatively, it may appear as multiple focal "punched-out" lesions.
- Location/course: Chordomas almost invariably occur in the midline and often lie in the lower sacrum. Giant cell tumors, by contrast, are usually eccentric in location and may abut or traverse the sacroiliac joints. They tend to occur in the proximal sacrum. Sacral myeloma may appear anywhere within the sacrum but rarely cross disk spaces.
- Bone involvement: Chordomas uniformly present with heterogeneous osseous destruction, often traversing cartilaginous disks in the spine and involving consecutive levels. Giant cell tumors often present with cortical breakthrough. Multiple myeloma often occurs in the setting of diffuse osteopenia.

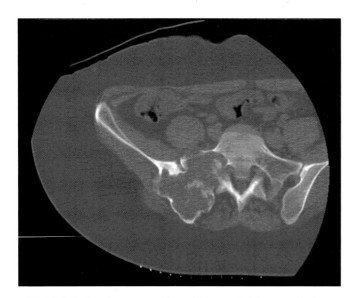

• **Fig. 51.2** A chondrosarcoma. An axial computed tomography image illustrates a large, destructive lytic lesion centered about the right sacroiliac joint, with a characteristic ring-and-arc matrix typical of cartilaginous lesions.

- Enhancement: Contrast enhancement is variable and not a strong differentiating factor.
- Calcification: Sacral chordomas typically exhibit amorphous internal calcifications. Conversely, giant cell tumors often exhibit a conspicuous absence of calcification or osseous matrix. Chondrosarcomas may have a ring-and-arc pattern of calcification typical of cartilaginous lesions. Calcification is rare in persons with multiple myeloma.
- Demographics: The mean age of patients with a chordoma is 50 years. Men are affected twice as often as women. Giant cell tumors occur in patients between 20 and 40 years of age and affect women more frequently than men. The peak age of multiple myeloma diagnosis is 64 years.

Signs and Complications

The most common initial symptom of sacral tumors is local pain. Other neurologic symptoms such as numbness, weakness, radicular pain, and incontinence can ensue from nerve root compression or infiltration.

Sacral chordomas are slowly growing tumors that may present with distant metastases in the lung, liver, lymph nodes, or bone. Symptoms may exist for up to 2 years before diagnosis. En bloc surgical resection with adjuvant radiotherapy is a mainstay of treatment. However, local recurrence is seen in up to 90% of cases.

Sacral giant cell tumors are benign entities. However, local malignant transformation occurs in up to 2%, often after radiotherapy is administered. These lesions are complicated by a pathologic fracture in up to 30% of cases. Traditionally, wide excision with adjuvant cryotherapy or thermocoagulation has been the treatment of choice for resectable lesions. More recently, the chemotherapeutic agent denosumab, a human monoclonal antibody that inhibits osteolysis, has been adopted as a supplement to surgical resection and as a standalone treatment in cases where surgical resection is not feasible. Lung, liver, or bony metastases may be present in up to 13% of cases.

Multiple myeloma often occurs in the setting of osteopenia and is frequently complicated by a pathologic fracture. Additional complications, such as infection and anemia, may result from marrow failure. Chemotherapy and local radiation are preferred treatments for persons with multiple myeloma, though surgery is often indicated for patients with neurologic involvement or tumor-related spinal instability. Median survival with chemotherapy is approximately 3 to 5 years. Plasmacytoma, the unifocal form of multiple myeloma, carries a more favorable prognosis.

Suggested Readings

Althausen PL, Schneider PD, Bold RJ, et al: Multimodality management of a giant cell tumor arising in the proximal sacrum: case report, *Spine* 27:361–365, 2002.

Bloem JL, Reidsma II: Bone and soft tissue tumors of hip and pelvis, *Eur J Radiol* 81:3793–3801, 2012.

Chakarun CJ, Forrester DM, Gottsegen CJ, et al: Giant cell tumor of bone: review, mimics, and new developments in treatment, *Radiographics* 33(1):197–211, 2013.

Dimopoulos MA, Moulopoulos LA, Maniatis A, et al: Solitary plasmacytoma of bone and asymptomatic multiple myeloma, *Blood* 96(6): 2037–2044, 2000.

Disler DG, Miklic D: Imaging findings in tumors of the sacrum, *AJR Am J Roentgenol* 173:1699–1706, 1999.

Farsad K, Kattapuram SV, Sacknoff R, et al: Sacral chordoma, *Radiographics* 29(5):1525–1530, 2009.

Huang WY, Tan WL, Geng DY, et al: Imaging findings of the spinal peripheral Ewing's sarcoma family of tumours, *Clin Radiol* 69(2):179–185, 2014.

Kwon JW, Chung HW, Cho EY, et al: MRI findings of giant cell tumors of the spine, *AJR Am J Roentgenol* 189(1):246–250, 2007.

Llauger J: Primary tumors of the sacrum: diagnostic imaging, *AJR Am J Roentgenol* 174(2):417–424, 2000.

Murphey MD, Andrews CL, Flemming DJ, et al: From the archives of the AFIP. Primary tumors of the spine: radiologic pathologic correlation, *Radiographics* 16(5):1131–1158, 1996.

Ravindra VM, Eli IM, Schmidt MH, et al: Primary osseous tumors of the pediatric spinal column: review of pathology and surgical decision-making. *Neurosurg Focus* 41(2):E3, 2016.

Sung MS, Lee GK, Kang HS, et al: Sacrococcygeal chordoma: MR imaging in 30 patients, *Skeletal Radiol* 34:87–94, 2005.

Thornton E, Krajewski KM, O'Regan KN, et al: Imaging features of primary and secondary malignant tumours of the sacrum. *Br J Radiol* 85(1011):279–286, 2012.

52

Disk Infection Versus Inflammatory/Degenerative Changes

JUAN E. SMALL, MD, MSC

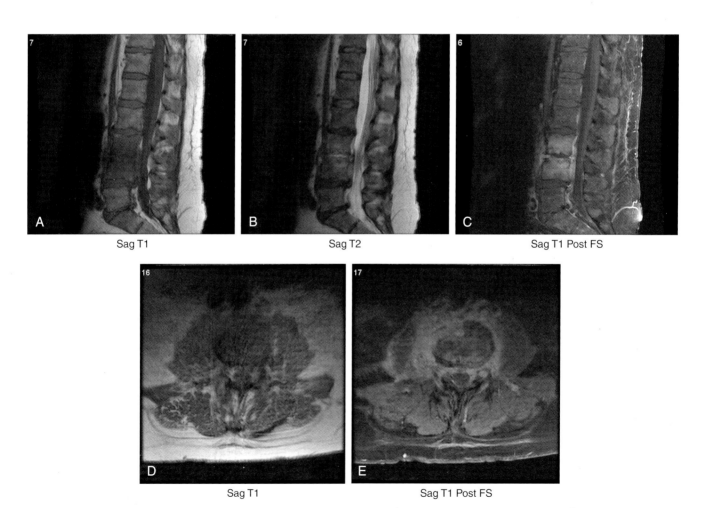

Sag T1   Sag T2   Sag T1 Post FS

Sag T1   Sag T1 Post FS

CASE A: A 58-year-old with a history of heavy alcohol use, gastrointestinal bleeding, and prior bowel resection presenting with low back pain. *FS*, fat saturated; *Sag*, sagittal.

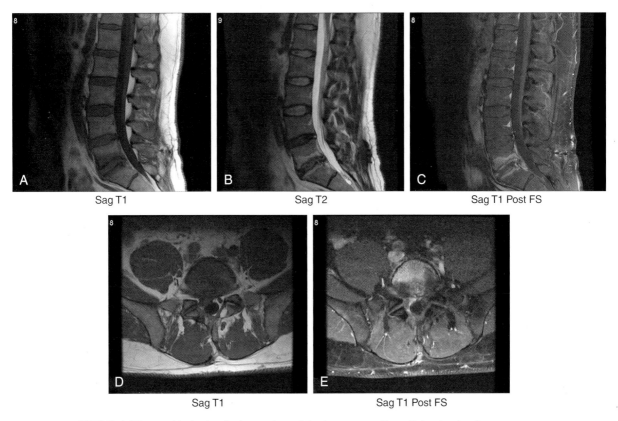

Sag T1   Sag T2   Sag T1 Post FS

Sag T1   Sag T1 Post FS

CASE B: A 36-year-old who has had a previous diskectomy, presenting with low back pain.
FS, Fat saturated; *Sag*, sagittal.

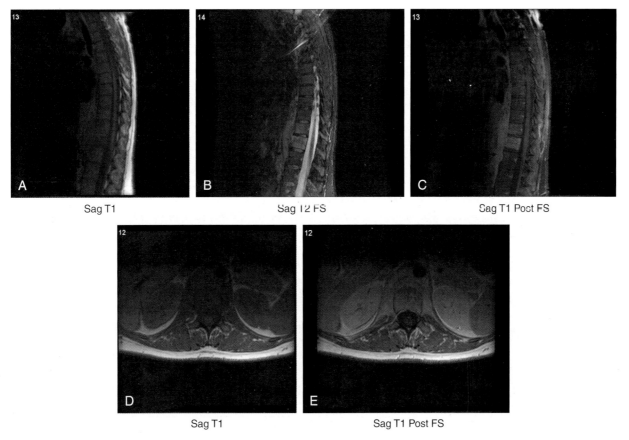

Sag T1   Sag T2 FS   Sag T1 Post FS

Sag T1   Sag T1 Post FS

CASE C: A 42-year-old presenting with back pain of several months' duration. *FS*, fat saturated; *Sag*,
sagittal.

DESCRIPTION OF FINDINGS

- Case A: At the L3/L4 level prominent, T2 hyperintense signal is present in the disk space, with enhancement of the disk periphery, erosion of enhancing adjacent endplates, and phlegmonous paraspinal and psoas muscle inflammation.
- Case B: At the L5/S1 level, edematous, enhancing endplate changes are present with mild T2 hyperintense signal and lack of central enhancement in the disk space. Enhancement is noted along the surgical tract, most likely representing postoperative granulation tissue.
- Case C: Visible are large prevertebral phlegmon, anterior subligamentous edema/enhancement, prominent vertebral marrow edema, and enhancement with relative preservation of the intervertebral disk.

Diagnosis

Case A: Bacterial diskitis/osteomyelitis
Case B: Postoperative edematous/inflammatory endplate changes
Case C: Tuberculous osteomyelitis

Summary

Distinguishing between infectious and inflammatory etiologies affecting the disk space and adjacent endplate often can be difficult. Imaging findings supportive of a pyogenic infectious etiology, such as *Staphylococcus aureus* infection involving the disk space, include the presence of paraspinal and/or epidural inflammation and phlegmonous change, disk enhancement, T2 hyperintensity in the disk space, and erosion or destruction of the adjacent endplates.

One of the most valuable signs of infection is the identification of paraspinal or epidural inflammatory/phlegmonous change, although it is not entirely sensitive, especially in early infection. Infected disks almost always enhance; in particular, rim enhancement of the disk appears to be more specific for infection than partial or diffuse disk enhancement. Lack of enhancement is very rare, but has been reported in the literature. Disk infection classically involves the two adjacent vertebrae, which should demonstrate an MRI edema pattern (T1 hypointensity and T2 hyperintensity) and enhance with contrast administration. Destruction or erosion of the endplates is considered a typical finding. However, lack of endplate involvement does not exclude infection. Partial or heterogeneous vertebral marrow involvement beyond the endplates can be seen and even involve the entire vertebral body. Collapse of the vertebral body may be seen in infection, but is uncommon.

Early infection may not demonstrate these classic imaging features; therefore the presence of T2 isointensity or hypointensity within the disk does not exclude infection. Conversely, although T2 hyperintensity of the disk suggests infection, it is not a specific sign and may also be seen in inflammatory conditions.

Several features help distinguish pyogenic from tuberculous spinal infection. Imaging features seen with tuberculous spinal infections include subligamentous spread, marked paraspinous inflammatory change, paraspinal abscesses with thick peripheral enhancement, calcifications within the paraspinous inflammatory change, and fragmentary osseous destruction. A relatively preserved disk space in the setting of such findings is an especially strong marker of tuberculous infection.

Tuberculous spinal infections tend to involve the thoracic spine more often than the lumbar spine. In addition, they tend to start anteriorly and progress posteriorly. Slow progression and chronic symptoms suggest tuberculous rather than pyogenic infection. In severe and/or chronic cases, progression to kyphotic angulation, vertebral body destruction, or even vertebra plana may be seen. Although two or three adjacent vertebral bodies often are involved, noncontiguous vertebral body involvement may be seen.

Because tuberculous spinal infection may involve multiple noncontiguous vertebral bodies and spare the disk space, it may be confused with metastatic disease. However, paravertebral abscesses/phlegmonous change and subligamentous spread are strong indicators of tuberculous infection.

Spectrum of Disease

It can be very challenging to distinguish between postsurgical disk inflammation and inflammation seen in infectious spondylodiscitis. General guidelines favoring noninfectious inflammation include a relative paucity of vertebral endplate edema, intervertebral disk enhancement, and paraspinal signal abnormality. However, given the imaging overlap between these two states, correlation with clinical markers of infection is essential. This can include a suggestive physical examination and a set of patient symptoms, fever, and blood test results, such as elevated erythrocyte sedimentation rate, C-reactive protein, and white blood cell count.

Differential Diagnosis

1. A guideline for the differential diagnosis is provided in Table 52.1.

Pearls

- The following findings are suggestive of a pyogenic infectious etiology involving the disk space:
  - Paraspinal and/or epidural inflammation and phlegmonous change
  - Disk enhancement
  - T2 hyperintensity in the disk space
  - Erosion or destruction of the adjacent endplates
- The following findings are suggestive of a tuberculous spinal infection:

TABLE 52.1	Differential Diagnosis of Spinal Infections
Spinal Abnormality	**Imaging Features**
Charcot spine	subchondral osteopenia, formation of debris/fragmentation, periosteal bone formation.
Ankylosing spondylitis	syndesmophytes, Anderssen lesion, bamboo spine, shiny corners
Acute Schmorl's node	focal globular morphology with involvement of a single enplate and surrounding edema

- Subligamentous spread
- Vertebral marrow involvement and relative preservation of the intervertebral disk
- Marked paraspinous inflammatory change with a thick, enhancing rim
- Calcification within the paraspinous inflammatory change and fragmentary osseous destruction

Signs and Complications

Complications of infectious spondylodiscitis include vertebral destruction and paraspinal and epidural abscess formation.

Suggested Readings

Hong SH, Choi JY, Lee JW, et al: MR imaging assessment of the spine: infection or an imitation?, *Radiographics* 29(2):599–612, 2009.

Joseffer SS, Cooper PR: Modern imaging of spinal tuberculosis, *J Neurosurg Spine* 2(2):145–150, 2005.

Ledermann HP, Schweitzer ME, Morrison WB, et al: MR imaging findings in spinal infections: rules or myths?, *Radiology* 228(2):506–514, 2003.

Mendonça RA: Spinal infection and inflammatory disorders. In Atlas SW, editor: *Magnetic resonance imaging of the brain and spine*, ed 4, Philadelphia, 2008, Lippincott Williams & Wilkins, 2008.

Stabler A, Reiser MF: Imaging of spinal infection, *Radiol Clin North Am* 39(1):115–135, 2001.

53

Vertebral Compression Fractures

KENNETH S. ALLISON, MD

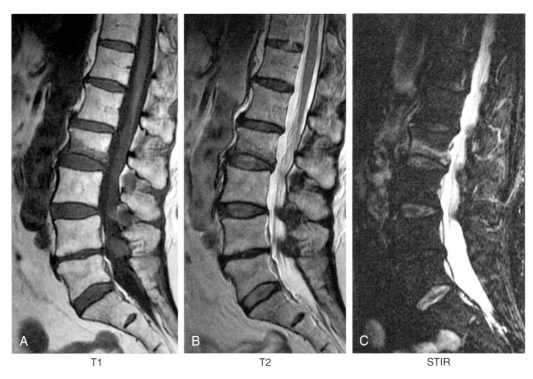

T1   T2   STIR

CASE A: An 83-year-old presenting with back pain. *STIR*, Short T1 inversion recovery.

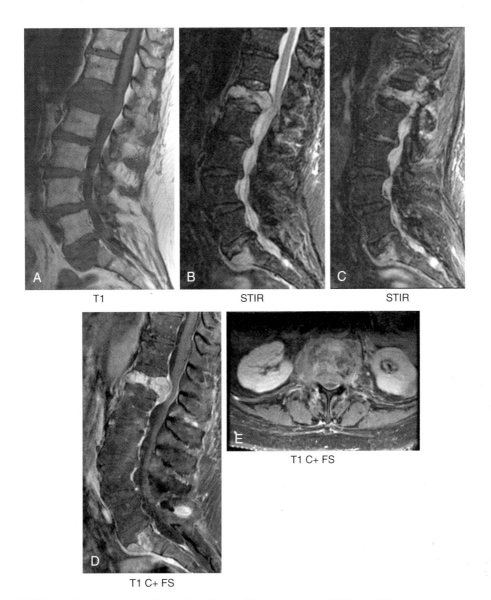

T1

STIR

STIR

T1 C+ FS

T1 C+ FS

CASE B: A 77-year-old presenting with back pain. *FS,* Fat saturated; *STIR,* short T1 inversion recovery.

DESCRIPTION OF FINDINGS

- Case A: Approximately one-third loss of height of the L2 vertebral body is present from compression deformity of the inferior L2 endplate. Hypointense signal abnormality partially replaces the normal marrow signal in the lower half of the vertebral body on T1-weighted images, with corresponding hyperintense signal abnormality on STIR images. A hypointense fracture line can be seen parallel to the inferior L2 endplate on T1 and T2 images, and there is mild retropulsion of a small fracture fragment from the posteroinferior corner of the vertebral body.
- Case B: Compression deformities of both the superior and inferior endplates of the L1 vertebral body are present, with convex bowing of the posterior vertebral body margin into the spinal canal. Low signal completely replaces the normal T1 bright marrow signal on T1-weighted imaging. STIR images demonstrate diffusely hyperintense signal abnormality within the vertebral body as well as the pedicle. On contrast-enhanced imaging, diffuse heterogeneous enhancement of the vertebral body is present with confluent paraspinal and epidural soft tissue extension. Additional enhancing lesions can be seen in the S1 vertebral body and the L5 spinous process.

Diagnosis

Case A: Benign (osteoporotic) compression fracture
Case B: Malignant compression fracture

Summary

Acute vertebral compression fractures are commonly encountered radiologic findings and can pose an etiologic dilemma. Causes of benign compression fractures include osteoporosis, trauma, eosinophilic granuloma, Paget disease, and hemangioma. Malignant compression fractures can arise from metastatic disease or from primary neoplasms such as multiple myeloma, lymphoma, leukemia, and primary bone tumors. Distinguishing benign from malignant fractures is sometimes difficult and may have important implications for patient treatment and prognosis.

Several findings on MRI can be helpful in making the distinction. Diffuse homogeneous replacement of normal bone marrow signal with low signal on T1-weighted images suggests a malignant fracture, whereas benign fractures often demonstrate partial or more inhomogeneous marrow replacement. Other features that suggest a malignant etiology include involvement of the pedicles and/or posterior elements, a diffuse convex bulge of the posterior vertebral body cortex, and a paraspinal and/or epidural mass. Malignant fractures usually show diffuse or patchy heterogeneous enhancement of the vertebral body on postcontrast images, and additional metastases may be visualized elsewhere in the spine (with or without associated fractures) in many cases. Signs that support benign osteoporotic fractures include the presence of fluid signal adjacent to the fractured endplate (fluid sign), a retropulsed fracture fragment, a low signal intensity band adjacent to the fractured endplate corresponding to the fracture line, and an intravertebral vacuum cleft.

On CT, the most reliable evidence of malignancy is lytic osseous destruction, particularly of the anterolateral and/or posterior vertebral body cortices, of cancellous bone, or of the pedicles. Other malignant signs include a paraspinal mass larger than 5 mm or an epidural mass. Visualization of distinct fracture lines (as opposed to destruction), diffuse vertebral sclerosis, or an intravertebral vacuum cleft are features suggestive of a benign etiology.

In some cases, diffusion-weighted imaging (DWI) also can be used to distinguish malignant tumor infiltration (high signal) from benign edema (low signal) in acute compression fractures. In addition, fluorodeoxyglucose positron emission tomography ((FDG-PET) may be helpful in distinguishing benign from malignant lesions in equivocal cases. Malignant compression fractures tend to demonstrate increased FDG uptake, whereas benign fractures do not.

The presence of multiple compression fractures does not allow generalization about their etiology, so the features of each fracture should be individually evaluated. In addition, the above criteria are not reliable in acute traumatic compression fractures, which can resemble malignant fractures, or in fractures associated with multiple myeloma, which can mimic benign fractures. In ambiguous cases, follow-up imaging or biopsy may be indicated.

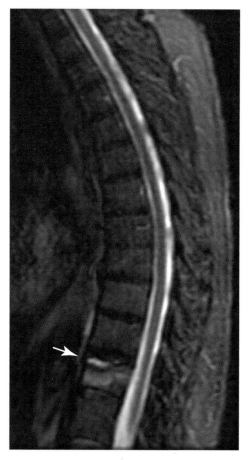

• **Fig. 53.1** The fluid sign in a 78-year-old male with an acute compression fracture of the T12 vertebral body. A sagittal short T1 inversion recovery (STIR) image demonstrates linear hyperintense signal adjacent to the fractured superior endplate *(arrow)*. This patient later underwent a vertebral augmentation procedure, and a bone biopsy obtained during that procedure confirmed the benign, osteoporotic nature of the fracture.

Differential Diagnosis

1. Benign compression fracture (osteoporosis, eosinophilic granuloma, hemangioma, and Paget disease)
2. Malignant compression fracture (metastatic disease, multiple myeloma, lymphoma, leukemia, primary bone tumors)
3. Traumatic compression fracture
4. Compression fracture associated with infection

Pearls

- Multiple myeloma may mimic a benign fracture.
- Trauma may mimic a malignant fracture.

Signs and Complications

The fluid sign refers to hyperintense signal on STIR images, which is isointense to CSF, within an acutely collapsed vertebral body (Fig. 53.1). The fluid sign can support a benign, osteoporotic etiology for a compression fracture and is rarely seen in malignant fractures.

Suggested Readings

Baker LL, Goodman SB, Perkash I, et al: Benign versus pathologic compression fractures of vertebral bodies: assessment with conventional spin-echo, chemical-shift, and STIR MR imaging, *Radiology* 174(2): 495–502, 1990.

Baur A, Stäbler A, Arbogast S, et al: Acute osteoporotic and neoplastic vertebral compression fractures: fluid sign at MR imaging, *Radiology* 225(3):730–735, 2002.

Bredella MA, Essary B, Torriani M, et al: Use of FDG-PET in differentiating benign from malignant compression fractures, *Skeletal Radiol* 37(5):405–413, 2008.

Kubota T, Yamada K, Ito H, et al: High-resolution imaging of the spine using multidetector-row computed tomography: differentiation between benign and malignant vertebral compression fractures, *J Comput Assist Tomogr* 29(5):712–719, 2005.

Raya JG, Dietrich O, Reiser MF, et al: Methods and applications of diffusion imaging of vertebral bone marrow, *J Magn Reson Imaging* 24(6):1207–1220, 2006.

Uetani M: Malignant and benign compression fractures: differentiation and diagnostic pitfalls on MRI, *Clin Radiol* 59(2):124–131, 2004.

Yuh WT, Zachar CK, Barloon TJ, et al: Vertebral compression fractures: distinction between benign and malignant causes with MR imaging, *Radiology* 172(1):215–218, 1989.

54

Periauricular Cystic Lesions

BRIAN ZIPSER, MD AND PAUL M. BUNCH, MD

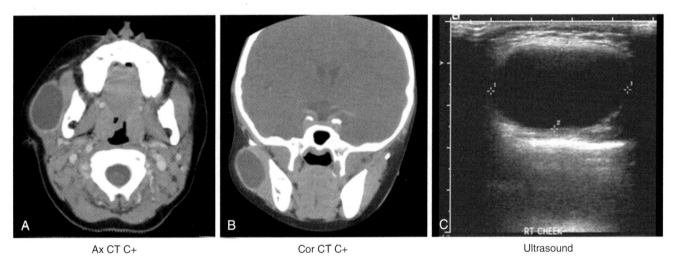

A	B	C
Ax CT C+	Cor CT C+	Ultrasound

CASE A: A 5-year-old male presenting with painful right facial swelling after recent ear infection. *Ax,* Axial; *Cor,* coronal; *CT,* Computed tomography.

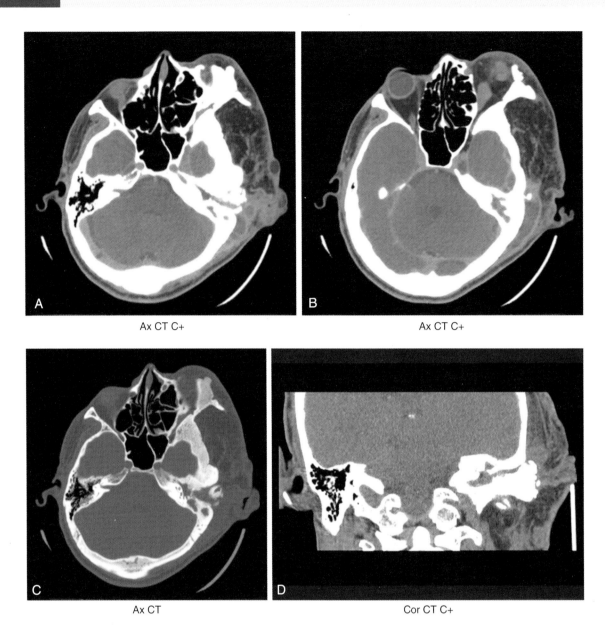

Ax CT C+

Ax CT C+

Ax CT

Cor CT C+

CASE B: A 40-year-old male with neurofibromatosis type 1 and known facial dysmorphism resulting from left facial plexiform neurofibromas and multiple surgeries, now presenting with a fluctuant mass posterior to the left ear, ear pain for the past 2 to 3 weeks, fever, headache, nausea, and vomiting. *Ax*, Axial; *Cor*, coronal; *CT*, Computed tomography.

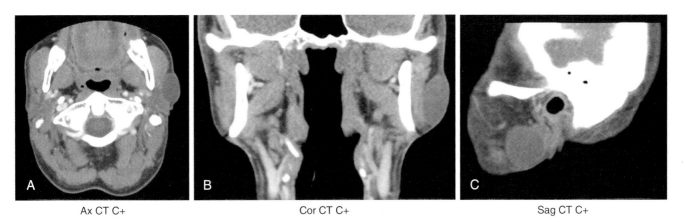

Ax CT C+   Cor CT C+   Sag CT C+

CASE C: A 51-year-old male presenting with a left cheek mass. *Ax*, Axial; *Cor*, coronal; *CT*, Computed tomography; *Sag*, sagittal.

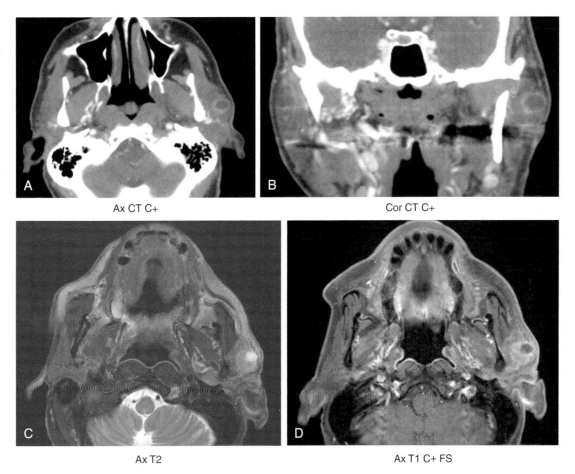

Ax CT C+   Cor CT C+

Ax T2   Ax T1 C+ FS

CASE D: An 84-year-old male with a history of multiple cutaneous squamous cell carcinomas of the head and neck. *Ax*, Axial; *Cor*, coronal; *CT*, Computed tomography; *FS*, fat saturated.

DESCRIPTION OF FINDINGS

- Case A: The CT images demonstrate a circumscribed, homogeneously hypodense mass within the superficial lobe of the right parotid gland with a thick, enhancing rim and mild surrounding fat stranding. An ultrasound confirms the presence of a unilocular cystic mass.
- Case B: The CT images demonstrate a peripherally enhancing fluid collection within the soft tissues posterior and inferior to the left ear and communicating with the left external auditory canal. Adjacent osseous permeative lytic changes are noted within the left temporal bone and mastoid air cells. Intracranial extension of the fluid collection into the left temporal epidural space is demonstrated, with mass effect on the adjacent left temporal lobe.
- Case C: The CT images demonstrate a circumscribed hypodense ovoid mass within the subcutaneous fat superficial to the left parotid gland, with a broad margin contiguous with the skin.
- Case D: The CT images demonstrate a peripherally enhancing, centrally hypodense lesion within the superficial left parotid gland. On MRI, this lesion peripherally enhances and is heterogeneously T2 hyperintense with a central, nonenhancing cystic component.

Diagnosis

Case A: First branchial cleft cyst

Case B: Coalescent otomastoiditis complicated by subperiosteal and epidural abscesses

Case C: Epidermal inclusion cyst

Case D: Cutaneous squamous cell carcinoma metastatic to an intraparotid lymph node

Summary

First branchial cleft cysts have a characteristic periauricular location associated with the parotid gland and seventh cranial nerve that directly relates to their embryologic origin. It is this typical location that suggests the diagnosis and helps differentiate first branchial anomalies from other head and neck cystic masses, including other branchial apparatus lesions.

First branchial apparatus anomalies are congenital anomalies that occur during the development and differentiation of the mesodermal arches, ectodermal cleft, and endodermal pouch. Externally, the first and second branchial arches are separated by an ectodermally lined cleft, which is the only branchial cleft to give rise to an anatomic structure, the external auditory canal. Internally, the first and second arches are separated by an endodermally lined pouch that gives rise to the Eustachian tube and middle ear cavity. Either failure of the cleft/pouch to be completely obliterated or the presence of cell rests or remnants of the branchial apparatus can result in an external or internal sinus, a fistula, and/or an isolated cyst.

Consistent with the embryologic origin, first branchial apparatus lesions are most commonly located near the external auditory canal in a preauricular or postauricular location. Because the posterior migration of the parotid gland and the anterior migration of the facial nerve (which arises from the second branchial arch) occur after the development of the first branchial cleft structures, first branchial cleft anomalies have a variable association with the parotid gland and facial nerve (Fig. 54.1).

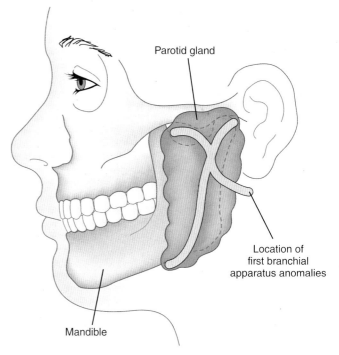

- **Fig. 54.1** Possible locations of first branchial apparatus anomalies. (Modified from Koch BL: Cystic malformations of the neck in children, *Pediatr Radiol* 35:463–477, 2005; and Benson MT, Dalen K, Mancuso AA, et al: Congenital anomalies of the branchial apparatus: embryology and pathologic anatomy, *Radiographics* 12(5):943–960, 1992.)

Clinically, these anomalies typically present acutely in children following an upper respiratory tract infection, most commonly as a cystic inflammatory neck mass or abscess in or near the parotid gland. They also may present as a nontender neck mass in the absence of acute infection. Recurrent or chronic otorrhea in the absence of chronic otitis should also raise the suspicion for a first branchial apparatus anomaly.

Infected lesions appear as an inflammatory mass or abscess on cross-sectional imaging, typically within the parotid gland or adjacent to the external auditory canal. Noninfected first branchial cleft cysts appear as a simple anechoic mass on ultrasound or as a unilocular cystic lesion on contrast-enhanced CT, respecting the adjacent structures and fascial planes, with minimal or no rim enhancement. These lesions have a variable association with the facial nerve. Sinus tracts and fistulae may be small and difficult to visualize on cross-sectional imaging, but may be characterized with CT or fluoroscopic fistulograms to further aid in surgical planning. Treatment involves complete surgical excision, often with a partial parotidectomy and facial nerve monitoring; otherwise, recurrence is common. The variable location of first branchial apparatus lesions that are lying superficial, deep, or even between branches of the facial nerve may complicate surgical resection.

Other causes of a periauricular cystic lesion to consider include suppurative or metastatic lymph node, cystic parotid neoplasm, lymphatic malformation, dermoid/epidermoid cyst, lymphoepithelial cyst, and abscess. In an adult patient, a cystic or necrotic nodal metastasis from a primary cutaneous malignancy is a primary differential consideration, particularly involving the frontal and temporal skin, eyelid, anterior auricle, and external auditory canal. Although the imaging features of some of these entities overlap, clinical clues are often helpful for narrowing the differential diagnosis.

Spectrum of Disease

First branchial apparatus anomalies may present as cysts, sinuses, or fistulae, reflecting their embryologic origin. They may be contiguous with or have a sinus tract opening to the external auditory canal (in approximately 44% of cases) or, rarely, to the tympanic membrane or middle ear.

First branchial cleft cysts are almost always a single lesion. Multiple cysts or lesions within a similar location should raise suspicion for other pathology, including parotid neoplasms, lymphoepithelial cysts in persons with HIV, Sjögren syndrome, or sialoceles. In older patients presenting with a cystic-appearing periauricular lesion, cystic parotid neoplasm and nodal metastases (most commonly from cutaneous squamous cell carcinoma or melanoma) should be suspected.

The Work classification divides first branchial cleft cysts into two types, which may affect the surgical approach (Fig. 54.2). Type 1 lesions are thought to be of ectodermal origin and are considered to be duplications of the membranous external auditory canal. Type 1 lesions lie superior and lateral to the facial nerve, extend medial to the conchal cartilage, and are oriented parallel to the external auditory canal. These lesions may be removed with a retroauricular incision, keeping the skin of the external auditory meatus intact. Type 2 lesions may have both mesodermal and ectodermal components and may present as

cysts, sinuses, or fistulae. Type 2 lesions may lie more inferiorly than type 1 lesions, extending below the angle of the mandible, deeper within the parotid gland, and anterior to the sternocleidomastoid muscle. A tract from Work type 2 lesions may course superficial or deep to the facial nerve with sites of possible openings including the skin of the suprahyoid neck near the angle of the mandible, the skin just inferior to the external auditory canal, and within the external auditory canal near the osseocartilaginous junction. To safely remove Work type 2 lesions, the surgeon must first identify the facial nerve in relation to the lesion at the stylomastoid foramen and trace the nerve distally. Work type 2 lesions also may involve the tympanic membrane or middle ear structures, which will affect the surgical approach.

First branchial apparatus lesions may rarely lie between the nasopharynx and middle ear or as inferiorly as the angle of the mandible. The first branchial pouch anomaly most commonly manifests as a short Eustachian tube, clinically presenting in children with recurrent otitis media. A rare lateral nasopharyngeal cyst also may represent a first, or possibly a second, branchial pouch remnant, lying between the posterior tonsillar pillar and the pharyngeal opening of the Eustachian tube.

Differential Diagnosis

Lymphatic Malformation

On MR imaging, lymphatic malformations are typically T2 hyperintense with rim enhancement and/or thin enhancing septae. T1 hyperintense and T2 hypointense components may be seen in the setting of hemorrhage or otherwise proteinaceous fluid (Fig. 54.3).

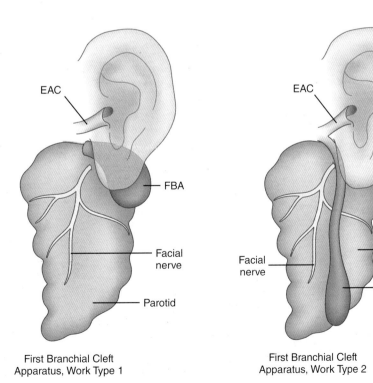

First Branchial Cleft
Apparatus, Work Type 1

First Branchial Cleft
Apparatus, Work Type 2

• **Fig. 54.2** Work classification of first branchial apparatus anomalies. *EAC,* External auditory canal; *FBA,* first branchial apparatus anomaly. (Modified from Acierno SP, Waldhausen JHT: Congenital cervical cysts, sinuses, and fistulae, *Otolaryngol Clin North Am* 40(1):161–176, 2007.)

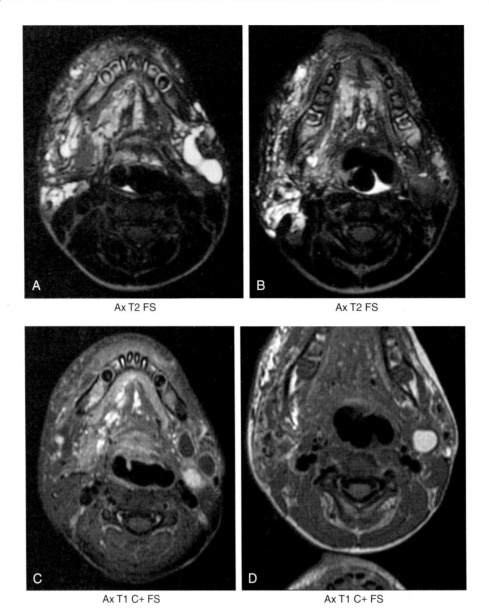

Ax T2 FS

Ax T2 FS

Ax T1 C+ FS

Ax T1 C+ FS

• **Fig. 54.3** A 3-year-old male presenting with facial swelling and bleeding after minor trauma. *FS,* fat saturated. The MR images demonstrate a large, trans-spatial, multicystic mass involving the bilateral parotid, pharapharyngeal, masticator, submandibular, and sublingual spaces, consistent with a lymphatic malformation. Although most of the malformation is T1 hypointense and T2 hypointense, a component along the posterior aspect of the left mandibular angle exhibits T1 hyperintensity (D) and T2 hypointensity (B), consistent with hemorrhage or other proteinaceous content. *Ax,* Axial.

Fluid-fluid levels may also be seen. Rarely, a unilocular lymphatic malformation may mimic a branchial cleft cyst.

Dermoid/Epidermoid Cyst

The presence of fat and restricted diffusion are imaging features that favor dermoid/epidermoid cyst.

Dilated Parotid Duct and Postobstructive Sialoceles

A sialocele is a cystic space containing saliva and arising within a salivary gland. Sialoceles are uncommon but may occur after traumatic or iatrogenic injury to a salivary duct or in the setting of obstructing sialolith or stricture. Consider sialocele in the

setting of periauricular cystic lesion with a dilated parotid duct. With impaired ductal drainage, parotid inflammatory changes may also be seen (Fig. 54.4).

Sjögren Syndrome

Parotid findings in Sjögren syndrome include multiple small bilateral cystic lesions. Fatty replacement of the parotid parenchyma may also be seen.

Cystic-Appearing Parotid Neoplasms

Parotid neoplasms may be partially cystic (Fig. 54.5) or exhibit signal characteristics that mimic a cyst (Fig 54.6), particularly if post-contrast imaging is not acquired or not carefully examined.

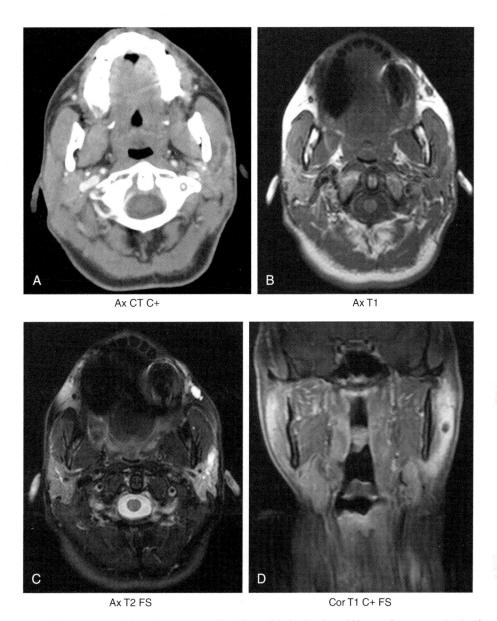

Ax CT C+

Ax T1

Ax T2 FS

Cor T1 C+ FS

• **Fig. 54.4** A 55-year-old female presenting with left parotid gland pain and history of a recent episode of acute left parotid gland swelling. Axial CT image (A) demonstrates a tubular, fluid-filled structure coursing within the anterior aspect of the left parotid gland and along the superficial aspect of the left masseter muscle, consistent with a dilated left parotid duct. Thickening and hyperenhancement of the duct walls suggest superimposed inflammation. No radiopaque sialolith is identified. Axial T2-weighted (C) and coronal gadolinium-enhanced T1-weighted images (D) respectively demonstrate asymmetric T2 hyperintensity and hyperenhancement of the left parotid gland, consistent with superimposed left parotitis. Ax, Axial; Cor, coronal; *CT,* Computed tomography; *FS,* fat saturated.

Warthin tumors are frequently located in the parotid tail and are commonly partially cystic. The solid components enhance poorly and often exhibit relative T2 hypointensity. The cystic components are typically T1 hypointense but may exhibit T1 hyperintensity in the setting of proteinaceous content.

Some parotid neoplasms, including pleomorphic adenomas, exhibit marked T2 hyperintensity and a delayed enhancement pattern. On T2-weighted images, the marked T2 hyperintensity may mimic a cyst, and if post-contrast T1-weighted images are acquired shortly after gadolinium injection, solid enhancement may be difficult to appreciate. As such, delayed (e.g., 10 minutes)

post-contrast imaging can be useful to decrease the risk of mistaking a cystic-appearing parotid neoplasm for a cyst.

In contrast to first branchial cleft anomalies, cystic or cystic-appearing parotid gland neoplasms are typically found in an older population and usually also have solid components or enhancing septations.

Benign Lymphoepithelial Lesions

Benign lymphoepithilial lesions result from lymphocytic infiltration of the major salivary glands and are most frequently

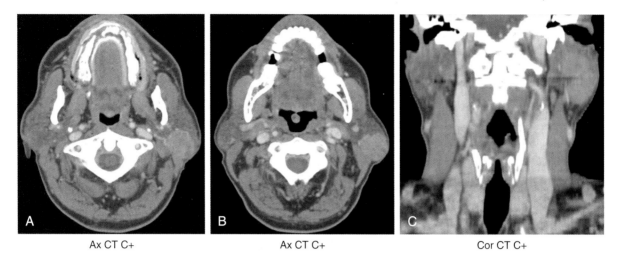

Ax CT C+   Ax CT C+   Cor CT C+

• **Fig. 54.5** A 51-year-old male with history of a palpable left facial mass for 3 to 4 years. Axial (A, B) and coronal (C) contrast-enhanced CT images demonstrate ovoid masses involving the superficial left parotid gland and left parotid tail. Although the masses appear predominantly solid, some small, hypoattenuating, cystic components are present in these pathologically-proven Warthin tumors. *Ax,* Axial; *Cor,* coronal; *CT,* Computed tomography.

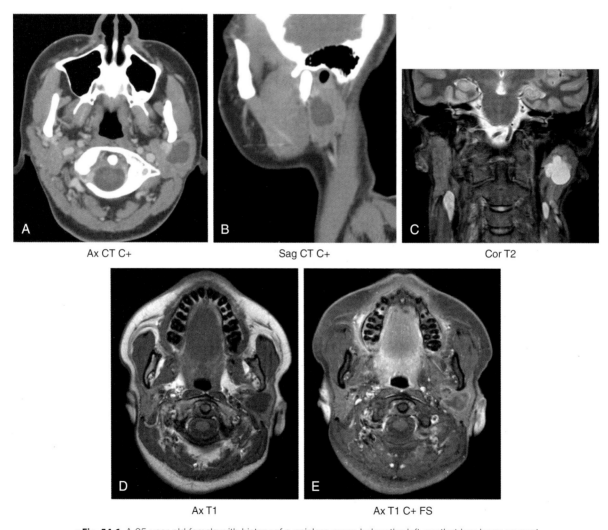

Ax CT C+   Sag CT C+   Cor T2

Ax T1   Ax T1 C+ FS

• **Fig. 54.6** A 25-year-old female with history of a painless mass below the left ear that has been present for years. Axial (A) and sagittal (B) contrast-enhanced CT images demonstrate a well-defined, multilobulated, hypoattenuating mass within the left parotid gland. On the coronal T2-weighted image (C), the mass exhibits marked T2 hyperintensity. Given the CT attenuation and T2 signal similar to fluid, this mass could be mistaken for a cyst. However, the axial gadolinium-enhanced T1-weighted image (E) demonstrates internal enhancement in this pathologically-proven pleomorphic adenoma. *Ax,* Axial; *Cor,* coronal; *CT,* Computed tomography; *FS,* fat saturated; *Sag,* sagittal.

associated with HIV infection but also occur in autoimmune diseases (e.g., Sjögren syndrome) and sporadically. These lesions typically affect the parotid glands (bilateral in approximately 20%) but can rarely involve the submandibular, sublingual, and minor salivary glands. On CT and MR imaging, benign lymphoepithelial lesions typically manifest as multiple well-circumscribed cysts. Thin rim enhancement is expected after administration of contrast. Internal septations and small mural nodules may also be seen.

Suppurative Lymphadenitis

Suppurative lymph nodes within the parotid gland or along the cervical lymph node chain may be a differential diagnosis for infected first and second through fourth branchial cleft cysts, respectively. Similar to infected branchial apparatus lesions, suppurative lymphadenopathy may develop following a recent head and neck infection, beginning as reactive nodes and developing into an intranodal abscess.

Cold Abscess

Tuberculous or nontuberculous mycobacterial infection may present as cystic-appearing necrotic lymph nodes, often without significant surrounding inflammatory change.

Cystic or Necrotic Lymph Node Metastases

Most parotid lymph node metastases are from cutaneous squamous cell carcinomas or melanomas of the upper face or scalp.

Pearls

- In a child, first branchial apparatus lesions should be the primary consideration for a sinus tract, cystic, or inflammatory neck mass associated with the parotid gland near the external auditory canal.
- First branchial apparatus lesions may lie anywhere from the external auditory canal to below the angle of the mandible and often are intimately associated with the parotid gland and facial nerve. A cystic lesion in this area should prompt a careful search for a sinus tract, either internally to the external auditory canal or externally at a level inferior to the angle of the mandible or at a level anterior to the sternocleidomastoid muscle.
- Cystic or necrotic metastases from cutaneous squamous cell carcinoma or melanoma are the primary differential

considerations in adult patients older than 40 years, and an appropriate diagnostic workup for a primary lesion should be performed.
- Multiple cystic lesions in or adjacent to the parotid gland suggest a diagnosis other than first branchial cleft anomaly, such as abscesses, Sjögren syndrome, multiple primary parotid neoplasms (e.g., Warthin), benign lymphoepithelial lesions in the setting of HIV, sialoceles, or cystic or necrotic nodal metastases.

Signs and Complications

Incomplete excision of a sinus tract associated with a branchial cleft cyst may result in lesion recurrence.

The intimate and complex association of first branchial anomalies with the facial nerve increases the risk of iatrogenic nerve injury during surgical excision.

Suggested Readings

Acierno SP, Waldhausen JHT: Congenital cervical cysts, sinuses and fistulae, *Otolaryngol Clin North Am* 40(1):161–176, 2007.

Adams A, Mankad K, Offiah C, et al: Branchial cleft anomalies: a pictorial review of embryological development and spectrum of imaging findings, *Insights Imaging* 7(1):69–76, 2016.

Pomar Blanco P, Martín Villares C, San Román Carbajo J, et al: Metastases to the parotid gland, *Acta Otorrinolaringol Esp* 57(1):47–50, 2006.

Chun RH, Choi SS: First branchial cleft cyst: a rare presentation with mesotympanic extension, *Int J Pediatr Otorhinolaryol Extra* 4:80–83, 2009.

Guarisco JL, Fatakia A: Intraoperative fistulograms in the management of branchial apparatus abnormalities in children, *Int J Pediatr Otorhinolaryngol* 72(12):1777–1782, 2008.

Myers LL, Ahn C: Cutaneous squamous cell carcinoma metastasis to the parotid region lymph nodes, *Laryngoscope* 129(7):1579–1586, 2019.

Sujatha D, Babitha K, Prasad RS, et al: Parotid lymphoepithelial cysts in human immunodeficiency virus: a review, *J Laryngol Otol* 127(11):1046–1049, 2013.

Sun Z, Zhang Z, Fu K, et al: Diagnostic accuracy of parotid CT for identifying Sjögren's syndrome, *Eur J Radiol* 81(10):2702–2709, 2012.

Takita H, Takeshita T, Shimono T, et al: Cystic lesions of the parotid gland: radiologic-pathologic correlation according to the latest World Health Organization 2017 Classification of Head and Neck Tumours, *Jpn J Radiol* 35(11):629–647, 2017.

Tham YS, Low WK: First branchial cleft anomalies have relevance in otology and more, *Ann Acad Med Singapore* 34:335–338, 2005.

Whetstone J, Branstetter BF 4th, Hirsch BE: Fluoroscopic and CT fistulography of the first branchial cleft, *AJNR Am J Neuroradiol* 27(9):1817–1819, 2006.

55

Cystic Lateral Neck Masses

BRIAN ZIPSER, MD AND PAUL M. BUNCH, MD

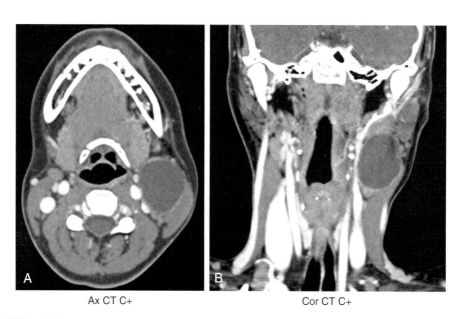

Ax CT C+   Cor CT C+

CASE A: A 22-year-old female presenting with swelling in the left side of the neck. *Ax*, Axial; *Cor*, coronal; *CT*, Computed tomography.

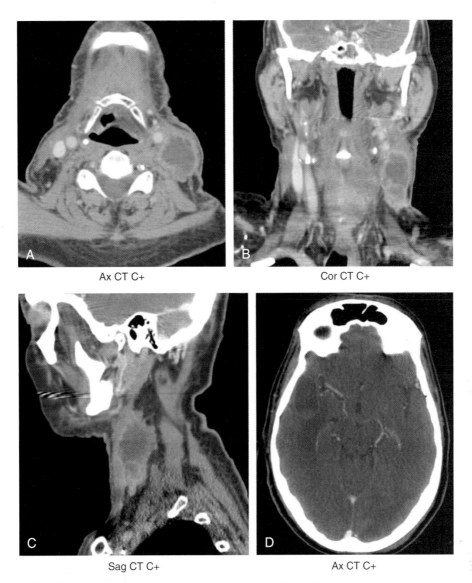

Ax CT C+

Cor CT C+

Sag CT C+

Ax CT C+

CASE B: A 61-year-old male with squamous cell carcinoma of the oral tongue and lung cancer. *Ax*, Axial; *Cor*, coronal; *CT,* Computed tomography; *Sag*, sagittal.

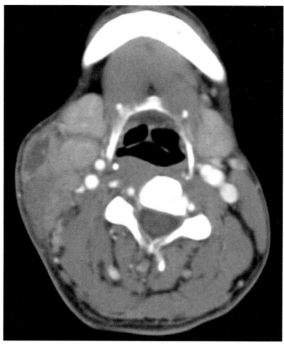

Ax CT C+

CASE C: A 35-year-old male who recently traveled to Cambodia now presents with a mass in the right side of the neck. *Ax*, Axial; *CT*, Computed tomography.

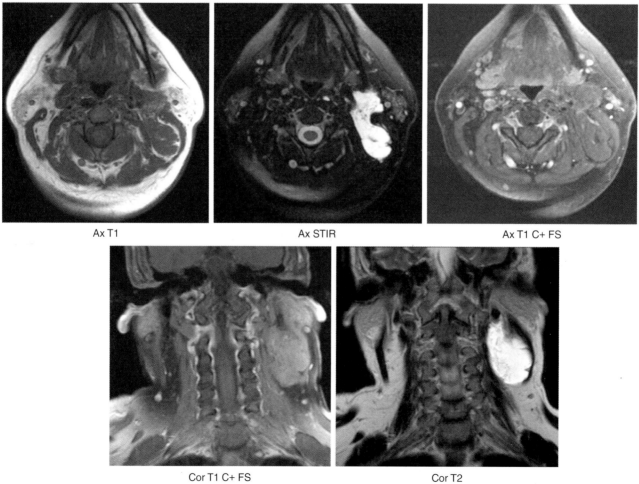

Ax T1   Ax STIR   Ax T1 C+ FS

Cor T1 C+ FS   Cor T2

CASE D: A 54-year-old female with left neck fullness since childhood. *Ax*, Axial; *Cor*, coronal; *FS*, fat saturated; *STIR*, short tau inversion recovery.

DESCRIPTION OF FINDINGS

Images from four different patients with cystic lesions along the lateral aspect of the neck are presented.

- Case A features a rim-enhancing, homogeneous, low-attenuation cystic lesion in the left side of the neck between the submandibular gland and the left sternocleidomastoid muscle that is displacing the left common carotid artery bifurcation medially and abutting the parotid gland along the lesion's superolateral margin.
- Case B features a thick-rimmed, peripherally enhancing mass with central low attenuation in the left side of the neck at the junction of levels II and III that is elevating the sternocleidomastoid muscle, abutting the left common carotid artery anteromedially, and narrowing the left internal jugular vein. A ring-enhancing lesion involving the right temporal lobe and right insula is also present.
- Case C features a large, centrally hypodense mass in the right side of the neck involving the right sternocleidomastoid muscle at a level just inferior to the parotid gland. The right sternocleidomastoid muscle is edematous, and there are inflammatory changes in the adjacent fat. Multiple enlarged right jugulodigastric nodes are present. Narrowing of the right internal jugular vein is observed medially.
- Case D features an extensive, well-marginated, multiseptated, T2 hyperintense, trans-spatial mass insinuating among structures of the left neck deep soft tissues and involving the left carotid space, left submandibular region, and deep left parotid region. Enhancement is present along the rim of the lesion and within some internal septations.

Diagnosis

Case A: Second branchial cleft cyst (typically requires histopathologic confirmation in an adult because a cystic nodal metastasis cannot be excluded by imaging alone)

Case B: Necrotic left cervical lymph node metastasis and brain metastasis

Case C: Tuberculosis (scrofula)

Case D: Lymphatic malformation

Summary

Second branchial apparatus lesions are the most common of the branchial apparatus anomalies, accounting for approximately 95%. As with other branchial apparatus lesions, they occur in a characteristic, predictable location, reflecting their embryologic origin. This characteristic location helps differentiate branchial apparatus lesions from other congenital abnormalities (e.g., lymphatic malformation, dermoid cyst) among pediatric patients. However, in adults, tissue sampling is often necessary to definitively differentiate a second branchial apparatus lesion from more sinister pathology, including necrotic or cystic lymph node metastases from squamous cell or papillary thyroid carcinoma.

The branchial apparatus is a developmental structure composed of pairs of mesodermal arches that are separated externally by paired ectodermally lined clefts and separated internally by paired endodermally lined pouches, all of which form structures of the head and neck. Either cell rests or remnants of the first through fourth branchial clefts and pouches may result in three congenital pathologies in the neck: a sinus opening as an external cleft or internal pouch, an internal-external fistula, or a cyst without an internal or external connection. The anomalies are named for their embryologic cleft or pouch of origin. Sinuses and fistulae may be lined by ciliated columnar respiratory epithelium of branchial pouch origin, whereas cysts and some external sinuses are lined by squamous epithelium of branchial cleft origin.

The second branchial cleft, along with the third and fourth branchial clefts as part of the cervical sinus of His, normally are obliterated during development. The second branchial arch forms the muscles of facial expression, the stylohyoid muscle, the stapedius muscle, the hyoid body and lesser horn, the styloid process, the stapes, and cranial nerve VII. The second branchial pouch forms the palatine tonsils. Therefore the tract of second branchial apparatus lesions may extend from an external opening along the anterior border of the junction of the mid to lower third of the sternocleidomastoid muscle, extending deep to the platysma, ascending along the carotid sheath, above the hypoglossal and glossopharyngeal nerves, between the internal and external carotid arteries, and ultimately opening internally into the tonsillar fossa or supratonsillar region (Fig. 55.1).

Clinically, second branchial apparatus anomalies most often present in children as a nontender neck mass or an inflammatory neck mass or abscess that often develops acutely after an upper respiratory tract infection. Some lesions may present as torticollis or, because of their close proximity to the pharynx, as dysphagia or respiratory distress, especially in neonates.

Second branchial cleft cysts most commonly appear as anechoic masses on ultrasound or as a unilocular cystic lesion on contrast-enhanced computed tomography (CT) or magnetic resonance imaging (MRI). These lesions may displace adjacent

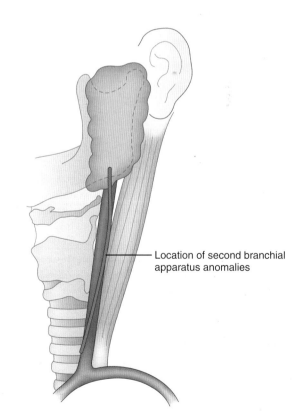

Location of second branchial apparatus anomalies

• **Fig. 55.1** Possible locations of second branchial apparatus anomalies. (Modified from Koch BL: Cystic malformations of the neck in children, *Pediatr Radiol* 35:463–477, 2005.)

structures but typically respect normal fascial planes, except in the setting of infection or after invasive procedure. Cysts may derive from remnants of the branchial cleft, arch, or pouch and may therefore vary in their location in the neck, ranging from between the skin surface and the cervical sinus of His to the pharyngeal wall as a pharyngeal pouch remnant and characterized by the Bailey classification of second branchial apparatus cysts (see the Spectrum of Disease section of this chapter). Most second branchial apparatus cysts lie in the anterolateral neck along the anterior border of the sternocleidomastoid muscle at the angle of the mandible. Fistula openings extend more inferiorly in the lower anterolateral neck at the junction of the middle and lower third of the sternocleidomastoid muscle. Sinus tracts to the pharynx may be small and difficult to identify with CT or MRI, especially in the acute phase when inflammation and edema may obstruct the sinus tract. Therefore most patients undergo direct evaluation of the tonsillar fossa or supratonsillar region with laryngoscopy. Once inflammation has subsided, fluoroscopic esophagram, CT esophagram, and/or fluoroscopic or CT fistulograms (for external sinuses) may further delineate the course of a fistula or sinus, which can help guide the surgical approach. Treatment involves complete surgical excision, with unresected or incompletely resected lesions having a high rate of infection and recurrence. The proximity of the tract to the glossopharyngeal, hypoglossal, spinal accessory, and vagus nerves may complicate surgical resection.

It is extremely important to consider cystic or necrotic lymph node metastases in the differential diagnosis. Metastases most commonly originate from head and neck squamous cell carcinoma (often oropharyngeal) or papillary thyroid carcinoma. In an adult patient who presents with a cystic neck lesion, even if a primary malignancy is not visualized on imaging, an occult primary lesion should be suspected. This is true even in young adult patients because both human papillomavirus (HPV)–related oropharyngeal cancer and papillary thyroid cancer may affect this patient group. The rare development of branchiogenic carcinoma, a squamous cell carcinoma arising de novo within a branchial apparatus anomaly, is controversial.

In contrast to uncomplicated second branchial apparatus lesions, metastases and granulomatous nodal disease often cross fascial planes and may disrupt adjacent structures. However, infected branchial apparatus lesions may similarly disrupt and cross tissue planes. If a primary neoplastic lesion is not identified by imaging in an adult patient, additional workup should include fine-needle aspiration or excisional biopsy of the cystic neck lesion, If histopathology shows squamous cell carcinoma, pan-endoscopy, directed biopsies of the Waldeyer ring, and/or bilateral tonsillectomy may be performed in an attempt to identify the site of primary malignancy. If a primary carcinoma arising from a branchial cleft cyst is suspected, lesions are treated with wide resection and modified radical neck dissection with possible postoperative radiation and/or adjuvant chemotherapy.

Spectrum of Disease

Branchial apparatus anomalies may present as cysts, sinuses, or fistulae, reflecting their embryologic origin. Second branchial apparatus lesions most commonly present as an enlarging cystic, frequently infected mass along the anterolateral neck at the angle of the mandible.

The four Bailey types of second branchial cleft cysts reflect the different possible locations along the embryologic tract (Fig. 55.2):
- Type I cysts are superficial, lying deep to the platysma and anterior to the sternocleidomastoid muscle, and do not contact the carotid sheath.
- Type II cysts, the most common type, are located anterior to the sternocleidomastoid muscle, lateral to the carotid sheath, and posterior to the submandibular gland. Type II cysts are sometimes adherent to the internal jugular vein.
- Type III cysts lie between the internal carotid artery and external carotid artery and extend medially toward the lateral wall of the pharynx; they sometimes are associated with a dilated pharyngeal pouch and may extend superiorly to the skull base.
- Type IV cysts are located medial to the carotid sheath against the pharyngeal wall and tonsillar fossa and possibly are pharyngeal pouch remnants.

Differential Diagnosis

1. **Cystic or necrotic lymph node metastases:** Most cystic or necrotic lymph node metastases are from head and neck squamous cell carcinomas or papillary thyroid carcinomas and should be the primary consideration in a cystic-appearing neck mass in an adult patient.
2. **Lymphatic malformation:** These lesions commonly are multiloculated, are trans-spatial, and have fluid-fluid levels on MRI. A rare unilocular lymphatic malformation may appear similar to a branchial cleft cyst.
3. **Dermoid/epidermoid cyst:** The presence of fat and restricted diffusion are imaging features that favor dermoid/epidermoid cyst.
4. **Teratoma:** Teratomas often are diagnosed prenatally in the second trimester.
5. **Suppurative lymphadenitis:** Suppurative lymph nodes within the parotid gland or along the cervical lymph node chain may be included in the differential diagnosis for infected first and second through fourth branchial cleft cysts, respectively. Suppurative lymphadenopathy is similar to infected branchial apparatus lesions in that it may develop after another head and neck infection, beginning as reactive nodes and developing into an intranodal abscess.
6. **Cold abscess:** Tuberculous or nontuberculous mycobacterial infection may present as cystic-appearing necrotic lymph nodes, often without significant surrounding inflammatory change.

Pearls

- Second branchial cleft cysts characteristically lie along the anterior border of the sternocleidomastoid muscle, posterior to the submandibular gland, and lateral to the carotid sheath at the angle of the mandible.
- Cystic or necrotic metastases should be the primary differential consideration in adult patients with particular consideration

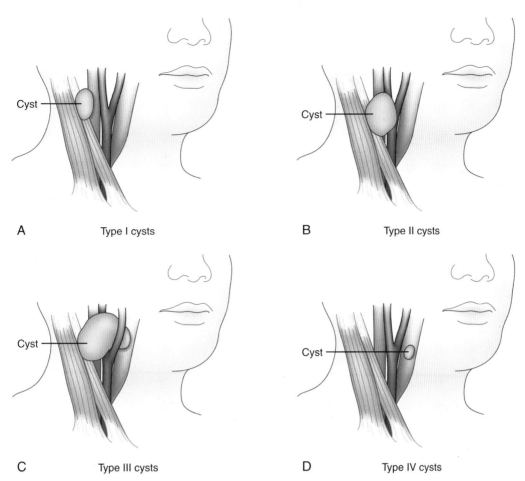

A   Type I cysts

B   Type II cysts

C   Type III cysts

D   Type IV cysts

• **Fig. 55.2** Bailey classification of second branchial cleft cysts. (A) Type I cysts are superficial, anterior to the sternocleidomastoid muscle, and separate from the carotid sheath. (B) Type II cysts (the most common) are anterior to the sternocleidomastoid muscle, lateral to and along the carotid sheath, and posterior to the submandibular gland. (C) Type III cysts are between the internal carotid artery and external carotid artery, extending toward the lateral wall of the pharynx. (D) Type IV cysts are medial to the carotid sheath and abut the pharyngeal wall and tonsillar fossa.

given to HPV-associated oropharyngeal squamous cell carcinoma and papillary thyroid carcinoma. An appropriate diagnostic workup for a primary lesion should be performed. Occasionally, these cancers also occur in teenagers. Metastases should also be considered in patients with more than one cystic neck mass.

- Although not always apparent on cross-sectional imaging, in patients with second branchial apparatus anomalies, a sinus tract may open internally into the tonsillar fossa or supratonsillar region and externally along the anterior border of the sternocleidomastoid muscle in the lower third of the neck.
- An esophagram and fistulogram with or without accompanying CT may confirm the presence of a sinus tract and subsequently aid surgical planning.
- Tuberculous infection may appear similar to suppurative lymphadenitis or infected branchial cleft cysts, but with a relative paucity of surrounding inflammatory changes. On

imaging of the neck, always inspect the visualized upper lungs for signs of tuberculous infection. Raising the suspicion for this differential diagnosis is important because these lesions are treated medically or with complete resection rather than with drainage, which would inadequately treat the infection and may unnecessarily expose others.

Signs and Complications

Cystic lateral neck masses may produce airway compromise, especially in neonates.

Incomplete excision of a sinus tract associated with a branchial cleft cyst may result in lesion recurrence.

Postsurgical complications may relate to superior laryngeal, glossopharyngeal, spinal accessory, hypoglossal, or facial nerve injury, depending on the lesion type and location.

Suggested Readings

Acierno SP, Waldhausen JHT: Congenital cervical cysts, sinuses and fistulae, *Otolaryngol Clin North Am* 40:161–176, 2007.

Adams A, Mankad K, Offiah C, et al: Branchial cleft anomalies: a pictorial review of embryological development and spectrum of imaging findings, *Insights Imaging* 7:69–76, 2016.

Black CJ, O'Hara JT, Berry J, et al: Magnetic resonance imaging of branchial cleft abnormalities: illustrated cases and literature review, *J Laryngol Otol* 124:213–215, 2010.

Devaney KO, Rinaldo A, Ferlito A, et al: Squamous carcinoma arising in a branchial cleft cyst: have you ever treated one? Will you?, *J Laryngol Otol* 122:547–550, 2008.

Guarisco JL, Fatakia A: Intraoperative fistulograms in the management of branchial apparatus abnormalities in children, *Int J Pediatr Otorhinolaryngol* 72:1777–1782, 2008.

Koch BL: Cystic malformations of the neck in children, *Pediatr Radiol* 35:463–477, 2005.

Kumar R: *Textbook of human embryology*, New Delhi, 2008, I.K. International.

Onoue K, Fujima N, Andreu-Arasa VC, et al: Cystic cervical lymph nodes of papillary thyroid carcinoma, tuberculosis and human papillomavirus positive oropharyngeal squamous cell carcinoma: comparative CT analysis for their differentiation, *Eur J Radiol* 132: 109310, 2020.

Pietarinen-Runtti P, Apajalahti S, Robinson S, et al: Cystic neck lesions: clinical, radiological and differential diagnostic considerations, *Acta Otolaryngol* 130:300–304, 2010.

Quintanilla-Dieck L, Penn EB Jr: Congenital neck masses, *Clin Perinatol* 45:769–785, 2018.

Stone ME, Link DT, Egelhoff JC, et al: A new role for computed tomography in the diagnosis and treatment of pyriform sinus fistula, *Am J Otolaryngol* 21:323–325, 2000.

Whetstone J, Branstetter BF: 4th, Hirsch BE: Fluoroscopic and CT fistulography of the first branchial cleft, *AJNR Am J Neuroradiol* 27: 1817–1819, 2006.

56
Infrahyoid Neck Cystic Lesions

BRIAN ZIPSER, MD AND PAUL M. BUNCH, MD

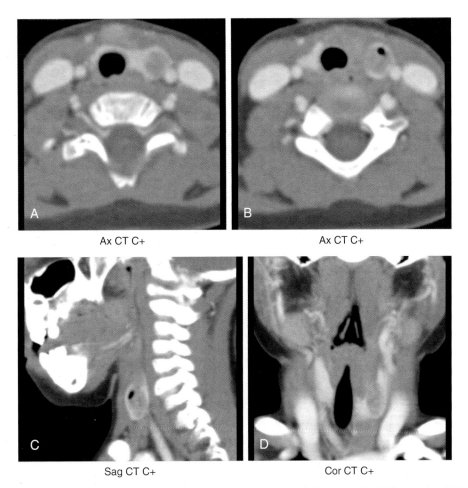

Ax CT C+

Ax CT C+

Sag CT C+

Cor CT C+

CASE A: A 2-year-old female presenting with fever and a mass in her neck for 24 hours. *Ax,* Axial; *Cor,* coronal; *CT,* Computed tomography; *Sag,* sagittal.

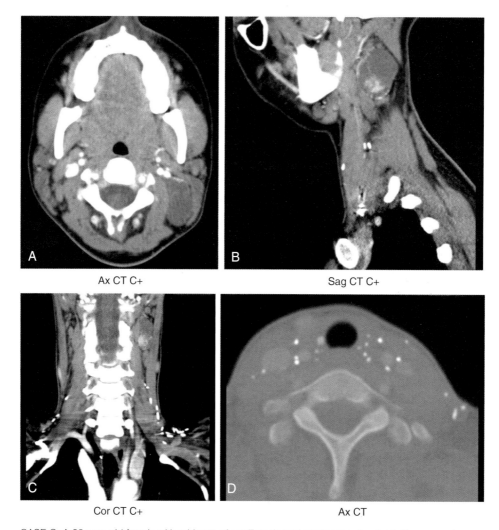

Ax CT C+   Cor CT C+   Sag CT C+

CASE B: A 2-month-old female presenting with swelling in the left side of the neck, a mass, and firm induration. *Ax,* Axial; *Cor,* coronal; *CT,* Computed tomography; *Sag,* sagittal.

Ax CT C+   Sag CT C+

Cor CT C+   Ax CT

CASE C: A 23-year-old female with a history of papillary thyroid carcinoma. *Ax,* Axial; *Cor,* coronal; *CT,* Computed tomography; *Sag,* sagittal.

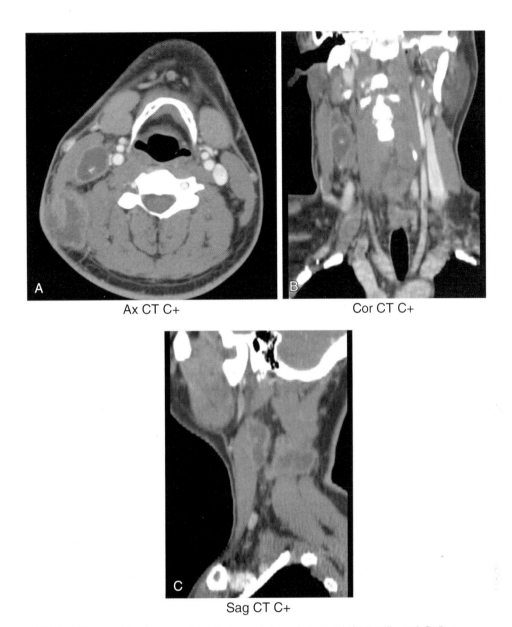

Ax CT C+

Cor CT C+

Sag CT C+

CASE D: A 29-year-old male presenting with hemoptysis and abnormal chest radiograph findings. *Ax,* Axial; *Cor,* coronal; *CT,* Computed tomography; *Sag,* sagittal.

DESCRIPTION OF FINDINGS

- Case A: Round, low-attenuation lesion centered within the left lobe of the thyroid gland with peripheral ring enhancement and containing air.
- Case B: Large, irregularly shaped, heterogeneously enhancing mass with central hypodensity in the left side of the neck that extends from the base of the skull to the supraclavicular region. The mass anteriorly displaces and is inseparable from the left sternocleidomastoid muscle and is closely associated with the left parotid gland. Surrounding fat stranding and fascial thickening are present.
- Case C: Cystic mass with an avidly enhancing nodule and a few foci of calcification located in the left posterolateral neck deep to the left sternocleidomastoid muscle and inferior to the left parotid gland. Multiple surgical clips and calcifications are noted in the lower anterior neck in the expected location of the thyroid gland.
- Case D: Multiple large, low-density masses with thick, peripheral enhancement are located along the right posterior cervical lymph node chain. One of the masses has a central calcification.

Diagnosis

Case A: Thyroid abscess from a third or fourth branchial apparatus remnant or fistula

Case B: Suppurative lymphadenitis (the clinical and imaging differential diagnosis also included infected branchial cleft cyst)

Case C: Lymph node metastasis from a papillary thyroid carcinoma

Case D: Scrofula, active/reactivation tuberculosis (additional images through the upper chest demonstrated calcified granulomas, apical scarring, and calcification in bilateral hilar and mediastinal lymph nodes)

Summary

Third and fourth branchial apparatus anomalies are often indistinguishable from each other because they originate in very similar locations along their embryologic paths. Although these lesions are less common than other branchial apparatus anomalies, their characteristic locations (based on their embryologic origins) may raise suspicion of this diagnosis and help differentiate them from other cystic neck lesions. Both third and fourth branchial apparatus lesions present similarly, often as acute suppurative thyroiditis, more commonly on the left. Recurrent low neck abscesses, cutaneous draining fistulae, or an inflammatory mass may also occur.

The branchial apparatus is composed of pairs of mesodermal arches separated externally by paired ectodermally lined clefts and separated internally by paired endodermally lined pouches.

The third branchial arch forms the stylopharyngeus muscle, the common and internal carotid arteries, cranial nerve IX, and the greater horn and lower body of the hyoid (Fig. 56.1). The fourth branchial arch forms the laryngeal muscles, aortic arch, right subclavian artery, cranial nerve X, and the thyroid, cricoid, arytenoid, corniculate, and cuneiform cartilages (Fig. 56.2). The third branchial pouch forms the base of the pyriform sinus, the inferior parathyroid glands, and the thymus, whereas the fourth branchial pouch forms the apex of the pyriform sinus, the superior parathyroid glands, and

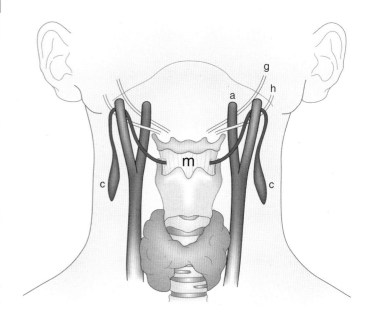

• **Fig. 56.1** Potential locations of third branchial apparatus lesions. *g,* Glossopharyngeal nerve; *h,* hypoglossal nerve; *a,* internal carotid artery; *m,* thyrohyoid membrane; *c,* potential locations of third branchial apparatus lesions.

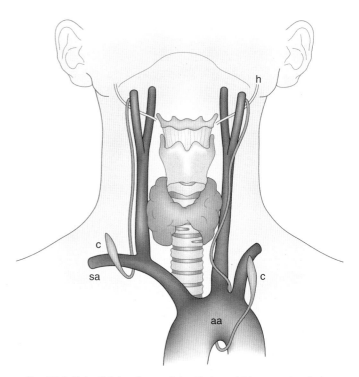

• **Fig. 56.2** Potential locations of fourth branchial apparatus lesions. *h,* Hypoglossal nerve; *aa,* aortic arch; *sa,* right subclavian artery; *c,* potential locations of fourth branchial apparatus lesions.

the ultimobranchial body, which gives rise to the calcitonin-secreting cells (parafollicular or C cells) of the thyroid gland.

Based on embryology, third branchial apparatus anomalies are expected to lie along a tract that extends from the base of the pyriform sinus and courses above the internal branch of the superior laryngeal nerve before turning inferiorly posterior to the sternocleidomastoid muscle, posterior to the common and internal carotid arteries, and lateral to the vagus nerve. Their expected openings lie lateral to the thyroid gland along the anterior margin of the middle and lower third of the sternocleidomastoid muscle.

In comparison, fourth branchial apparatus anomalies are expected to lie along a tract from the pyriform sinus apex extending around the inferior cornu of the thyroid cartilage and coursing beneath the superior laryngeal nerve to descend in the tracheoesophageal groove posterior to the thyroid gland and into the mediastinum. The pathway differs on the right compared with the left. On the right, the tract loops around the subclavian artery, whereas on the left, the tract loops under the aortic arch, medial to the ligamentum arteriosum. On both sides, the tracts ascend posterior to the common carotid artery to pass superior to the hypoglossal nerves before turning anteriorly and descending along the medial border of the sternocleidomastoid muscle.

Fourth branchial apparatus lesions may present as acute suppurative thyroiditis, likely because of the close association of a sinus tract to the thyroid gland, although suspected third branchial apparatus lesions also have been associated with suppurative thyroiditis. Third and fourth branchial apparatus lesions also may present as recurrent lower neck abscesses or a single externally draining cutaneous sinus along the lower anterior third of the neck. Infections of third and fourth branchial apparatus elements are most common in the first portion of the tract before they enter the mediastinum. Both third and fourth branchial apparatus lesions may result in airway compression if a rapid increase in size occurs. These lesions may appear as cold nodules on thyroid scans.

Because tracts may be small and difficult to identify by computed tomography (CT) or magnetic resonance imaging (MRI), most patients undergo direct evaluation of the pyriform sinus with laryngoscopy for an associated sinus or pit. In the acute phase, inflammation and edema usually obstruct the sinus tract. Once inflammation has subsided, a barium swallow, postbarium swallow CT, and/or fluoroscopic or CT fistulogram (for external sinuses) may further delineate the course of a fistula or sinus and help guide the surgical approach. The addition of a Valsalva or trumpet maneuver during a barium swallow may increase sinus tract patency.

Treatment depends on the type of branchial apparatus anomaly (cyst, thyroid abscess, sinus or fistula), and may include traditional open resection with or without heimthyroidectomy, endoscopic cauterization of an internal opening, or a combination of internal cauterization and external fistula resection.

When evaluating a cystic lower neck mass, especially in adults, it is important to consider lymph node metastases, which most commonly arise from head and neck squamous cell carcinoma or papillary thyroid carcinoma. Very rarely, ectopic thyroid tissue in a third or fourth branchial cleft cyst may develop into a papillary thyroid carcinoma.

Spectrum of Disease

Differentiating between third and fourth branchial cleft cysts and fistulas by imaging is very difficult. This distinction often is made surgically by identifying the relationship to the superior laryngeal nerve, with the third lying superiorly and the fourth lying inferiorly. The origin of lesions from the base or apex of the pyriform sinus cannot be used reliably to differentiate third and fourth branchial apparatus lesions because some overlap has been observed.

An internal fistula or sinus tract may be found extending from the pyriform sinus to the thoracic inlet, anterior and medial to the sternocleidomastoid muscle. Although traditionally a third branchial apparatus sinus tract or a pit is thought to be associated with the base of the pyriform sinus and the fourth branchial apparatus sinus tract from the apex, recently this relationship has been considered to be controversial. Many fistulas, in fact, may be pseudofistulas from infection or prior surgery rather than a true congenital fistula. Presence of air within an infected branchial anomaly is considered diagnostic of an associated sinus.

Both third and fourth branchial apparatus lesions may be associated with thyroid abscesses (Fig. 56.3). Third branchial apparatus lesions tend to be centered at the superior pole of the thyroid, whereas fourth branchial apparatus lesions tend to lie

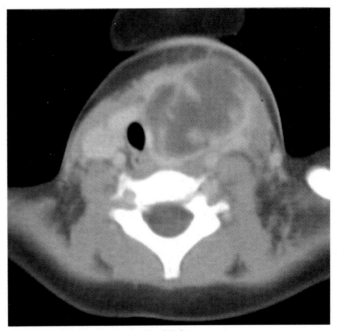

Ax CT C+

• **Fig. 56.3** A 2-year-old female presenting with fever and a painful mass in the neck. Axial CT image demonstrates an irregular rim-enhancing fluid collection consistent with abscess in the left lobe of the thyroid gland. A thyroid abscess should raise suspicion for an underlying third or fourth branchial apparatus anomaly. *Ax,* Axial; *CT,* Computed tomography.

more anterior to the thyroid gland. However, reliable differentiation for individual cases is not possible on this basis. Thyroid, thymic, or parathyroid tissue may be found in both third and fourth branchial apparatus anomalies.

Third branchial cleft cysts classically lie in the posterior cervical compartment, posterior to the sternocleidomastoid muscle and common or internal carotid arteries, but they also may lie along the lower, anterior border of the sternocleidomastoid muscle. Fourth branchial cysts more often lie within or adjacent to the left thyroid lobe. Rare reports have described mediastinal abscesses from fourth branchial apparatus origin.

Differential Diagnosis

1. **Bacterial abscess:** Among patients with a history of intravenous drug use, bacterial abscesses typically correspond to sites of attempted injection (e.g., near the external and anterior jugular veins) and are often located superficial to the sternocleidomastoid muscle (Fig. 56.4).
2. **Lymphatic malformation:** These lesions commonly are multiloculated, transspatial, and may have fluid-fluid levels on MRI. Rarely, a unilocular lymphatic malformation may have an appearance similar to that of a branchial cleft cyst.
3. **Dermoid/epidermoid cysts:** The presence of fat and restricted diffusion are imaging features that favor dermoid/epidermoid cyst.
4. **Teratoma:** Teratomas often are diagnosed prenatally, in the second trimester.
5. **Thyroglossal duct cysts:** In contrast to third and fourth branchial cleft cysts, thyroglossal duct cysts most commonly occur closer to the midline, from the tongue base to the thyroid gland, and arise from remnants of the thyroid diverticulum.

They are typically associated with the hyoid bone and/or embedded in the strap muscles and clinically elevate with swallowing or tongue protrusion. When located above the level of the hyoid, a midline location is typical. However, a paramedian location is common for infrahyoid lesions. Thyroglossal duct cysts may contain ectopic thyroid tissue.

6. **Thymic cysts:** Thymic cysts are remnants of the thymopharyngeal duct from the third branchial pouch that courses from the angle of the mandible to the upper mediastinum and typically is associated with the carotid sheath. Approximately half of thymic cysts are continuous with the thymus gland.
7. **Parathyroid cysts:** The inferior and superior parathyroid glands derive from the third and fourth branchial pouches, respectively, and the anatomic distribution of parathyroid cysts matches the anatomic distribution of the parathyroid glands.
8. **Bronchogenic cysts:** Bronchogenic cysts are a developmental anomaly from abnormal budding of the ventral foregut. They appear as well-defined, usually solitary cystic masses typically located in the paratracheal region or subcarinal region and rarely in the neck (Fig. 56.5).
9. **Midline cervical cleft:** A rare lesion present at birth, a midline cervical cleft is located in the anterior lower midline neck with a cutaneous ulceration and a sinus tract to the sternum, mandible, or a blind pouch.
10. **Saccular cysts:** Saccular cysts may be considered in the differential diagnosis of third and fourth branchial apparatus anomalies because of their close proximity to the pyriform sinus. Whereas a laryngocele represents an air-filled dilatation of the laryngeal ventricular appendix that communicates with the laryngeal lumen (Fig. 56.6), a saccular cyst is

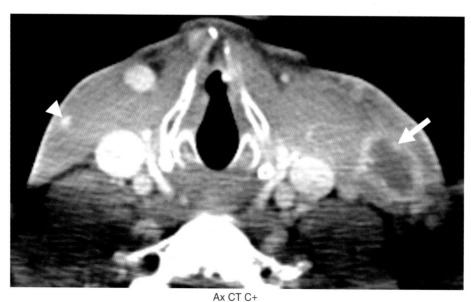

Ax CT C+

• **Fig. 56.4** A 36-year-old male with history of intravenous drug use presents to the emergency department with left neck swelling. The axial contrast-enhanced CT image demonstrates a rim-enhancing fluid collection consistent with abscess in the left neck along the superficial and lateral aspects of the left sternocleidomastoid muscle. The patient underwent incision and drainage of the abscess, and cultures grew Staphylococcus aureus. Note that the left external jugular vein *(arrow)* courses along the anterior aspect of the abscess. The normal right external jugular vein is marked with an *arrowhead* for comparison.

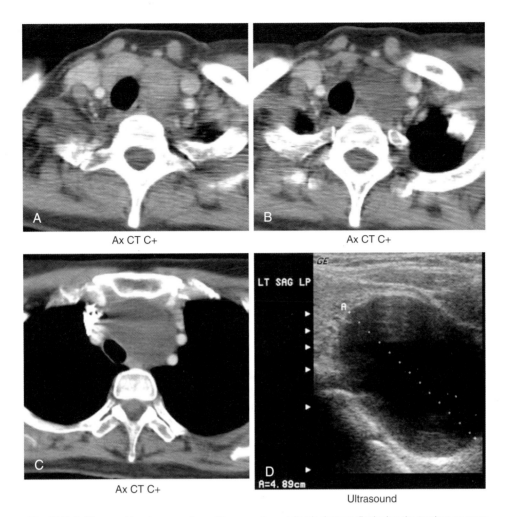

Ax CT C+   Ax CT C+

Ax CT C+   Ultrasound

• **Fig. 56.5** A 48-year-old male presenting with a superior mediastinal mass displacing the trachea as seen on an upper gastrointestinal series. A bronchogenic cyst was proven by pathology. *Ax,* Axial; *Cor,* coronal; *CT,* computed tomography.

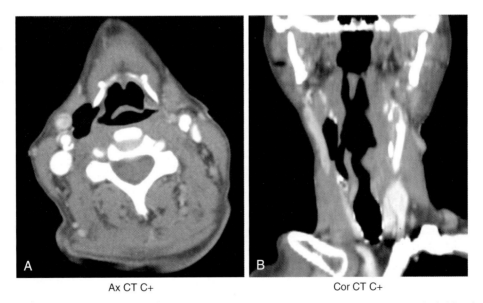

Ax CT C+   Cor CT C+

• **Fig. 56.6** An 81-year-old female presenting with dysphagia and a feeling of a lump in the neck. Axial and coronal CT images demonstrate the dilated, air-filled right laryngeal ventricular appendix, which communicates with the lumen of the supraglottic larynx and which extends lateral to the laryngeal cartilages into the right neck. These findings are consistent with an external laryngocele. *Ax,* Axial; *Cor,* coronal; *CT,* Computed tomography.

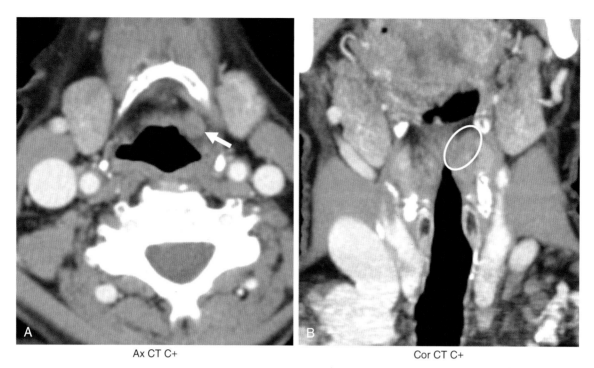

Ax CT C+   Cor CT C+

• **Fig. 56.7** (A) Axial and (B) coronal CT images demonstrate a dilated, fluid-filled left laryngeal ventricular appendix (*arrow*, A; *oval*, B) consistent with a saccular cyst. *Ax*, Axial; *Cor*, coronal; *CT*, Computed tomography.

a fluid- or mucous-filled dilatation of the ventricular appendix that typically does not communicate with the laryngeal lumen (Fig. 56.7).

11. **Suppurative lymphadenitis:** Suppurative lymph nodes within the parotid gland or along the cervical lymph node chain may be included in the differential for infected first and second through fourth branchial cleft cysts, respectively. In a similar fashion to infected branchial apparatus lesions, suppurative lymphadenopathy may develop after another head and neck infection, beginning as reactive nodes and developing into an intranodal abscess.

12. **Cold abscess:** A tuberculous or nontuberculous mycobacterial infection may present as cystic-appearing necrotic lymph nodes, often without significant surrounding inflammatory change.

13. **Cystic or necrotic lymph node metastases:** Most cystic and necrotic lymph node metastases are from head and neck squamous cell carcinomas or papillary thyroid carcinomas and should be the primary consideration in an adult patient.

Pearls

• Third and fourth branchial cysts, fistulae, and sinuses have similar clinical presentations and are difficult to distinguish from each other. Both may open into the pyriform sinus and may result in suppurative thyroiditis.

• Consider a thyroid abscess to represent a third or fourth branchial anomaly until proven otherwise, especially recurrent abscesses.

• Third branchial cleft cysts may lie posterior to the sternocleidomastoid muscle. An expected sinus tract may originate from the base of the pyriform sinus.

• Fourth branchial cleft cysts should be considered in lesions within or adjacent to the left thyroid lobe. An expected sinus tract may originate from the apex of the pyriform sinus.

• Cystic or necrotic nodal metastasis from head and neck squamous cell carcinoma or papillary thyroid carcinoma is the primary differential consideration in adult patients, and an appropriate diagnostic workup for a primary lesion should be performed.

• An esophagram (pharyngogram) and fistulogram with or without accompanying CT may confirm the presence of a sinus tract and aid surgical planning.

Signs and Complications

Cystic infrahyoid neck masses may produce airway compromise, especially in neonates.

Incomplete excision of a sinus tract associated with a branchial cleft cyst may result in lesion recurrence.

Postsurgical complications may relate to superior laryngeal, glossopharyngeal, spinal accessory, hypoglossal, or facial nerve injury, depending on the lesion type and location.

Although often not apparent on imaging, always look for an associated sinus tract contiguous with the lesion or originating from the expected location of an internal opening in the setting of a suspected branchial anomaly.

Consider cystic or necrotic nodal metastases in cases with more than one cystic-appearing neck mass.

Suggested Readings

Acierno SP, Waldhausen JHT: Congenital cervical cysts, sinuses and fistulae, *Otolaryngol Clin North Am* 40:161–176, 2007.

Adams A, Mankad K, Offiah C, et al: Branchial cleft anomalies: a pictorial review of embryological development and spectrum of imaging findings, *Insights Imaging* 7(1):69–76, 2016.

Black CJ, O'Hara JT, Berry J, et al: Magnetic resonance imaging of branchial cleft abnormalities: illustrated cases and literature review, *J Laryngol Otol* 124:213–215, 2010.

Devaney KO, Rinaldo A, Ferlita A, et al: Squamous carcinoma arising in a branchial cleft cyst: have you ever treated one? Will you? *J Laryngol Otol* 122:547–550, 2008.

Guarisco JL, Fatakia A: Intraoperative fistulograms in the management of branchial apparatus abnormalities in children, *Int J Pediatr Otorhinolaryngol* 72:1777–1782, 2008.

Joshi MJ, Provenzano MJ, Smith RJ, et al: The rare third branchial cleft cyst, *AJNR Am J Neuroradiol* 30:1804–1806, 2009.

Koch BL: Cystic malformations of the neck in children, *Pediatr Radiol* 35:463–477, 2005.

Li Y, Mashhood A, Mamlouk MD, et al: Prenatal diagnosis of third and fourth branchial apparatus anomalies: case series and comparison with lymphatic malformation, *AJNR Am J Neuroradiol* 42(11):2094–2100, 2021.

Nicoucar K, Giger R, Jaecklin T, et al: Management of congenital third branchial arch anomalies: a systematic review, *Otolaryngol Head Neck Surg* 142:21–28, 2010.

Nicoucar K, Giger R, Pope HG Jr., et al: Management of congenital fourth branchial arch anomalies: a review and analysis of published cases, *J Pediatr Surg* 44:1432–1439, 2009.

Pietarinen-Runtti P, Apajalahti S, Robinson S, et al: Cystic neck lesions: clinical, radiological, and differential diagnostic considerations, *Acta Otolaryngol* 130(2):300–304, 2010.

Quintanilla-Dieck L, Penn EB Jr: Congenital neck masses, *Clin Perinatol* 45(4):769–785, 2018.

Rea PA, Hartley BE, Bailey CM, et al: Third and fourth branchial pouch anomalies, *J Laryngol Otol* 118:19–24, 2004.

Renukaswamy GM, Soma MA, Hartley BE: Midline cervical cleft: a rare congenital anomaly, *Ann Otol Rhinol Laryngol* 118:786–790, 2009.

Stone ME, Link DT, Egelhoff JC, et al: A new role for computed tomography in the diagnosis and treatment of pyriform sinus fistula, *Am J Otolaryngol* 21(5):323–325, 2000.

Thomas B, Shroff M, Forte V, et al: Revisiting imaging features and the embryologic basis of third and fourth branchial anomalies, *AJNR Am J Neuroradiol* 31:755–760, 2010.

Whetstone J, Branstetter BF 4th, Hirsch BE: Fluoroscopic and CT fistulography of the first branchial cleft, *AJNR Am J Neuroradiol* 27:1817–1819, 2006.

57

Parapharyngeal Space Masses

PAUL M. BUNCH, MD AND GUL MOONIS, MD

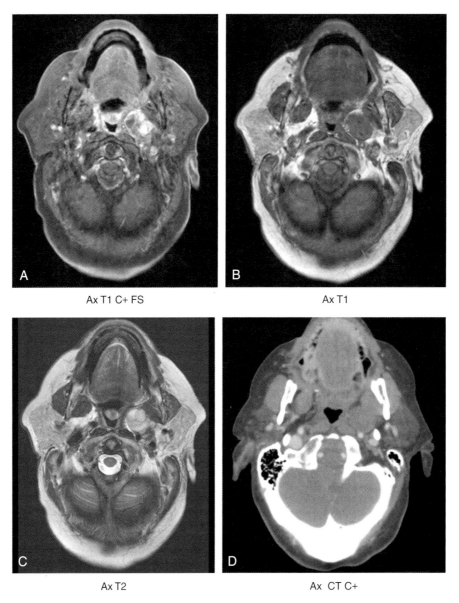

A	B
Ax T1 C+ FS	Ax T1
C	D
Ax T2	Ax CT C+

CASE A: A 71-year-old female with a mass discovered incidentally in the left parapharyngeal space. *Ax,* Axial; *CT,* Computed tomography; *FS,* fat saturated.

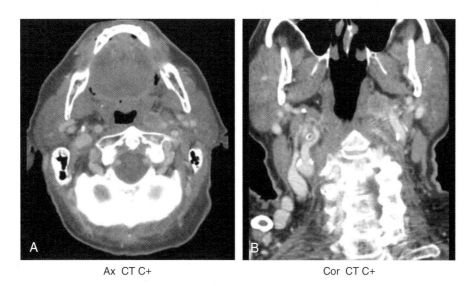

Ax CT C+ Cor CT C+

CASE B: Surveillance neck imaging for a 73-year-old male with a history of medullary thyroid cancer revealed a mass. *Ax,* Axial; *Cor,* coronal; *CT,* Computed tomography.

DESCRIPTION OF FINDINGS

- Case A: Contrast-enhanced CT demonstrates a homogeneously enhancing ovoid mass in the left parapharyngeal space. MRI demonstrates the ovoid mass to be sharply marginated with uniform intermediate signal intensity on T1-weighted images, intermediate to high signal intensity on T2-weighted images, and heterogeneous enhancement on postcontrast T1-weighted images.
- Case B: Axial and coronal contrast-enhanced CT images demonstrate a mass in the left retropharyngeal space with a hypodense center and mild peripheral enhancement. The lesion is located medial to the left internal carotid artery and lateral to the prevertebral musculature.

Diagnosis

Case A: Pleomorphic adenoma

Case B: Lateral retropharyngeal nodal metastasis from medullary thyroid carcinoma

Summary

The parapharyngeal space is a compartment in the deep neck extending from the base of the skull to the hyoid bone. The parapharyngeal space is subdivided by the tensor-vascular-styloid fascia, which extends from the styloid process and styloid musculature to the tensor veli palatini, into the prestyloid parapharyngeal compartment anteriorly (more commonly called the parapharyngeal space) and the poststyloid parapharyngeal compartment posteriorly (more commonly called the carotid space). Confidently determining the space of origin (i.e., parapharyngeal versus carotid) for lesions in this region is important for diagnosis and treatment planning, as the two spaces are associated with distinct differential diagnoses. The relationship of a mass to the internal carotid artery helps differentiate parapharyngeal space lesions (anterior to the internal carotid artery) from carotid space lesions (at the level of or posterior to the internal carotid artery). Tumors originating in the parapharyngeal space often are asymptomatic and thus cross-sectional imaging plays an important role in identification and characterization. The normal contents of the parapharyngeal space include fat, salivary tissue, blood vessels, and small nerve branches.

Salivary Gland Tumors

The vast majority of parapharyngeal space lesions are salivary gland neoplasms, most commonly benign pleomorphic adenoma. Most of these salivary gland neoplasms arise from the parapharyngeal process of the deep lobe of the parotid gland and protrude into the parapharyngeal space, often widening the stylomandibular tunnel (Fig. 57.1).

Occasionally a lesion may arise from embryonic salivary gland rests in the parapharyngeal space. Malignant salivary gland tumors, such as mucoepidermoid carcinoma or adenoid cystic carcinoma, are less common. Imaging alone is insufficient for definitive determination of salivary gland neoplasm subtype; however, typical MR features of pleomorphic adenoma (Fig. 57.2) include marked T2 hyperintensity, "bosselated" (i.e.,

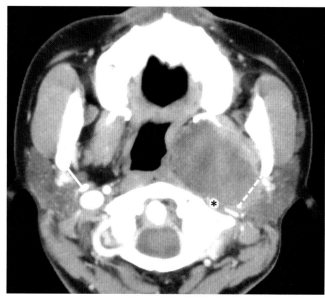

Ax CT

- **Fig. 57.1** Axial *(Ax)* contrast-enhanced computed tomography *(CT)* image demonstrates a large mass arising from the deep lobe of the left parotid gland and extending medially to involve the left parapharyngeal space. Note that the mass is located anterior to the left internal carotid artery *(asterisk)* and widens the left stylomandibular tunnel *(dashed line)*. For reference, the normal right stylomandibular tunnel is marked by the *solid line*. This mass was resected and shown to represent a pleomorphic adenoma.

slightly undulating) margins, and progressive enhancement (i.e., relatively little enhancement on early postcontrast imaging that gradually fills in over time).

Miscellaneous Lesions

Because the parapharyngeal space contains fat, blood vessels, and small nerve branches, lipomas (Fig. 57.3), vascular malformations, neurogenic tumors, and branchial cleft anomalies may also occur here. Sarcoma should be considered for a rapidly growing or otherwise aggressive-appearing lesion, particularly in a pediatric patient.

Lymph Nodes

Lymph nodes do not normally occur in the parapharyngeal space. However, enlarged lymph nodes of the retropharyngeal space can mimic a parapharyngeal space lesion by bulging anteriorly to compress the parapharyngeal fat. Abnormal retropharyngeal lymph nodes may be solid or cystic appearing, depending on the etiology, size, and extent of internal necrosis. Nodal enlargement may be related to neoplastic etiologies (e.g., nasopharyngeal carcinoma, non-Hodgkin lymphoma, or thyroid metastasis) or infectious etiologies.

Spectrum of Disease

The spectrum of disease is detailed in the preceding sections.

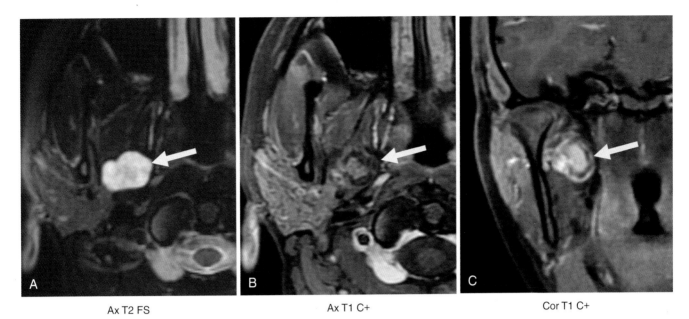

Ax T2 FS   Ax T1 C+   Cor T1 C+

• **Fig. 57.2** Axial *(Ax)* T2-weighted, fat-suppressed image demonstrates a markedly T2 hyperintense right parapharyngeal space mass with bosselated margins *(arrow, A)*. The (B) initial axial and (C) delayed coronal *(Cor)* gadolinium-enhanced images demonstrate progressive enhancement of the lesion *(arrows, B and C)*. This mass was resected and shown to represent a pleomorphic adenoma. *FS*, fat saturated.

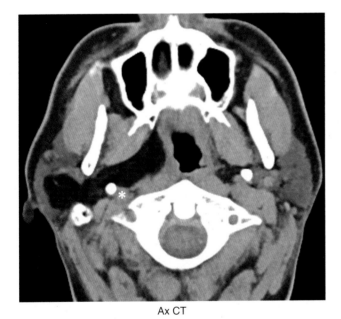

Ax CT

• **Fig. 57.3** Axial *(Ax)* noncontrast computed tomography *(CT)* demonstrates a homogeneous fat-attenuation mass consistent with lipoma involving the right parotid gland and the right parapharyngeal space. Note that the lipoma passes through and widens the right stylomandibular tunnel and that the lipoma is located anterior to the right internal carotid artery *(asterisk)*.

Differential Diagnosis

1. Salivary gland neoplasm
2. Lipoma
3. Venous malformation
4. Neurogenic tumor
5. Branchial cleft anomaly
6. Sarcoma

Pearls

• The majority of lesions in the parapharyngeal space are of salivary gland origin. These lesions displace the internal carotid artery posteriorly, whereas retropharyngeal lesions displace the internal carotid artery laterally (Case B). Carotid space masses push the carotid artery anteriorly.

• Salivary gland neoplasms: Pleomorphic adenoma is the most common salivary gland neoplasm in the parapharyngeal space. These lesions usually have an intermediate signal on T1-weighted images and high signal on T2-weighted images with moderate homogenous or patchy enhancement. A hypointense rim often is present around the lesion. The lesion may be characteristically "bosselated" with slight undulation of the margin.

• Widening of the stylomandibular tunnel is a clue that a parapharyngeal space is arising from the deep lobe of the parotid gland (Fig. 57.4). Additionally, the facial nerve passes just lateral to the stylomandibular tunnel, such that the tunnel is an important landmark.

Signs and Complications

Most lesions in this space are asymptomatic and are found incidentally. Malignant degeneration of a pleomorphic adenoma can occur and is clinically manifested by a rapid increase in the size of a preexisting adenoma. The risk of

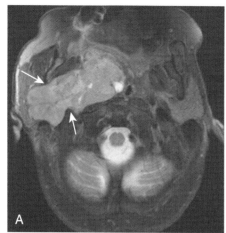

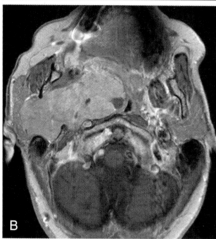

• **Fig. 57.4** (A) Axial T2-weighted and (B) gadolinium-enhanced axial T1-weighted images demonstrate a large, enhancing, mildly T2 hyperintense mass involving the right parotid and the right parapharyngeal space with widening of the stylomandibular tunnel *(arrows)*.

carcinoma-ex-pleomorphic adenoma increases with time. The tumor can recur after surgery and rarely metastasizes to distant locations.

Suggested Readings

Gupta A, Chazen JL, Phillips CD: Imaging evaluation of the parapharyngeal space, *Otolaryngol Clin North Am* 45(6):1223–1232, 2012.

Matsuki T, Miura K, Tada Y, et al: Classification of tumors by imaging diagnosis and preoperative fine-needle aspiration cytology in 120 patients with tumors in the parapharyngeal space, *Head Neck* 41(5):1277–1281, 2019.

Shin JH, Lee HK, Kim SY, et al: Imaging of parapharyngeal space lesions: focus on the prestyloid compartment, *Am J Roentgenol* 177(6):1465–1470, 2001.

Tomblinson CM, Fletcher GP, Lidner TK, et al: Parapharyngeal space venous malformation: an imaging mimic of pleomorphic adenoma, *AJNR Am J Neuroradiol* 40(1):150–153, 2019.

58

Carotid Space Masses

PAUL M. BUNCH, MD AND GUL MOONIS, MD

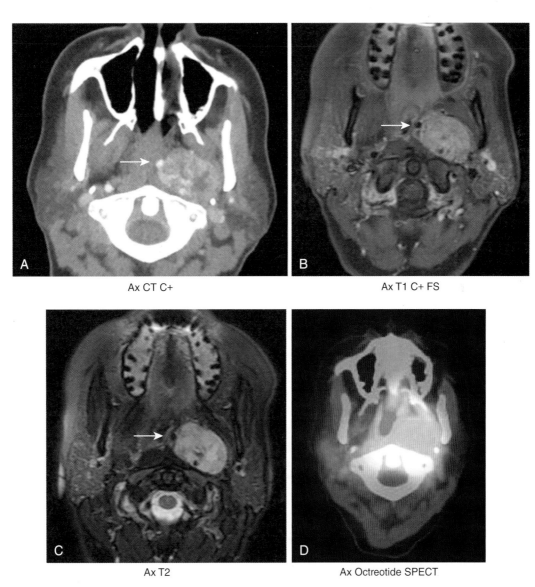

Ax CT C+

Ax T1 C+ FS

Ax T2

Ax Octreotide SPECT

CASE A: A 46-year-old female with an incidentally detected left neck mass. *Ax,* Axial; *CT,* Computed tomography; *FS,* fat saturated; *SPECT,* single-photon emission computed tomography.

Ax T1 C+ FS   Ax T2

CASE B: A 61-year-old female presenting with a mass in the left neck. *Ax,* Axial; *FS,* fat saturated.

DESCRIPTION OF FINDINGS

- Case A: Axial contrast-enhanced CT (A), gadolinium-enhanced, fat-suppressed, T1-weighted (B), and fat-suppressed T2-weighted (C) images demonstrate an avidly enhancing, T2 hyperintense mass displacing the left internal carotid artery anteromedially *(arrow)*. Note the internal flow voids on the T2-weighted image. The octreotide single-photon emission computed tomography (SPECT)-CT image (D) demonstrates intense indium-111 octreotide uptake in the mass.
- Case B: Axial fat-suppressed T2-weighted and contrast-enhanced T1-weighted images (A and B) demonstrate a mildly enhancing, T2 hyperintense mass that displaces the left internal carotid artery anteromedially *(arrow)*. There are no internal flow voids.

Diagnosis

Case A: Vagal paraganglioma (formerly glomus vagale)
Case B: Vagal schwannoma

Summary

The parapharyngeal space is a region or compartment in the deep neck extending from the base of the skull to the hyoid bone. As discussed in the previous chapter, the parapharyngeal space can be divided into two portions—the prestyloid compartment anteriorly and the poststyloid compartment posteriorly—by the tensor-vascular-styloid fascia running obliquely from the styloid process and styloid musculature to the tensor veli palatini. The prestyloid and poststyloid terminology are more anatomically accurate and commonly used in the anatomic and surgical literature. However, most radiologists favor the terms "parapharyngeal space" for the prestyloid compartment and "carotid space" for the poststyloid compartment. Confidently determining the space of origin (i.e., parapharyngeal space vs. carotid space) for lesions in this region is important for diagnosis and treatment planning, as the two spaces are associated with distinct differential diagnoses. The relationship of a mass to the internal carotid artery helps differentiate carotid space lesions (at the level of or posterior to the internal carotid artery) from parapharyngeal space lesions (anterior to the internal carotid artery). Tumors originating in the carotid space often are asymptomatic and thus cross-sectional imaging plays an important role in identification and characterization. The normal contents of the carotid space include the internal carotid artery, the internal jugular vein, cranial nerves IX, X, XI, and XII, the sympathetic chain, and the ansa cervicalis.

Neurogenic tumors are the most common type of tumors arising within the carotid space, with the majority representing schwannomas, although neurofibromas may be considered in patients with neurofibromatosis. Malignant neurogenic tumors are very rare in this location. Nerves within the carotid space that may give rise to neurogenic tumors include cranial nerves IX, X, XI, and XII as well as the sympathetic plexus. The most common carotid space neurogenic tumors are schwannomas arising from the vagus nerve or from the sympathetic chain. Because the vagus nerve is located between the internal carotid artery medially and the internal jugular vein laterally, vagal schwannomas will displace the internal carotid artery medially and the internal jugular vein laterally (Fig. 58.1A). In contrast, the sympathetic chain runs along the medial aspect of the internal carotid artery, such that sympathetic chain schwannomas will displace both the internal carotid artery and the internal jugular vein laterally (Fig. 58.1B). On MR imaging, schwannomas typically demonstrate increased signal on T2-weighted images with a variable enhancement pattern.

Paragangliomas are neuroendocrine tumors arising from chromaffin cells within paraganglionic tissues of the autonomic

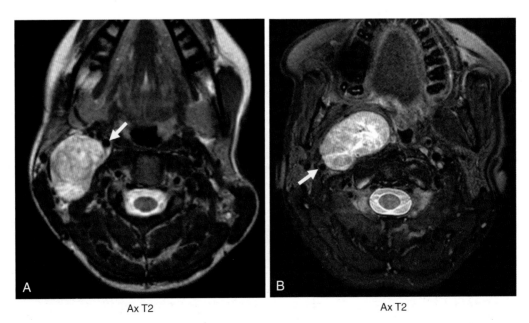

A   Ax T2   B   Ax T2

• **Fig. 58.1** Axial T2-weighted images obtained in two different patients with right carotid space schwannomas. The schwannoma in (A) displaces the right internal carotid artery medially *(arrow)*, most consistent with a right vagal schwannoma. The schwannoma in (B) displaces the right internal carotid artery laterally *(arrow)*, as would be expected from a tumor arising from the sympathetic chain. *Ax,* axial.

nervous system. Most head and neck paragangliomas arise from nonsecretory parasympathetic ganglia (as opposed to secretory sympathetic ganglia) and therefore tend to lack endocrine activity. Historically, head and neck paragangliomas have been referred to by various terms, including glomus tumors and chemodectomas; however, the World Health Organization has indicated that these alternative names should no longer be used when referring to these tumors. Approximately 35% to 40% of head and neck paragangliomas are associated with familial disease. The most common site of paraganglioma origin in the carotid space is the nodose ganglion of the vagus nerve, which is located between the internal carotid artery and internal jugular vein approximately 1 cm below the skull base. These hypervascular masses exhibit avid enhancement on both CT and MR imaging, and flow voids are commonly identifiable on MR imaging. The classic "salt and pepper" appearance on T1-weighted

images refers to high signal foci of subacute hemorrhage or slow flow (salt) and low signal vascular flow voids (pepper) interspersed within the tumor stroma. In addition to anatomic (e.g., CT, MR) imaging, there has been increasing interest in functional imaging of head and neck paragangliomas, most commonly with somatostatin receptor imaging such as [68]gallium-DOTATATE, which has been shown to have very high sensitivity for head and neck paragangliomas and can aid differentiation of a paraganglioma from a schwannoma. Additionally, dynamic contrast-enhanced MR imaging parameters show promise in differentiating paragangliomas from schwannomas.

Meningiomas may occur in the carotid space, either primarily or as a result of direct extension from the intracranial compartment through the skull base foramina (e.g., jugular foramen, hypoglossal canal). Mineralization and relatively low T2 signal may suggest meningioma (Fig. 58.2), as schwannomas

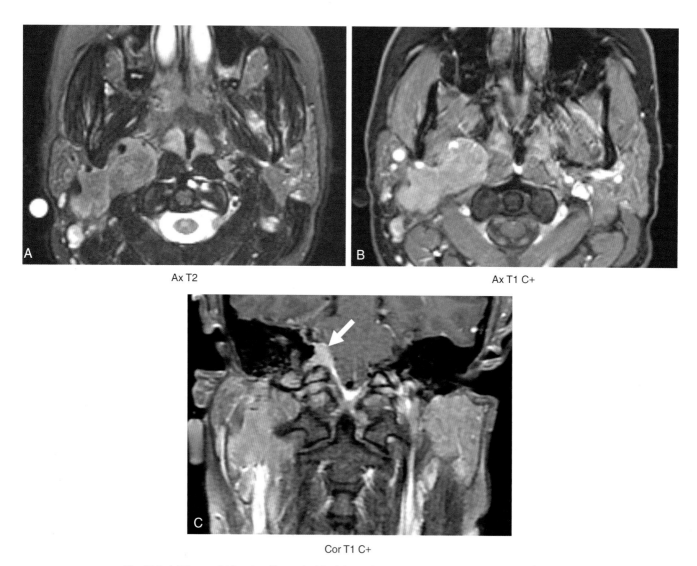

Ax T2

Ax T1 C+

Cor T1 C+

• **Fig. 58.2** A 25-year-old female with a palpable right neck mass, which was subsequently resected and shown to represent a meningioma. Note the relatively low T2 signal of the right carotid space mass (A) relative to the schwannomas and paraganglioma shown earlier in this chapter. The axial (B) and coronal (C) gadolinium-enhanced images demonstrate homogeneous enhancement of the mass, and the coronal image shows an intracranial component (*arrow*, C) with inferior extension to the right carotid space via the right jugular foramen. *Ax*, axial; *Cor*, coronal.

and paragangliomas both rarely mineralize and are typically T2 hyperintense.

The superior cervical ganglion is a normal anatomic structure that can be mistaken for pathology (e.g., metastatic lateral retropharyngeal lymph node), particularly in the posttreatment neck because the ganglion may enlarge following radiotherapy. Location along the medial aspect of the internal carotid artery at the level of the oropharynx (as opposed to the level of the nasopharynx as would be expected for a lateral retropharyngeal lymph node), a central "black dot" sign (Fig. 58.3), and an elongated configuration with tapered margins in the coronal plane are typical of the ganglion. Additionally, careful correlation with pretreatment imaging will show the structure to have been present previously (i.e., rather than new).

Lymph nodes are not typically present within the carotid space. However, lateral retropharyngeal lymph nodes are located more medially in the retropharyngeal space between the prevertebral musculature medially and the internal carotid artery laterally. The lateral retropharyngeal lymph nodes may be involved by various malignancies; however, metastases from nasopharyngeal carcinoma are most common.

Spectrum of Disease

Although nerve sheath tumors and head and neck paragangliomas are most commonly benign, malignant tumors occasionally occur, and differentiating between benign and malignant lesions on an imaging basis can be difficult. The presence of distant metastasis is an indication of malignancy, regardless of the primary tumor histology.

Differential Diagnosis

1. The differential diagnosis is detailed in the preceding sections.

Pearls

- Relationship of a mass to the internal carotid artery helps differentiate carotid space lesions (at the level of or posterior to the internal carotid artery) from parapharyngeal space lesions (anterior to the internal carotid artery).
- Schwannomas are smoothly marginated, have low to intermediate intensity on T1-weighted images, and have high signal intensity on T2-weighted images with either homogeneous or heterogeneous enhancement. Schwannomas arising from the vagus nerve displace the internal carotid artery medially, whereas schwannomas arising from the sympathetic chain displace the internal carotid artery laterally.
- Paragangliomas are hypervascular lesions with prominent vessels and avid enhancement. Vagal paragangliomas arise from the nodose ganglion of the vagus nerve located

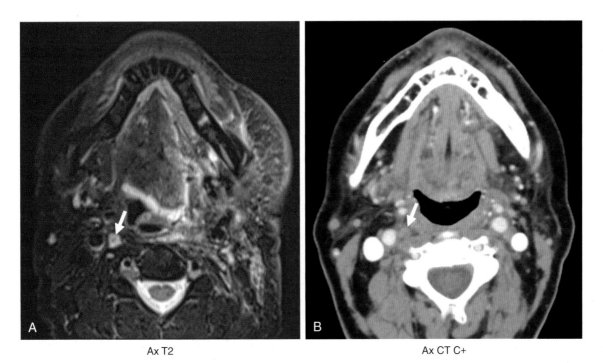

Ax T2   Ax CT C+

• **Fig. 58.3** A 49-year-old male with history of multiple previously treated head and neck cancers, now presenting with left face pain and left hypoglossal palsy. The axial T2-weighted image demonstrates findings of left neck swelling and edema as well as left hypoglossal palsy. A large left neck recurrence (not shown) was also demonstrated. In the right neck, there is a T2 hyperintense nodule (*arrow*, A) with a central "black dot" located along the medial aspect of the right internal carotid artery. Although a metastatic lateral retropharyngeal lymph node is a differential consideration, the location at the level of the oropharynx (rather than the nasopharynx), the central "black dot" sign, and the fact that the structure appears unchanged from a prior neck CT obtained 3 years earlier (*arrow*, B) all favor the structure to represent the superior cervical ganglion rather than a nodal metastasis.

approximately 1 cm below the skull base, whereas carotid body paragangliomas arise from the carotid body located at the medial aspect of the common carotid bifurcation.

- Somatostatin receptor imaging (e.g., octreotide scintigraphy or ^{68}gallium-DOTATATE PET/CT) is often positive in paragangliomas and can be useful in differentiating these lesions from schwannoma. However, meningiomas can also demonstrate uptake on octreotide and DOTATATE imaging.
- Lymph nodes are not typically located within the carotid space. However, lateral retropharyngeal lymph nodes are present within the adjacent retropharyngeal space along the medial aspect of the internal carotid artery.

Suggested Readings

Cleere EF, Martin-Grace J, Gendre A, et al: Contemporary management of paragangliomas of the head and neck, *Laryngoscope Investig Otolaryngol* 7(1):93–107, 2021.

Loke SC, Karandikar A, Ravanelli M, et al: Superior cervical ganglion mimicking retropharyngeal adenopathy in head and neck cancer patients: MRI features with anatomic, histologic, and surgical correlation, *Neuroradiology* 58(1):45–50, 2016.

Malla SR, Bhalla AS, Manchanda S, et al: Dynamic contrast-enhanced magnetic resonance imaging for differentiating head and neck paraganglioma and schwannoma, *Head Neck* 43(9):2611–2622, 2021.

Nguyen RP, Shah LM, Quigley EP, et al: Carotid body detection on CT angiography, *AJNR Am J Neuroradiol* 32(6):1096–1099, 2011.

Ota Y, Liao E, Capizzano AA, et al: Diagnostic role of diffusion-weighted and dynamic contrast-enhanced perfusion MR imaging in paragangliomas and schwannomas in the head and neck, *AJNR Am J Neuroradiol* 42(10):1839–1846, 2021.

Ravanelli R, Tononcelli E, Leali M, et al: Magnetic resonance imaging features of the superior cervical ganglion and expected changes after radiation therapy to the head and neck in a long-term follow-up, *Neuroradiology* 62(4):519–524, 2020.

Shirakura S, Tsunoda A, Akita K, et al: Parapharyngeal space tumors: anatomical and image analysis findings, *Auris Nasus Larynx* 37(5):621–625, 2010.

Som PM, Curtin HD: Fascia and spaces of the neck. In Som PM, Curtin HD, editors: *Head and neck imaging*, St. Louis, 2011, Mosby.

Valero C, Ganly I: Paragangliomas of the head and neck, *J Oral Pathol Med* 51(10):897–903, 2022.

Zheng X, Guo K, Wang H, et al: Extracranial schwannoma in the carotid space: a retrospective review of 91 cases, *Head Neck* 39(1):42–47, 2017.

59

Floor of Mouth Lesions

NICHOLAS A. TELISCHAK, MD, MS, PAUL M. BUNCH, MD, AND GUL MOONIS, MD

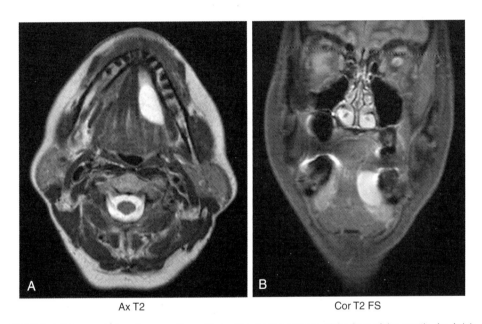

Ax T2   Cor T2 FS

CASE A: A 53-year-old female presenting with swelling on the left side of the floor of the mouth. *Ax*, Axial; *Cor*, coronal; *FS*, fat saturated.

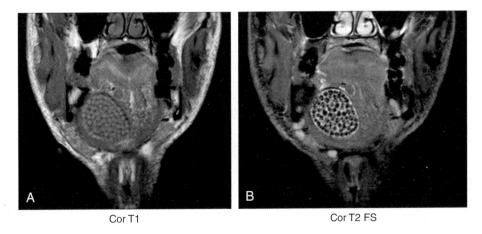

Cor T1   Cor T2 FS

CASE B: A 60-year-old male presenting with a slowly enlarging, nontender mass in the right anterior neck. *Cor*, Coronal; *FS*, fat saturated.

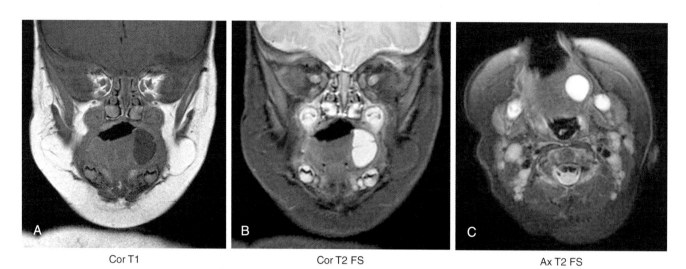

<table>
<tr><td>Cor T1</td><td>Cor T2 FS</td><td>Ax T2 FS</td></tr>
</table>

CASE C: A 2-month-old child presenting with a mass at the root of the tongue. *Ax*, Axial; *Cor*, coronal; *FS*, fat saturated.

DESCRIPTION OF FINDINGS

- Case A: Axial T2-weighted and coronal T2-weighted, fat-suppressed images demonstrate a fluid signal mass centered along the posterior aspect of the left sublingual gland in the left sublingual space. Note on the axial image that the anterior aspect of the lesion comes to a point along the posterior aspect of the left sublingual gland.
- Case B: Coronal T1-weighted and coronal T2-weighted, fat-suppressed images demonstrate a spherical mass centered in the right sublingual space containing numerous T1 hyperintense nodules surrounded by fluid. Note the hypointensity of these nodules on the fat-suppressed T2-weighted image.
- Case C: Coronal T1-weighted and fat-suppressed coronal and axial T2-weighted images demonstrate a fluid signal mass centered in the left root of tongue.

Diagnosis

Case A: Ranula
Case B: Dermoid cyst
Case C: Foregut duplication cyst

Summary

Cystic lesions in the floor of the mouth include simple or diving ranulas, dermoid cysts, and foregut duplication cysts. These lesions can often be differentiated based on imaging appearance and supporting clinical information.

A ranula is a benign cystic mass most commonly produced by extravasation of saliva from a damaged salivary duct (i.e., traumatic pseudocyst), in which case the lesion is not lined by epithelium. Less commonly, a ranula may be congenital, in which case it is classified histopathologically as a retention cyst lined by stratified squamous epithelium. A "simple" ranula refers to a lesion confined to the sublingual space above and medial to the paired mylohyoid muscles. A simple ranula presents clinically as an intraoral mass lesion. A "plunging" ranula refers to a ranula extending either through a defect in the mylohyoid muscle or around the muscle's posterior margin to involve the submandibular space. A plunging ranula most often presents as a submandibular neck mass; however, a "tail" can be seen communicating with the sublingual space (Fig. 59.1). Because both simple and plunging ranulas are formed by saliva, a tapering connection to the sublingual gland is expected and can be a useful clue to the diagnosis.

Although dermoid cysts are congenital lesions, they may not manifest clinically until late childhood or early adulthood because of their slow increase in size. Dermoid cysts are on a spectrum of true dermoid cyst, epidermoid cyst, and teratoid cyst, depending on the types of tissues found histologically and the embryologic layers represented. When located in the floor of mouth, dermoid cysts are typically midline lesions. On MRI, fat globules within the fluid matrix of the cyst may give the pathognomonic appearance of a sack of marbles. Occasionally, they can take on an hourglass shape on coronal images, a finding reported to be specific for dermoid cysts.

Foregut duplication cysts arise from persistent heterotopic rests of embryonic foregut that normally contribute to the pharynx, lower respiratory tract, and upper gastrointestinal tract during development. The oral cavity is the most common site of foregut duplication cysts within the head and neck. The

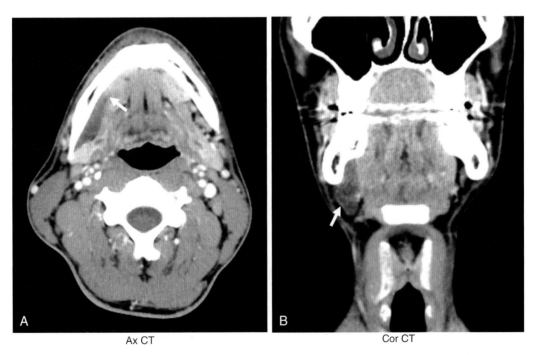

Ax CT   Cor CT

• **Fig. 59.1** A 19-year-old male with a mass in the right side of the neck has a plunging ranula. (A) Axial and (B) coronal CT images demonstrate a fluid attenuation lesion along the posterior aspect of the right sublingual gland (*arrow*, A) with extension into the right submandibular space (*arrow*, B) via the free posterior edge of the mylohyoid muscle. *Ax,* Axial; *Cor,* coronal; *CT,* Computed tomography.

majority of oral cavity lesions are asymptomatic, but associated symptoms can include feeding or speech-related problems. Foregut duplication cysts appear on CT and MRI as simple, thin-walled cysts. Most patients present with these cysts before they are 7 years of age and often in the first year of life.

MRI can readily distinguish a ranula from a dermoid cyst in most cases. The key is to look for a close relationship to the sublingual gland for a ranula or the presence of fat, often with a sack-of-marbles appearance, within a dermoid. In pediatric patients, consider the possibility of a foregut duplication cyst.

Spectrum of Disease

A plunging ranula is shown in Fig. 59.1.

Differential Diagnosis

1. Ranula
2. Dermoid
3. Foregut duplication cyst
4. Lymphatic malformation
5. Abscess

Pearls

- Smooth tapering of a cystic lesion to the posterior aspect of the sublingual gland is highly suggestive of a ranula.
- The differentiation between a simple and plunging ranula is important for surgical planning. Simple ranulas are confined to the sublingual space (above the mylohyoid muscle), whereas plunging ranulas extend below the mylohyoid muscle to also involve the submandibular space.

- A sack of marbles appearance due to intralesional fat globules is pathognomonic for a dermoid cyst.
- Foregut duplication cysts are relatively uncommon, but should be considered in the pediatric population.

Signs and Complications

Infection is a complication of the cystic lesions discussed in this chapter; in addition, an estimated 1% to 2% of dermoid cysts undergo malignant degeneration to squamous cell carcinoma.

Suggested Readings

Brown RE, Harave S: Diagnostic imaging of benign and malignant neck masses in children – a pictorial review, *Quant Imaging Med Surg* 6(5):591–604, 2016.

Edwards RM, Chapman T, Horn DL, et al: Imaging of pediatric floor of mouth lesions, *Pediatr Radiol* 43(5):523–535, 2013.

Fujimoto N, Fujii N, Nagata Y, et al: Dermoid cyst with magnetic resonance image of sack-of-marbles, *Br J Dermatol* 158:415–417, 2008.

Harrison JD: Modern management and pathophysiology of ranula: literature review, *Head Neck* 32(10):1310–1320, 2010.

Ikeda K, Koseki T, Maehara M, et al: Hourglass-shaped sublingual dermoid cyst: MRI features, *Radiat Med* 25:306–308, 2007.

Kieran SM, Robson CD, Nosé V, et al: Foregut duplication cysts in the head and neck: presentation, diagnosis, and management, *Arch Otolaryngol Head Neck Surg* 136(8):778–782, 2010.

Kurabayashi T, Ida M, Yasumoto M, et al: MRI of ranulas, *Neuroradiology* 42:917–922, 2000.

Patel S, Bhatt AA: Imaging of the sublingual and submandibular spaces, *Insights Imaging* 9(3):391–401, 2018.

Yadav R, Tewari V: Ranula, its etiopathogenesis and management; a systematic review, *ENT Updates* 11(1):56–61, 2021.

60
Thyroglossal Duct Abnormalities

NICHOLAS A. TELISCHAK, MD, MS, PAUL M. BUNCH, MD, AND GUL MOONIS, MD

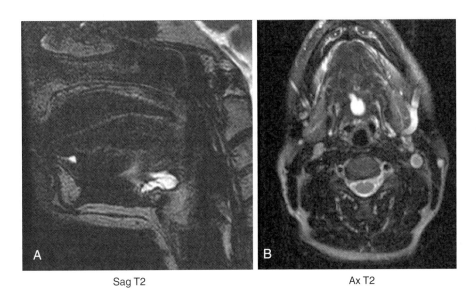

Sag T2   Ax T2

CASE A: A 41-year-old male with left arm paresthesias. *Ax*, Axial; *Sag*, sagittal.

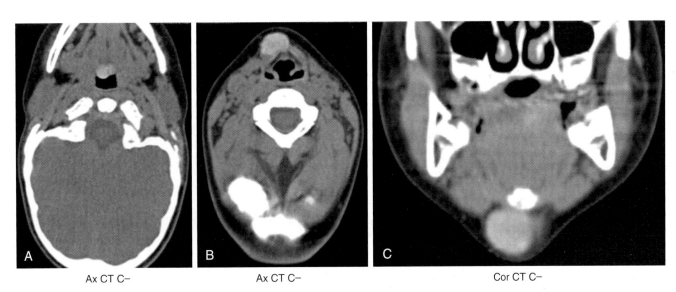

Ax CT C–   Ax CT C–   Cor CT C–

CASE B: A 4-year-old female with a palpable anterior neck mass. *Ax*, Axial; *Cor*, coronal; *CT*, Computed tomography.

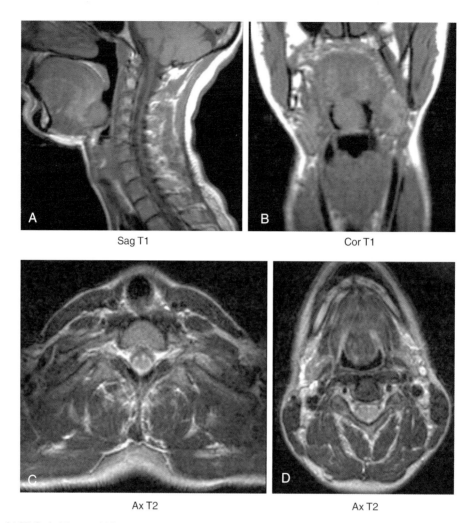

Sag T1

Cor T1

Ax T2

Ax T2

CASE C: A 45-year-old female with dysphagia and hypothyroidism. *Ax*, Axial; *Cor*, coronal; *Sag*, sagittal.

DESCRIPTION OF FINDINGS

- Case A: A hyperintense cystic structure lying within the root of the tongue is incidentally noted on sagittal and axial T2-weighted images of the cervical spine. No mass effect, mural nodularity, or surrounding inflammatory change is noted.
- Case B: Axial and coronal noncontrast computed tomography (CT). A midline lingual lesion lies at the expected locale of the foramen cecum and involves the midline tongue base, extends inferiorly to but not into the vallecula, and spares the hyoepiglottic ligament. A second right paramedian mass consistent with ectopic thyroid abuts the right aspect of the hyoid body superiorly, descends exolaryngeally along the anteromedial margin of the right thyroid lamina, splays the right sternohyoid and sternothyroid muscles, and does not significantly compromise the airway. No normal orthotopic thyroid tissue is seen.
- Case C: Sagittal and coronal T1-weighted and axial T2-weighted images demonstrate an isointense mass on both T1- and T2-weighted sequences that protrudes from the root of the tongue posteriorly into the vallecular recess and narrows the oropharynx. No orthotopic thyroid tissue is seen.

Diagnosis

Case A: Thyroglossal duct cyst (TGDC) at the root of tongue
Case B: Ectopic thyroid gland—CT findings
Case C: Ectopic thyroid gland—MRI findings

Summary

The thyroglossal duct forms as the thyroid primordium migrates from the foramen cecum, penetrates the underlying mesoderm of the tongue and floor of mouth musculature, and passes anterior to the hyoid bone. After wrapping around to attach to the posterior hyoid, the primordium descends along the lateral aspect of the thyroid cartilage to the lower neck. The duct normally involutes by the 8th to 10th gestational week.

The TGDC is the most common congenital neck mass (with an incidence of approximately 7%). This cyst is more common in women than in men and typically diagnosed in childhood. TGDCs form as the result of failure of involution of the duct and usually are located at the level of the hyoid bone or in the strap muscles immediately inferior to the hyoid (80%). When located above the hyoid bone, TGDCs usually are in a midline location; when below the hyoid bone, they usually are slightly off midline, but not by more than 2 cm. TGDCs appear as a smoothly marginated cyst with capsular enhancement (Case A) and can be complicated by infection (Fig. 60.1). A high signal on T2-weighted images is the rule, and 50% demonstrate isointense to high signal intensity on T1-weighted MRI as a result of high protein content. Surgical excision is performed by the Sistrunk procedure, which involves removal of the thyroglossal remnant, as well as the central portion of the hyoid bone and the cuff of tissue around the tract from the hyoid to the foramen cecum.

TGDC carcinoma complicates about 1% to 2% of TGDCs, among which more than 90% are papillary thyroid carcinomas (Fig. 60.2). This complication usually occurs in adults. Suspicious imaging findings include mural nodularity and enhancement, and in one-third of these patients, the thyroid also is involved. Diagnosis is made by fine-needle aspiration.

Lingual thyroid is a developmental anomaly in which the thyroid anlage arising from the ventral pharynx between the first and second pharyngeal pouches fails to descend to its normal position. The lingual thyroid tissue is located between the circumvallate papillae and the epiglottis at the base of the tongue and may be the only functioning thyroid tissue in the body in 70% of cases. Lingual thyroid can present at a young age or in adults. Symptomatic lingual thyroid is more common in adults and can present with dysphagia, dysphonia, bleeding, or dyspnea as well as with hyperthyroidism or hypothyroidism. On noncontrast CT, the lingual thyroid is hyperattenuating due to intrinsic iodine content, and on MR imaging, the lingual thyroid tissue is isointense to hyperintense to muscle on both T1- and T2-weighted images and enhances homogeneously.

Radionuclide scanning with use of radioactive iodine or 99mTc pertechnetate also may be performed to locate the functioning thyroid tissue. Thyroid function tests are also indicated. The differential diagnosis of a midline mass at the root and base of tongue includes epidermoid/dermoid, teratoma, carcinoma, and soft tissue sarcoma. In symptomatic patients, the lingual thyroid can be removed surgically. Prior to removal, it is important to determine whether thyroid tissue is present in the normal location in the lower neck. In patients who are unfit for surgery or unwilling to undergo surgery, symptomatic lingual thyroid tissue also can be treated with radioactive thyroid ablation.

Spectrum of Disease

The spectrum of TGDC disease is illustrated in Figs. 60.1, 60.2, and 60.3.

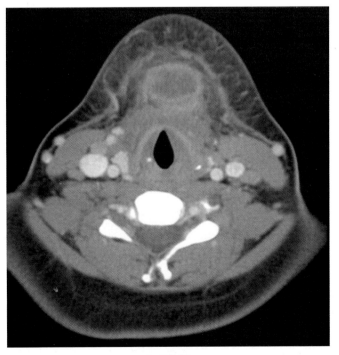

Ax CT C+

• **Fig. 60.1** A 24-year-old female with neck pain, swelling, and fever. The image demonstrates a cystic structure in the midline neck with a thick, enhancing wall, surrounding inflammatory fat stranding, and thickening of the overlying platysma muscle, consistent with an infected thyroglossal duct cyst. *Ax,* Axial; *CT,* Computed tomography.

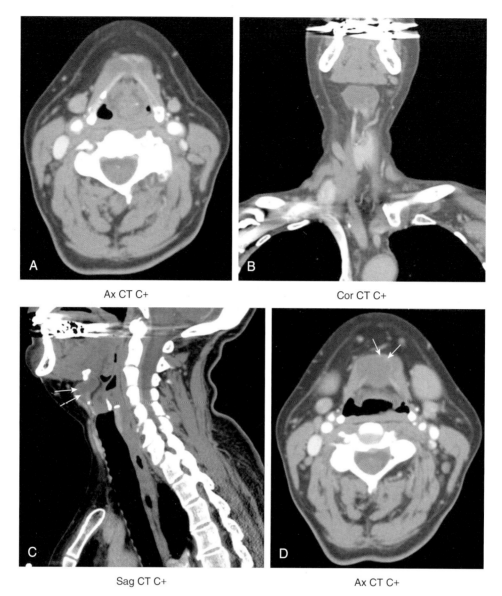

Ax CT C+   Cor CT C+

Sag CT C+   Ax CT C+

• **Fig. 60.2** A 56-year-old female smoker presenting with dysphagia. These images demonstrate a midline cystic structure within the neck that extends inferiorly from the expected location of the foramen cecum. Nodularity is seen along the cyst wall (*arrows*, C and D) which proved to represent papillary thyroid carcinoma arising within a thyroglossal duct cyst. *Ax,* Axial; *Cor,* coronal; *CT,* Computed tomography; *Sag,* sagittal.

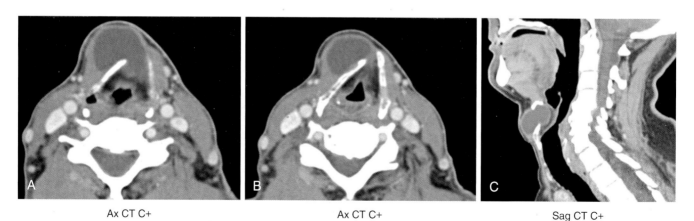

Ax CT C+   Ax CT C+   Sag CT C+

• **Fig. 60.3** A 65-year-old female with a history of resection of a mass in the neck. The images demonstrate a low-density cystic structure with a thin rim of peripheral enhancement just lateral to midline at the level of the thyroid cartilage and projecting into the preepiglottic space, consistent with a thyroglossal duct cyst. *Ax,* Axial; *CT,* Computed tomography; *Sag,* sagittal.

Differential Diagnosis

1. TGDC
2. Lingual thyroid
3. Dermoid cyst
4. Venolymphatic malformation
5. Foregut duplication cyst

Pearls

- A cystic lesion in the midline neck (or just off midline) is characteristic of a thyroglossal duct remnant lesion. If the lesion becomes infected, the cyst wall can thicken and enhance. If nodularity or calcification develops within an existing TGDC, papillary thyroid carcinoma should be suspected.

Signs and Complications

TGDC carcinoma
Infection

Suggested Readings

Ahuja AT, Wong KT, King AD, et al: Imaging for thyroglossal duct cyst: the bare essentials, *Clin Radiol* 60:141–148, 2005.

Bayram F, Külahli I, Yüce I, et al: Functional lingual thyroid as unusual cause of progressive dysphagia, *Thyroid* 14(4):321–324, 2004.

Forest VI, Murali IR, Clark JR: Thyroglossal duct cyst carcinoma: case series, *J Otolarnygol Head Neck Surg* 40(2):151–156, 2011.

Oomen KP, Modi VK, Maddalozzo J: Thyroglosal duct cyst and ectopic thyroid: surgical management, *Otolaryngol Clin North Am* 48:15–27, 2015.

61

Primary Hyperparathyroidism

PAUL M. BUNCH, MD AND HILLARY R. KELLY, MD

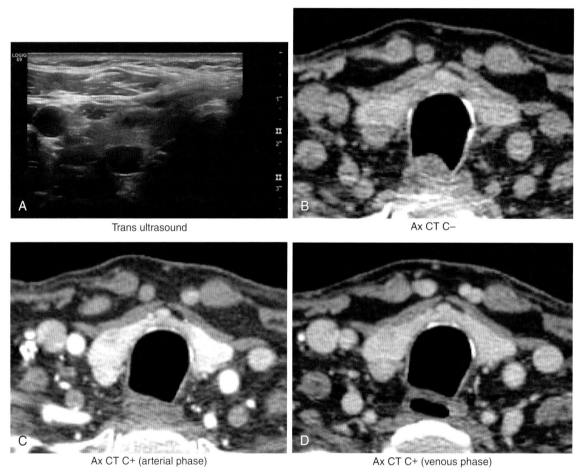

Trans ultrasound

Ax CT C–

Ax CT C+ (arterial phase)

Ax CT C+ (venous phase)

CASE A: A 65-year-old male with primary hyperparathyroidism. Ultrasound (A) demonstrates a candidate parathyroid lesion along the posterior aspect of the right thyroid lobe. *Ax*, Axial; *CT*, Computed tomography; *Trans*, transverse.

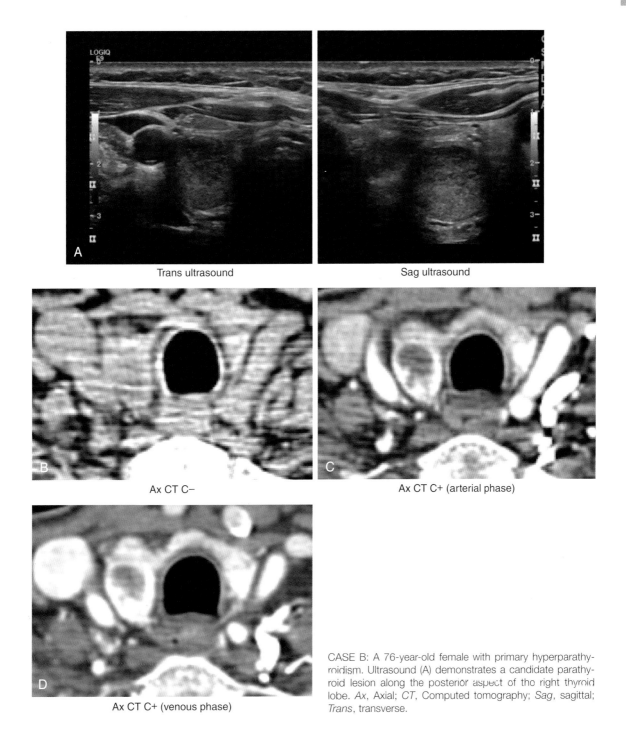

Trans ultrasound

Sag ultrasound

Ax CT C−

Ax CT C+ (arterial phase)

Ax CT C+ (venous phase)

CASE B: A 76-year-old female with primary hyperparathyroidism. Ultrasound (A) demonstrates a candidate parathyroid lesion along the posterior aspect of the right thyroid lobe. *Ax*, Axial; *CT*, Computed tomography; *Sag*, sagittal; *Trans*, transverse.

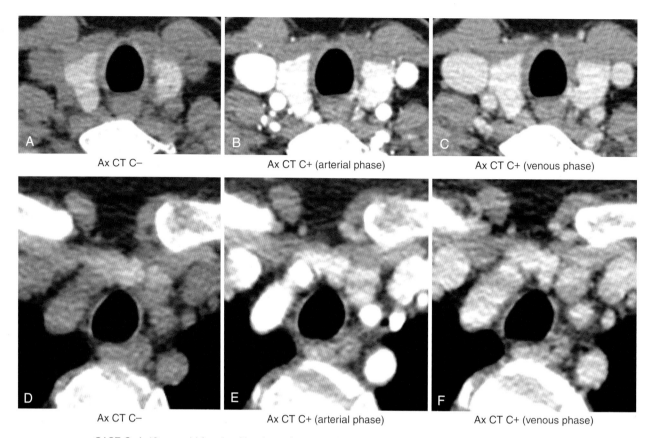

CASE C: A 42-year-old female with primary hyperparathyroidism. No candidate parathyroid lesions were identified by surgeon-performed ultrasound (not shown). *Ax*, Axial; *CT*, Computed tomography.

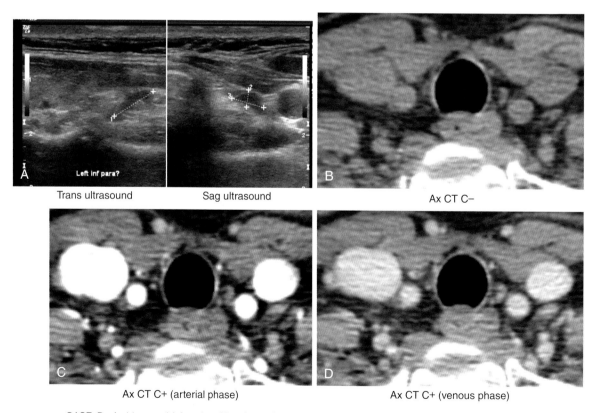

CASE D: A 44-year-old female with primary hyperparathyroidism. Surgeon-performed ultrasound (A) demonstrated a candidate parathyroid lesion along the inferior aspect of the left thyroid lobe and medial to the left common carotid artery. *Ax*, Axial; *CT*, Computed tomography; *Sag*, sagittal; *Trans*, transverse.

- Case A: Ultrasound demonstrates a homogeneously hypoechoic candidate lesion along the posterior aspect of the right thyroid lobe. On parathyroid CT, the candidate lesion is hypoattenuating relative to the thyroid gland on the noncontrast phase, isoattenuating on the arterial phase, and hypoattenuating on the venous phase.
- Case B: Ultrasound demonstrates a candidate lesion along the posterior aspect of the right thyroid lobe that appears isoechoic to slightly hypoechoic relative to the normal thyroid gland. On the parathyroid CT noncontrast phase, the periphery of the candidate lesion is isoattenuating relative to the thyroid gland.
- Case C: Parathyroid CT demonstrates a large candidate lesion along the inferior aspect of the left thyroid lobe lying anterior to the left common carotid artery. The lesion is hypoattenuating relative to the thyroid gland on the noncontrast phase, arterial phase, and venous phase. Additional smaller candidate lesions are present along the posterior aspects of the right and left thyroid lobes, both hypoattenuating relative to the thyroid gland on the noncontrast phase. The right candidate is isoattenuating and the left slightly hypoattenuating to the thyroid on the arterial phase, and both are hypoattenuating on the venous phase.
- Case D: Ultrasound demonstrates a candidate lesion with a hyperechoic hilum along the inferior aspect of the left thyroid lobe. On parathyroid CT, the candidate exhibits minimal enhancement on the arterial phase when compared to the noncontrast phase with progressive increase in attenuation on the venous phase. A fatty hilum is also present medially.

Diagnosis

Case A: Parathyroid adenoma (single gland disease)
Case B: Thyroid nodule
Case C: Multigland disease
Case D: Lymph node

Summary

Primary hyperparathyroidism refers to a parathyroid glandular abnormality producing increased parathyroid hormone. Primary hyperparathyroidism is the most common cause of hypercalcemia. The risk increases with age, and women are affected by the disease more commonly than men. Primary hyperparathyroidism is cured by surgical removal of the hyperfunctioning parathyroid tissue (most commonly one gland; less frequently multiple glands). The disease is diagnosed by serum biochemical testing, and the role of imaging is localization of the abnormal parathyroid gland(s), which in turn informs operative planning.

Multiple imaging modalities and techniques are available for parathyroid imaging, each with various advantages and disadvantages. There is no universally accepted algorithm for preoperative localization, and multiple imaging studies may be utilized in combination to maximize localization accuracy and confidence via concordant imaging results. This chapter discusses ultrasound and multiphase (so-called "4D") parathyroid CT.

Ultrasound is a widely available modality for parathyroid localization and the optimal modality for assessing concurrent thyroid pathology. Additional advantages of ultrasound include low cost and lack of ionizing radiation. Overall, ultrasound has good sensitivity and positive predictive value for localizing parathyroid lesions, but it is less sensitive for mediastinal, retropharyngeal, and retroclavicular lesions (no acoustic window), mildly enlarged glands, and multigland disease.

Parathyroid CT refers to multiphase CT of the neck, most commonly including noncontrast, arterial, and venous phases. Although the enhancement patterns of parathyroid adenomas are variable, scrutiny of the multiple CT phases usually allows for confident differentiation of parathyroid lesions from common mimics—exophytic thyroid nodules or thyroid parenchyma and lymph nodes. Key advantages of parathyroid CT include exceptional spatial and anatomic detail, relative sensitivity for multigland disease, and superior performance in several challenging clinical situations, including patients with nonlocalizing, inconclusive, or discordant other imaging results and patients with a previous failed operation. Disadvantages include the need for ionizing radiation and iodinated contrast media. A comprehensive economic analysis concluded that ultrasound followed by parathyroid CT if necessary represents the most cost-effective primary hyperparathyroidism imaging approach.

Regardless of the imaging modality or modalities employed, the key information that the surgeon wants to know from localization is the number, size, and location of candidate lesions, what the radiologist thinks each candidate most likely represents, and the presence or absence of supernumerary or ectopic parathyroid tissue, concurrent thyroid pathology, and arterial anomalies (e.g., aberrant right subclavian artery) associated with a nonrecurrent laryngeal nerve. The focus of this chapter is utilizing ultrasound and parathyroid CT to determine what a candidate lesion most likely represents.

Spectrum of Disease

Parathyroid Adenoma

Parathyroid adenoma (single gland disease) is the cause of primary hyperparathyroidism in approximately 80% of patients. Localization of a single parathyroid adenoma facilitates minimally invasive parathyroidectomy (single gland surgery), which is the preferred operation when appropriate. Single gland disease is most likely when there is a single candidate lesion larger than 13 mm in maximum dimension.

On ultrasound, parathyroid adenomas are usually homogeneously hypoechoic (Fig. 61.1), and an echogenic capsule separating the adenoma from the thyroid gland is often seen. A polar vessel is typical of a parathyroid lesion—as opposed to the hilar blood supply of a lymph node—and can be seen on ultrasound or CT (Fig. 61.2).

On parathyroid CT, parathyroid adenomas will always be hypoattenuating relative to the normal thyroid parenchyma on the noncontrast phase. However, chronic thyroid disease (e.g., Hashimoto) commonly coexists with primary hyperparathyroidism and can result in abnormal hypoattenuation of the thyroid gland due to diminished iodine content, in turn complicating confident discrimination of parathyroid lesions from thyroid tissue. Because an element's CT attenuation is maximal near its K-edge (33.2 keV for iodine), dual-energy parathyroid CT 40 keV virtual monoenergetic images can be utilized to improve differentiation of parathyroid adenomas from thyroid tissue by disproportionately increasing the attenuation of thyroid iodine (Fig. 61.3).

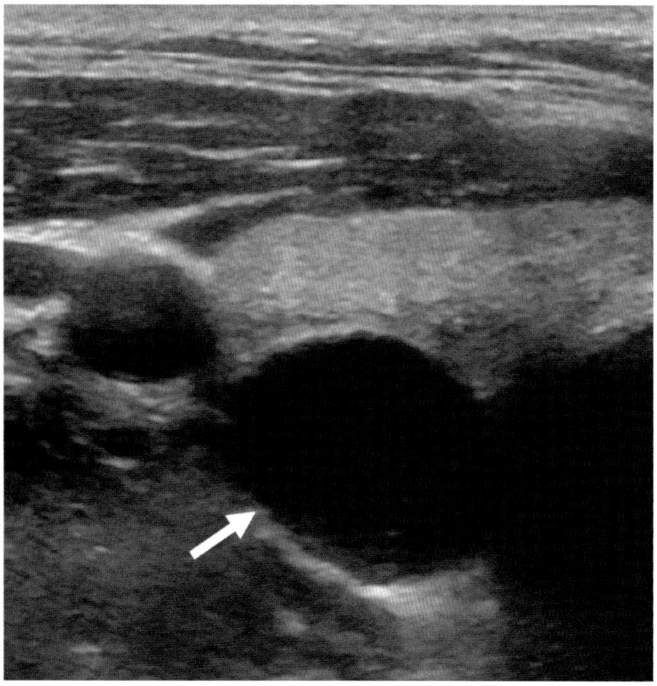

Although the classic parathyroid adenoma enhancement pattern (hyperattenuating relative to thyroid on the arterial phase; hypoattenuating or "washed out" on the venous phase) is well described, this classic pattern is seen in only 20% of adenomas. As such, a pitfall in interpreting parathyroid CT is overreliance on enhancement patterns to decide parathyroid lesion likelihood (Fig. 61.4). Furthermore, parathyroid adenomas may exhibit cystic foci, fat deposition, or calcification. For these reasons, it is most prudent to describe any structure as a candidate parathyroid lesion that is not clearly thyroid, lymph node, or vascular.

Multigland Disease

A substantial minority of primary hyperparathyroidism patients have multigland disease. For primary hyperparathyroidism patients with more than one abnormal parathyroid gland, the preferred operation is bilateral neck exploration, in which the surgeon physically examines all parathyroid glands and resects the diseased glands. If all 4 glands are diseased, the surgeon will typically choose to leave a small amount of parathyroid tissue (either by resecting the 3 largest diseased glands or resecting 3.5 diseased glands) in an effort to avoid postoperative hypoparathyroidism.

Trans US

• **Fig. 61.1** Transverse ultrasound *(Trans US)* image demonstrates a homogeneously hypoechoic parathyroid adenoma *(arrow)* along the posterior aspect of the right thyroid lobe.,

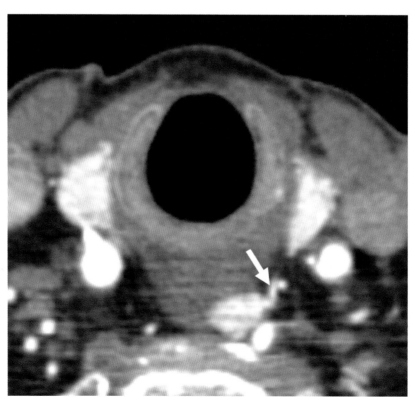

Ax CT C+ (arterial phase)

• **Fig. 61.2** Axial parathyroid CT arterial phase image demonstrates a left superior parathyroid adenoma in left retroesophageal location. Note the polar vessel *(arrow)* along the lateral aspect of the adenoma. *Ax,* Axial; *CT,* computed tomography.

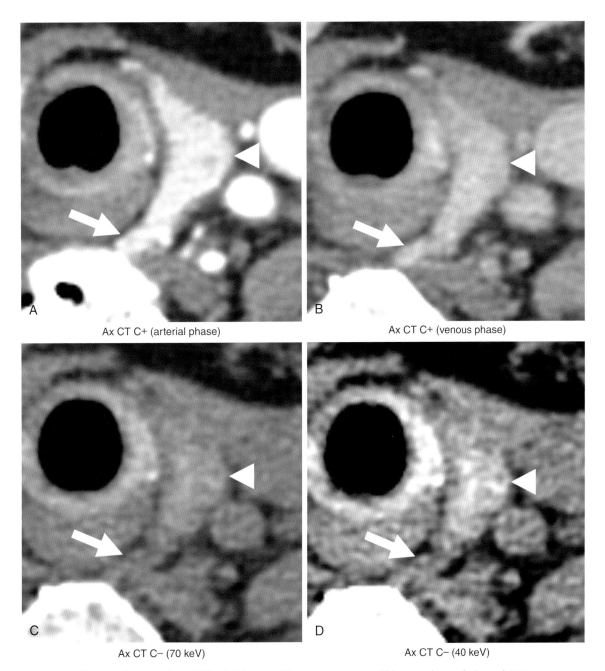

Ax CT C+ (arterial phase)

Ax CT C+ (venous phase)

Ax CT C− (70 keV)

Ax CT C− (40 keV)

• **Fig. 61.3** Axial parathyroid CT arterial phase (A) and venous phase (B) images demonstrate a left superior parathyroid adenoma (*arrows*, A and B) along the posterior aspect of the left thyroid lobe. Because the adenoma abuts and is isoattenuating to the adjacent thyroid gland (*arrowheads*, A and B), it could be easily overlooked on the contrast-enhanced phases. Careful examination of the standard (70 keV) dual-energy CT noncontrast image (C) shows the adenoma *(arrow)* to be hypoattenuating relative to the adjacent iodine-containing thyroid gland *(arrowhead)*. The 40 keV dual-energy CT noncontrast image (D) accentuates the difference in attenuation between the thyroid gland and adjacent parathyroid adenoma. The window (400 HU) and level (40 HU) settings are identical in both noncontrast images. *Ax,* Axial; *CT,* computed tomography.

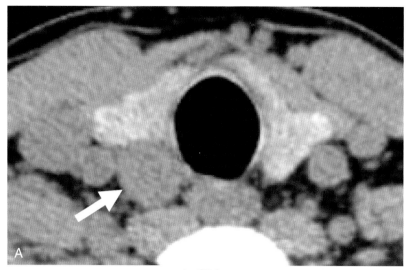

Ax CT C–

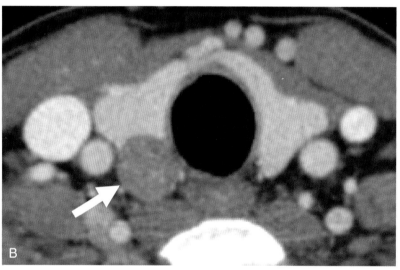

Ax CT C+ (arterial phase)

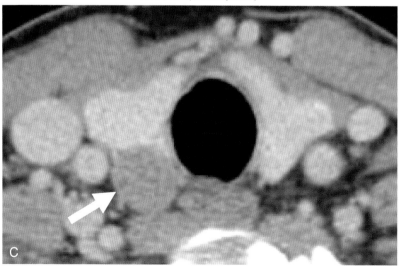

Ax CT C+ (venous phase)

• **Fig. 61.4** Axial parathyroid CT images demonstrate a right superior parathyroid adenoma (*arrows*, A, B, and C) along the posterior aspect of the right thyroid lobe. Ultrasound of the same lesion is shown in Fig. 61.1. Hypoattenuation of the parathyroid adenoma relative to the thyroid gland on the arterial phase (*arrow*, B) defies the classic enhancement pattern and illustrates the importance of not overemphasizing enhancement characteristics when determining the likelihood that a candidate lesion is of parathyroid origin. *Ax*, Axial; *CT*, computed tomography.

Although patients with multigland disease do not stand to benefit from minimally invasive parathyroidectomy, preoperative localization of the abnormal glands is nevertheless a valuable aid to bilateral neck exploration planning.

Ultrasound is insensitive for detecting multigland disease, whereas parathyroid CT performs relatively well. On parathyroid CT, multigland disease is more likely when there are either zero or multiple candidate lesions or when the largest candidate lesion (even if single) is less than 7 mm in maximum dimension.

Given the potential for multigland disease, it is important to avoid the satisfaction of search pitfall and continue looking for additional parathyroid glands even after identifying the first candidate lesion, despite the fact that single gland disease is far more common (Fig. 61.5). In many institutions, the primary operative approach is to initially attempt minimally invasive parathyroidectomy of the largest, highest confidence candidate lesion, regardless of the number of candidate lesions identified on parathyroid CT. The parathyroid hormone level is then checked intraoperatively, and if there is a 50% or greater decrease from the preoperative parathyroid hormone level then the operation is considered biochemically successful and ended. Any additional candidate lesions identified preoperatively with parathyroid CT are presumed to represent a combination of normal parathyroid glands, lymph nodes, thyroid nodules, exophytic thyroid tissue, and vasculature. If the intraoperative parathyroid hormone level does not decrease by at least 50% after removal of the first candidate lesion

(evidence of persistent parathyroid disease) or if the first candidate lesion examined at surgery is found to represent a mimic (e.g., thyroid nodule or lymph node), then the surgeon converts the operation to bilateral neck exploration.

Thus by meticulously describing the presence and location of all candidate parathyroid lesions and ranking them according to size and confidence, the radiologist enables the surgeon to develop a comprehensive and contingency-laden operative plan, potentially first attempting minimally invasive parathyroidectomy of the highest confidence lesion followed by imaging-directed conversion to bilateral neck exploration when necessary. When interpreting parathyroid CT and faced with a large, high-confidence lesion as well as smaller, lower-confidence lesions, it is far better to alert the surgeon to the presence and exact location of the additional, lower-confidence lesions that may or may not require surgical removal. Neglecting to describe a lesion that the surgeon ultimately must locate and remove to achieve biochemically successful parathyroidectomy risks withholding the important benefits of preoperative imaging.

Exophytic Thyroid

Ultrasound is the optimal modality for assessing the thyroid gland. Whereas parathyroid adenomas are typically homogeneously hypoechoic on ultrasound, exophytic thyroid parenchyma will be identical to the adjacent thyroid parenchyma. Although thyroid nodules can be hypoechoic relative to normal thyroid parenchyma, they are typically not as hypoechoic as a parathyroid gland and demonstrate a somewhat stippled or heterogeneous echotexture. Some thyroid nodules will be isoechoic or hyperechoic (Fig. 61.6) relative to the thyroid gland. As such, although parathyroid adenomas may rarely appear isoechoic or hyperechoic to the thyroid related to intralesional fibrosis, hemorrhage, calcification, or fat deposition, it is most often prudent to consider such isoechoic or hyperechoic candidate lesions to more likely represent thyroid nodules and to continue the search for a parathyroid lesion elsewhere within the neck.

On parathyroid CT, exophytic thyroid nodules and exophytic thyroid parenchyma can mimic parathyroid lesions, particularly if the noncontrast phase is either not acquired or not carefully reviewed. Unlike parathyroid lesions, thyroid tissue exhibits hyperattenuation on the noncontrast CT phase due to glandular iodine content. As described above, the attenuation of thyroid iodine can be accentuated by utilizing dual-energy CT 40 keV virtual monoenergetic images (Fig. 61.7). Intrathyroidal parathyroid adenomas may be surrounded by a rim of hyperattenuating thyroid tissue on the noncontrast phase of parathyroid CT. However, such intrathyroidal lesions are uncommon and should only be considered after an exhaustive search for parathyroid lesions elsewhere within the neck is unrevealing.

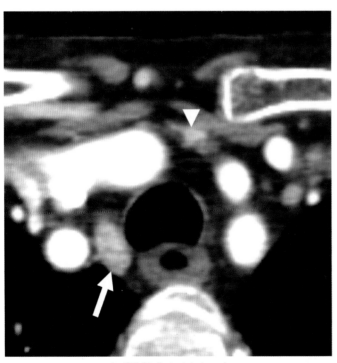

Ax CT C+ (arterial phase)

• **Fig. 61.5** Axial parathyroid CT arterial phase image demonstrates a larger candidate parathyroid lesion in the right tracheoesophageal groove *(arrow)* and a smaller candidate parathyroid lesion along the anteromedial aspect of the left common carotid artery *(arrowhead)*. Surgical removal of both parathyroid lesions was necessary to achieve the desired intraoperative decrease in parathyroid hormone level. *Ax,* Axial, *CT,* computed tomography.

Lymph Node

Lymph nodes can also mimic parathyroid lesions both morphologically and on noncontrast images, as both are hypoattenuating relative to the thyroid gland. A fatty hilum is characteristic,

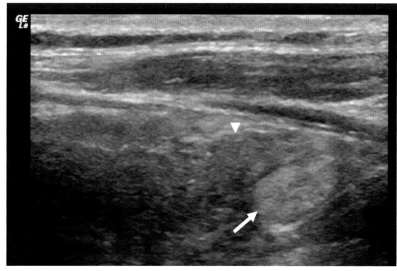

Sag ultrasound

• **Fig. 61.6** Sagittal ultrasound image demonstrates a hyperechoic candidate lesion *(arrow)* along the posteroinferior aspect of the right thyroid lobe *(arrowhead)*. Although parathyroid adenomas may occasionally appear hyperechoic relative to the thyroid parenchyma, this appearance is much more typical of a thyroid nodule. Continued search identified a parathyroid adenoma elsewhere in the neck in this patient.

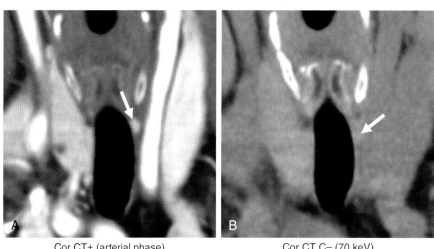

Cor CT+ (arterial phase)　　Cor CT C− (70 keV)

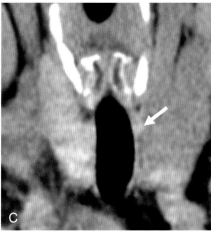

Cor CT C− (40 keV)

• **Fig. 61.7** Coronal parathyroid CT arterial phase image (A) obtained in a patient with primary hyperparathyroidism and prior left hemithyroidectomy demonstrates an avidly enhancing left paratracheal nodule *(arrow)*. On the arterial phase image alone, it is unclear whether this nodule represents residual thyroid tissue or a parathyroid adenoma. Careful examination of the standard (70 keV) dual-energy CT noncontrast image (B) shows the nodule *(arrow)* to be isoattenuating to the right thyroid lobe and faintly hyperattenuating relative to the other soft tissue structures in the neck, consistent with residual thyroid tissue; however, these findings are more conspicuous on the 40 keV dual-energy CT noncontrast image (C). The window (400 HU) and level (40 HU) settings are identical in both noncontrast images. *Cor,* Coronal; *CT,* computed tomography.

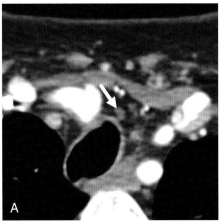

Ax CT C+ (arterial phase)

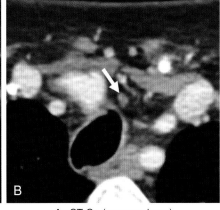

Ax CT C+ (venous phase)

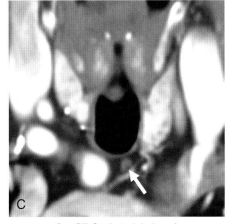

Cor CT C+ (arterial phase)

• **Fig. 61.8** Axial parathyroid CT arterial (A) and venous (B) phase images and coronal arterial phase image (C) demonstrate a left pretracheal candidate lesion *(arrows)*. The progressive enhancement pattern (hyperattenuating on venous phase relative to arterial phase) and fatty hilum *(arrow, C)* are typical of a lymph node.

although is often best appreciated on ultrasound. Lymph nodes also exhibit a progressive enhancement (Fig. 61.8) pattern (hyperattenuating on the venous phase relative to the arterial phase), which would be unusual for a parathyroid lesion. If in doubt as to whether a candidate lesion is a lymph node or not, it is often helpful to compare the candidate in question to jugular chain lymph nodes on both the arterial and venous phases.

If the enhancement of the candidate appears identical to jugular chain lymph nodes on both phases, the candidate is most likely a lymph node. Otherwise, a parathyroid lesion should be strongly considered.

Differential Diagnosis

IMAGING CHARACTERISTICS

Diagnosis	Ultrasound	CT
Parathyroid Adenoma (single gland disease)	Homogeneously hypoechoic Echogenic capsule separating adenoma from thyroid gland often seen	Always hypoattenuating relative to normal thyroid parenchyma on the noncontrast phase Variable enhancement on arterial and venous phases but almost always hyperattenuating relative to cervical lymph nodes on the arterial phase Most likely when there is a single candidate lesion larger than 13 mm in maximum dimension
Multigland disease	Poor sensitivity	More likely when there are no candidate lesions identified, multiple candidate lesions identified, or when the largest candidate lesion (even if single) is less than 7 mm in maximum dimension
Exophytic Thyroid Parenchyma	Isoechoic to other areas of the thyroid gland	Isoattenuating to other areas of the thyroid gland on all CT phases Attention to the noncontrast phase is particularly helpful, as thyroid parenchyma is normally hyperattenuating relative to other soft tissue structures due to glandular iodine content

IMAGING CHARACTERISTICS

Diagnosis	Ultrasound	CT
Thyroid Nodule	Variable echotexture (i.e., may be hypoechoic, isoechoic, or hyperechoic relative to normal thyroid parenchyma), though typically similar in quality to the thyroid gland.	Variable CT attenuation; however, on noncontrast CT surrounding hyperattenuation (i.e., iodine-containing thyroid parenchyma) indicates intrathyroidal location
	Hypoechoic thyroid nodules are typically less homogeneous and less hypoechoic than parathyroid adenomas.	
Lymph Node	Echogenic (fatty) hilum	Fatty hilum
		Progressive enhancement pattern (hyperattenuating on the venous phase relative to the arterial phase)
		Identical enhancement to jugular chain lymph nodes

Pearls

- Parathyroid lesions are always hypoattenuating relative to the normal thyroid gland.
- Iodine (hyperattenuating on noncontrast CT) within a candidate lesion is definitive for an exophytic thyroid nodule or thyroid parenchyma.
- Dual-energy CT low keV virtual monoenergetic imaging can be utilized to accentuate iodine attenuation and aid differentiation of parathyroid lesions from thyroid tissue.
- Given that only patients with biochemically proven primary hyperparathyroidism should undergo parathyroid imaging (100% pretest probability of disease), all candidate lesions that are not definitively thyroid, lymph node, or vascular should be considered suspicious for a parathyroid lesion.
- Utilize all available imaging information for localization interpretation, including other parathyroid imaging studies as well as remote prior imaging including the area of interest.

Signs and Complications

Spontaneous hemorrhage is a rare presentation of parathyroid adenomas with clinical symptoms related to associated mass effect. Consider biochemical evaluation for primary hyperparathyroidism in patients with spontaneous hemorrhage into the central compartment or upper mediastinum.

Parathyroid carcinoma is a very rare cause of primary hyperparathyroidism. Although uncommonly diagnosed preoperatively, young patient age, markedly elevated parathyroid hormone, and parathyroid calcifications should raise suspicion of malignancy.

Suggested Readings

Bahl M, Sepahdari AR, Sosa JA, et al. Parathyroid Adenomas and Hyperplasia on Four-dimensional CT Scans: Three Patterns of Enhancement Relative to the Thyroid Gland Justify a Three-Phase Protocol, *Radiology* 277(2):454–462, 2015.

Bahl M, Muzaffar M, Vij G, et al. Prevalence of the Polar Vessel Sign in Parathyroid Adenomas on the Arterial Phase of 4D CT, *AJNR Am J Neuroradiol* 35(3):578–581, 2014.

Bunch PM, Kelly HR. Preoperative Imaging Techniques in Primary Hyperparathyroidism: A Review, *JAMA Otolaryngol Head Neck Surg* 144(10):929–937, 2018.

Bunch PM, Randolph GW, Brooks JA, et al. Parathyroid 4D CT: What the Surgeon Wants to Know, *RadioGraphics* 40(5):1383–1394, 2020.

Bunch PM, Pavlina AA, Lipford ME, et al. Dual-Energy Parathyroid 4D CT: Improved Discrimination of Parathyroid Lesions from Thyroid Tissue Using Noncontrast 40 keV Virtual Monoenergetic Images, *AJNR Am J Neuroradiol* 42(11):2001-2008, 2021.

Hoang JK, Sung WK, Bahl M, et al. How to Perform Parathyroid 4D CT: Tips and Traps for Technique and Interpretation, *Radiology* 270(1):15–24, 2014.

Lubitz CC, Stephen AE, Hodin RA, et al. Preoperative Localization Strategies for Primary Hyperparathyroidism: An Economic Analysis, *Ann Surg Oncol* 19(13):4202–4209, 2012.

Rodgers SE, Hunter GJ, Hamberg LM, et al. Improved Preoperative Planning for Directed Parathyroidectomy with 4-Dimensional Computed Tomography, *Surgery* 140(6):932–940, 2006.

Sho S, Yilma M, Yeh MW, et al. Prospective Validation of Two 4D-CT-Based Scoring Systems for Prediction of Multigland Disease in Primary Hyperparathyroidism, *AJNR Am J Neuroradiol* 37(12):2323–2327, 2016.

Tessler I, Adi M, Diment J, et al. Spontaneous Neck Hematoma Secondary to Parathyroid Adenoma: A Case Series, *Eur Arch Otorhinolaryngol* 277(9):2551–2558, 2020.

62

Masses Involving the Anterior Cranial Fossa

GIRISH KORI, MD, PAUL M. BUNCH, MD, AND HILLARY R. KELLY, MD

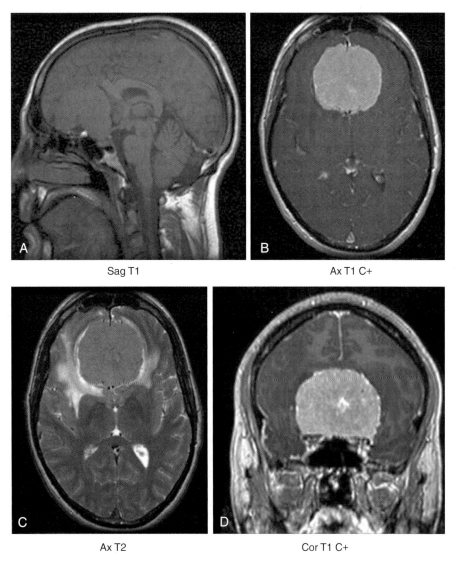

Sag T1

Ax T1 C+

Ax T2

Cor T1 C+

CASE A: A 46-year-old male with a history of progressive personality change for 1.5 years. *Ax*, Axial; *Cor*, coronal; *Sag*, sagittal.

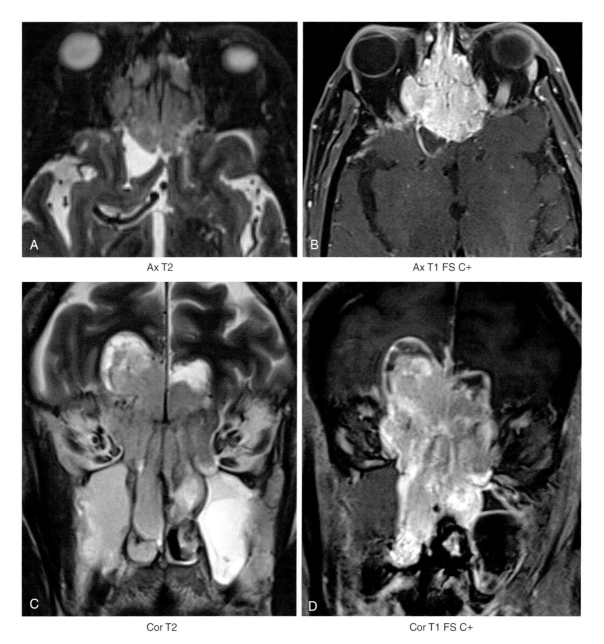

Ax T2

Ax T1 FS C+

Cor T2

Cor T1 FS C+

CASE B: A 69-year-old male with nasal mass and hyposmia. *Ax*, Axial; *Cor*, coronal; *FS*, fat saturated.

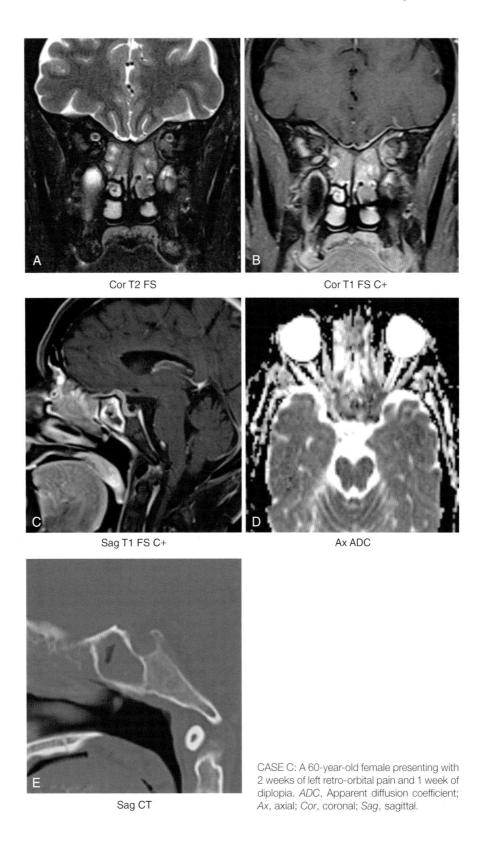

A — Cor T2 FS

B — Cor T1 FS C+

C — Sag T1 FS C+

D — Ax ADC

E — Sag CT

CASE C: A 60-year-old female presenting with 2 weeks of left retro-orbital pain and 1 week of diplopia. *ADC*, Apparent diffusion coefficient; *Ax*, axial; *Cor*, coronal; *Sag*, sagittal.

Sag T1

Ax T1 C+

Ax T2

Cor T1 C+

CASE D: A 68-year-old male with history of colon cancer. *Ax*, Axial; *Cor*, coronal; *Sag*, sagittal.

DESCRIPTION OF FINDINGS

Tumors Involving the Anterior Skull Base
- Magnetic resonance (MR) images demonstrate multiple masses of the anterior skull base with varying intrinsic signal properties, morphologies, and patterns of enhancement.
- Case A features a broad-based, avidly enhancing extraaxial mass centered at the floor of the anterior cranial fossa along the fovea ethmoidalis and extending posteriorly along the planum sphenoidale. Mass effect and superior displacement of the overlying gyrus recti and orbitofrontal cortex are present. Cerebrospinal fluid clefting confirms the extraaxial origin of the tumor. Also note the posterior displacement of the anterior cerebral arteries without evidence of vascular encasement.
- Case B features a T2 hypointense, heterogeneously enhancing mass centered within the superior nasal cavity and extending into the right orbit and into the anterior cranial fossa. The intracranial component of the tumor exerts mass effect on the inferior frontal lobes, and there are marginal cysts along the superior and posterior aspects of the intracranial tumor component.
- Case C features a T2 hypointense, homogeneously enhancing, low diffusivity mass centered in the nasal cavity and ethmoid air cells but also involving the left orbit, floor of the anterior cranial fossa, and sella. Despite the tumor involving both the sinonasal and intracranial compartments, the intervening bone appears intact rather than destroyed.
- Case D features a heterogeneously enhancing, markedly T2 hypointense, intraaxial mass centered within the orbitofrontal parenchyma. Inferiorly, the mass involves the meninges along the floor of the left anterior cranial fossa. Examination of the remainder of the brain parenchyma revealed multiple additional enhancing intraaxial lesions (not shown).

Diagnosis

Case A: Meningioma
Case B: Esthesioneuroblastoma
Case C: Diffuse large B-cell lymphoma
Case D: Colorectal cancer with intracranial metastases

Summary

General

Distinction between the multiple possible lesions that affect the anterior cranial fossa can be further delineated with consideration of the morphologic appearance, violation of surrounding anatomic boundaries, and transcompartmental extension of disease. Consideration also must be given to the pattern of aggressive, destructive bony cortical involvement (as is often seen with sinonasal malignancies) and the presence of sclerotic or hyperostotic bone reaction (as seen with meningiomas). The enhancement pattern and the presence of calcification also may provide clues to the diagnosis. Extraaxial intracranial tumors such as meningioma may involve the anterior cranial fossa primarily. Alternatively, the anterior cranial fossa can be involved secondarily by sinonasal malignancies extending superiorly or (much more rarely) by intraaxial malignancies (e.g., metastasis, glioblastoma) extending inferiorly.

Meningioma

A common diagnostic consideration for an anterior cranial fossa mass is a meningioma. Classic imaging findings associated with this tumor include a broad-based, smoothly marginated, extraaxial mass lesion abutting and arising from the dural surface with uniform or slightly heterogenous enhancement. Of biopsy-proven intracranial meningiomas, 12% to 22% are within the anterior cranial fossa and typically arise from the meningeal coverings of the olfactory groove/cribriform plate, fovea ethmoidalis, planum sphenoidale, or tuberculum sellae. On computed tomography, the mass may demonstrate a slightly hyperdense appearance, with internal foci of calcification (approximately 20%). On MR imaging, the majority of these lesions are T1 isointense and T2 isointense or hyperintense to gray matter. On postcontrast images, avid and relatively homogenous enhancement is seen routinely—however, not without exception. In 60% of cases, a dural tail—linear enhancement extending along the dura away from the tumor—is present, raising confidence in the diagnosis. Pneumosinus dilatans refers to expansion of an aerated paranasal sinus (Fig. 62.1) and represents an additional characteristic feature of anterior cranial fossa meningiomas. Brain parenchymal invasion is not seen in grade 1 meningiomas and thus represents a feature of higher grade (grade 2 or grade 3) lesions. Otherwise, reliable grading of meningiomas based on imaging features alone is not possible. Solitary fibrous tumor (hemangiopericytoma) and dural metastasis can mimic meningioma on imaging. Dural metastases are most commonly associated with primary cancers of the breast, prostate, and lung, and it is rare for the primary malignancy to be unknown at the time of brain imaging.

Sinonasal Malignancies

Malignancies arising in the sinonasal cavities are an important diagnostic consideration because they frequently invade the anterior cranial fossa. Aggressive sinonasal tumors that may invade the anterior cranial fossa include squamous cell carcinoma, adenocarcinoma, esthesioneuroblastoma, adenoid cystic carcinoma, sinonasal undifferentiated carcinoma, melanoma, and lymphoma. In a pediatric patient, rhabdomyosarcoma (Fig. 62.2) should also be considered. Although anatomic location and imaging characteristics may help to narrow the differential diagnosis, these tumors often exhibit a nonspecific imaging appearance. However, these lesions are also typically amenable to endoscopic transnasal biopsy. Therefore, the role of imaging is primarily to define the anatomic extent in order to determine if a lesion is resectable, to identify which structures may need to be sacrificed to achieve a surgical cure, and to aid in radiation therapy planning. CT and MR are complementary when evaluating aggressive sinonasal lesions with particular focus paid to detection of intracranial invasion, orbital invasion, and involvement of cranial nerves.

Sinonasal malignancies that *may* (but do not necessarily) have characteristic imaging appearances allowing for correct prospective imaging diagnosis include esthesioneuroblastoma, lymphoma, and melanoma. Esthesioneuroblastoma represents a malignancy of neural crest origin that typically arises from the basal stem cells of the olfactory neuroepithelium located in the superior nasal cavity. Rare cases of "ectopic" esthesioneuroblastoma have been

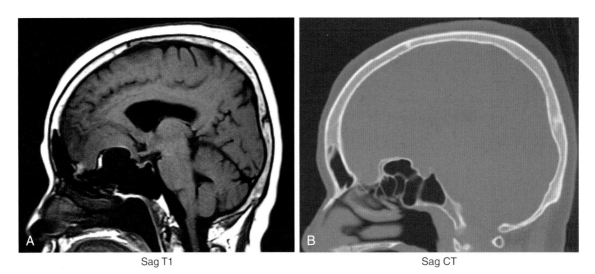

Sag T1

Sag CT

• **Fig. 62.1** A 51-year-old female with fatigue and progressive balance problems. Sagittal T1-weighted image demonstrates an extraaxial mass centered along the floor of the anterior cranial fossa. The sagittal T1-weighted MR and CT images demonstrate abnormal enlargement of the ethmoid air cells (i.e., pneumosinus dilatans) subjacent to the extraaxial mass. The presence of pneumosinus dilatans in association with an adjacent skull base mass strongly favors meningioma. *Sag*, Sagittal.

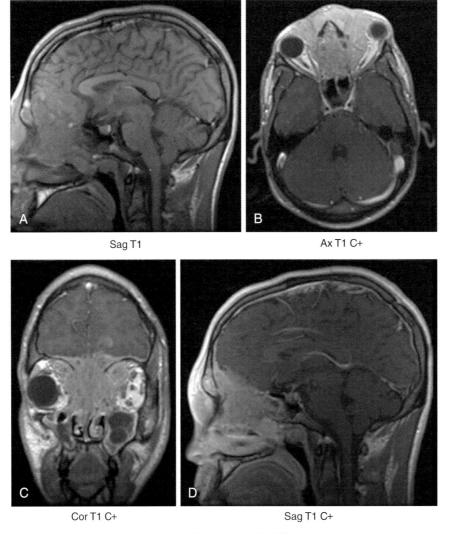

Sag T1

Ax T1 C+

Cor T1 C+

Sag T1 C+

• **Fig. 62.2** A 17-year-old male with swelling of the forehead. The MR images demonstrate a large enhancing sinonasal mass (biopsy-proven rhabdomyosarcoma) extending to involve the anterior cranial fossa, the orbits, and the soft tissues of the face. *Ax*, Axial; *Cor*, coronal; *Sag*, sagittal.

described in the maxillary sinus, nasopharynx, and sella turcica. The classic imaging appearance is a bilobed, dumbbell-shaped mass with central "waisting" at the cribriform plate. These lesions usually present relatively late in the course of the malignancy and typically are large with regional osseous changes that may or may not appear aggressive. When seen in the early form, this lesion appears as a small superior nasal cavity polypoid soft tissue mass. On MR imaging, the mass exhibits variable T1 and T2 signals with avid enhancement (comparable to the enhancement of the nasal turbinates) often seen on postgadolinium images. The presence of high T2 signal cysts at the margins of the intracranial tumor components has been described as diagnostic of this malignancy; however, this reportedly pathognomonic manifestation is rarely seen. Internal foci of calcification have also been described, although this finding is also seen in other skull base and nasal cavity tumors, including meningioma, inverted papilloma, and chondrosarcoma.

Imaging features that favor sinonasal lymphoma include homogeneous T2 hypointensity, homogeneous restricted diffusion, and permeative extension through bone with little if any associated osseous destruction. Although the imaging features of sinonasal melanoma are often nondescript, the presence of intrinsic T1 hyperintensity related to intratumoral melanin is a relatively specific imaging feature that may be seen (Fig. 62.3). Otherwise, the sinonasal malignancies described in this section typically present as a nonspecific sinonasal soft tissue mass with bone destruction. The lesions will most commonly exhibit intermediate to hypointense signal on T2-weighted images (when compared to fluid or normal mucosa) and demonstrate heterogeneous intermediate enhancement on postcontrast T1-weighted imaging (relative to

normal sinonasal mucosa). An example of a large sinonasal undifferentiated carcinoma is shown in Fig. 62.4.

Intraaxial Malignancies

One of the most common etiologies for intraaxial masses is hematogenous dissemination of metastatic disease. Of the known biopsy-proven neoplasms, lung cancer leads the list (as high as 80% in some series), followed by other common primary neoplasms, including breast cancer and melanoma. The example presented in Case D is a biopsy-proven colon cancer metastasis to the orbitofrontal region. Metastatic disease is a primary differential consideration for multiple intraaxial masses with or without a known cancer history. High-grade primary glial neoplasms (e.g., glioblastoma) may also involve the anterior cranial fossa by direct extension and warrant particular consideration in the absence of a known cancer history.

Spectrum of Disease

The spectrum of pathology affecting the anterior cranial fossa is detailed in the previous section.

Differential Diagnosis

Masses involving the anterior cranial fossa include:
1. **Intracranial extraaxial**
   - Meningioma
   - Solitary fibrous tumor (hemangiopericytoma)
   - Dural metastasis
2. **Sinonasal with intracranial extension**
   - Squamous cell carcinoma
   - Esthesioneuroblastoma
   - Lymphoma
   - Melanoma
   - Adenocarcinoma
   - Adenoid cystic carcinoma
   - Sinonasal undifferentiated carcinoma
   - Rhabdomyosarcoma (pediatric population)
3. **Intraaxial with extraaxial extension**
   - Metastasis
   - High-grade glial neoplasm (e.g., glioblastoma)

Pearls

- The keys to differentiating lesions of the floor of the anterior cranial fossa include location (intraaxial or extraaxial), site of mass origin, transcompartmental characteristics, regional mass effect, changes to surrounding soft tissues and bone, and pattern of enhancement.
- In almost all tumors, the final diagnosis is made by biopsy. Imaging is done to define the anatomic extent and margins.
- A smoothly marginated, dural-based, homogeneously enhancing mass lesion with accompanying adjacent calvarial hyperostosis and pneumosinus dilatans most likely represents a meningioma.
- A mass centered along the upper nasal cavity and cribriform plate with a bilobed configuration and a pattern of marginal

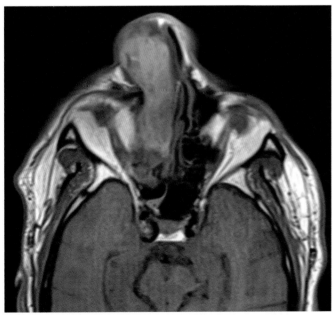

Ax T1

- **Fig. 62.3** A 69-year-old male with epistaxis. Axial T1-weighted image demonstrates intrinsic T1 hyperintensity within a large right nasal cavity mass, which was subsequently biopsied and shown to represent sinonasal melanoma. *Ax*, Axial.

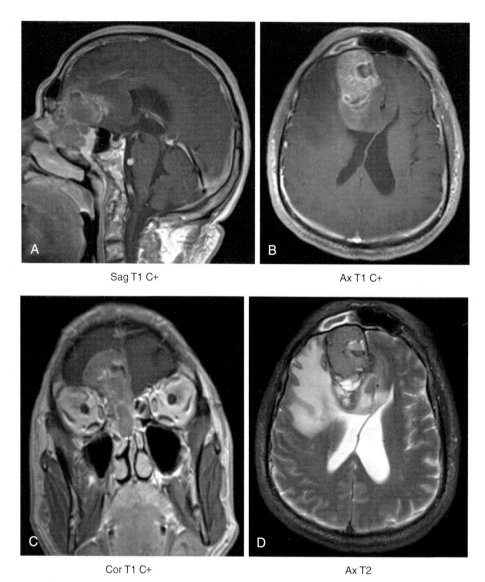

A	B
Sag T1 C+	Ax T1 C+
C	D
Cor T1 C+	Ax T2

• **Fig. 62.4** A 67-year-old male with lethargy, lack of motivation, and disorganization. The MR images demonstrate a large, heterogeneous mass (biopsy-proven sinonasal undifferentiated carcinoma) involving the right superior nasal cavity and anterior cranial fossa. The irregular enhancement and poorly defined margin along the posterior aspect of the mass as well as the extensive vasogenic edema within the right frontal lobe raise concern for direct brain parenchymal invasion by the mass. *Ax,* Axial; *Cor,* coronal; *Sag,* sagittal.

cysts along the interface between the mass and the brain cortical mantle is suggestive of esthesioneuroblastoma.
- Homogeneous T2 hypointensity, homogeneous enhancement, restricted diffusion, and relatively little if any bone destruction are characteristics suggestive of lymphoma.
- Intrinsic T1 hyperintensity is an imaging feature of melanoma.
- Imaging features of sinonasal malignancies are most often nonspecific, and biopsy is often necessary for definitive diagnosis. The role of imaging is primarily to define the anatomic extent, to identify which adjacent structures are involved, and to aid in radiation therapy planning.

Signs and Complications

Local mass effect related to anterior skull base masses can result in sensory deficits, including vision loss or diplopia from direct orbital invasion or the effect of the mass on the optic nerve or extraocular muscles. Anosmia can occur from invasion of the olfactory bulb or nerves or from blockage of air flow to the superior nasal cavity. Direct tumor invasion of the cavernous sinus can result in thrombosis and encasement of the traversing cranial nerves. Cranial nerve deficits may also result from skull base foraminal involvement by tumor.

Suggested Readings

Agarwal M, Policeni B: Sinonasal neoplasms, *Semin Roentgenol* 54(3): 244–257, 2019.
Bunch PM, Kelly HR: Esthesioneuroblastoma. In Small JE, Noujaim DL, Ginat DT, Kelly HR, Schaefer PW, editors: *Neuroradiology: spectrum and evolution of disease,* ed 1. Philadelphia, 2018, Elsevier, 346–356.

Dean KE, Shatzkes D, Phillips CD: Imaging review of new and emerging sinonasal tumors and tumor-like entities from the fourth edition of the World Health Organization Classification of Head and Neck Tumors, *AJNR Am J Neuroradiol* 40(4):584–590, 2019.

Hirano H, Yokoyama S, Yunoue, et al: MRI T2 hypointensity of metastatic brain tumors from gastric and colonic cancers, *Int J Clin Oncol* 19(4):643–648, 2014.

Louis DN, Perry A, Wesseling P, et al: The 2021 WHO classification of tumors of the central nervous system: a summary, *Neuro Oncol* 23(8):1231–1251, 2021.

Parmar HA, Ibrahim M: Imaging of anterior skull base, *Semin Ultrasound CT MR* 42(3):281–294, 2021.

Som PM, Lidov M, Brandwein M, et al: Sinonasal esthesioneuroblastoma with intracranial extension: marginal tumor cysts as a diagnostic MR finding, *AJNR Am J Neuroradiol* 15(7):1259–1262, 1994.

Som PM, Lidov M: The significance of sinonasal radiodensities: ossification, calcification, or residual bone? *AJNR Am J Neuroradiol* 15(5):917–922, 1994.

63

Petrous Apex Lesions

NINO BOALS, MD AND HILLARY R. KELLY, MD

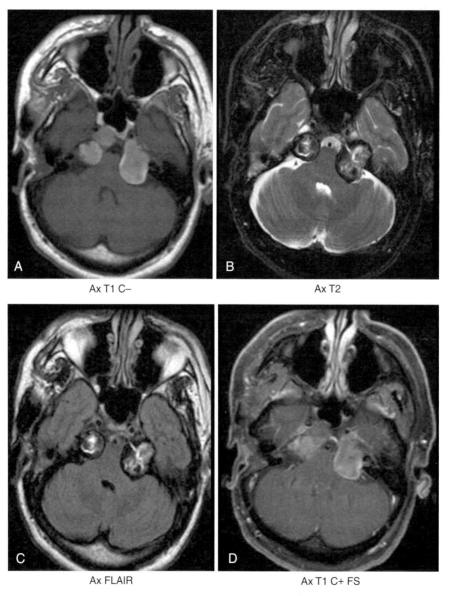

Ax T1 C−

Ax T2

Ax FLAIR

Ax T1 C+ FS

CASE A: A 67-year-old male with hearing loss and headache. *Ax,* Axial; *FS,* fat saturated; *FLAIR,* fluid-attenuated inversion recovery.

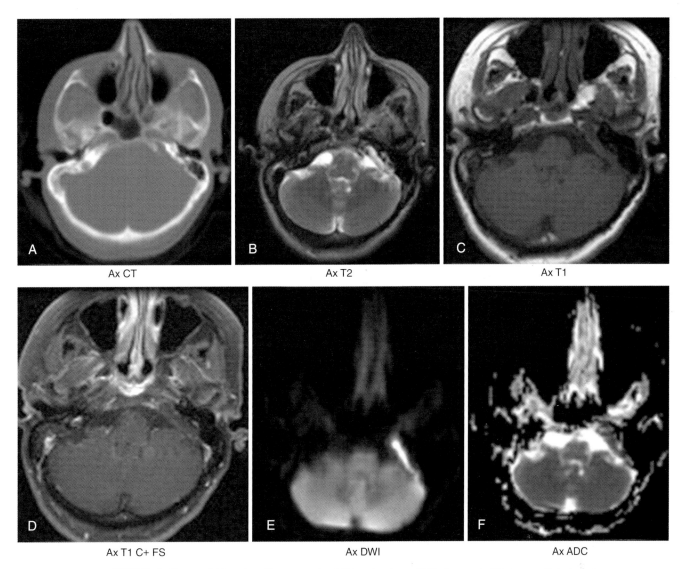

Ax CT

Ax T2

Ax T1

Ax T1 C+ FS

Ax DWI

Ax ADC

CASE B: A 53-year-old female with progressive left hearing loss. *ADC*, Apparent diffusion coefficient; *Ax*, Axial; *CT*, Computed tomography; *DWI*, diffusion-weighted imaging; *FS*, fat saturated.

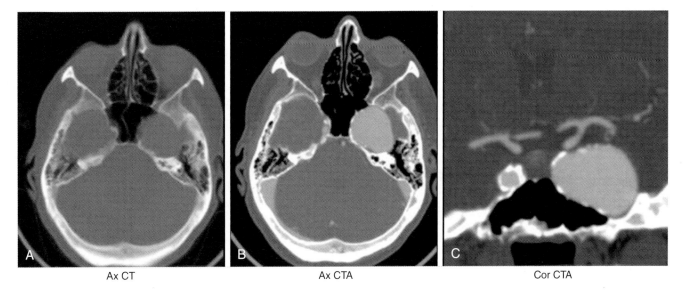

Ax CT

Ax CTA

Cor CTA

CASE C: A 49-year-old female presenting with a throbbing sensation in her head. *Ax*, Axial; *Cor*, coronal; *CT*, Computed tomography; *CTA*, CT angiography.

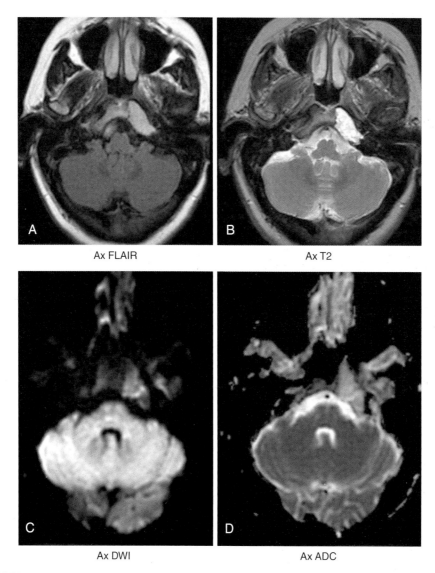

Ax FLAIR

Ax T2

Ax DWI

Ax ADC

CASE D: A 56-year-old male presenting with a headache. *Ax,* Axial; *ADC,* Apparent diffusion coefficient; *DWI,* diffusion-weighted imaging; *FLAIR,* fluid-attenuated inversion recovery.

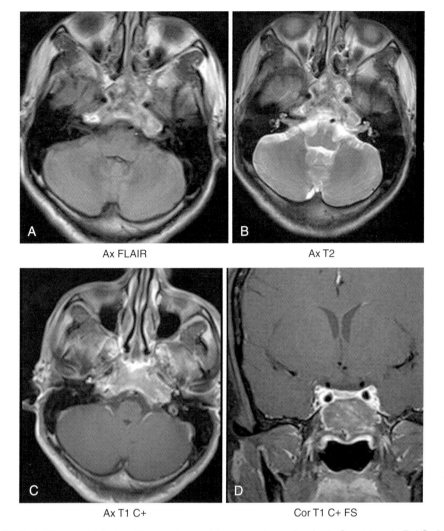

Ax FLAIR

Ax T2

Ax T1 C+

Cor T1 C+ FS

CASE E: A 69-year-old male with multiple cranial nerve palsies. *Ax,* Axial; *Cor,* coronal; *FLAIR,* fluid attenuated inversion recovery.

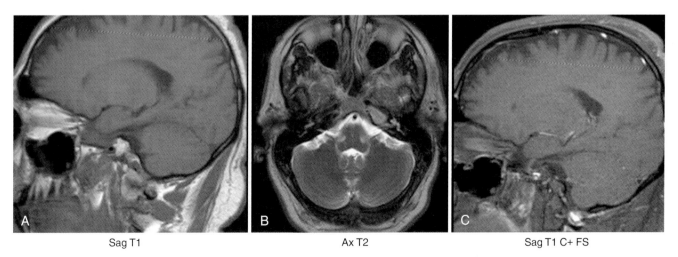

Sag T1

Ax T2

Sag T1 C+ FS

CASE F: An asymptomatic 32-year-old female. *Ax,* Axial; *FS,* fat saturated; *Sag,* sagittal.

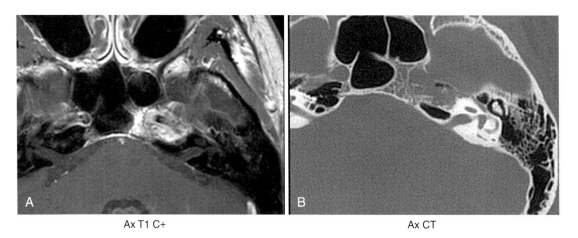

Ax T2 | Ax T1 | Ax SSFP

Ax DWI | Ax ADC

CASE G: A 53-year-old female with incidental findings on magnetic resonance imaging. *ADC*, Apparent diffusion coefficient; *Ax*, Axial; *DWI*, diffusion-weighted imaging; *SSFP*, steady state free precession.

Ax T1 C+ | Ax CT

CASE H: A 39-year-old male with otalgia and left cranial nerve VI palsy. *Ax*, Axial; *CT*, Computed tomography.

DESCRIPTION OF FINDINGS

- Case A: Demonstrates bilateral T1 and T2 hyperintense petrous apex lesions with rims of T2 hypointense signal suggestive of hemosiderin.
- Case B: Features a T1 hypointense, T2 hyperintense, mildly expansile lesion along the left petrous ridge that has minimal peripheral enhancement and demonstrates restricted diffusion.
- Case C: A well-circumscribed skull base lesion results in erosive changes of the left petrous apex and demonstrates similar enhancement to the adjacent and intimately associated left internal carotid artery.
- Case D: A homogenously T2-hyperintense expansile lesion is centered at the left petroclival synchondrosis. The lesion exhibits facilitated diffusion.
- Case E: An expansile, T2 hyperintense, heterogeneously enhancing mass appears to involve the basiocciput and basisphenoid in an infiltrative fashion.
- Case F: Demonstrates a T1 hyperintense, relatively T2 isointense lesion in the left petrous apex that does not enhance and "disappears" with the fat saturation technique.
- Case G: Features lobulated, T2 hyperintense lesions in both petrous apices that do not show restricted diffusion and appear to be contiguous with Meckel caves bilaterally.
- Case H: Shows avid enhancement within the left petrous apex with corresponding destructive bony changes on computed tomography (CT).

Diagnosis

Case A: Bilateral cholesterol granulomas (cholesterol cysts)
Case B: Cholesteatoma (epidermoid)
Case C: Internal carotid artery aneurysm eroding the left petrous apex
Case D: Myxoid chondrosarcoma
Case E: Plasmacytoma
Case F: Asymmetric bone marrow
Case G: Petrous apex meningoceles
Case H: Petrous apicitis

Summary

Lesions involving the petrous apex vary in presentation depending on the size and underlying etiology. Symptoms may include headaches, hearing loss, vestibular dysfunction, facial paralysis, or diplopia. However, many abnormalities are asymptomatic.

Most benign processes are related to the presence of petrous apex pneumatization, a normal physiologic variant that occurs in up to 30% of the population. The nonneoplastic category can be subdivided into the "leave me alone" lesions, which consist of asymmetric bone marrow and petrous air cell effusion; obstructive processes, giving rise to the spectrum of mucoceles and cholesterol granulomas (also known as cholesterol cysts); congenital lesions, such as congenital cholesteatomas (also called epidermoids); infectious processes, such as petrous apicitis; and miscellaneous lesions, including aneurysms of the petrous internal carotid artery, fibrous dysplasia, Paget disease, and apical meningocele/cephaloceles.

The neoplastic processes include benign entities, such as meningiomas and schwannomas of the facial, trigeminal, or abducens nerves and their branches, and malignant processes consisting of primary neoplasms (e.g., chordoma,

chondrosarcoma, osteosarcoma, and plasmacytoma) and metastases. Neoplasms that can arise in multiple locations, including schwannomas, paragangliomas, and meningiomas, are covered in other chapters and will not be further discussed here.

Spectrum of Disease

Care must be taken to diagnose nonsurgical "do not touch" lesions, such as asymmetric pneumatization/marrow and trapped petrous apex fluid, with relative certainty.

Asymmetric pneumatization of the petrous apices is commonly observed, but can be misconstrued as a pathologic process. The pneumatized apex will be hypointense on T1-weighted imaging, leading to asymmetric T1 hyperintense fat signal in the bone marrow of the contralateral nonpneumatized petrous apex. The presence of fat can be further confirmed with fat saturation techniques and comparison of the signal intensity in the petrous apex with that of orbital fat. On CT, the lack of bony erosion or expansion confirms the nonpathologic character of this variant.

The presence of fluid signal within the otherwise normally developed petrous apex cells and the absence of expansion or destructive changes in the adjacent bone suggest the diagnosis of trapped fluid in the petrous apex. Some centers continue to monitor these lesions with imaging to ensure stability and to exclude more aggressive entities. The presence of intermediate or hyperintense T1 signal suggests either proteinaceous fluid or a developing cholesterol granuloma, in which case correlation with clinical history and consideration of imaging follow-up is warranted.

Cholesterol granulomas (or cholesterol cysts) are expansile, T1- and T2 hyperintense lesions of the petrous apex that may demonstrate peripheral enhancement. These lesions are believed to result from air cell obstruction in a pneumatized petrous apex. Negative pressure develops within the obstructed air cells, leading to mucosal engorgement and hemorrhage. Cholesterol crystals result from red cell degradation and incite a foreign body reaction, leading to further hemorrhage and development of inflammatory granulation tissue. In addition to central T1 and T2 hyperintensity, a low-signal hemosiderin rim is also commonly seen. The combination of MRI and CT offers the best means of imaging diagnosis, with the latter modality revealing expansion and smooth scalloping of the surrounding bone.

Cholesteatomas (or epidermoids) of the petrous apex are rare. They are expansile, T1 hypointense, and T2/FLAIR hyperintense nonenhancing lesions that may demonstrate subtle peripheral enhancement. Mucoceles are even rarer than cholesteatomas in the petrous apex. Petrous apex cholesteatomas and mucoceles may have an identical appearance on CT and on T1- and T2-weighted MR images but may be differentiated by means of diffusion-weighted imaging (DWI), which demonstrates restricted diffusion within cholesteatomas.

The pathogenesis of the apical meningocele/cephalocele is thought to stem from congenital or acquired protrusion of the floor of Meckel cave into the petrous apex. These lesions follow signal and attenuation characteristics of cerebrospinal fluid (CSF) and demonstrate direct communication with Meckel cave. They can be bilateral and have been associated with idiopathic intracranial hypertension. Additional imaging features include expansion and smooth scalloping of the adjacent bony margins and absence of enhancement. Occasional "prolapse" of the normally mildly enhancing Gasserian ganglion into the meningocele/cephalocele should not be mistaken for enhancement.

The presence of trabecular breakdown in opacified petrous air cells with concurrent mastoid air cell opacification and rim-like enhancement of the fluid-filled cells is highly suspicious for petrous apicitis. The clinical setting usually includes otorrhea and deep facial/retroorbital pain or otalgia with or without cranial nerve palsies of cranial nerves V through VIII. Cranial nerve VI is particularly at risk because of its course through Dorello canal at the apex of the petrous bone. Advanced cases of petrous apicitis may demonstrate thickening and enhancement of the adjacent meninges, venous sinus thrombosis, fistulization into the labyrinth, petrous carotid pseudoaneurysm, and findings of skull base osteomyelitis.

The presence of osseous destruction and nodular or masslike soft tissue components should raise concern for one of the neoplastic processes that specifically involve the petrous apex, such as a chordoma or chondrosarcoma, or those that can arise in any osseous structure, such as plasmacytoma or metastatic disease. In a child, histiocytosis and various sarcomas (e.g., Ewing, rhabdomyosarcoma) also can arise in or involve the petrous apex.

Differential Diagnosis

1. Asymmetric pneumatization/marrow should not present a diagnostic dilemma in adults. Observation of fat signal intensity in the petrous apex, similar to that of orbital fat and the absence of enhancement or destructive changes, suggests this diagnosis, which can be confirmed with fat saturation techniques. In children, the marrow may not have converted to fat, but the lack of bony expansion or erosion and stability over time can suggest the diagnosis.
2. Petrous apex effusion is trapped fluid within petrous air cells that usually results in a unilateral T2 hyperintense signal, with T1 signal following fluid or mucous. As with asymmetric pneumatization/marrow, the lack of bony destruction or expansion on CT usually resolves the diagnostic dilemma.
3. Cholesterol granulomas (cholesterol cysts) are T1- and T2 hyperintense expansile lesions that can demonstrate peripheral enhancement but no internal enhancement. These lesions also often have a peripheral, T2 hypointense hemosiderin rim.
4. Cholesteatomas (epidermoids) are T1 hypointense and T2 hyperintense expansile lesions that may demonstrate peripheral enhancement and often demonstrate restricted diffusion on DWI.
5. Mucoceles also are expansile T1-hypointense and T2-hyperintense lesions that can be indistinguishable from a

cholesteatoma on CT imaging and on T1- and T2-weighted MR sequences but may be differentiated by the absence of restricted diffusion. Some consider mucoceles to be part of a spectrum with cholesterol granulomas (cysts) rather than a distinct entity.
6. Petrous apicitis is a T1 hypointense/T2 hyperintense lesion with associated trabecular destruction. Peripheral enhancement in the appropriate clinical setting (e.g., face pain, abducens palsy, and otitis media) should suggest this diagnosis; however, aggressive neoplasms could have a similar radiologic appearance.
7. Meningoceles/cephaloceles follow CSF attenuation/intensity and demonstrate smooth bony scalloping, a connection with Meckel cave, and no enhancement.
8. Internal carotid artery aneurysms on MR imaging often exhibit pulsation artifact and may have alternating areas of T1 and T2 hyperintensity with a central flow void that is most consistent with a partially thrombosed aneurysm. Head CT angiography (CTA) or MR angiogram (MRA) usually confirms the diagnosis.
9. Paget disease features enlarged bone and thickened trabeculae with the appropriate clinical history.
10. Fibrous dysplasia has heterogeneous signal on T1- and T2-weighted sequences and is often avidly enhancing on postcontrast MR images. Given the enhancement on MR imaging, this lesion may be mistaken for malignancy; however, the observation of a "ground glass" matrix without aggressive features on CT imaging is usually diagnostic.
11. Chordoma and chondrosarcoma are both malignant neoplasms of the skull base and may demonstrate similar imaging characteristics, appearing T1 hypointense and T2 hyperintense with various patterns of contrast enhancement. However, chordomas tend to arise in the midline (originating from notochord remnants) and exhibit relatively low apparent diffusion coefficient (ADC) values, whereas chondroid tumors usually emanate from the petrooccipital synchondrosis and exhibit relatively high ADC values. The presence of chondroid matrix is an additional imaging feature suggestive of a chondroid neoplasm.

Pearls

- Imaging plays a crucial role in evaluation and diagnosis of the lesions involving the petrous apex because this area is not amenable to direct inspection by a clinician. The combination of imaging findings with clinical signs and symptoms results in a correct diagnosis in most cases.

Signs and Complications

Petrous apicitis is a potentially fatal condition that should not be overlooked and must be suspected in the appropriate clinical setting. On the other hand, care must be taken in diagnosing benign findings, such as fluid or asymmetric bone marrow, to avoid aggressive or incorrect management. Although cholesterol granulomas and cholesteatomas are benign lesions, they can result in hearing loss and fistulous communications. Neoplasms and aneurysms must be differentiated from other entities affecting the petrous apex because they may lead to devastating consequences if incorrectly managed.

Suggested Readings

Bialer OY, Rueda MP, Bruce BB, et al: Meningoceles in idiopathic intracranial hypertension, *AJR Am J Roentgenol* 202(3):608–613, 2014.

Boardman JF, Rothfus WE, Dulai HS: Lesions and pseudolesions of the cavernous sinus and petrous apex, *Otolaryngol Clin North Am* 41:195–213, 2008.

Downs DM, Damiano TR, Rubinstein D: Gasserian ganglion: appearance on contrast enhanced MR, *Am J Neuroradiol* 17:237–241, 1996.

Isaacson B, Kutz WJ, Roland PS: Lesions of the petrous apex: diagnosis and management, *Otolaryngol Clin North Am* 40:479–519, 2007.

Moore KR, Fischbein NJ, Harnsberger RH, et al: Petrous apex cephaloceles, *AJNR Am J Neuroradiol* 22:1867–1871, 2001.

Moore KR, Harnsberger HR, Shelton C, et al: 'Leave me alone' lesions of the petrous apex, *Am J Neuroradiol* 19:733–738, 1998.

Potter GM, Siripurapu R: Imaging of petrous apex lesions, *Neuroimaging Clin N Am* 31(4):523–540, 2021.

Razek AA, Huang BY: Lesions of the petrous apex: classification and findings at CT and MR imaging, *Radiographics* 32(1):151–173, 2012.

Tsang Juliano AF, et al: Temporal and cerebellopontine angle lesions. In Som PM, Curtin HD, editors: *Head and neck imaging*, St Louis, 2011, Mosby.

Yeom KW, Lober RM, Mobley BC, et al: Diffusion-weighted MRI: distinction of skull base chordoma from chondrosarcoma, *AJNR Am J Neuroradiol* 34(5):1056–1061, 2013.

64
Lesions of the External Auditory Canal

NINO BOALS, MD AND PAUL M. BUNCH, MD

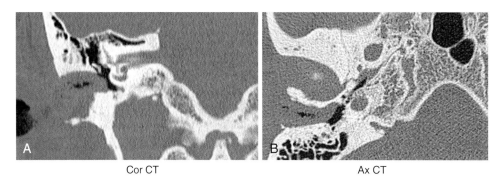

Cor CT Ax CT

CASE A: A 35-year-old male presenting with unilateral otalgia, otorrhea, and mild conductive hearing loss. *Ax*, Axial; *Cor*, coronal; *CT*, Computed tomography.

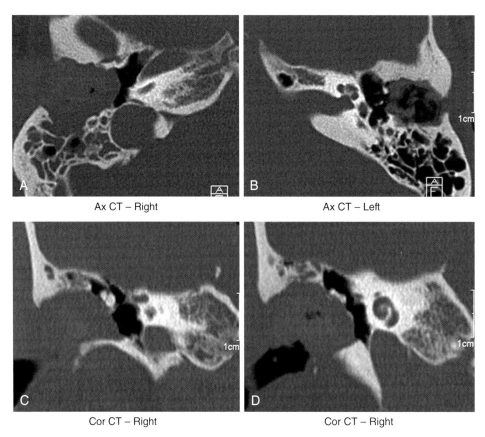

Ax CT – Right Ax CT – Left

Cor CT – Right Cor CT – Right

CASE B: A patient with chronically draining ears. *Ax*, Axial; *Cor*, coronal; *CT*, Computed tomography.

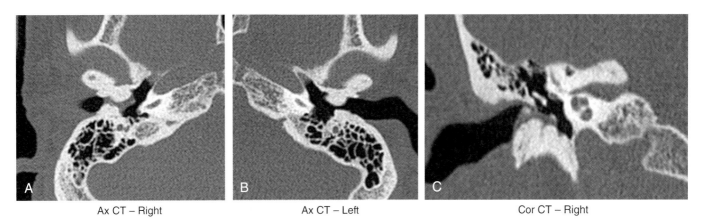

Ax CT – Right   Ax CT – Left   Cor CT – Right

CASE C: A 30-year-old patient with narrowing of the external auditory canals. *Ax*, Axial; *Cor*, coronal; *CT*, Computed tomography.

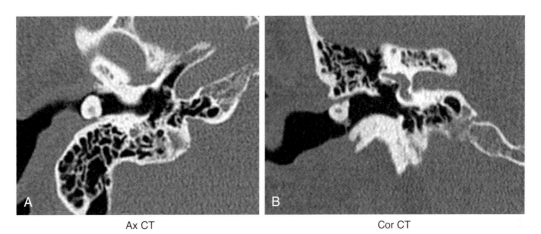

Ax CT   Cor CT

CASE D: A patient with a mass in the right ear canal covered by skin. *Ax*, Axial; *Cor*, coronal; *CT*, Computed tomography.

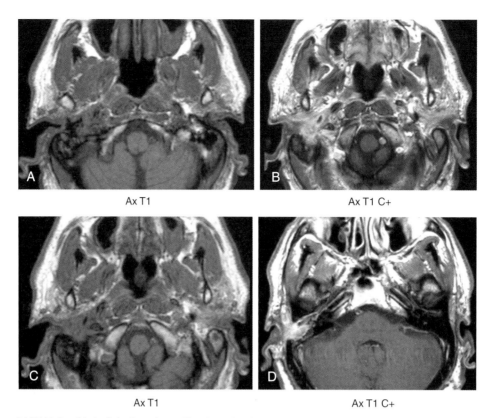

CASE E: An elderly diabetic patient with pain and a draining right ear who now has right facial paralysis. *Ax*, Axial.

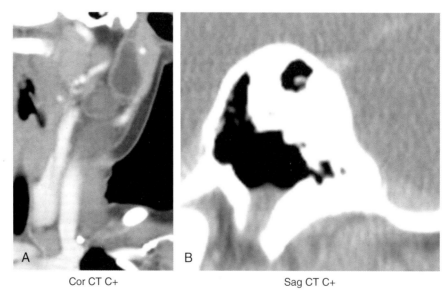

CASE F: A 34-year-old male presenting with a fluctuant periauricular mass. *CT,* Computed tomography; *Cor*, coronal; *Sag*, sagittal.

DESCRIPTION OF FINDINGS

- Case A: Coronal and axial CT images of the right temporal bone demonstrate soft tissue density in the right external auditory canal (EAC), resulting in bony erosion, most pronounced along the inferior aspect of the EAC.
- Case B: Axial and coronal CT images demonstrate soft tissue density in both EACs, resulting in expansion and bony remodeling.
- Case C: Axial and coronal CT images demonstrate broad-based ossific masses along the walls of both bony EACs.
- Case D: Axial and coronal CT images demonstrate an ossific density projecting from the wall of the right EAC without an associated soft tissue mass or erosive bony changes.
- Case E: Axial T1-weighted images of the temporal bone before and after the administration of gadolinium contrast reveal soft tissue thickening and diffuse enhancement in the right EAC extending into the bone and soft tissue inferior to the temporal bone with associated obliteration of adjacent fat planes, including at the right stylomastoid foramen.
- Case F: Contrast-enhanced coronal CT image of the neck demonstrates a cystic, rim-enhancing mass spanning the left periauricular region to the angle of the mandible. Contrast-enhanced sagittal CT image demonstrates communication of the cystic mass with the left EAC floor.

Diagnosis

Case A: EAC cholesteatoma (although squamous cell carcinoma [SCC] could have an identical imaging appearance)

Case B: Keratosis obturans

Case C: Bilateral EAC exostoses

Case D: EAC osteoma

Case E: Necrotizing otitis externa

Case F: Type II first branchial cleft cyst

Summary

The disorders affecting the EAC range from cerumen impaction to malignancy. Some of these entities have distinguishing characteristics, whereas others share overlapping imaging appearances.

Dermatologic lesions affecting the pinna are not discussed and are better evaluated by visual inspection.

Spectrum of Disease

Although acquired cholesteatomas most commonly arise in the middle ear, cholesteatomas may also arise primarily in the EAC, either spontaneously or as a result of prior surgery or trauma. These lesions are composed of stratified squamous epithelium and exfoliated keratinous material. The most common presenting symptoms of EAC cholesteatomas are otorrhea and otalgia.

On imaging, the hallmark of cholesteatomas is osseous erosion, and internal osseous fragments ("flecks") may also be seen. These lesions demonstrate restricted diffusion and do not enhance on postcontrast imaging. EAC cholesteatomas are typically unilateral with a propensity for posterior and inferior EAC wall involvement. Extension into the middle ear and mastoid may occur. Importantly, the imaging appearance of EAC cholesteatoma and EAC squamous cell carcinoma can be identical, such that correlation with direct inspection is necessary.

Keratosis obturans is believed to result from sympathetic reflex stimulation of EAC ceruminous glands, which leads to hyperemia and epidermal plugging from accumulation of exfoliated keratin without an enclosing sac of stratified squamous epithelium. On imaging, keratosis obturans appears as a homogenous soft tissue density/intensity mass that commonly expands and remodels, but classically does not erode, the surrounding bone. Sometimes, mild rim enhancement is observed. Keratosis obturans usually affects young male patients, is frequently bilateral, and may lead to conductive hearing loss or otalgia. Sinus infections and bronchiectasis may be concurrent. EAC cholesteatomas, conversely, are usually unilateral and generally affect elderly persons.

Medial canal fibrosis usually presents in the setting of chronic otitis externa, with symptoms ranging from otorrhea to conductive hearing loss. This entity is bilateral in up to 60% of cases and appears as crescent-shaped fibrous tissue in the medial portion of the EAC, overlying the tympanic membrane. The lesion conforms to the surrounding structures without bony remodeling or erosive changes. CT demonstrates homogenous soft tissue density within the EAC, inseparable from the tympanic membrane. On MRI, signal characteristics reflect the fibrous composition of the lesion, which tends to be hypointense on T1-weighted imaging and isointense to hypointense on T2-weighted sequences. Mild peripheral enhancement may occur early in the course, reflecting inflammation and edema.

EAC exostoses represent benign overgrowth of the bony portion of the EAC and are thought to occur as a result of repeated and prolonged exposure to cold water (although they also are seen in patients without this history). These lesions almost always are bilateral and result in variable degrees of EAC narrowing. The overlying soft tissues are normal in appearance, with no associated destructive changes. On CT, these lesions appear as broad-based or lobulated bony excrescences within the EAC without associated soft tissue masses, abnormal enhancement, or erosive bony changes. MRI is not useful for diagnosis, but when it is performed, low-signal exostoses are seen within the EAC.

EAC osteomas are less common than exostoses. They are benign, well-circumscribed, pedunculated lesions of the EAC that frequently are unilateral and solitary and often are found incidentally. As with exostoses, these lesions can be found in persons with a history of prolonged exposure to cold water, and although an association appears to exist with cholesteatomas and prior surgery, many lesions are found in patients without these predisposing factors. On imaging, they demonstrate attenuation/signal characteristics consistent with bony matrix, without aggressive features.

Necrotizing otitis externa (also known as malignant otitis externa) is an invasive infection typically caused by *Pseudomonas aeruginosa* or, less commonly, by *Aspergillus fumigatus* and primarily affecting elderly diabetic or otherwise immunocompromised patients. The infection begins in the EAC but quickly spreads to adjacent tissues, classically inferiorly into the soft tissues beneath the temporal bone and then medially beneath the skull base, where multiple cranial nerves can be affected. Extension into and through the bone can occur as well. CT of the temporal bones may demonstrate abnormal enhancing soft tissue, destructive changes in the adjacent bone, and surrounding edema with obliteration of the fat planes beneath the skull base. MRI findings can be variable, but the extension beneath the skull base and obliteration of the fat planes may be more obvious. As progressive involvement of the skull base occurs, adjacent dural venous and cavernous sinuses should be evaluated for thrombosis. Other potential complications are related to intracranial extension, including meningitis and abscess. A three-phase technetium-99m methylene diphosphonate bone scan is more sensitive than CT for early detection of skull base osteomyelitis. Both gallium-67 citrate and technetium-labeled white blood cell scans can be used, often in conjunction with MR, to assess treatment response. Of note, osseous changes may persist on CT for more than 1 year, even in the absence of active infection.

SCC is the most common malignancy of the EAC and is associated with chronic inflammatory states, such as chronic otitis media. In early stages, SCC involves primarily the EAC, but it can spread into the adjacent soft tissues and middle ear. On imaging, SCC can appear as a lobular or infiltrating soft tissue mass and may resemble medial canal fibrosis, cholesteatoma, keratosis obturans, or malignant otitis externa. It is T1 hypointense and isointense or hypointense on T2-weighted imaging, demonstrating various degrees of enhancement. CT is best for evaluating the extension and degree of bone destruction and for staging the disease relative to the external canal, but MRI is better for defining extension into the mastoid or dura.

Schwannomas are slow-growing, benign tumors that very rarely involve the EAC but can arise from the sensory branches of cranial nerves V, VII, IX, X, and the cervical plexus. Clinically, these lesions may present with recurrent otitis externa, pain, otorrhea, and/or mild conductive hearing loss. On imaging, EAC schwannomas appear as lobulated enhancing masses without invasive or destructive features.

First branchial cleft anomalies are rare, constituting fewer than 1% of all branchial cleft lesions. They are thought to arise as a result of incomplete obliteration of the first branchial cleft, leading to cyst, fistula, or sinus development. A type I lesion is derived from ectoderm and essentially represents a duplication anomaly of the membranous EAC, usually located posteromedial to the ear concha and lateral to cranial nerve VII. Type II anomalies are composed of both ectoderm and mesoderm and often are associated with cranial nerve VII in the parotid gland. They can extend into the anterolateral part of the neck and often demonstrate a tract that crosses the parotid gland and extends to the bony-cartilaginous EAC junction, resulting in direct communication with the EAC.

Differential Diagnosis

1. Cholesteatoma, keratosis obturans, medial canal fibrosis, osteoma, and EAC exostosis
2. Malignant otitis externa
3. Malignant neoplasms, such as SCC, melanoma, and metastasis
4. First branchial cleft anomalies
5. Schwannoma of the EAC

Pearls

• The clinical history is very helpful in arriving at the correct diagnosis. Age, gender, duration of symptoms, laterality, and the presence of comorbid conditions should aid greatly in the radiographic evaluation of the conditions affecting the EAC.

Signs and Complications

Whereas most pathologies affecting the EAC are not life-threatening, others, such as SCC and malignant otitis externa, can lead to devastating consequences and even death.

Suggested Readings

Bunch PM, Kelly HR: Cholesteatoma. In Small JE, Noujaim DL, Ginat DT, Kelly HR, Schaefer PW, editors: *Neuroradiology: spectrum and evolution of disease*, Philadelphia, 2018, Elsevier.

Chapman PR, Choudhary G, Singhal A: Skull base osteomyelitis: a comprehensive imaging review, *AJNR Am J Neuroradiol* 42(3):404–413, 2021.

Harnsberger HR, Hudgins P, Wiggins R, et al: *Diagnostic imaging head and neck*, Salt Lake City, 2006, Amirsys.

Harris KC, Conley SF, Kerschner JE: Foreign body granuloma of the external auditory canal, *Pediatrics* 113(4):371–373, 2004.

Mahdyoun P, Pulcini C, Gahide I, et al: Necrotizing otitis externa: a systematic review, *Otol Neurotol* 34(4):620–629, 2013.

Persaud RA, Hajioff DM, Thevasagayam MJ: Keratosis obturans and external ear canal cholesteatoma: how and why we should distinguish between these conditions, *Clin Otolaryngol* 29:577–581, 2007.

Salzman KL, Glastonbury CM, Harnsberger HR: External auditory canal cholesteatoma: clinical and imaging spectrum, *AJNR Am J Neuroradiol* 24(4):751–756, 2003.

Swartz JD, Hagiwara M: Inflammatory diseases of the temporal bone. In Som PM, Curtin HD, editors: *Head and neck imaging*, St Louis, 2011, Mosby.

Topal O, Erbek S, Erbek S: Schwannoma of the external auditory canal: a case report, *Head Face Med* 3:6, 2007.

Tsuno NSG, Tsuno MY, Neto CAFC, et al: Imaging the external ear: practical approach to normal and pathologic conditions, *Radiographics* 42(2):522–540, 2022.

65
Cochlear Promontory Lesions

MAI-LAN HO, MD, PAUL M. BUNCH, MD, AND GUL MOONIS, MD

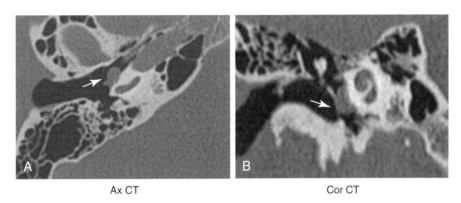

| Ax CT | Cor CT |

CASE A: A 39-year-old female presenting with pulsatile tinnitus. *Ax,* Axial; *Cor,* coronal; *CT,* Computed tomography.

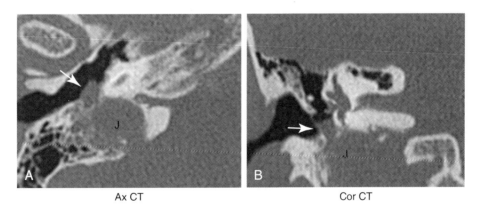

| Ax CT | Cor CT |

CASE B: A 33-year-old female presenting with pulsatile tinnitus. *Ax,* Axial; *Cor,* coronal; *CT,* Computed tomography.

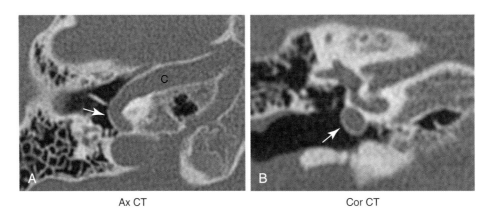

Ax CT   Cor CT

CASE C: A 27-year-old female presenting with otalgia and pulsatile tinnitus. *Ax*, Axial; *Cor*, coronal; *CT*, Computed tomography.

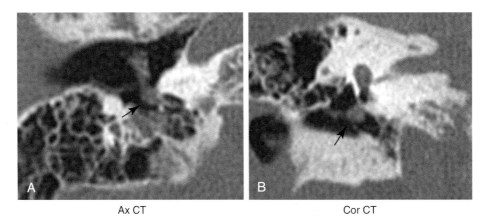

Ax CT   Cor CT

CASE D: A 2-year-old male presenting with otalgia and conductive hearing loss. *Ax*, Axial; *Cor*, coronal; *CT*, Computed tomography.

DESCRIPTION OF FINDINGS

- Case A: CT of the temporal bone demonstrates a soft tissue mass *(arrow)* centered on the cochlear promontory and extending laterally to abut the tympanic membrane. The mass contacts the tip of the malleus manubrium. No communication with the carotid artery or jugular vein is seen.
- Case B: CT of the temporal bone demonstrates an irregular, infiltrative, soft tissue mass centered within the right jugular foramen *(J)*, with superolateral extension *(arrow)* into the right middle ear and mastoid air cells. There is associated permeative bony destruction.
- Case C: CT of the temporal bone demonstrates a so-called "aberrant" course of the right internal carotid artery *(C, arrow)* through the right middle ear. The distal C1 (cervical) segment is absent, with an anomalous connection passing laterally and anteriorly over the cochlear promontory to join the C2 (petrous) segment in the carotid canal. The carotid artery abuts the tip of the malleus manubrium at its lateral aspect.
- Case D: CT of the temporal bone demonstrates a well-circumscribed, rounded, soft tissue opacity *(arrow)* within the middle ear. This opacity projects just posterior and inferior to the cochlear promontory and contacts the tympanic membrane. The auditory ossicles are laterally displaced but intact. The Prussak space and the remainder of the middle ear cavity are spared.

Diagnosis

Case A: Paraganglioma tympanicum
Case B: Jugulotympanic paraganglioma
Case C: Aberrant internal carotid artery
Case D: Congenital cholesteatoma

Summary

Middle ear masses at the cochlear promontory include paraganglioma, aberrant internal carotid artery, and congenital cholesteatoma.

Paragangliomas can involve the middle ear in one of two ways, and the associated terminology is potentially confusing. Historically, head and neck paragangliomas have been referred to by various terms, including glomus tumors and chemodectomas; however, the World Health Organization has indicated that these alternative names should no longer be used. A paraganglioma may originate in the middle ear along the cochlear promontory, in which case it is referred to as a paraganglioma tympanicum (formerly "glomus tympanicum"). Alternatively, a jugular foramen paraganglioma (formerly "glomus jugulare") may secondarily involve the middle ear by direct extension, in which case it is referred to as a jugulotympanic paraganglioma (formerly "glomus jugulotympanicum"). On CT, jugular foramen paragangliomas appear as masses that progressively erode and destroy the surrounding bone, eventually extending into the middle ear. MRI demonstrates T2 hyperintense masses with intense contrast enhancement. Larger lesions (>1 to 2 cm) may demonstrate a "salt and pepper" appearance on T1-weighted imaging, with high-signal foci of subacute hemorrhage or slow flow (salt) and low-signal vascular flow voids (pepper) interspersed within the tumor stroma.

An "aberrant" internal carotid artery refers to the compensatory enlargement of two small arteries—the inferior tympanic artery (a branch of the ascending pharyngeal artery) and the caroticotympanic artery (a branch of the petrous segment of the internal carotid artery)—in the setting of failed development or involution of the cervical (C1) segment of the internal carotid artery. In the absence of the normal cervical (C1) segment of the internal carotid artery, blood flows through an anastomosis between the inferior tympanic and caroticotympanic arteries to reach the horizontal petrous internal carotid artery. Thus, the aberrant vessel enters the middle ear through an enlarged inferior tympanic canaliculus and passes lateral to the cochlear promontory before joining the horizontal portion of the petrous internal carotid artery in the carotid canal. CT and MRI demonstrate a tubular structure coursing laterally through the middle ear cavity from posterior to anterior. Expansion of the inferior tympanic canaliculus occurs, and the normal vertical portion of the petrous carotid canal is absent.

A congenital cholesteatoma or epidermoid cyst represents a collection of desquamated epithelium arising from residual ectodermal rests in the middle ear. These lesions usually are seen in children and present with conductive hearing loss or a white mass behind an intact eardrum in a child with no history of otitis or prior middle ear surgery. Lesions vary in size and invasiveness, depending on the stage of development. They most commonly occur in the middle ear adjacent to the cochlear promontory, but also can be present in the peristapedial region and posterior tympanum; they are rarely present within the mastoid. Growing lesions can rupture and obstruct the eustachian tube and erode the auditory ossicles and surrounding bony walls. Because the lesions are avascular, no contrast enhancement is seen. Cholesteatomas demonstrate restricted diffusion on diffusion-weighted imaging sequences.

Spectrum of Disease

Paragangliomas are benign neoplasms that arise from neural crest derivatives. They can originate in several typical locations, including the cochlear promontory (paraganglioma tympanicum), jugular fossa (jugular paraganglioma; Fig. 65.1), nodose ganglion of the vagus nerve (vagal paraganglioma; Fig. 65.2), carotid body (carotid body paraganglioma; Fig. 65.3), and facial nerve (facial nerve paraganglioma). Contrast enhancement is avid because of hypervascularity. In large lesions (>1 to 2 cm), foci of hemorrhage, slow flow, and vascular flow voids (salt and pepper appearance) may be present, and the presence of permeative bony destruction differentiates a jugular foramen paraganglioma from a schwannoma. Paragangliomas are usually solitary but can be multifocal in conditions such as multiple endocrine neoplasia type IIA/B, neurofibromatosis type 1, von Hippel–Lindau disease, Carney triad (gastrointestinal stromal tumors, pulmonary chondromas, and extraadrenal paragangliomas), and hereditary paraganglioma-pheochromocytoma syndromes.

Differential Diagnosis

1. Paraganglioma
2. Aberrant internal carotid artery
3. Congenital cholesteatoma

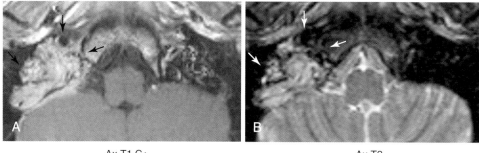

Ax T1 C+   Ax T2

• **Fig. 65.1** Jugular foramen paragangliomas can arise from the jugular bulb at the lateral plate of the jugular fossa. Magnetic resonance images demonstrate a T2 hyperintense, intensely enhancing lesion with internal flow voids *(arrows)* centered in the right jugular fossa and extending posteromedially into the cerebellopontine angle cistern. The anteriormost *arrows* on both images point to the carotid artery. There is surrounding bony destruction and extension into the middle ear. The vector of growth is superolateral, extending into the floor of the middle ear cavity (paraganglioma jugulotympanicum). *Ax,* Axial.

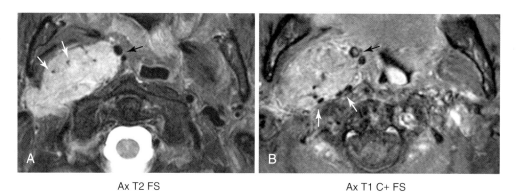

Ax T2 FS   Ax T1 C+ FS

• **Fig. 65.2** Vagal paragangliomas arise from the nodose ganglion of the vagus nerve, 1 to 2 cm below the jugular foramen. Magnetic resonance images show a T2 hyperintense, heterogeneously enhancing mass with internal flow voids *(white arrows)*. This mass originates in the right carotid space (also referred to as the poststyloid parapharyngeal space). Because the vagus nerve is positioned between the internal carotid artery and the internal jugular vein, lesions arising from the vagus nerve will displace the internal carotid artery medially *(black arrows)* and the internal jugular vein laterally. *Ax,* Axial; *FS,* fat saturated.

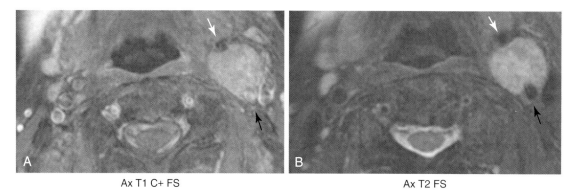

Ax T1 C+ FS   Ax T2 FS

• **Fig. 65.3** Carotid body paragangliomas arise from the carotid body at the common carotid bifurcation. Magnetic resonance images illustrate a T2 hyperintense, avidly enhancing mass that arises from the left carotid bifurcation, just above the level of the hyoid bone. The external carotid artery *(white arrow)* is displaced anteromedially. The internal carotid artery *(black arrow)* is displaced posterolaterally and is partially surrounded by the mass. *Ax,* Axial; *FS,* fat saturated.

Pearls

- Signal: Paragangliomas show increased signal on T2-weighted images, with foci of hemorrhage, slow flow, and vascular flow voids (salt and pepper appearance) in lesions larger than 1 to 2 cm. Cholesteatomas are heterogeneously T2 hyperintense with restricted diffusion.
- Enhancement: Paragangliomas are hypervascular and demonstrate avid contrast enhancement. Cholesteatomas demonstrate no contrast enhancement or only thin rim enhancement.
- Morphology: Cholesteatoma and paraganglioma tympanicum tumors are well-circumscribed lesions. Jugular foramen paragangliomas appear infiltrative with associated bone destruction. An aberrant internal carotid artery is a tubular and curvilinear structure that courses laterally over the cochlear promontory.
- Course: An aberrant internal carotid artery is formed by inferior tympanic and caroticotympanic collateralization to reach the petrous internal carotid artery. The aberrant vessel passes through the middle ear, lateral to the cochlear promontory, before joining the posterolateral margin of the horizontal petrous internal carotid artery. Expansion of the inferior tympanic canaliculus occurs, and the normal carotid foramen and vertical petrous carotid canal are absent.

Signs and Complications

Clinical signs of middle ear pathology include otalgia, conductive hearing loss, and pulsatile tinnitus with vascular lesions. Radiologist recognition of an aberrant internal carotid artery as the cause of a red mass behind the tympanic membrane is of critical importance to avoid catastrophic hemorrhage from biopsy or attempted resection.

Suggested Readings

Cunnane MB: Imaging of tinnitus, *Neuroimaging Clin N Am* 29(1): 49–56, 2019.

Maroldi R, Farina D, Palvarini L, et al: Computed tomography and magnetic resonance imaging of pathologic conditions of the middle ear, *Eur J Radiol* 40(2):78–93, 2001.

McEachen JC, Obrzut M, Bokhari SJ: A rare combination of carotid artery congenital abnormalities: understanding the embryology and clinical associations, *Emerg Radiol* 16(5):411–414, 2009.

Richter GT, Lee KH: Contemporary assessment and management of congenital cholesteatoma, *Curr Opin Otolaryngol Head Neck Surg* 17(5):339–345, 2009.

Shah LM, Wiggins RH 3rd: Imaging of hearing loss, *Neuroimaging Clin N Am* 19(3):287–306, 2009.

Woolen S, Gemmete JJ: Paragangliomas of the head and neck, *Neuroimaging Clin N Am* 26(2):259–278, 2016.

66

Incomplete Partition and Other Cochlear Anomalies

KEVIN D. HIATT, MD

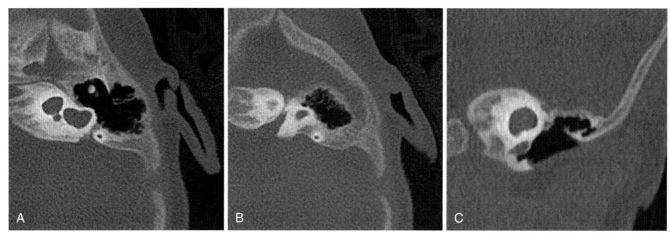

Ax CT   Ax CT   Cor CT

CASE A: A 6-week-old female with sensorineural hearing loss. *Ax*, Axial; *Cor*, coronal; *CT*, Computed tomography.

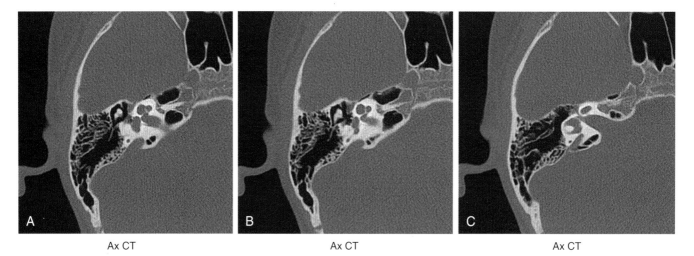

Ax CT   Ax CT   Ax CT

CASE B: A 9-year-old female with sensorineural hearing loss. *Ax*, Axial; *CT*, Computed tomography.

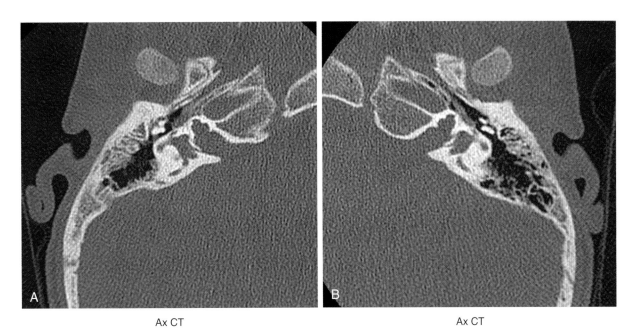

Ax CT   Ax CT

CASE C: A 3-year-old male with mixed hearing loss. *Ax,* Axial; *CT,* Computed tomography.

DESCRIPTION OF FINDINGS

- Case A: The cochlea has a cystic appearance resulting from absence of the modiolus and interscalar septum. The external dimensions of the cochlea are normal. There is also a cystic appearance of the vestibule (seen in image A), which is separate from the cochlea.
- Case B: There is fusion of the apical and middle turns of the cochlea with normal appearance of the basal turn. There is also enlargement of the vestibular aqueduct and mild dilation of the vestibule.
- Case C: There is a corkscrew appearance of the cochlea with present interscalar septum but absent modiolus. The internal auditory canal (IAC) is dilated.

Diagnosis

Case A: Cochlear incomplete partition type I
Case B: Cochlear incomplete partition type II
Case C: Cochlear incomplete partition type III

Summary

Congenital sensorineural hearing loss most commonly results from abnormalities of the membranous labyrinth, which are occult by imaging and include abnormalities of cochlear hair cells. A minority (20% to 40%) exhibit abnormalities of the bony labyrinth that can be identified by CT or MRI. Cochlear malformations can be separated into cochlear hypoplasias and cochlear incomplete partitions. Unlike cochlear hypoplasias, which are thought to exist on a continuum of severity, incomplete partitions represent unique entities that differ in etiopathogenesis. Correctly describing and classifying cochlear malformations is important for directing appropriate management, predicting risk of cerebrospinal fluid (CSF) gusher and facial nerve abnormalities, and predicting underlying genetic mutations.

Imaging assessment of the temporal bones is best accomplished with standardized imaging protocols, including thin slice bone algorithm CT and thin slice T2-weighted steady-state free precession MRI sequences like Fast imaging employing steady-state acquisition (FIESTA) and constructive interference in steady state (CISS). Using a standardized imaging plane (e.g., orienting axial images parallel to the lateral semicircular canal) facilitates comparison between studies.

Assessment of the cochlea on CT should include an evaluation of overall cochlear size, the number and morphology of the cochlear turns, the presence of the interscalar septum, the presence of the modiolus, and the patency and width of the cochlear aperture (Fig. 66.1). MRI offers the clear advantage over CT for nerve assessment (Fig. 66.2).

When approaching cases of suspected cochlear malformation, answering the following questions will help the imaging interpreter choose the correct classification and include information needed for both medical and surgical patient management:
1. *Is the cochlea normal in size?*
2. *Is the cochlea separate from the vestibule?*
3. *Is the modiolus present?*
4. *Is the interscalar septum present? If so, does it fully separate the basal, middle, and apical turns of the cochlea?*
5. *Is the vestibular aqueduct enlarged?*

Regardless of patient age, the cochlear height should measure greater than 4.3 mm (Fig. 66.3). This measurement is performed in the coronal plane. If the cochlea is abnormally small, then the case should be classified as cochlear hypoplasia, rather than incomplete partition.

If the cochlea is inseparable from the vestibule (Fig. 66.4A), then the case should be classified as a common cavity malformation. The incomplete partition classification is reserved for cases where the cochlea is normal in size and separate from the vestibule (Fig. 66.4B).

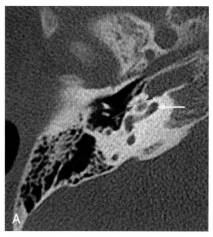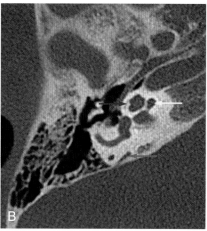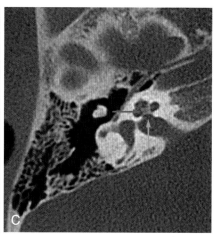

• **Fig. 66.1** (A) An inferior axial slice through the cochlea demonstrates the normal interscalar septum *(red arrows)* clearly separating the middle and apical turns, which are distinct from the basal turn *(yellow arrow)*. (B) More superiorly, the normal interscalar septum is again evident, resulting in a notch at its lateral attachment between the middle and apical turns *(red arrow)*. The normal basal turn of the cochlea *(yellow arrow)* and vestibular aqueduct *(blue arrow)* are also seen on this slice. (C) Further cephalad, the normal modiolus is visualized *(blue arrow)* with the cochlear aperture at its base *(green arrow)* arising at the anteroinferior aspect of the fundus of the internal auditory canal.

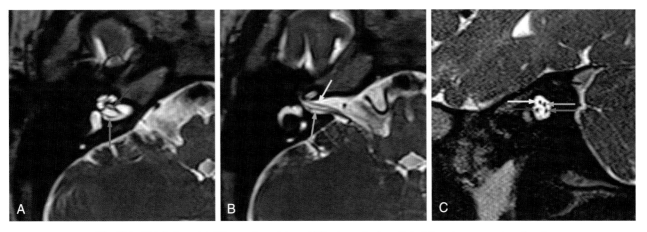

• **Fig. 66.2** (A) Inferior axial, (B) superior axial, and (C) reformatted sagittal oblique images centered on the normal right internal auditory canal (IAC) demonstrate the facial nerve superiorly and anteriorly *(yellow arrows)*, the cochlear nerve inferiorly and anteriorly *(red arrows)*, and the superior and inferior vestibular nerves posteriorly (*green and blue arrows*, respectively).

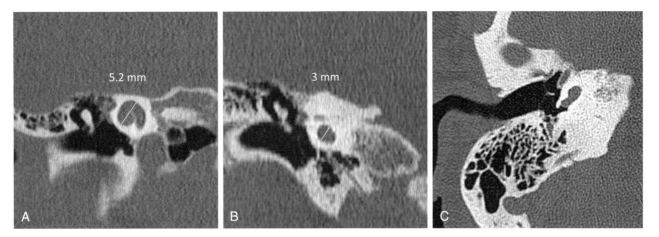

• **Fig. 66.3** (A) Normal cochlear height, as measured on a coronal image from Case B. (B) Decreased cochlear height in a patient with right cochlear hypoplasia. In the same patient with right cochlear hypoplasia, (C) the axial image demonstrates a flattened appearance of the apical portion of the hypoplastic right cochlea.

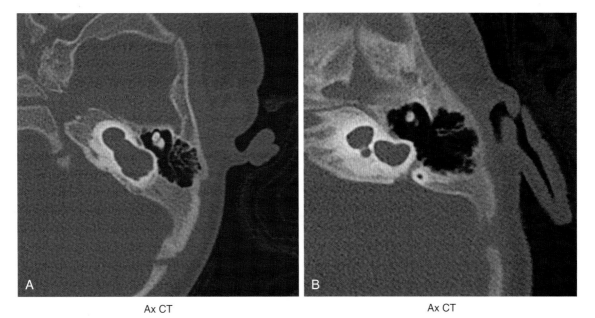

Ax CT   Ax CT

• **Fig. 66.4** (A) Fused left cochlea and vestibule in a patient with common cavity malformation. (B) Separate left cochlea and vestibule in a patient with left cochlear incomplete partition type I. *Ax,* Axial; *CT,* Computed tomography. (A, Courtesy Benjamin Huang, MD, University of North Carolina School of Medicine.)

Cochlear incomplete partition type I (IP-I), also called cystic cochleovestibular malformation, results from failure of formation of the modiolus and interscalar septum, resulting in a single cochlear cavity that is similar in external dimensions to a normally formed cochlea. The lamina cribrosa (at the base of the modiolus) is deficient, leading to a gaping communication between the cochlea and internal auditory canal (IAC). This defect allows for an anomalous communication between the subarachnoid space in the IAC and the perilymphatic fluid in the cochlea. The vestibule is usually markedly dilated but remains separate from the cochlea, leading to a "figure 8" appearance of these two adjacent structures. In addition, the stapes footplate is characteristically defective, allowing communication between the cochlea and middle ear through the oval window.

Cochlear incomplete partition type II (IP-II) results from deficiency of the apical portions of the modiolus and interscalar septum, leading to fusion of the middle and apical turns with normal separation of the basal turn. These abnormalities produce a characteristic "baseball cap" appearance of the cochlea (Fig. 66.5). Importantly, this appearance should not be described as a cochlea with one and a half turns, as this description is reserved for cochlear hypoplasia. IP-II is usually associated with an enlarged vestibular aqueduct (due to an enlarged endolymphatic duct and sac) and mild dilation of the vestibule. The presence of all three of these findings has historically been referred to as the "Mondini triad" or "Mondini malformation;" however, these eponymous terms are no longer preferred. As measured in the axial plane, the vestibular aqueduct should measure no greater than 0.9 mm at the midpoint or 1.9 mm at the operculum. As measured in the

Pöschl plane, the midpoint should also measure no greater than 0.9 mm.

The morphologic diagnosis of IP-II can be challenging on MRI because a band of low signals representing the dysplastic spiral lamina–basilar membrane neural complex extending from the lateral modiolus to the lateral wall of the cochlea can mimic the normal lateral attachment of the interscalar septum. However, in IP-II, the distance ("distance X") between the osseous spiral lamina–basilar membrane complex of the upper basal turn and the first T2 hypointense linear band (in normal circumstances corresponding to the interscalar septum separating the middle and apical turns; in IP-II corresponding to the dysplastic osseous spiral lamina–basilar membrane neural complex) is abnormally increased (Fig. 66.6). An abnormal distance X is defined as ≥ 1.2 mm on axial images oriented parallel to the lateral semicircular canal.

Cochlear incomplete partition type III (IP-III), also known as X-linked deafness and X-linked stapes gusher, is a genetic inner ear malformation (X-linked recessive inheritance) with characteristic findings including absence of the modiolus, a thin otic capsule, and bulbous appearance of the IAC (Fig. 66.7). The lamina cribrosa is deficient, similar to IP-I. Though the modiolus is absent, the interscalar septum forms normally, resulting in a characteristic appearance of the cochlea unique to IP-III. Though an abnormally thin otic capsule develops, endosteal development is preserved, which includes formation of a normal stapes footplate (unlike IP-I). The labyrinthine segment of the facial nerve typically takes an abnormal course superior to the cochlea.

In IP-I, the cochlear nerve may be hypoplastic or absent. The cochlear aperture should normally measure at least 2 mm

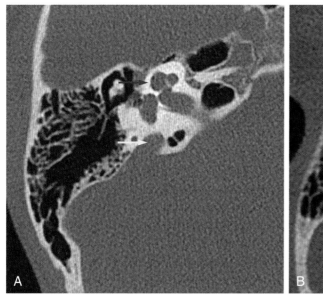
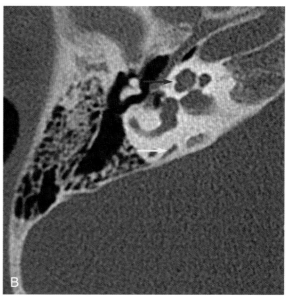

Ax CT   Ax CT

• **Fig. 66.5** (A) Absent apical portion of the interscalar septum (and modiolus) from case B. Note the convex lateral margin of the fused middle and apical turns producing the characteristic "baseball cap" appearance of the left cochlea *(red arrow)*. Note that the vestibular aqueduct is also enlarged *(yellow arrow)*. (B) For comparison, image B demonstrates the normal appearance of the interscalar septum, which results in a notched appearance laterally between the middle and apical turns of the cochlea *(red arrow)*. The vestibular aqueduct is also normal *(yellow arrow)*. *Ax,* Axial; *CT,* Computed tomography.

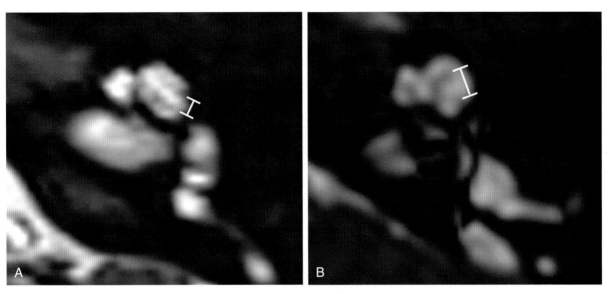

• **Fig. 66.6** (A) Normal cochlear partitioning demonstrated on an axial thin section, T2-weighted steady-state free precession MR image, with distance X measuring 0.9 mm. (B) Abnormally increased distance X, measuring 1.7 mm, in a patient with cochlear incomplete partition type II. (B, Courtesy Asha Sarma, MD, Vanderbilt University School of Medicine.)

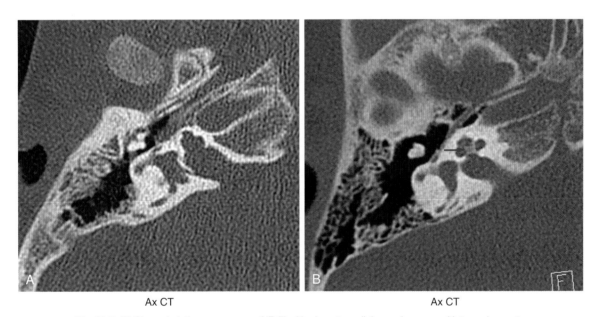

Ax CT   Ax CT

• **Fig. 66.7** (A) Characteristic appearance of IP-III with absent modiolus and preserved interscalar septum producing a "corkscrew cochlea." (B) For comparison, image B demonstrates the normal appearance of the modiolus *(red arrow)*. *Ax,* Axial; *CT,* Computed tomography.

in diameter (Fig. 66.8). Stenosis or absence of the cochlear aperture is concerning for cochlear nerve hypoplasia or aplasia and should prompt MR imaging to assess the status of the cochlear nerve. If the cochlear nerve is absent, a cochlear implant will not be effective, and an auditory brainstem implant should instead be considered.

Spectrum of Disease

The cochlear incomplete partitions are *not* a spectrum of a single disease; rather, they are distinct entities with different

genetic associations and different developmental pathogenesis. IP-I has no known genetic cause and is thought to result from abnormal vascular supply traveling through the IAC. IP-II has been linked to *SLC26A* mutations. The *SLC26A* gene encodes the protein pendrin, and *SLC26A* pathogenic variants can also cause Pendred syndrome, which is characterized by sensorineural hearing loss, goiter, and enlarged vestibular aqueduct. A proposed mechanism for IP-II is increased endolymphatic pressure transmitted to the cochlea and vestibule during development as a result of an enlarged endolymphatic sac and duct, though this mechanism is not universally agreed upon. IP-III

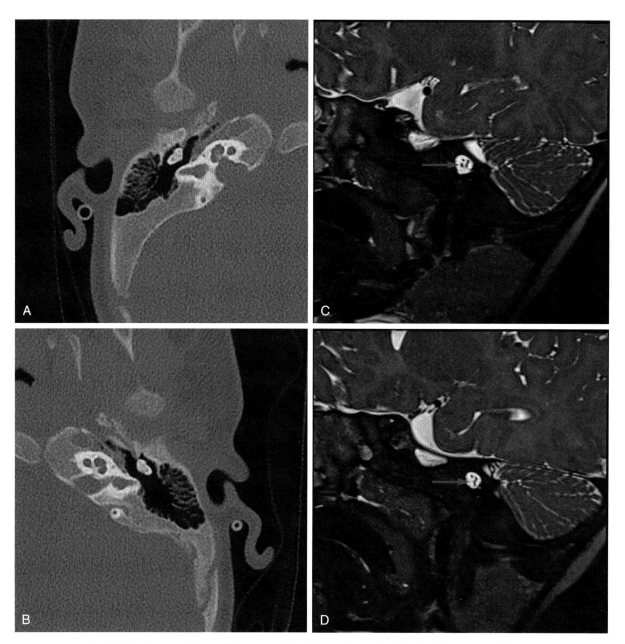

• **Fig. 66.8** Axial temporal bone CT images obtained from a 3-month-old male with profound left senso-rineural hearing loss and normal hearing in the right ear demonstrate (A) a normal cochlear aperture on the right and (B) a markedly stenotic cochlear aperture on the left. Sagittal oblique T2-weighted steady-state free precession images of the (C) right and (D) left internal auditory canals demonstrate the normal right cochlear nerve (C, *red arrow*) and absent left cochlear nerve (D, *red arrow*).

has been linked to *POU3F4* and *COL4A6* mutations. IP-III is thought to result from abnormal vascular supply from the middle ear mucosa.

Differential Diagnosis

The primary differential considerations for IP-I are common cavity malformation and cochlear hypoplasia. Although the cochlea and vestibule are cystic in appearance in both IP-I and common cavity malformation, they are clearly separate from each other in IP-I, creating a "figure 8" appearance, and form a single cavity in common cavity malformation. The external

dimensions of the cochlea (including cochlear height >4.3 mm) should be normal in IP-I, but abnormally small in cochlear hypoplasia.

The primary differential consideration for IP-II is cochlear hypoplasia. The external dimensions of the cochlea should be normal in IP-II, but abnormally small in cochlear hypoplasia. Branchio-oto-renal (BOR) syndrome often demonstrates dysmorphic, abnormally segmented middle and apical cochlear turns. An unwound cochlear morphology with abnormally increased separation of the middle and basal turns laterally is pathognomonic for the *EYA1* genotype of BOR (Fig. 66.9), whereas patients with the *SIX1* genotype typically have a

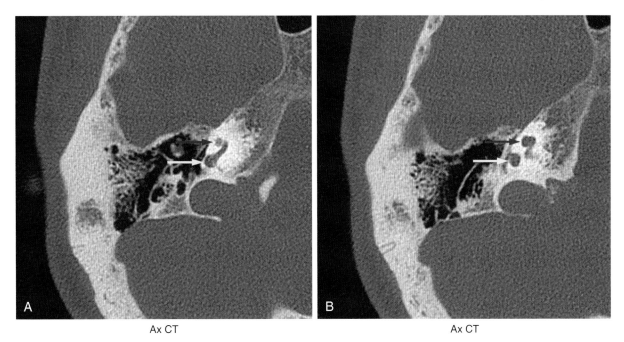

Ax CT   Ax CT

• **Fig. 66.9** (A and B) Unwound appearance of the right cochlea in a 36-year-old male with branchio-oto-renal syndrome. Note the increased separation between the basal *(yellow arrows)* and middle *(red arrows)* turns. *Ax,* Axial; *CT,* Computed tomography.

shortened, irregular appearance of the apical turn without abnormal separation of the middle and basal turns.

IP-III has a unique imaging appearance, for which there is no differential diagnosis (Table 66.1).

Pearls

- A cochlear incomplete partition *must* have normal external cochlear dimensions, and the cochlea *must* be separate from the vestibule. The cochlear height should measure >4.3 mm.
- IP-I results in an empty cochlea with a "figure 8" appearance of the cochlea and dilated vestibule.
- IP-II results in fusion of the middle and apical turns of the cochlea, commonly paired with an enlarged vestibular aqueduct and mildly dilated vestibule.

- IP-III results in an absent modiolus and thinned otic capsule.

Signs and Complications

The risk for meningitis and spontaneous CSF leak is increased with a defective stapes footplate and therefore greater in IP-I than in IP-II or IP-III. The defective lamina cribrosa in IP-I and IP-III allows an anomalous communication between CSF (in the IAC) and perilymphatic fluid and places patients at high risk for CSF gusher during stapedotomy or cochlear implantation. Enlarged vestibular aqueduct is a minor risk factor for CSF gusher, and IP-II patients more commonly have oozing of perilymphatic fluid rather than gusher during these procedures.

TABLE 66.1 Differentiating Features, Complications, and Genetics of Cochlear Incomplete Partitions (IPs)

	Modiolus	Lamina Cribrosa	Interscalar Septum	Stapes Footplate	Vestibule	Vestibular Aqueduct	Risk for CSF Gusher	Risk for Meningitis and CSF Leak	Cochlear Nerve	Genetic Associations
IP-I	Absent	Deficient	Absent	Deficient	Markedly dilated	Not enlarged	+++	+++	Possibly absent	None known
IP-II	Deficient at apex	Intact	Deficient at apex	Intact	Usually mildly dilated	Often enlarged	+	+	Present	SLC26A
IP-III	Absent	Deficient	Normal	Intact	Often dilated	Not enlarged	+++	+	Present	POU3F4 COL4A6

Suggested Readings

Boston M, Halsted M, Meinzen-Derr J, et al: The large vestibular aqueduct: a new definition based on audiologic and computed tomography correlation, *Otolaryngol Head Neck Surg* 136(6):972–977, 2007.

D'Arco F, Sanverdi E, O'Brien WT, et al: The link between inner ear malformations and the rest of the body: what we know so far about genetic, imaging and histology, *Neuroradiology* 62(5):539–544, 2020.

Hsu A, Desai N, Paldino MJ: The unwound cochlea: a specific imaging marker of branchio-oto-renal syndrome, *AJNR Am J Neuroradiol* 39(12):2345–2349, 2018.

Juliano AF, Ting EY, Mingkwansook V, et al: Vestibular aqueduct measurements in the 45° oblique (Pöschl) plane, *AJNR Am J Neuroradiol* 37(7):1331–1337, 2016.

Mazón M, Pont E, Montoya-Filardi A, et al: Inner ear malformations: a practical diagnostic approach, *Radiologia* 59(4):297–305, 2017.

Pao J, D'Arco F, Clement E, et al: Re-examining the cochlea in branchio-oto-renal syndrome: genotype-phenotype correlation, *AJNR Am J Neuroradiol* 43(2):309–314, 2022.

Reinshagen KL, Curtin HD, Quesnel AM, et al: Measurement for detection of incomplete partition type II anomalies on MR imaging, *AJNR Am J Neuroradiol* 38(10):2003–2007, 2017.

Sennaroğlu L: Histopathology of inner ear malformations: do we have enough evidence to explain pathophysiology?, *Cochlear Implants Int* 17(1):3–20, 2016.

Sennaroğlu L, Bajin MD: Classification and current management of inner ear malformations, *Balkan Med J* 34(5):397–411, 2017.

67
Lucent Otic Capsule Lesions

BHAVANA BUDIGI, MBBS, MD AND PAUL M. BUNCH, MD

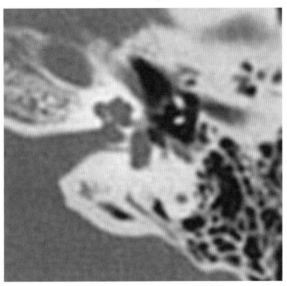

Ax CT bone

CASE A: A 51-year-old female with progressive left conductive hearing loss. *Ax*, Axial; *CT*, Computed tomography.

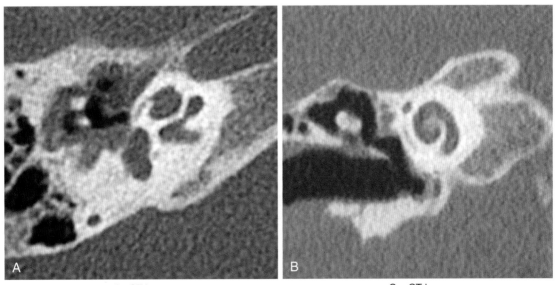

Ax CT bone   Cor CT bone

CASE B: A 3-year-old male imaged for suspected otomastoiditis. *Ax*, Axial; *Cor*, coronal; *CT*, Computed tomography.

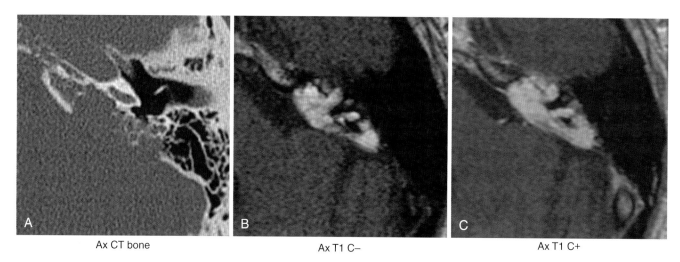

Ax CT bone

CASE C: A 79-year-old male imaged for right temporal bone fracture. *Ax,* Axial; *CT,* Computed tomography.

Ax CT bone   Ax T1 C−   Ax T1 C+

CASE D: A 41-year-old female presenting with tinnitus and left hearing loss. *Ax,* Axial; *CT,* Computed tomography.

DESCRIPTION OF FINDINGS

- Case A: Axial CT image of the left temporal bone demonstrates focal lucency along the anterior aspect of the oval window in the region of the fissula ante fenestram.
- Case B: Axial and coronal CT images of the right temporal bone demonstrate a curvilinear lucency in the otic capsule that parallels the basal turn of the cochlea, anterior to the oval window (axial image), and medial to the cochleariform process (coronal image).
- Case C: Axial CT image of the left temporal bone demonstrates a small focal lucency along the anteroinferior aspect of the internal auditory canal.
- Case D: Axial CT image of the left temporal bone demonstrates an infiltrative, destructive, lucent lesion centered along the posterior petrous ridge in the expected location of the endolymphatic sac. Corresponding axial T1-weighted pre- and postcontrast magnetic resonance (MR) images demonstrate areas of intrinsic T1 hyperintensity and other areas of superimposed enhancement, respectively.

Diagnosis

Case A: Fenestral otospongiosis
Case B: Cochlear cleft
Case C: Internal auditory canal diverticulum
Case D: Endolymphatic sac tumor

Summary

Lucent lesions involving the otic capsule may represent normal variants (e.g., cochlear cleft) or result from a variety of pathologic processes, including primary bone disorders (e.g., otospongiosis) and neoplasm (e.g., endolymphatic sac tumor). Knowledge of temporal bone anatomy and careful attention to the anatomic site(s) of lucent lesion involvement will often facilitate a confident diagnosis, as the different processes underlying these lucent lesions exhibit predilections for specific sites within the petrous temporal bone.

For example, otospongiosis (also referred to as otosclerosis) almost always begins along the anterior aspect of the oval window (Fig. 67.1) in the region of the fissula ante fenestram, which is a small cleft in the otic capsule that is filled with connective tissue and typically not visible on CT. Endolymphatic sac tumors arise along the posterior petrous ridge within the endolymphatic duct and sac (Fig. 67.1). Internal auditory canal diverticula affects the anteroinferior aspect of the internal auditory canal, and a cochlear cleft parallels the basal turn of the cochlea. Radiologists familiar with the normal appearance of these respective structures are more likely to detect associated pathology when it is encountered.

Spectrum of Disease

Otospongiosis

Otospongiosis refers to a progressive primary bone disease resulting from abnormal bone resorption and deposition. Although osteoclastic resorption and osteoblastic deposition are normal processes that allow for remodeling of most bones, this kind of osteoclastic and osteoblastic activity is abnormal within the otic capsule. The active, vascular, spongiotic phase

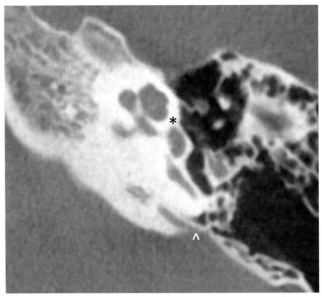

Ax CT bone

• **Fig. 67.1** Axial CT image of a normal left temporal bone demonstrates the location *(*)* where otospongiosis almost always begins along the anterior aspect of the oval window in the region of the fissula ante fenestram. The image also demonstrates the expected location of the endolymphatic sac *(^)*, which is the site of origin of endolymphatic sac tumors. *Ax,* Axial; *CT,* Computed tomography.

is characterized by abnormal osteoclast activity, which ultimately results in the lucent appearance of otospongiosis on CT. The vascular nature of the spongiotic phase can manifest on otoscopy as a reddish or pinkish discoloration overlying the oval window and cochlear promontory (Schwartze sign) and on MRI as an area of focal enhancement (Fig. 67.2).

The inactive, sclerotic phase is characterized by the predominance of osteoblasts, ultimately resulting in obliteration by bone of the dilated vascular spaces from the spongiotic phase. The sclerotic phase may be more difficult to detect on CT in the absence of the characteristic lucency; however, otic capsule thickness >2.3 mm is a sensitive and specific indicator of otospongiosis (Fig. 67.3). In this context, otic capsule thickness is defined as the distance between the posterolateral margin of the junction of the basal and middle turns of the cochlea and the apex of the convex contour of the otic capsule at the level of the cochleariform process and anterior margin of the oval window. Otic capsule thickness should be measured on axial images reformatted parallel to the plane of the lateral semicircular canal.

Otospongiosis almost always (95+%) begins in a characteristic location along the anterior aspect of the oval window in the region of the fissula ante fenestram, as shown in Case A and Fig. 67.2. Disease limited to this locale is classified as "fenestral" otospongiosis and produces conductive hearing loss secondary to fixation of the adjacent stapes footplate. The disease may progress to involve additional otic capsule sites (e.g., perichlear) beyond the region of the fissula ante fenestram, in which case the disease is classified as "retrofenestral" otospongiosis (Fig. 67.4). Typically coexisting with fenestral otospongiosis, retrofenestral disease may produce sensorineural or

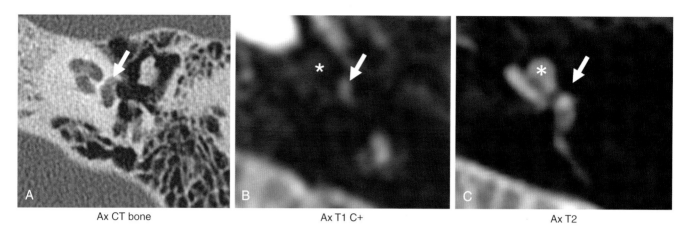

Ax CT bone   Ax T1 C+   Ax T2

• **Fig. 67.2** Axial CT image of the left temporal bone (A) demonstrates fenestral otospongiosis *(arrow)*. Corresponding axial T1-weighted, gadolinium-enhanced image (B) of the brain demonstrates a small focus of enhancement *(arrow)* corresponding to the fenestral otospongiosis seen on CT and consistent with the active, vascular, spongiotic phase. The cochlea is denoted with an *asterisk* in B. For purpose of orientation, an axial T2-weighted image (C) of the brain is also provided with the cochlea denoted by the *asterisk* and the anterior margin of the oval window by the *arrow*. *Ax*, Axial; *CT*, Computed tomography.

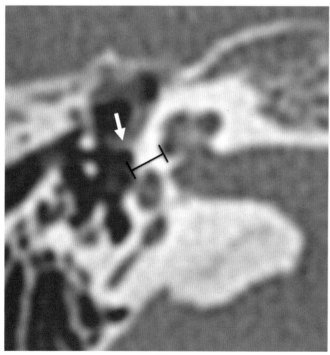

Ax CT bone

• **Fig. 67.3** Axial CT image of the right temporal bone at the level of the cochleariform process *(arrow)* and oval window demonstrates abnormally increased otic capsule thickness (2.6 mm) in this 49-year-old female patient with surgically proven fenestral otospongiosis. Absence of lucency on CT indicates the sclerotic phase of the disease. *Ax*, Axial; *CT*, Computed tomography.

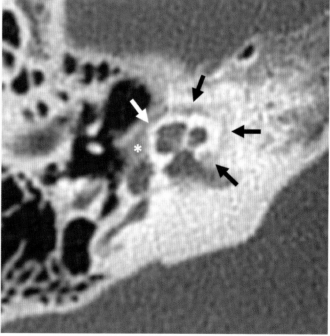

Ax CT bone

• **Fig. 67.4** Axial CT image of the right temporal bone demonstrates pericochlear lucency *(white and black arrows)* consistent with retrofenestral otospongiosis. Fenestral disease *(*)* is also present. *Ax*, Axial; *CT*, Computed tomography.

mixed hearing loss as well as vestibular symptoms, depending on the sites of retrofenestral involvement.

The second most common site (~30%) of otospongiosis involvement is the round window (Fig. 67.5), and isolated round window disease is occasionally seen. Round window involvement is important to identify for the otologist because it may decrease the effectiveness of a stapes prosthesis to treat

conductive hearing loss and may complicate the placement of a cochlear implant in the setting of profound sensorineural hearing loss.

Cochlear Cleft

Cochlear cleft refers to a thin curvilinear area of pericochlear hypoattenuation located just anterior to the oval window and

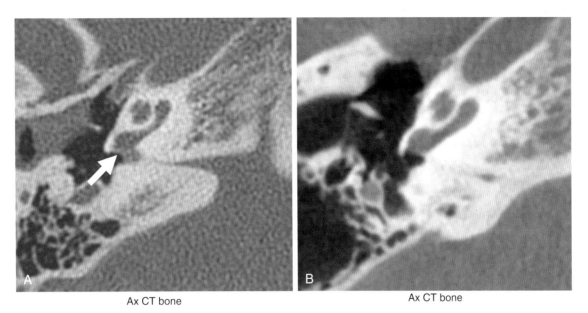

Ax CT bone   Ax CT bone

• **Fig. 67.5** Axial CT image of (A) the right temporal bone demonstrates obliteration of the round window by otospongiosis *(arrow)*. For comparison, the normal appearance of the round window is shown in (B). *Ax,* Axial; *CT,* Computed tomography.

paralleling the basal turn of the cochlea. On coronal CT images, the cochlear cleft typically extends superiorly to the level of the cochleariform process (Fig. 67.6). On histopathology, the cochlear cleft corresponds to residual fatty marrow in the setting of incomplete ossification. The cochlear cleft represents a "do not touch" finding of no clinical significance. Whereas otospongiosis is rare among pediatric patients, the cochlear cleft is commonly seen in young children (~40%), but may persist into adulthood. Unlike otospongiosis, the cochlear cleft

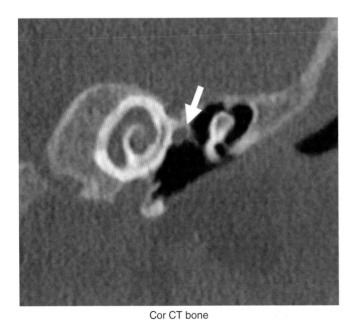

Cor CT bone

• **Fig. 67.6** Coronal CT image obtained in a 4-month-old male demonstrates the typical appearance of the cochlear cleft, which extends superiorly to the level of the cochleariform process *(arrow)*. *Cor,* Coronal; *CT,* Computed tomography.

does not produce thickening or expansion of the otic capsule at the anterior margin of the oval window.

Internal Auditory Canal Diverticulum

Internal auditory canal diverticula are well-demarcated, focal lucencies along the anteroinferior aspect of the internal auditory canal fundus. Internal auditory canal diverticula most commonly occur in isolation (~5% of adults and ~15% of children), and isolated internal auditory canal diverticula are considered a normal anatomic variant of no clinical significance. However, internal auditory canal diverticula have also been identified in >30% of otospongiotic temporal bones (Fig. 67.7), suggesting a predilection for otospongiosis to involve the anteroinferior aspect of the internal auditory canal fundus in addition to the region of the fissula ante fenestram. As such, it is worth looking for clinical and imaging evidence of otospongiosis before concluding that a finding represents an isolated internal auditory canal diverticulum.

Endolymphatic Sac Tumor

Endolymphatic sac tumor is an aggressive papillary adenomatous neoplasm that originates from the epithelium of the endolymphatic sac and duct. Clinical symptoms commonly include gradual-onset, low-frequency hearing loss, tinnitus, and vertigo. Labyrinthine hemorrhage can be a presenting manifestation of endolymphatic sac tumor, in which case there may be an acute onset of clinical symptoms. Location along the endolymphatic sac and duct is characteristic. On CT, endolymphatic sac tumors exhibit an aggressive, infiltrative, erosive appearance. On MRI, intrinsic T1 hyperintensity and magnetic susceptibility effect are typical (Fig. 67.8), both relating to intralesional hemorrhage within this vascular neoplasm. Although sporadic

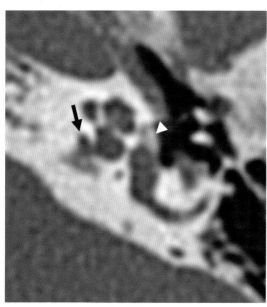

Ax CT bone

• **Fig. 67.7** Axial CT image of the left temporal bone obtained in a 41-year-old male with conductive hearing loss demonstrates an internal auditory canal diverticulum *(arrow)* in the setting of fenestral otospongiosis *(arrowhead)*. *Ax*, Axial; *CT*, Computed tomography.

tumors are more common, these lesions may also occur in the setting of von Hippel–Lindau syndrome. As such, careful attention to the endolymphatic sac and duct on surveillance imaging of von Hippel–Lindau patients is prudent.

Differential Diagnosis

1. Attention to the anatomic site(s) of involvement is often sufficient for differentiating among the lucent otic capsule lesions discussed in this chapter; however, there are a few differential considerations worth mentioning.

2. For example, osteogenesis imperfecta, Paget disease, and other disorders of bone may cause abnormal lucency within the otic capsule that may appear similar to otospongiosis. However, these diseases typically exhibit more extensive involvement of the temporal bone (or beyond) and have no predilection for the region of the fissula ante fenestram that is characteristic of otospongiosis.

3. Glomus jugulare paragangliomas can exhibit permeative and destructive osseous changes similar to those seen with endolymphatic sac tumors and may involve the otic capsule by direct extension. However, these paragangliomas are centered in the jugular foramen rather than along the endolymphatic sac. Meningiomas may occur along the posterior petrous ridge, but intralesional hemorrhage and lytic osseous changes would not be expected.

Pearls

• Location, location, location—careful attention to sites(s) of involvement informs the diagnosis of lucent otic capsule lesions.

• Otospongiosis almost always begins anterior to the oval window in the region of the fissula ante fenestram, but the round window (second most common site of involvement) should also be included in the search pattern, given the surgical implications.

• In isolation, internal auditory canal diverticula may be considered a normal variant of no clinical significance. However, careful scrutiny for associated otospongiosis is prudent.

• Thin curvilinear hypoattenuation paralleling the basal turn of the cochlea is characteristic of cochlear cleft, a normal variant most commonly seen in young children.

• Scrutinize the endolymphatic sac and duct when interpreting surveillance imaging of von Hippel–Lindau patients.

• Consider endolymphatic sac tumor as an underlying cause of labyrinthine hemorrhage.

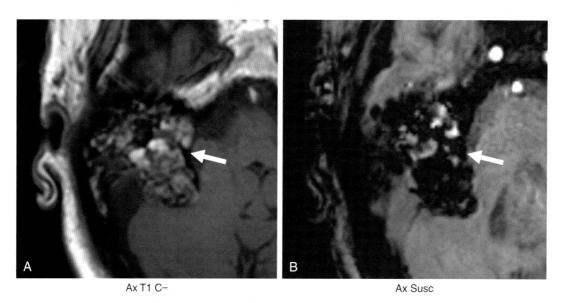

Ax T1 C–   Ax Susc

• **Fig. 67.8** Axial T1-weighted, unenhanced (A) and susceptibility weighted (B) magnetic resonance images demonstrate intrinsic T1 hyperintensity and magnetic susceptibility effect in a right endolymphatic sac tumor *(arrows)* due to intralesional hemorrhage. *Ax*, Axial; *Susc*, susceptibility weighted.

Signs and Complications

Diagnosis		Location	Imaging Characteristics	Clinical Features
Otospongiosis	Fenestral	Anterior to the oval window in the region of the fissula ante fenestram	Spongiotic phase—ill-defined lucency	Conductive hearing loss
	Retrofenestral	Pericochlear, most commonly	Sclerotic phase—difficult to detect with CT because approximates the density of normal bone, increased otic capsule thickness a clue to diagnosis	Sensorineural or mixed hearing loss
Cochlear cleft		Parallels the basal turn of the cochlea between the cochleariform process and the anterior aspect of the oval window	Thin curvilinear hypoattenuation. No thickening or expansion	Asymptomatic normal variant
Internal auditory canal diverticulum		Anteroinferior aspect of the internal auditory canal	Focal, well-defined lucency	Asymptomatic normal variant in isolation
Endolymphatic sac tumor		Endolymphatic sac (along the posterior petrous ridge)	CT—infiltrative, destructive, lucent lesion MR—intrinsic T1 hyperintensity and magnetic susceptibility artifact from intralesional hemorrhage	Hearing loss, vertigo, tinnitus. Although more commonly gradual and progressive, acute symptoms may occur in the setting of labyrinthine hemorrhage.

Suggested Readings

Bunch PM, Zapadka ME, Lack CM, et al: Internal auditory canal diverticula among pediatric patients: prevalence and assessment for hearing loss and anatomic associations, *AJNR Am J Neuroradiol* 41(9):1712–1717, 2020.

Chadwell JB, Halsted MJ, Choo DI, et al: The cochlear cleft, *AJNR Am J Neuroradiol* 25(1):21–24, 2004.

Curtin HD: Imaging of conductive hearing loss with a normal tympanic membrane, *AJR Am J Roentgenol* 206(1):49–56, 2016.

Jagannathan J, Butman JA, Lonser RR, et al: Endolymphatic sac tumor demonstrated by intralabyrinthine hemorrhage, *J Neurosurg* 107(2):421–425, 2007.

Juliano AF, Ginat DT, Moonis G: Imaging review of the temporal bone: part II. Traumatic, postoperative and noninflammatory nonneoplastic conditions, *Radiology* 276(3):655–672, 2015.

Mihal DC, Feng Y, Kodet ML, et al: Isolated internal auditory canal diverticula: a normal anatomic variant not associated with sensorineural hearing loss, *AJNR Am J Neuroradiol* 39(12):2340–2344, 2018.

Puac P, Rodriguez A, Lin HC, et al: Cavitary plaques in otospongiosis: CT findings and clinical implications, *AJNR Am J Neuroradiol* 39(6):1135–1139, 2018.

Pucetaite M, Quesnel AM, Juliano AF, et al: The cochlear cleft: CT correlation with histopathology, *Otol Neurotol* 41(6):745–749, 2020.

Reinshagen KL, Kelly HR: Otospongiosis. In Small JE, Noujaim DL, Ginat DT, Kelly HR, Schaefer PW, editors: *Neuroradiology: spectrum and evolution of disease*. ed 1, Philadelphia, PA: Elsevier, 363–368, 2018.

Sanghan N, Chansakul T, Kozin ED, et al: Retrospective review of otic capsule contour and thickness in patients with otosclerosis and individuals with normal hearing on CT, *AJNR Am J Neuroradiol* 39(12):2350–2355, 2018.

68

Lesions of the Facial Nerve

MAI-LAN HO, MD, PAUL M. BUNCH, MD, AND GUL MOONIS, MD

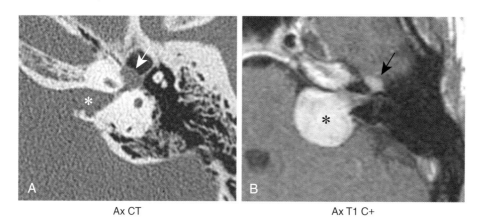

| Ax CT | Ax T1 C+ |

CASE A: A 51-year-old male presenting with facial weakness and sensorineural hearing loss. *Ax,* Axial; *CT,* Computed tomography.

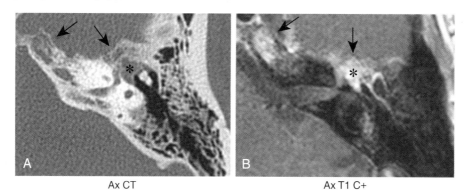

| Ax CT | Ax T1 C+ |

CASE B: A 39-year-old female presenting with otalgia and facial palsy. *Ax,* Axial; *CT,* Computed tomography.

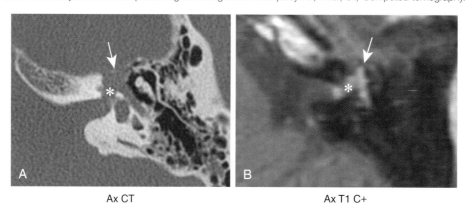

| Ax CT | Ax T1 C+ |

CASE C: A 67-year-old male with a parotid malignancy and progressive facial paralysis. *Ax,* Axial; *CT,* Computed tomography.

DESCRIPTION OF FINDINGS

- Case A: CT of the temporal bone demonstrates smooth expansion of the left internal auditory canal *(asterisk)*, with extension into the labyrinthine segment and geniculate ganglion *(arrow)* of the facial nerve. T1-weighted postcontrast MRI shows a homogeneously enhancing mass *(asterisk)* involving the left cerebellopontine angle cistern, the internal auditory canal, and the intracanalicular, labyrinthine, and geniculate *(arrow)* segments of the facial nerve.
- Case B: CT of the temporal bone demonstrates irregular bone along the labyrinthine segment, anterior genu, and proximal tympanic *(asterisk)* portions of the left facial nerve. Associated expansion, thickening, and sclerosis of the adjacent tegmen tympani and petrous air cells *(arrows)* is noted, producing a "speckled bone" appearance. T1-weighted postcontrast MRI demonstrates corresponding heterogeneous enhancement of the labyrinthine, geniculate, and proximal tympanic segments *(asterisk)* of the left facial nerve and the adjacent bone. Enhancement is also present in the tegmen tympani and petrous apex *(arrows)* with associated dural thickening.
- Case C: CT of the temporal bone depicts asymmetric expansion of the tympanic, geniculate, labyrinthine *(asterisk)*, and lateral intracanalicular segments of the left facial nerve. There is also expansion of the left facial hiatus *(arrow)*. T1-weighted postcontrast MRI shows corresponding enhancement of the involved facial nerve segments *(asterisk)* and extension to the facial hiatus *(arrow)*.

Diagnosis

Case A: Facial nerve schwannoma
Case B: Facial nerve venous malformation
Case C: Perineural spread of tumor (adenoid cystic carcinoma)

Summary

Facial nerve lesions of the middle and inner ear may be primary or secondary. Primary facial nerve lesions include schwannomas, venous malformations, neurofibromas, epidermoids, and paragangliomas (glomus faciale). Secondary lesions may result from perineural or hematogenous dissemination of malignancy. Perineural extension into the facial canal is most commonly seen with parotid and cutaneous malignancies. Hematogenous spread may occur with leukemic infiltration or metastatic carcinoma.

Schwannomas are benign encapsulated tumors of Schwann cells, which surround the peripheral portion of the facial nerve. These tumors most frequently originate from the geniculate ganglion, but they can arise anywhere along the course of the facial nerve and often involve multiple contiguous segments. CT shows smooth fusiform enlargement of the facial canal. Extension into the middle cranial fossa, middle ear cavity, and mastoid air cells can be seen with involvement of the greater superficial petrosal nerve, tympanic segment, and mastoid segment of the facial nerve, respectively. On MRI, lesions are T1 hypointense to isointense and T2 hyperintense. Smaller lesions typically enhance homogeneously, whereas larger lesions may demonstrate internal heterogeneity as a result of cystic changes.

Venous malformations of the facial nerve (previously hemangioma) are benign, nonencapsulated lesions that arise from anastomotic perineural vessels within the temporal bone. They can arise in the bone adjacent to the nerve and invade the nerve secondarily, or they can arise along the nerve itself. These lesions occur most commonly in the region of the geniculate fossa and less frequently in the internal auditory canal or posterior genu of the facial nerve. Capillary, cavernous, and ossifying histologies have been described. On CT, facial nerve venous malformations appear amorphous with spiculated margins and reactive osteitis, producing a "honeycomb" or speckled matrix. MRI demonstrates a poorly circumscribed, irregular mass with a mixed T1 and high T2 signal, as well as avid heterogeneous contrast enhancement.

Perineural spread of tumor has been described in persons with adenoid cystic carcinoma, squamous cell carcinoma, mucoepidermoid carcinoma, non-Hodgkin lymphoma, rhabdomyosarcoma, melanoma, and other malignancies. Common primary sites include the parotid gland and skin. Disease from the parotid gland first passes through the stylomastoid foramen to involve the distal mastoid portion of the facial nerve. Over time, the tumor extends into more proximal segments of the facial nerve and may ascend as far as the root exit zone at the inferolateral pons. On CT, findings include asymmetric widening of the facial canal and obliteration of the fat in the stylomastoid foramen. Often the cortex of the facial nerve canal is intact, reflecting remodeling with slow growth. In cases of parotid malignancy, a mass in the parotid gland is frequently detectable. Associated opacification and destruction of mastoid air cells may be noted. MRI shows irregular infiltration extending along the nerve. Gadolinium contrast-enhanced MRI is better than CT for mapping the extent of facial nerve involvement, which is often relevant for treatment planning.

Spectrum of Disease

Facial nerve schwannomas vary widely in imaging appearance. They can arise anywhere along the course of the facial nerve, including the cisternal, intracanalicular, labyrinthine, geniculate, tympanic, mastoid, and extratemporal segments (Fig. 68.1). These lesions often extend along the nerve and involve multiple segments (Fig. 68.2). Smaller facial nerve schwannomas are well circumscribed with homogeneous contrast enhancement and may slightly expand the surrounding bone. Larger schwannomas may demonstrate internal heterogeneity. Multiple schwannomas may occur in association with neurofibromatosis type 2 (NF2). However, bilateral vestibular (rather than facial) schwannomas are typical in NF2.

Differential Diagnosis

1. Schwannoma
2. Venous malformation
3. Perineural spread of tumor
4. Leukemia
5. Metastasis
6. Paraganglioma
7. Meningioma

Pearls

- Morphology: Schwannomas are smooth and tubular. Venous malformations are poorly defined with intralesional

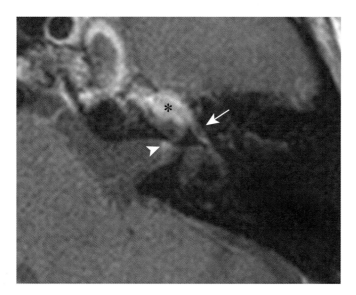

• **Fig. 68.1** A schwannoma of the geniculate ganglion. Axial T1-weighted postcontrast magnetic resonance imaging demonstrates an ovoid, homogeneously enhancing lesion centered in the geniculate ganglion *(asterisk)*, with thin projections along the labyrinthine *(arrowhead)* and proximal tympanic *(arrow)* segments of the facial nerve. This lesion has a well-circumscribed appearance, with minimal expansion of the surrounding bone.

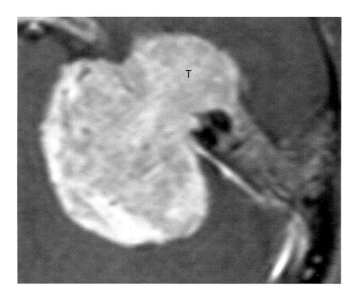

• **Fig. 68.2** A schwannoma involving multiple facial nerve segments. Axial T1-weighted postcontrast magnetic resonance imaging illustrates a large, heterogeneously enhancing lesion originating at the cerebellopontine angle that is markedly expanding the intracanalicular and labyrinthine segments and involves the geniculate ganglion and tympanic portion *(T)* of the facial nerve.

bone spicules. Perineural spread of tumor expands the canal and can have a similar appearance as a schwannoma; however, the presence of a parotid mass or history of local cutaneous malignancy should increase suspicion.

• **Location/course:** Schwannomas can arise anywhere along the course of the facial nerve and typically involve multiple contiguous segments. Venous malformations usually originate at the level of the geniculate ganglion. Perineural spread of malignancy begins at the level of the primary tumor in the parotid gland or adjacent skin and extends along nerve branches.

• **Bony involvement:** Schwannomas smoothly expand the surrounding bone, with possible erosion into the middle ear and mastoid air cells. Venous malformations show irregularity of adjacent bone with reactive osteitis, producing a honeycomb or speckled appearance. Perineural spread of malignancy usually causes expansion of the bony canal but can be more destructive. Changes may be first appreciated at the level of the stylomastoid foramen as effacement of the normal fat.

• **Enhancement:** Contrast enhancement is typically moderate and homogeneous in schwannomas; avid and heterogeneous in venous malformations; and mixed/variable in perineural spread of tumors.

• **Mineralization:** Intralesional mineralization is common in venous malformations and very rare in schwannomas and perineural spread of tumor.

Signs and Complications

Common symptoms of facial nerve tumors include unilateral facial paralysis and occasionally facial twitching. When located within the internal auditory canal, pressure on the adjacent vestibulocochlear nerve may produce sensorineural hearing loss, vertigo, and tinnitus. Lesions that expand the tympanic segment into the middle ear also can lead to conductive hearing loss by interfering with the ossicles. Symptomatic cases may require surgical excision with nerve transposition or grafting.

Suggested Readings

Casselman JW: Diagnostic imaging in clinical neuro-otology, *Curr Opin Neurol* 15(1):23–30, 2002.

Guerin JB, Takahashi EA, Lane JI, et al: Facial nerve venous malformation: a radiologic and histopathologic review of 11 cases, *Laryngoscope* 4(3):347–352, 2019.

Moonis G, Cunnane MB, Emerick K, et al: Patterns of perineural tumor spread in head and neck cancer, *Magn Reson Imaging Clin N Am* 20(3):435–446, 2012.

Raghavan P, Mukherjee S, Phillips CD: Imaging of the facial nerve, *Neuroimaging Clin North Am* 19(3):407–425, 2009.

Veillon F, Taboada LR, Eid MA, et al: Pathology of the facial nerve, *Neuroimaging Clin North Am* 18(2):309–320, 2008.

Wiggins RH III, Harnsberger HR, Salzman KL, et al: The many faces of facial nerve schwannoma, *AJNR Am J Neuroradiol* 27(3):694–699, 2006.

69
Labyrinthine Enhancement

PAUL M. BUNCH, MD AND HILLARY R. KELLY, MD

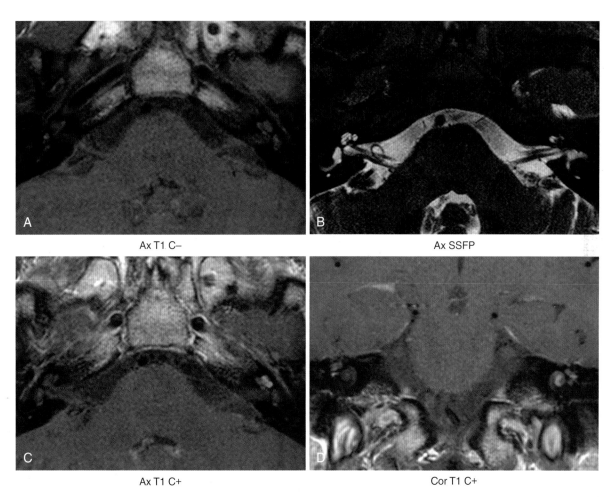

Ax T1 C−

Ax SSFP

Ax T1 C+

Cor T1 C+

CASE A: A 55-year-old male with asymmetric left sensorineural hearing loss. *Ax*, Axial; *Cor*, coronal; *SSFP*, steady-state free precession.

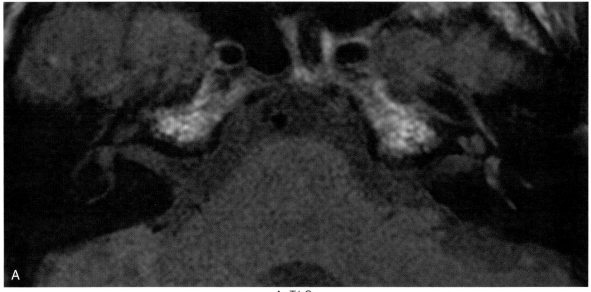

Ax T1 C−

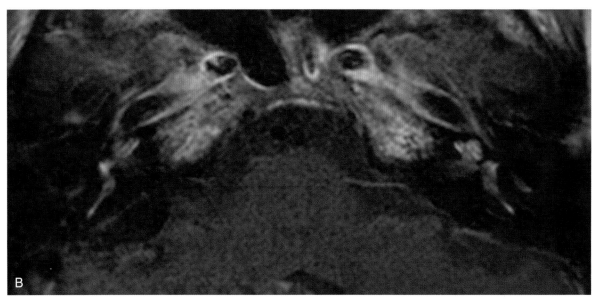

Ax T1 C+

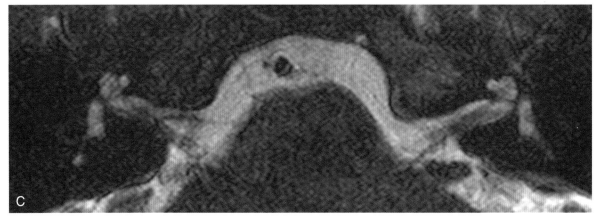

Ax SSFP

CASE B: A 52-year-old female with bacterial meningitis and hearing loss. *Ax*, Axial; *SSFP*, steady-state free precession.

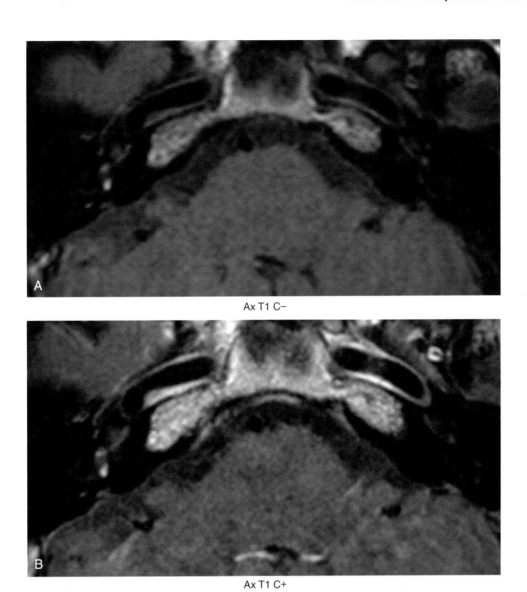

Ax T1 C−

Ax T1 C+

Ax T2 FLAIR

CASE C: A 42-year-old female with history of factor V deficiency presents with sudden onset vertigo and right hearing loss. *Ax,* Axial; *FLAIR,* fluid attenuated inversion recovery.

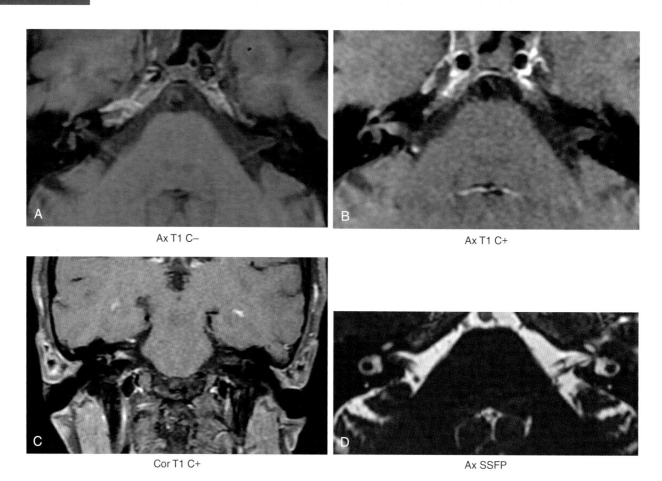

Ax T1 C–

Ax T1 C+

Cor T1 C+

Ax SSFP

CASE D: A 54-year-old female with sudden onset right hearing loss, imbalance, right facial paralysis, and right ear pain. *Ax*, Axial; *Cor*, coronal; *SSFP*, steady-state free precession.

DESCRIPTION OF FINDINGS

- Case A: Homogeneously enhancing lesion within the left cochlea with loss of the normal intracochlear fluid signal corresponding to the location of the enhancing abnormality.
- Case B: Avid enhancement of the bilateral membranous labyrinth structures with relative preservation of the normal membranous labyrinth fluid signal.
- Case C: Intrinsic T1 hyperintensity within the right vestibule and right posterior semicircular canals with corresponding fluid-attenuated inversion recovery (FLAIR) hyperintensity. No appreciable superimposed enhancement.
- Case D: Ill-defined enhancement involves the right internal auditory canal fundus, membranous labyrinth structures, and imaged portions of the right facial nerve. Although the fluid signal of the right lateral semicircular canal is preserved on the steady-state free precession (SSFP) image, there is abnormal soft tissue within the right internal auditory canal associated with the right facial and vestibulocochlear nerves.

Diagnosis

Case A: Intracochlear schwannoma
Case B: Acute infectious labyrinthitis
Case C: Labyrinthine hemorrhage
Case D: Herpes zoster oticus (Ramsay-Hunt syndrome)

Summary

Labyrinthine enhancement is always pathologic and may relate to infection, inflammation, or neoplasm. Furthermore, T1 hyperintense labyrinthine hemorrhage may be mistaken for labyrinthine enhancement if the precontrast T1-weighted images are not carefully reviewed in conjunction with the postcontrast images.

When confronted with labyrinthine enhancement, correlation with the clinical history (e.g., slow, progressive versus sudden onset of symptoms) and scrutiny of fluid-sensitive magnetic resonance (MR) sequences (e.g., T2, SSFP) in the context of the enhancing abnormality will usually enable the radiologist to determine the underlying cause. In cases where the underlying cause remains uncertain, a short-interval (e.g., 6 to 12 week) follow-up MRI without and with gadolinium contrast is often useful.

Spectrum of Disease

Schwannoma

Intralabyrinthine schwannomas are benign, slow-growing tumors of the terminal Schwann cells of the cochlear or vestibular nerves and arise within the structures of the membranous labyrinth, including the cochlea, vestibule, and semicircular canals. Previously considered very rare, modern high-resolution MR techniques have revealed these neoplasms to be more common than previously thought. Progressive hearing loss is the most frequent presenting symptom, though patients may also present with sudden hearing loss, tinnitus, imbalance, and vertigo. Intralabyrinthine schwannomas are most often centered in the cochlea, and some may extend through the modiolus into the internal auditory canal. Less commonly, intralabyrinthine schwannomas are centered in the vestibule or semicircular canals.

On MR imaging, intralabyrinthine schwannomas exhibit focal, well-defined, homogeneous, and contiguous enhancement on postcontrast T1-weighted images. On fluid-sensitive sequences (e.g., T2-weighted, SSFP) there will be a filling defect within the normal membranous labyrinth fluid corresponding precisely to the location of the enhancing lesion (Fig. 69.1). If in doubt, an intralabyrinthine schwannoma would not be expected

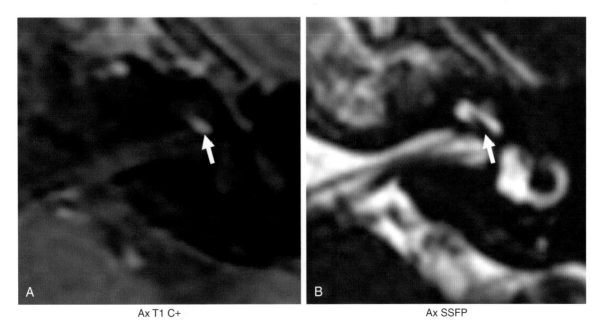

Ax T1 C+ Ax SSFP

• **Fig. 69.1** (A) Axial T1-weighted, gadolinium-enhanced image of the left temporal bone demonstrates a well-defined, homogeneously enhancing lesion (*arrow*) within the scala typani of the middle turn of the left cochlea. (B) Corresponding axial SSFP image demonstrates a focal filling defect (*arrow*) exactly matching the location of the enhancing abnormality in this 59-year-old female with a left cochlear schwannoma. *Ax*, Axial; *SSFP*, steady-state free precession.

to substantially change on short-interval follow-up imaging, whereas the other causes of labyrinthine enhancement (e.g., infectious, inflammatory) often will.

Labyrinthitis

Labyrinthitis can be subdivided into four stages: (1) serous, (2) purulent, (3) fibrous, and (4) osseous. Together, the serous and purulent stages are considered acute labyrinthitis, whereas the fibrous and osseous stages comprise chronic labyrinthitis.

Acute labyrinthitis, also referred to as acute otitis interna, is an inflammatory disorder of the inner ear that typically presents with sudden onset sensorineural hearing loss and vertigo. Causes may be classified by the mode of spread (e.g., tympanogenic, meningogenic, hematogenic, posttraumatic) or by causative agent (e.g., viral, bacterial, autoimmune, syphilitic), with viruses considered to be the most common underlying cause.

There are no CT findings of acute labyrinthitis. Temporal bone MR examinations are also normal in most patients. However, a minority of patients exhibit enhancement of the fluid-filled spaces of the membranous labyrinth on gadolinium-enhanced T1-weighted images. On corresponding fluid-sensitive sequence images, the normal hyperintense fluid signal is typically preserved (Fig. 69.2).

A substantial proportion of patients with acute labyrinthitis will progress to fibrous (begins approximately 2 weeks after the initial insult) and osseous (begins approximately 2 months after the initial insult) labyrinthitis. Familiarity with the imaging appearance and timing of the fibrous and osseous stages increases the utility of follow-up imaging when the underlying cause of labyrinthine enhancement remains uncertain.

As opposed to the acute phases in which the membranous labyrinth fluid signal may be diminished in intensity on fluid-sensitive sequences, but otherwise remains present in the fibrous stage, the normal high fluid signal is replaced by low signal-soft tissue, and this fibrous tissue enhances on gadolinium-enhanced T1-weighted images. The osseous stage of labyrinthitis—also known as labyrinthitis ossificans—is characterized by bone formation within the membranous labyrinth and represents the only stage with findings on CT. On MR imaging, labyrinthitis ossificans will appear as a low signal filling defect on fluid-sensitive sequences with minimal if any corresponding gadolinium enhancement (Fig. 69.3).

Postoperative labyrinthitis (Fig. 69.4) is a form of posttraumatic labyrinthitis. Following a translabyrinthine approach to the cerebellopontine angle cistern (e.g., vestibular schwannoma resection), labyrinthitis is an expected finding (rather than a complication) secondary to drilling through the labyrinth and should not be mistaken for residual or recurrent tumor.

Herpes Zoster Oticus

Herpes zoster oticus (also known as Ramsay-Hunt syndrome) results from reactivation of the varicella zoster virus affecting the facial nerve and resulting in facial paralysis. The vestibulocochlear nerve may also be involved, producing symptoms of vertigo, sensorineural hearing loss, or tinnitus. Anyone who has had chickenpox can develop herpes zoster oticus, but the disease most commonly affects adults over 60 years of age. External auditory canal vesicles are characteristic. Although vesicles typically precede or coincide with the onset of facial paralysis, clinical diagnosis is more challenging in the 15%

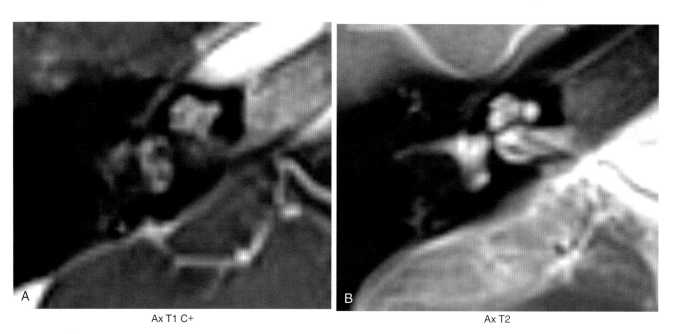

Ax T1 C+   Ax T2

• **Fig. 69.2** (A) Axial T1-weighted, gadolinium-enhanced image of the right temporal bone in a 2-year-old female with bacterial meningitis demonstrates enhancement of the cochlea, vestibule, and lateral semicircular canal. (B) Corresponding axial T2-weighted image demonstrates preservation of the normal fluid signal in the right cochlea and vestibule. The normal fluid signal in the lateral semicircular canal is not well seen due to volume averaging. *Ax,* Axial.

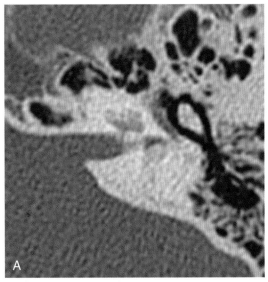

Ax CT bone

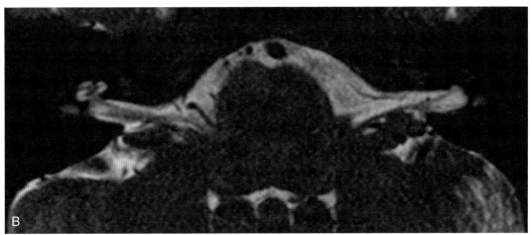

Ax SSFP

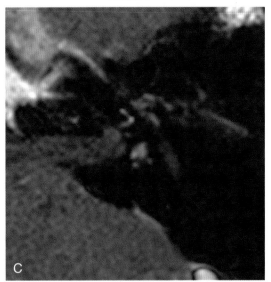

Ax T1 C+

• **Fig. 69.3** (A) Axial CT image of the left temporal bone demonstrates abnormal mineralization within the left cochlea, vestibule, and partially imaged posterior and lateral semicircular canals, consistent with labyrinthitis ossificans. Corresponding (B) axial SSFP and (C) T1-weighted, gadolinium-enhanced images demonstrate loss of the normal fluid signal in the left membranous labyrinth compared to the right (B) with minimal corresponding gadolinium enhancement (C). *Ax*, Axial; *CT*, Computed tomography; *SSFP*, steady-state free precession.

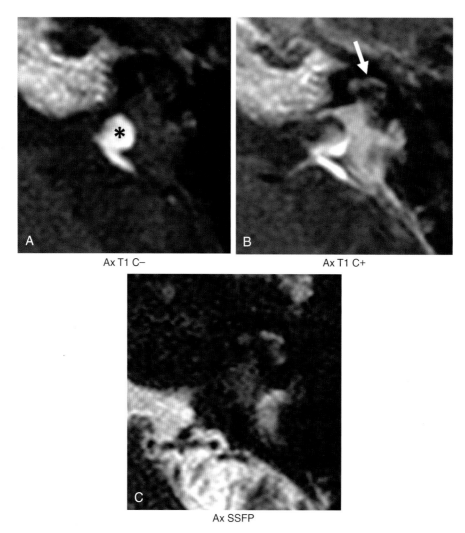

Ax T1 C−   Ax T1 C+

Ax SSFP

• **Fig. 69.4** (A) Axial T1-weighted, unenhanced image obtained in a 65-year-old female 3 months after left suboccipital craniotomy for translabyrinthine resection of a left vestibular schwannoma demonstrates postoperative changes to the left internal auditory canal and left labyrinth. A fat graft *(asterisk)* was used to close the surgical defect. Corresponding (B) axial T1-weighted, gadolinium-enhanced and (C) axial SSFP images demonstrate enhancement of the cochlea *(arrow,* B) with corresponding decrease in the normal fluid signal (C), consistent with the fibrous stage of labyrinthitis. These findings represent postoperative labyrinthitis, an expected finding after drilling of the labyrinth to facilitate tumor resection. *Ax,* Axial; *SSFP,* steady-state free precession.

to 35% of patients for whom vesicles do not appear until sometime after the onset of facial paralysis. On MR imaging, enhancement of cranial nerves VII and VIII, in addition to labyrinthine enhancement, is typical. External auditory canal and periauricular enhancement may also be seen.

Hemorrhage

Labyrinthine hemorrhage is rare but most commonly occurs in the setting of trauma, blood dyscrasias, and therapeutic anticoagulation. It has also been described in sickle cell disease and lupus, and labyrinthine hemorrhage may also be the presenting symptom of endolymphatic sac tumor. The clinical presentation is profound, unilateral, sudden sensorineural hearing loss with or without vertigo. In most patients, hearing does not recover.

On MR imaging, labyrinthine hemorrhage exhibits increased signal on both T1-weighted sequences and T2-weighted 3D FLAIR sequences. On T2-weighted images, low signal intensity may also be seen depending on the age of the blood products.

Differential Diagnosis

Diagnosis	Discriminating Feature(s)
Intralabyrinthine schwannoma	Focal, well-defined enhancement with corresponding filling defect on fluid-sensitive sequences
	Persists on follow-up imaging
Acute labyrinthitis	Ill-defined enhancement with preserved fluid signal
	On follow-up imaging, may resolve or progress to fibrous and ossific labyrinthitis
Fibrous labyrinthitis	Loss of normal fluid signal with corresponding enhancement in a patient with previous acute labyrinthitis
	Progresses to labyrinthitis ossificans on follow-up imaging
Labyrinthitis ossificans	Low signal filling defect on fluid-sensitive sequences with minimal if any corresponding enhancement
Postoperative/posttraumatic labyrinthitis	Prior translabyrinthine surgery or prior otic capsule-violating temporal bone fracture
	Imaging features will depend on the stage of labyrinthitis (i.e., acute, fibrous, ossific)
Herpes zoster oticus	Internal auditory canal enhancement involving cranial nerve VII +/- VIII
	External auditory canal vesicles
Labyrinthine hemorrhage	Labyrinthine T1 hyperintensity on noncontrast images

Pearls

In most cases of labyrinthine enhancement, correlation with the clinical history and scrutiny of fluid-sensitive MR sequences will enable confident determination of the underlying cause. Remember to carefully assess the precontrast T1-weighted images and to search for relevant findings outside of the labyrinth (e.g., facial nerve enhancement).

Signs and Complications

Deafness is a complication common to all causes of labyrinthine enhancement discussed in this chapter as well as to labyrinthine hemorrhage.

Labyrinthine hemorrhage can be the initial manifestation of an underlying endolymphatic sac tumor. Although uncommon, it is therefore prudent to scrutinize the region of the endolymphatic sac in the presence of labyrinthine hemorrhage.

Suggested Readings

Bunch PM, Kelly HR: Labyrinthitis. In Small JE, Noujaim DL, Ginat DT, Kelly HR, Schaefer PW, editors: *Neuroradiology: spectrum and evolution of disease*, ed 1, 331–338, 2018, Philadelphia, PA, Elsevier.

Chen XH, Zeng CJ, Fang ZM, et al: The natural history of labyrinthine hemorrhage in patients with sudden sensorineural hearing loss, *Ear Nose Throat J* 98(5):E13–E20, 2019.

Choudhury B, Carlson ML, Jethanamest J: Intralabyrinthine schwannomas: disease presentation, tumor management, and hearing rehabilitation, *J Neurol Surg B Skull Base* 80(2):196–202, 2019.

Jagannathan J, Butman JA, Lonser RR, et al: Endolymphatic sac tumor demonstrated by intralabyrinthine hemorrhage. Case report, *J Neurosurg* 107(2):421–425, 2007.

Kanerva M, Jones S, Pitkaranta A: Ramsay Hunt syndrome: characteristics and patient self-assessed long-term facial palsy outcome, *Eur Arch Otorhinolaryngol* 277(4):1235–1245, 2020.

Salzman KL, Childs AM, Davidson HC, et al: Intralabyrinthine schwannomas: imaging diagnosis and classification, *AJNR Am J Neuroradiol* 33(1):104–109, 2012.

Tieleman A, Casselman JW, Somers T, et al: Imaging of intralabyrinthine schwannomas: a retrospective study of 52 cases with emphasis on lesion growth, *AJNR Am J Neuroradiol* 29(5):898–905, 2008.

Vivas EX, Panella NJ, Baugnon KL: Spontaneous labyrinthine hemorrhage: a case series, *Otolaryngol Head Neck Surg* 159(5):908–913, 2018.

70

Lucent Jaw Lesions

MICHAEL T. PREECE, MD AND PAUL M. BUNCH, MD

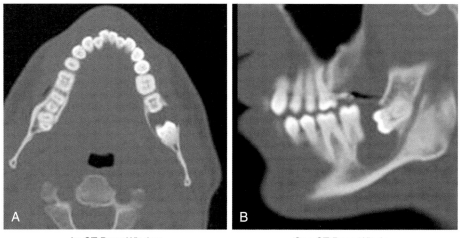

Ax CT Bone Window   Sag CT Bone Window

CASE A: A 33-year-old asymptomatic male with lucent lesion found on routine dental radiographs. *Ax*, Axial; *CT*, Computed tomography; *Sag*, sagittal.

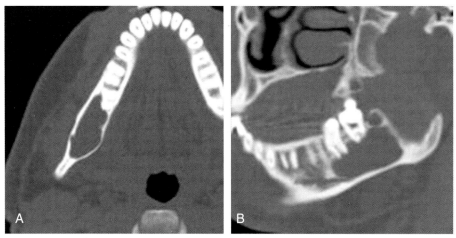

Ax CT Bone Window   Sag CT Bone Window

CASE B: A 31-year-old male with right lower jaw pain for 2 months. *Ax*, Axial; *CT*, Computed tomography; *Sag*, sagittal.

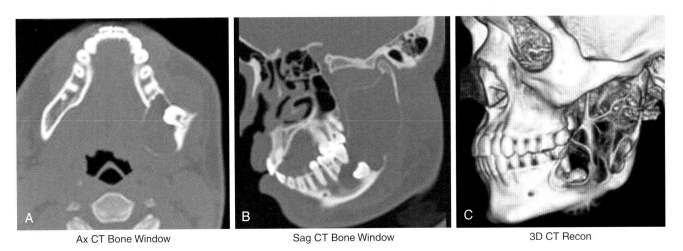

Ax CT Bone Window   Sag CT Bone Window   3D CT Recon

CASE C: A 20-year-old male presenting with progressive swelling of the left jaw for 8 months. *Ax,* Axial; *CT,* Computed tomography; *Recon,* reconstruction; *Sag,* sagittal.

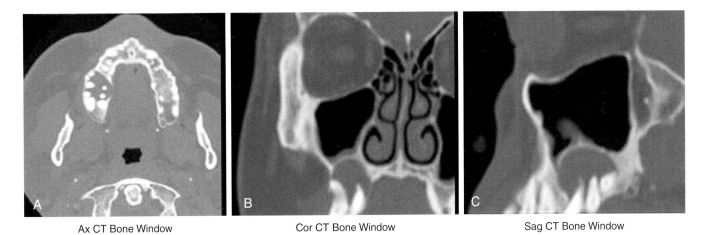

Ax CT Bone Window   Cor CT Bone Window   Sag CT Bone Window

CASE D: A 37-year-old male with upper jaw pain. *Ax,* Axial; *Cor,* coronal; *CT,* Computed tomography; *Sag,* sagittal.

DESCRIPTION OF FINDINGS

CT images from four patients demonstrate lucent jaw lesions without mineralization.

- Case A: There is a unilocular lesion involving the left posterior mandibular body that is associated with the crown of an unerupted left third mandibular molar. The lesion extends to the margin of the cemento-enamel junction of the unerupted tooth.
- Case B: There is an expansile unilocular lesion within the right posterior mandibular body that is associated with the roots of a normally erupted right third mandibular molar.
- Case C: There is a large, multilocular, expansile lesion involving the left mandibular body, ramus, coronoid process, and condylar neck with an associated displaced left third mandibular molar.
- Case D: There is a round lucent lesion associated with the roots of the normally erupted right first and second maxillary molars.

Diagnosis

Case A: Dentigerous cyst
Case B: Odontogenic keratocyst
Case C: Cystic ameloblastoma
Case D: Radicular cyst

Summary

Lucent lesions of the jaw often pose a diagnostic challenge for the neuroradiologist, in part because of limited familiarity with dental pathology, but also because of overlapping imaging features. One useful diagnostic approach is to divide pathologic entities into odontogenic lesions (i.e., those related to the teeth) and nonodontogenic lesions.

Lucent odontogenic lesions of the mandible can be further subdivided into lesions with and without mineralization. Lesions without mineralization include dentigerous cysts, odontogenic keratocysts, cystic ameloblastomas, and radicular cysts, as well as several other rare lesions. Although imaging features have significant overlap, an understanding of classic imaging findings is helpful in creating a properly weighted differential diagnosis. Odontogenic lesions with mineralization (i.e., most odontomas and other odontogenic tumors) and nonodontogenic cystic jaw lesions such as fissural cysts are beyond the scope of the current discussion.

A radicular (also known as periodontal, periapical, or dental) cyst is the most common jaw cyst. These lesions are associated with the root(s) of a nonvital tooth and represent the final step in an inflammatory cascade of events that begins as caries and pulpal necrosis and ends as an apical abscess. The abscess or cyst forms at the apex or tip of the root. The cyst typically measures less than 1 cm and is round or pear shaped. Unlike the other nonmineralized odontogenic lucent lesions, radicular cysts more commonly involve the maxillary rather than the mandibular teeth, particularly the incisors and canines.

Dentigerous (follicular) cysts represent the second most common odontogenic cyst and result from fluid accumulation between the follicular epithelium and the crown of a developing tooth. As the cyst enlarges, the wall of the cyst characteristically converges on the cemento-enamel junction, and these lesions are invariably associated with an impacted or unerupted tooth, most commonly an unerupted third molar. On imaging, a unilocular round or ovoid appearance is expected. The tooth roots are typically located outside of the cyst. There is no periosteal reaction or enhancing soft tissue component.

Odontogenic keratocysts represent the third most common cyst in the jaw and are the most aggressive of the jaw cysts. These lesions arise from remnants of the dental lamina and affect the mandible two to four times more often than the maxilla, exhibiting a predilection for the posterior jaw. Odontogenic keratocysts classically appear as expansile cystic lesions associated with the roots of normally erupted mandibular molars; however, they may also be located in a pericoronal position, a lateral root position, or without any discernible relationship to a dental structure. They are more often unilocular than multilocular and tend to grow within the medullary cavity in a predominantly anteroposterior orientation while causing minimal cortical expansion. On gadolinium-enhanced magnetic resonance imaging (MRI), only a thin peripheral rim of enhancement is expected, and restricted diffusion can be seen because of keratin within the lesion. Odontogenic keratocysts frequently recur after surgical excision, and multiplicity is suggestive of basal cell nevus (Gorlin) syndrome. The nomenclature of these lesions have been widely debated. In the 2005 World Health Organization classification, this lesion was classified as "keratocystic odontogenic tumor" because of its observed aggressive behavior and frequent association with a *PTCH1* mutation. However, despite these characteristics, the World Health Organization consensus group later concluded that there is insufficient evidence to support a neoplastic origin of this lesion. As such, the term "odontogenic keratocyst" was reinstated as the preferred term in the 2017 classification.

Ameloblastoma is a neoplasm typically originating from the epithelium of the dental lamina and less commonly from the lining of a dentigerous cyst. Although usually benign, these tumors are locally destructive, and extensive growth can be fatal. The most common location is the mandibular ramus and posterior body. On imaging, 80% appear as a multilocular "bubbly" or "honeycombed" lucent lesion devoid of mineralization, whereas 20% are unilocular. As opposed to the other lucent lesions discussed in this chapter, enhancing soft tissue components on contrast-enhanced CT or MRI are often identifiable. As opposed to the anteroposterior growth pattern of odontogenic keratocysts, ameloblastomas commonly exhibit buccallingual expansion. Recent molecular research has shown many tumors to be associated with a specific *BRAF* mutation, introducing the possibility of targeted therapy.

Spectrum of Disease

Although odontogenic keratocysts characteristically are associated with erupted teeth, they can cause tooth displacement and, therefore, mimic an unerupted tooth (Fig. 70.1A). Other nonodontogenic lesions such as cystic metastases (Fig. 70.1B) and posttraumatic cysts (Fig. 70.1C) also can mimic odontogenic lesions. Various odontogenic tumors that do not calcify also can appear as lucent lesions on CT, but they are uncommon, and gadolinium-enhanced MR imaging will often show

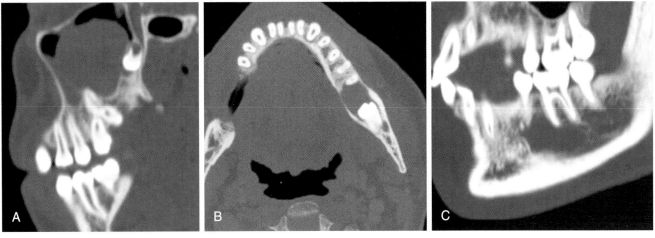

• **Fig. 70.1** (A) An odontogenic keratocyst with an unerupted tooth. (B) Metastasis mimicking a dentigerous cyst. (C) A posttraumatic cyst mimicking an odontogenic keratocyst. *Ax,* Axial; *CT,* Computed tomography; *Sag,* sagittal.

enhancing tissue within these lesions. Odontogenic myxomas are rare; they do not tend to calcify and usually have prominent but thin osseous ridges.

Differential Diagnosis

1. Dentigerous cyst
2. Odontogenic keratocyst
3. Cystic ameloblastoma
4. Radicular cyst
5. Posttraumatic cyst
6. Metastasis
7. Other rare noncalcified odontogenic tumors

Pearls

• Radicular cyst is the most common lucent jaw lesion and therefore should be the primary consideration for a periapical lucency associated with a carious tooth.
• Dentigerous cysts, cystic ameloblastomas, and odontogenic keratocysts have many overlapping imaging features and should be included routinely in the same differential diagnosis. In most cases, lesions must be removed and examined histopathologically to establish a definitive diagnosis.
• Dentigerous cysts should be the primary consideration for cystic lesions extending to the cemento-enamel junction in association with an unerupted tooth.
• Consider a cystic ameloblastoma if the lesion is multilocular or "bubbly" and remember that ameloblastomas can arise from the walls of dentigerous cysts.
• Odontogenic keratocyst should be the primary consideration for an expansile cystic lesion associated with roots of a normally erupted mandibular molar.

• Consider basal cell nevus (Gorlin) syndrome in the setting of multiple odontogenic keratocysts.

Signs and Complications

Most lucent jaw lesions are asymptomatic and discovered on routine dental radiography. Symptomatic lesions can be associated with pain, swelling, paresthesias, and tooth displacement.

Suggested Readings

Avril L, Lombardi T, Ailianou A, et al: Radiolucent lesions of the mandible: a pattern-based approach to diagnosis, *Insights Imaging* 5(1):85–101, 2014.

Bali A, Vanhoenacker FM, Vanhoenacker C, et al: Imaging of radiolucent jaw lesions, *Semin Musculoskelet Radiol* 24(5):549–557, 2020.

Devenny-Cakir B, Subramaniam RM, Reddy SM, et al: Cystic and cystic-appearing lesions of the mandible: review, *AJR Am J Roentgenol* 196 (6 Suppl):WS66–WS77, 2011.

Harmon M, Arrigan M, Toner M, et al: A radiological approach to benign and malignant lesions of the mandible, *Clin Radiol* 70(4):335–350, 2015.

Kaneda T, Weber AL, Scrivani SJ, et al: Cysts, tumors, and nontumorous lesions of the jaw. In Som PM, Curtin HD, editors: *Head and neck imaging*, St Louis, 2011, Mosby.

Siozopoulou V, Vanhoenacker FM: World Health Organization classification of odontogenic tumors and imaging approach of jaw lesions, *Semin Musculoskelet Radiol* 24(5):535–548, 2020.

Speight PM, Takata T: New tumour entities in the 4th edition of the World Health Organization classification of head and neck tumours: odontogenic and maxillofacial bone tumors, *Virchows Arch* 472(3):331–339, 2018.

71

Temporomandibular Joint Mineralized Lesions

ANDREW R. KING, MD AND PAUL M. BUNCH, MD

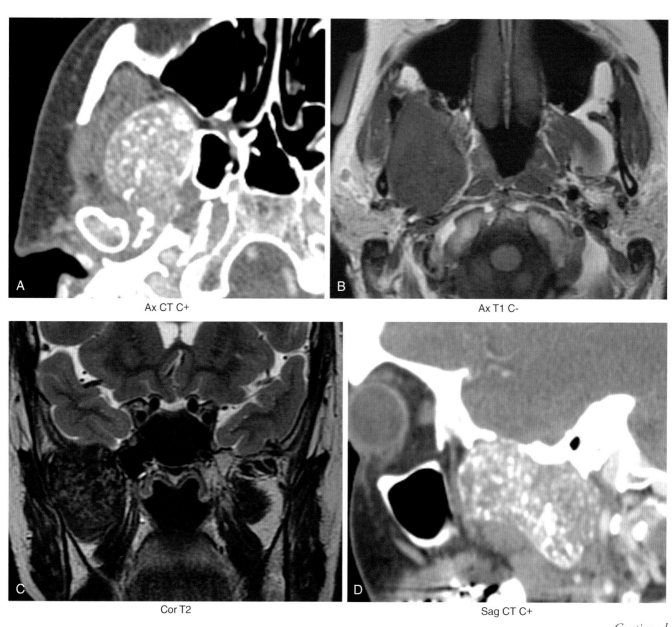

Ax CT C+

Ax T1 C-

Cor T2

Sag CT C+

Continued

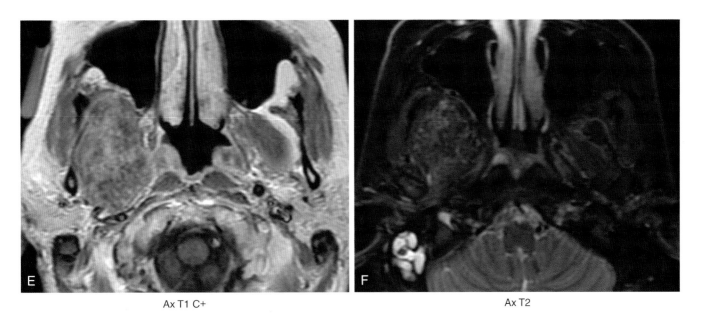

Ax T1 C+   Ax T2

CASE A: A 54-year-old female with new right hearing loss, years of right facial pressure, and history of multiple temporomandibular joint dislocations. *Ax*, Axial; *Cor*, coronal; *CT*, Computed tomography; *Sag*, sagittal.

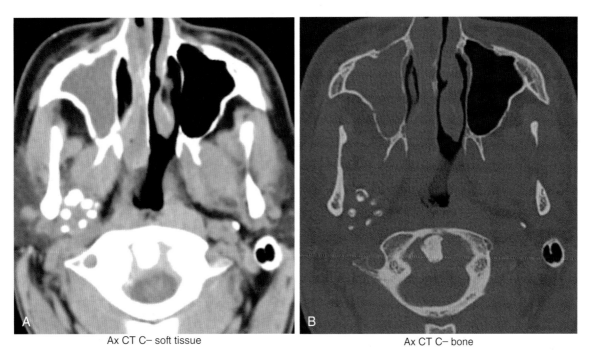

Ax CT C− soft tissue   Ax CT C− bone

CASE B: A 55-year-old male undergoing head CT after a fall. *Ax*, Axial; *CT*, Computed tomography.

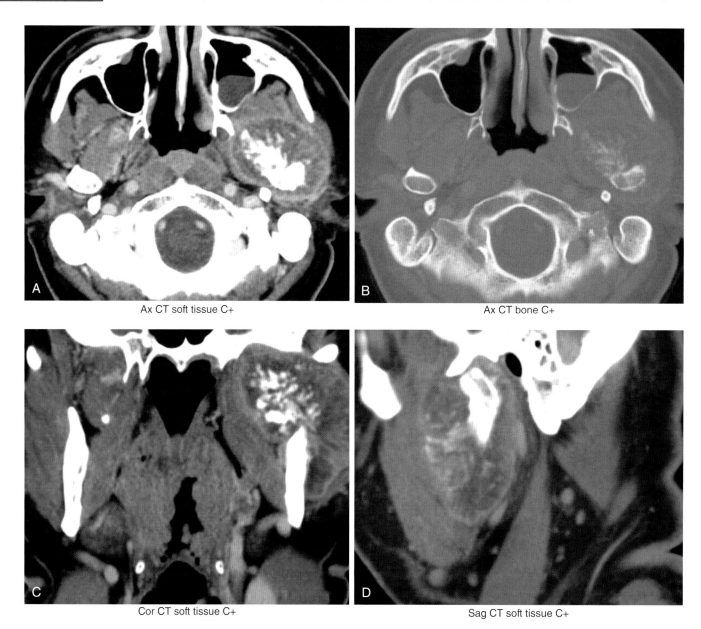

Ax CT soft tissue C+

Ax CT bone C+

Cor CT soft tissue C+

Sag CT soft tissue C+

CASE C: A 38-year-old male with progressive left face pain and swelling. *Ax*, Axial; *Cor*, coronal; *CT*, Computed tomography; *Sag*, sagittal.

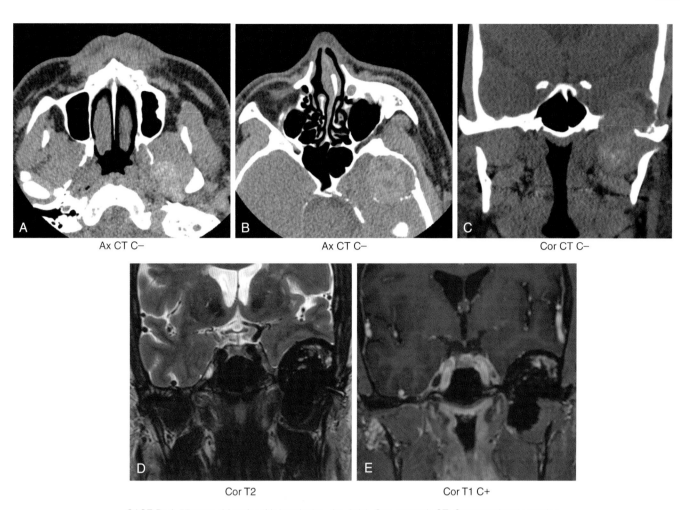

Ax CT C–

Ax CT C–

Cor CT C–

Cor T2

Cor T1 C+

CASE D: A 57-year-old male with headache. *Ax*, Axial; *Cor*, coronal; *CT*, Computed tomography.

DESCRIPTION OF FINDINGS

- Case A: A mineralized, T2 hypointense, heterogeneously enhancing right masticator space mass causes inferior displacement of the right lateral pterygoid muscle lower belly and insinuates between the right mandibular condyle and glenoid fossa.
- Case B: Multiple, small, discrete, round and ovoid calcified lesions along the medial aspect of the right mandibular ramus.
- Case C: A large, aggressive-appearing soft tissue mass with internal mineralization centered in the left mandibular ramus extends into the adjacent muscles of mastication and involves the left temporomandibular joint. There is left mandibular cortical destruction and periosteal reaction.
- Case D: Axial and coronal CT images demonstrate a soft tissue mass centered in the left temporomandibular joint with faint internal mineralization. The lesion erodes the floor of the left middle cranial fossa and extends intracranially. The mass exhibits marked hypointensity on coronal T2-weighted and coronal T1-weighted, gadolinium-enhanced images. Note the inferior displacement of the lower belly of the left lateral pterygoid muscle by the mass.

Diagnosis

Case A: Calcium pyrophosphate deposition disease (pseudogout)
Case B: Synovial osteochondromatosis
Case C: Osteosarcoma
Case D: Tenosynovial giant cell tumor (pigmented villonodular synovitis)

Summary

The temporomandibular joint is a synovial joint formed by the mandibular condyle and the glenoid fossa of the temporal bone. Mineralized lesions involving the temporomandibular joint may result from a variety of processes, including crystalline arthropathy (e.g., gout, calcium pyrophosphate deposition disease), benign neoplasm (e.g., osteochondromatosis, tenosynovial giant cell tumor), and malignancy (e.g., osteosarcoma, chondrosarcoma).

Detection of the mineralized abnormality on CT is often straightforward, but it is not always obvious that the lesion arises from the temporomandibular joint. Given the narrow space between the mandibular condyle and glenoid fossa as well as the relative distensibility of the joint capsule compared to the glenoid fossa, mandibular condyle, and external auditory canal (posterior joint wall), lesions arising from the temporomandibular joint are frequently centered anteroinferiorly with respect to the articular surfaces. The medial aspect of such temporomandibular joint lesions will inferiorly displace the lateral pterygoid lower belly (Figs. 71.1 and 71.2), whereas the lateral aspect of these lesions will laterally displace the masseter muscle (Fig. 71.3).

Although tissue sampling is typically warranted for definitive diagnosis, the differential diagnosis of lesions arising from the temporomandibular joint is relatively limited. Careful attention to several key imaging features may help further narrow the differential diagnosis and ensure appropriate pathologic evaluation (e.g., light microscopy to assess for possible crystalline arthropathy).

Spectrum of Disease

Calcium Pyrophosphate Deposition Disease

Calcium pyrophosphate deposition disease (pseudogout) is a benign crystalline arthropathy believed to result from a disorder

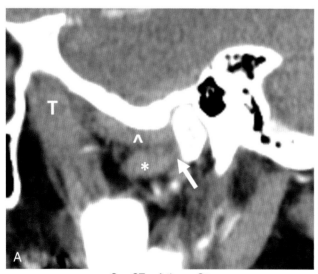

Sag CT soft tissue C+

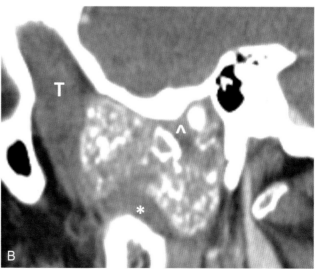

Sag CT soft tissue C+

• **Fig. 71.1** Sagittal CT images of the (A) normal left and (B) abnormal right temporomandibular joints in the 54-year-old female patient depicted in Case A with calcium pyrophosphate deposition disease demonstrate the anatomic basis for the utility of inferior displacement of the lower belly of the lateral pterygoid muscle for determining possible temporomandibular joint origin. On the normal left side (A), note the fat-filled potential space between the temporalis muscle *(T)*, the lateral pterygoid upper belly *(^)*, and the lateral pterygoid lower belly *(*)* as well as the attachment of the lower belly on the mandibular condyle *(arrow, A)* below the joint space. On the abnormal right side (B), the calcified mass inferiorly displaces the lateral pterygoid lower belly *(*)* and insinuates into the potential space between the temporalis muscle *(T)* and the lateral pterygoid upper belly *(^)*. *CT,* Computed tomography; *Sag,* sagittal.

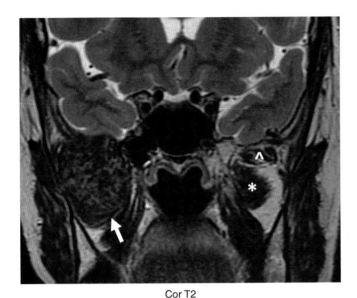

Cor T2

• **Fig. 71.2** Coronal T2-weighted image from the 54-year-old female with calcium pyrophosphate deposition disease depicted in Case A demonstrates the normal appearance of the left lateral pterygoid muscle upper (^) and lower (*) bellies in the coronal plane and inferior displacement of the right lateral pterygoid lower belly *(arrow)* by the right temporomandibular joint mass. *Cor,* Coronal.

of phosphate metabolism. The disease is uncommon before 50 years of age, and there is no sex predilection. The knee and wrist joints are most commonly involved, but the temporomandibular joint may also be affected, typically by the chronic form of the disease. On CT, a calcified intraarticular mass is typically seen with associated degenerative joint changes. Low T2 signal is expected on MRI, and heterogeneous gadolinium contrast

enhancement is often present. The diagnosis is confirmed through the detection of positively birefringent crystals on polarized light microscopy.

Synovial Osteochondromatosis

Synovial osteochondromatosis refers to a benign neoplastic proliferation of the synovium that most commonly involves the knee. Overall, males are affected 2 to 4 times more frequently than females by the disease; however, temporomandibular joint involvement is more common in women than men. Multiple round or oval loose bodies are characteristic (as shown in Case B); however, a single mineralized mass may also be seen (as shown in Fig. 71.3). MR will demonstrate enhancing synovium, and the loose bodies will exhibit T2 hypointensity. Surgical resection is the treatment of choice with low risk of recurrence.

Osteosarcoma

Osteosarcoma represents the most common malignant primary bone neoplasm, accounting for 40% to 60% of all primary bone malignancies. The defining characteristic of the tumor cells is production of osteoid (immature bone). Osteosarcoma of the jaw represents 7% of all osteosarcomas and 1% of all head and neck malignancies; a subset of these lesions involve the temporomandibular joint. Compared to long bone osteosarcomas, mandibular osteosarcomas occur in an older population (third to fourth decade compared to second decade) and have a better prognosis. Imaging features typical of osteosarcoma include bone destruction, aggressive periosteal reaction, and a large soft tissue mass containing mineralized

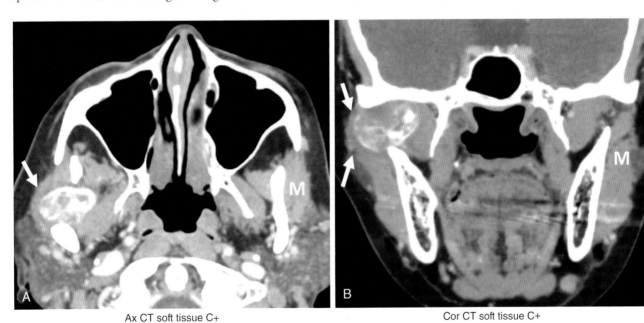

Ax CT soft tissue C+   Cor CT soft tissue C+

• **Fig. 71.3** (A) Axial and (B) coronal CT images of a 59-year-old female with synovial osteochondromatosis demonstrate a mineralized mass centered along the anteroinferior aspect of the right temporomandibular joint. The lateral aspect of the lesion laterally displaces the overlying right masseter muscle *(arrows).* The normal left masseter muscle *(M)* is shown for comparison. *Ax,* Axial; *Cor,* coronal; *CT,* Computed tomography.

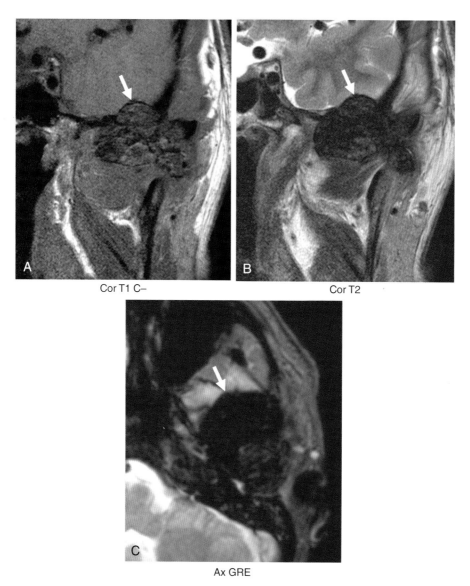

Cor T1 C−

Cor T2

Ax GRE

• **Fig. 71.4** (A) Coronal T1-weighted and (B) coronal T2-weighted MR images of a 42-year-old male with tenosynovial giant cell tumor of the left temporomandibular joint demonstrate a T1 and T2 hypointense mass *(arrows)* eroding through the roof of the left temporomandibular joint to involve the left middle cranial fossa. Note prominent magnetic susceptibility effect ("blooming," *arrow*) on (C) the axial GRE image. *Ax*, Axial; *Cor*, coronal; *GRE*, gradient recalled echo.

osteoid. Radical resection is the primary treatment of jaw osteosarcoma, which may be followed by adjuvant radiation and/or chemotherapy.

Tenosynovial Giant Cell Tumor

Tenosynovial giant cell tumor (pigmented villonodular synovitis) is a benign and locally aggressive neoplasm of the synovium and tendon sheath. The disease most commonly involves the knee, hip, and ankle, but may also affect the temporomandibular joint. On CT, tenosynovial giant cell tumor most commonly manifests as a hyperdense mass with associated osseous erosion. Although the disease is said to almost never calcify in other joints of the body, mineralization can occur in the temporomandibular joint, as shown in Case D. Low signal on all MR

sequences and pronounced magnetic susceptibility artifact (Fig. 71.4) are expected and the result of hemosiderin deposition from repetitive intralesional hemorrhage. As shown in Case D, intracranial extension is commonly seen (~35% of cases) due to this neoplasm's locally aggressive nature. Surgical removal of the affected synovium prevents further joint damage, alleviates pain, and improves function with a low risk of recurrence. Postoperative radiotherapy may be added in some cases, such as with recurrent disease or extensive disease with close surgical margins.

Differential Diagnosis

1. Additional mineralized lesions that may involve the temporomandibular joint include gout, chondrosarcoma, and chondroblastoma.

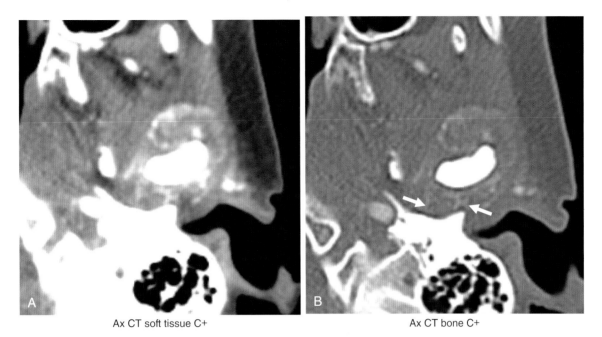

Ax CT soft tissue C+   Ax CT bone C+

• **Fig. 71.5** Axial CT images of a 53-year-old female with chondrosarcoma of the left temporomandibular joint demonstrate a circumferential mass surrounding the left mandibular condyle with areas of ring-and-arc mineralization (*arrows*, B). *Ax*, Axial; *CT*, Computed tomography.

2. Gout is a crystalline arthropathy caused by the deposition of monosodium urate crystals. Gout (negatively birefringent, needle-shaped crystals) is differentiated from calcium pyrophosphate deposition disease (weakly positively birefringent, rhomboid crystals) by polarized light microscopy—the imaging appearances of these two entities are identical.
3. Chondrosarcoma is a typical slow-growing primary bone malignancy characterized by tumor cell cartilage formation. Compared with osteosarcoma, chondrosarcoma is less common in the head and neck, and the imaging appearance is often less aggressive with less osseous destruction. A ring-and-arc pattern of mineralization is characteristic (Fig. 71.5).
4. Chondroblastoma is an uncommon benign cartilaginous neoplasm that very rarely involves the temporomandibular joint. On imaging, the lesion is typically lucent but may exhibit a mineralized internal matrix in approximately 50% of cases. Perilesional edema involving the surrounding bone and/or soft tissues is characteristic.

Pearls

• Temporomandibular joint origin of masticator space pathology may not be immediately obvious, as temporomandibular joint lesions are frequently eccentrically located with respect to the articular surfaces (anteroinferiorly, most commonly).
• In such cases, careful attention to the relationship of the medial aspect of the lesion to the lower belly of the lateral pterygoid muscle and the lateral aspect of the lesion to the masseter muscle can be useful for determining temporomandibular joint origin.

• Calcium pyrophosphate and gout exhibit identical imaging features and are distinguished with polarized light microscopy.
• Multiple, similarly sized, round or oval lesions favor synovial osteochondromatosis.
• Low signal on all MR sequences and prominent magnetic susceptibility artifact are typical of tenosynovial giant cell tumor (pigmented villonodular synovitis).
• Periosteal reaction, osseous destruction, and a mineralized soft tissue mass should raise concern for osteosarcoma.
• Tissue sampling is typically warranted for definitive diagnosis. However, careful attention to imaging features of mineralized temporomandibular joint lesions may narrow the differential diagnosis and ensure performance of appropriate pathologic tests.

Signs and Complications

Common clinical signs of temporomandibular joint lesions include pain, swelling, and trismus. Complications may relate to joint dysfunction and invasion of adjacent structures, including intracranial extension. Surgical resection is the treatment for most mineralized temporomandibular joint lesions with variable risk of recurrence.

Suggested Readings

Blancas C, Llauger J, Palmer J, et al: Imaging findings in chondroblastoma. *Radiologia* 50(5):416–423, 2008.
Ferrari D, Moneghini L, Allevi F, et al. Osteosarcoma of the jaw: classification, diagnosis and treatment. In Honoki K, Weiss KR, editors: *Osteosarcoma – biology, behavior, and mechanisms*, ed 1, Rijeka, Croatia 2017, InTech Open.

Giorgione C, Passali FM, Varakliotis T, et al: Temporo-mandibular joint chondrosarcoma: case report and review of the literature, *Acta Otorhinolaryngol Ital* 35(3):208–211, 2015.

Kwang-Jun K, Seok H, Jang-Ha L, et al: Calcium pyrophosphate dihydrate deposition disease in the temporomandibular joint: diagnosis and treatment, *Maxillofac Plast Reconstr Surg* 40(1):19, 2018.

Morales H, Cornelius R: Imaging approach to temporomandibular joint disorders, *Clinical Neuroradiol* 26(1):5–22, 2016.

Murphy MD, Vidal JA, Fanburg-Smith JC, et al: Imaging of synovial chondromatosis with radiologic-pathologic correlation, *Radiographics* 27(5):1465–1488, 2007.

Ochoa Escudero M, Juliano AF, Curtin HD: Inferior displacement of the lower belly of the lateral pterygoid muscle: a sign of temporomandibular joint lesions, *J Comput Assist Tomogr* 39(3):340–342, 2015.

Safaee M, Oh T, Sun MZ, et al: Pigmented villonodular synovitis of the temporomandibular joint with intracranial extension: a case series and systematic review, *Head Neck* 37(8):1213–1224, 2015.

Testaverde L, Perrone A, Caporali L, et al: CT and MR findings in synovial chondromatosis of the temporo-mandibular joint: our experience and review of literature, *Eur J Radiol* 78(3):414–418, 2011.

Wang S, Shi H, Yu Q: Osteosarcoma of the jaws: demographic and CT imaging features, *Dentomaxillofac Radiol* 41(1):37–42, 2012.

72

Jugular Foramen Lesions

JUAN E. SMALL, MD, MSC

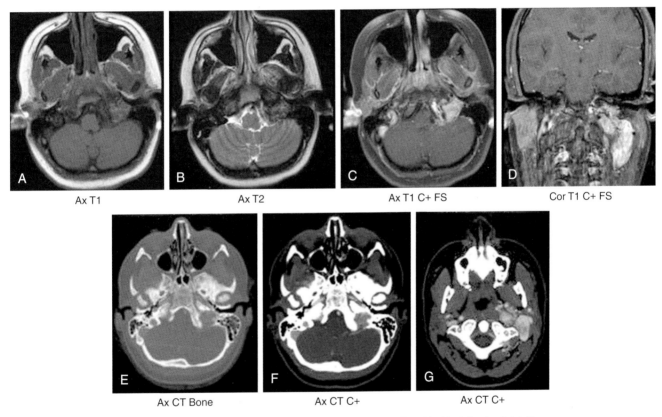

Ax T1   Ax T2   Ax T1 C+ FS   Cor T1 C+ FS

Ax CT Bone   Ax CT C+   Ax CT C+

CASE A: An 18-year-old who fell from a tree presents with a mass found incidentally. *Ax,* Axial; *Cor,* coronal; *CT,* Computed tomography; *FS,* fat saturated.

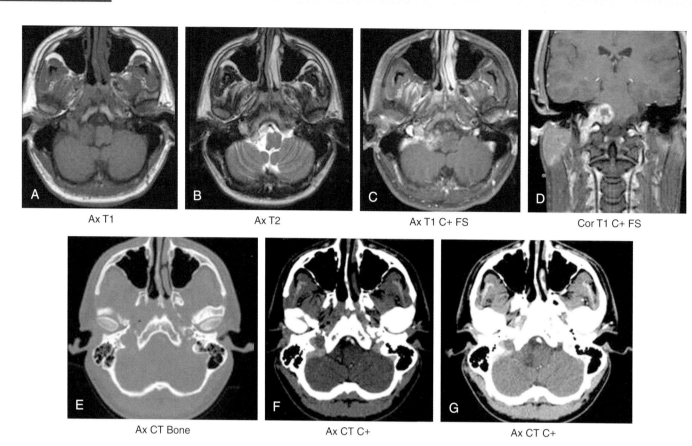

A   Ax T1   B   Ax T2   C   Ax T1 C+ FS   D   Cor T1 C+ FS

E   Ax CT Bone   F   Ax CT C+   G   Ax CT C+

CASE B: A 23-year-old presenting with dizziness and a 6-month history of decreased right-sided hearing. *Ax,* Axial; *Cor,* coronal; *CT,* Computed tomography; *FS,* fat saturated.

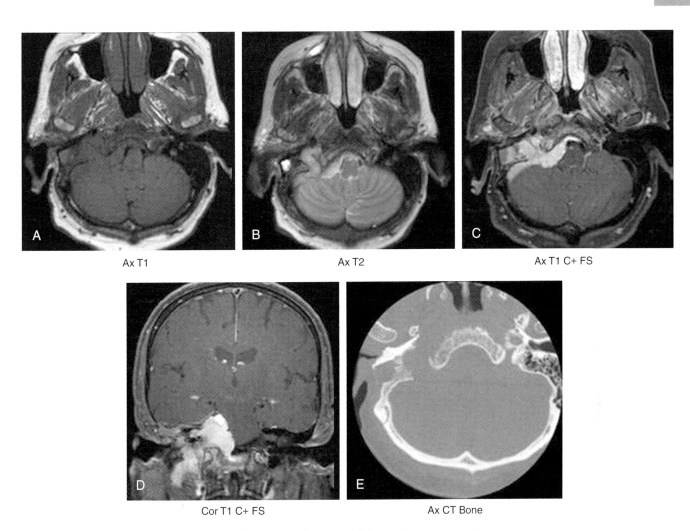

Ax T1

Ax T2

Ax T1 C+ FS

Cor T1 C+ FS

Ax CT Bone

CASE C: A 62-year-old with a history of a suboccipital craniotomy and mastoidectomy presents with a recurrent lesion. *Ax,* Axial; *Cor,* coronal; *CT,* Computed tomography; *FS,* fat saturated.

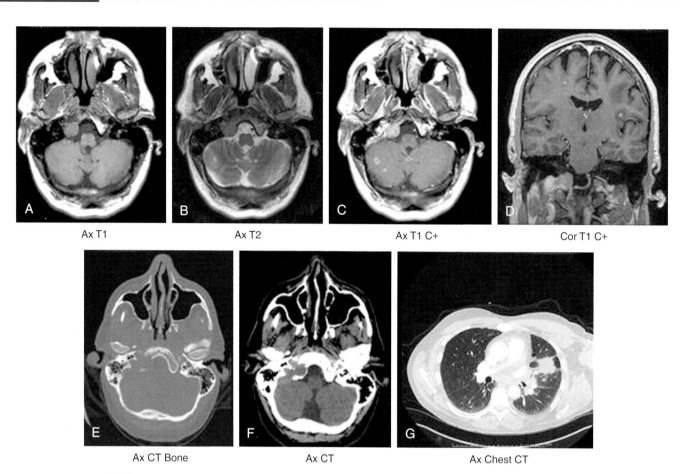

A Ax T1

B Ax T2

C Ax T1 C+

D Cor T1 C+

E Ax CT Bone

F Ax CT

G Ax Chest CT

CASE D: A 51-year-old with a history of a lung mass presenting with chest pain and weakness. *Ax,* Axial; *Cor,* coronal; *CT,* Computed tomography.

DESCRIPTION OF FINDINGS

- Case A: A heterogeneously enhancing mass centered within the left jugular foramen is noted. Close inspection demonstrates a "salt and pepper" imaging appearance resulting from internal flow voids most visible along the superior aspect of the lesion on the coronal postcontrast image. The axial T1 postcontrast image demonstrates a superolateral pattern of growth with extension to the hypotympanum and middle ear cavity. Attention to the CT images reveals an expanded left jugular foramen with irregular bony margins laterally and an erosive/permeative pattern of bony destruction. The postcontrast CT image inferior to the skull base clearly demonstrates invasion and expansion of the left jugular vein.

- Case B: A predominantly homogeneously enhancing, smoothly contoured mass centered within the right jugular foramen is seen. Of note, cystic degeneration is evident with a large intratumoral cyst along the superior aspect of the lesion, which is best evident on the coronal postcontrast image. A superomedial pattern of growth is noted, with mass effect on the medulla. On CT images, smooth cortical expansion of the jugular foramen is noted. Postcontrast CT images demonstrate the lesion compressing, but not invading, the adjacent jugular bulb.

- Case C: An avidly enhancing mass without internal flow voids is noted within a right dominant jugular foramen. Dural en-plaque growth and the presence of dural tails are clearly evident on the axial T1 postcontrast image. Infiltration/invasion of bone is noted in most directions with involvement of the temporal bone, clivus, mastoidectomy cavity, and C1 vertebral body (as seen on coronal postcontrast image). The axial CT image demonstrates a permeative-sclerotic pattern of bone involvement.

- Case D: An aggressive-appearing, enhancing mass is noted surrounding the right jugular foramen in a patient with a known history of lung cancer, as noted in the history and as evident on the chest CT scan. Multiple enhancing metastatic lesions are noted involving the right cerebellum and vermis (axial T1 postcontrast image), as well as the superior left insula and corona radiata (coronal T1 postcontrast image). Axial CT images demonstrate an aggressive, lytic pattern of bone destruction.

Diagnosis

Case A: Paraganglioma
Case B: Schwannoma
Case C: Meningioma
Case D: Metastases (lung cancer)

Summary

The first step in evaluating a jugular foramen lesion demands the exclusion of common pseudolesions including jugular foramen asymmetry, a high-riding jugular bulb, jugular bulb dehiscence, and jugular bulb diverticulum. Exclusion of these pseudolesions is achieved through experience and attention to this anatomic site in every healthy patient. Once a true jugular foramen lesion has been established, close inspection of the magnetic resonance imaging and CT findings often can lead to a diagnosis with a high degree of certainty.

Although the differential diagnosis of jugular foramen lesions is quite extensive, only three lesions account for the vast majority of enhancing neoplastic lesions centered within the jugular foramen. Of these, paragangliomas (glomus jugulare tumors) account for approximately 60% to 80% of lesions, schwannomas account for 15%, and meningiomas account for

approximately 10%. A less common differential diagnosis for this specific site is metastases, which often is suggested by a history of a primary malignancy or the multiplicity of lesions. Because rare lesions arising from the adjacent bone, bone marrow, or cartilaginous structures such as chondrosarcoma, plasmacytoma, lymphoma, or histiocytosis can secondarily involve the jugular foramen, they should at times (although sparingly) be entertained in the differential diagnosis.

Preoperative imaging differentiation often is of crucial importance because patients with highly vascular lesions, such as paragangliomas, benefit from preoperative embolization. Of the three most common lesions, two tumors (when large enough) generally are associated with enlargement/expansion of the jugular foramen: paragangliomas and schwannomas. Close inspection on CT of the bony margins of the expanded jugular foramen often yields the correct diagnosis. Irregular destruction of the cortical margins of the jugular foramen and erosive/permeative patterns of bony involvement are associated with paragangliomas. On the other hand, smooth cortical expansion of the jugular foramen by a well-demarcated, fusiform, smooth-contoured enhancing mass without associated osseous destruction is the hallmark of a schwannoma. It is important to note that these rules offer helpful guidelines that commonly yield the correct diagnosis, although the occasional aggressive schwannoma has been shown to result in irregular destruction. Therefore, other features of the lesion should be evaluated to lend further support for the suspected diagnosis. In particular, the internal structure of the lesions should be carefully scrutinized. Paragangliomas are highly vascular lesions, and as such they often demonstrate a speckled appearance referred to as a "salt and pepper" imaging pattern resulting from internal flow voids. Because schwannomas may demonstrate cystic degeneration/intratumoral cysts, the identification of cysts often is a reinforcing finding. Attention to the pattern of jugular vein involvement is helpful, because paragangliomas tend to invade the vein, whereas schwannomas tend to compress it. Lastly, when large lesions are being evaluated, the pattern of growth also can lend further support to the already suspected diagnosis. Paragangliomas tend to spread superolaterally and subsequently involve the hypotympanum and middle ear cavity, whereas jugular foramen schwannomas tend to spread superomedially toward the brainstem.

Meningiomas of the jugular foramen, on the other hand, rarely cause expansion of the jugular foramen and instead tend to infiltrate the bone or occasionally (but not commonly) result in hyperostosis. Of note, the margins of the nonexpanded jugular tend to appear irregular because of small areas of cortical loss. When meningiomas primarily arise in the jugular foramen, the extraaxial component of the lesion tends to demonstrate an en-plaque pattern of growth, and the pattern of underlying bony infiltration tends to be extensive. When bony invasion is evident, an enhancing permeative-sclerotic pattern may be seen. Internal or peripheral calcification of the tumor, when present, often can be a helpful key to diagnosis. Although meningiomas generally are avidly enhancing lesions, the absence of internal flow voids is another helpful feature differentiating them from jugular foramen paragangliomas. When the diagnosis of jugular foramen meningioma is being considered, attention to the dura may reveal important clues to this diagnosis, such as the identification of dural tails or the already mentioned en-plaque dural growth.

The diagnosis of jugular foramen metastasis can be entertained with a greater degree of suspicion when indicated by a history of a primary malignancy and/or the identification of multiple lesions. Metastatic involvement of the jugular foramen is most often associated with an aggressive permeative/destructive pattern of bone involvement.

Spectrum of Disease

The spectrum of disease is detailed in the preceding section.

Differential Diagnosis

1. Jugular foramen pseudolesions
2. Paraganglioma/glomus jugulare
3. Schwannoma
4. Meningioma
5. Metastasis
6. Secondary involvement of the jugular foramen from lesions such as chondrosarcoma, plasmacytoma, lymphoma, or histiocytosis arising from the adjacent bone, bone marrow, or cartilaginous structures

Pearls

- Paraganglioma/glomus jugulare: Irregular bony margins, erosive/permeative bony destruction, and a "salt and pepper" imaging appearance as a result of internal flow voids (Table 72.1)
- Schwannoma: Smooth cortical expansion of the jugular foramen without osseous destruction; fusiform shape; may demonstrate cystic degeneration with intratumoral cysts (see Table 72.1)
- Meningioma: Rarely expands the jugular foramen; invasion of bone with an enhancing permeative-sclerotic pattern may be evident; hyperostosis or internal calcification (when present) can be a helpful key to diagnosis; dural en-plaque growth or the presence of dural tails may be seen (see Table 72.1)
- Metastasis: History of a primary malignancy and/or multiplicity of lesions are strong indicators; aggressive permeative/destructive bony margins are the norm

TABLE 72.1

	Paraganglioma	Schwannoma	Meningioma
Jugular foramen expansion	Yes	Yes	No
Bony margins of the foramen	Irregular	Smooth	May be mildly irregular
Pattern of bony involvement	Erosive/ permeative	Not generally seen (i.e., intact cortex)	Permeative-sclerotic
Pattern of growth/ spread	Superolateral	Superomedial	En-plaque with bone infiltration
Internal flow voids	Yes	No	No
Intratumoral cysts	No	Yes	No
Internal calcification	No	No	Yes
Dural involvement/ growth	No	No	Yes

Signs and Complications

Signs and complications generally are related to involvement of the middle ear, mass effect on the brainstem, involvement of cranial nerves, or compression/thrombosis of venous structures.

Suggested Readings

Caldemeyer KS, Mathews VP, Azzarelli B, et al: The jugular foramen: a review of anatomy, masses, and imaging characteristics, *Radiographics* 17(5):1123–1139, 1997.

Christie A, Teasdale E: A comparative review of multidetector CT angiography and MRI in the diagnosis of jugular foramen lesions, *Clin Radiol* 65(3):213–217, 2010.

Eldevik OP, Gabrielsen TO, Jacobsen EA: Imaging findings in schwannomas of the jugular foramen, *AJNR Am J Neuroradiol* 21(6):1139–1144, 2000.

Löwenheim H, Koerbel A, Ebner FH, et al: Differentiating imaging findings in primary and secondary tumors of the jugular foramen, *Neurosurg Rev* 29(1):1–11, 2006.

Macdonald AJ, Salzman KL, Harnsberger HR, et al: Primary jugular foramen meningioma: imaging appearance and differentiating features, *AJR Am J Roentgenol* 182(2):373–377, 2004.

73
Optic Nerve Mass

JALIL AFNAN, MD, MRCS AND PAUL M. BUNCH, MD

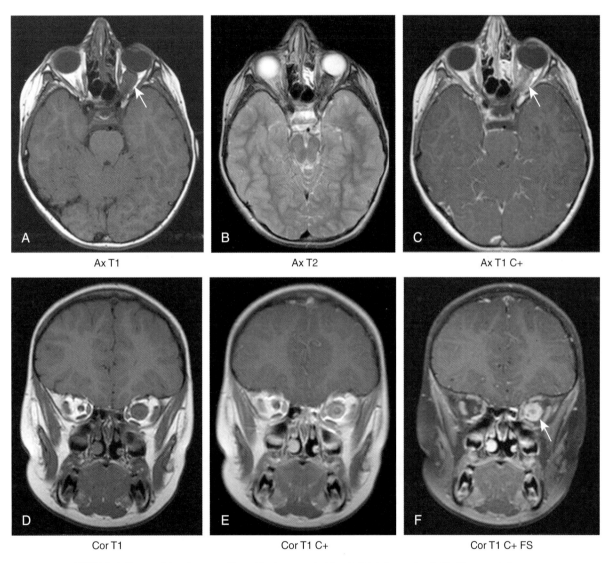

Ax T1 Ax T2 Ax T1 C+

Cor T1 Cor T1 C+ Cor T1 C+ FS

CASE A: A 6-year-old male presenting with decreased vision in the left eye. *Ax,* Axial; *Cor,* coronal; *FS,* fat saturated.

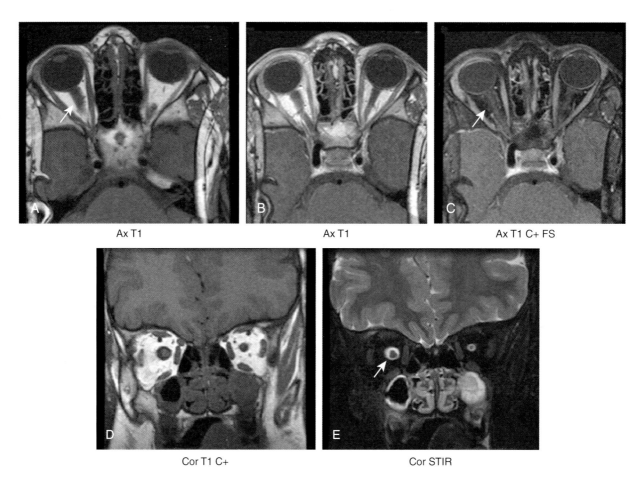

Ax T1   Ax T1   Ax T1 C+ FS

Cor T1 C+   Cor STIR

CASE B: A 6-year-old male presenting with decreased vision in the right eye. *Ax,* Axial; *Cor,* coronal; *FS,* fat saturated; *STIR,* short tau inversion recovery.

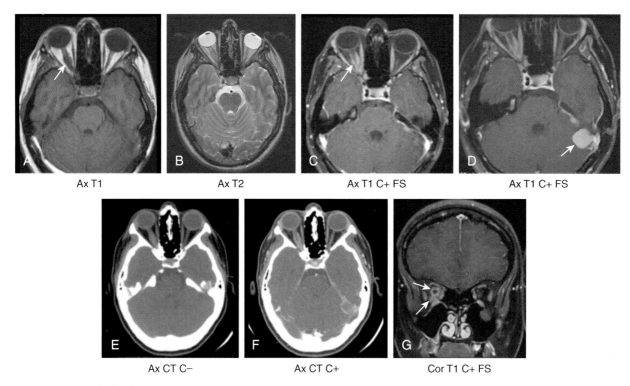

Ax T1   Ax T2   Ax T1 C+ FS   Ax T1 C+ FS

Ax CT C−   Ax CT C+   Cor T1 C+ FS

CASE C: A 24-year-old female presenting with blurred vision. *Ax,* Axial; *Cor,* coronal; *CT,* Computed tomography; *FS,* fat saturated.

DESCRIPTION OF FINDINGS

- Case A: Images demonstrate enlargement of the left optic nerve sheath with concentric avid enhancement evident on coronal postcontrast images (arrow, F), with a parallel "tram-track" appearance to the optic nerve sheath on axial postcontrast images (arrow, C); these features are consistent with an optic nerve meningioma.
- Case B: Asymmetric fusiform enlargement (arrows, A and E) of the right optic nerve with faint contrast enhancement (arrow, C). The appearance of the enlarged nerve indicates a lesion intrinsic to the optic nerve, such as an optic nerve glioma.
- Case C: Evidence of the tram-track sign, with avid enhancement of the thickened right optic nerve sheath (arrows, A and C; superior arrow, G) and an intrinsically normal-appearing optic nerve. A broad-based, extra-axial, homogeneously enhancing mass (arrow, D) is noted in the left posterior fossa, consistent with an additional meningioma. Precontrast CT does not demonstrate calcification in this case, although homogeneous enhancement and the tram-track sign are evident. Incidental note is made of an additional enhancing mass in the inferior aspect of the right orbit (inferior arrow, G), likely a schwannoma associated with the inferior division of the right oculomotor nerve. Findings are suggestive of neurofibromatosis (NF) type 2 (NF2).

Diagnosis

Case A: Left optic nerve sheath meningioma associated with NF2

Case B: Right optic nerve glioma associated with NF type 1 (NF1)

Case C: Right optic nerve sheath meningioma associated with NF2, with incidental left posterior fossa meningioma and incidental right oculomotor schwannoma

Summary

Optic nerve (also referred to as "optic pathway") gliomas are the most common primary neoplasm of the optic nerve. They can be divided into three broad subtypes: childhood tumors associated with NF1, childhood tumors not associated with NF1, and adult tumors. In children, optic pathway gliomas are almost always lowgrade, whereas in adults, they are typically malignant (e.g., grade 3 astrocytoma or glioblastoma) and convey a poor prognosis. NF1, also known as von Recklinghausen disease, is present in approximately one-third of children with an optic nerve glioma. Conversely, approximately 15% to 40% of children with NF1 will have an optic nerve glioma. Childhood tumors often present with proptosis and can present with vision loss, but they often are asymptomatic, especially in patients with NF1. In adult populations, the usual presenting symptom is rapidly progressive vision loss.

The classic imaging finding is tubular, noncalcified enlargement of the optic nerve. Characteristic kinking or buckling of the nerve may be noted. This lesion typically is isoattenuating on CT with a variable enhancement pattern due to areas of cystic degeneration. In patients with NF1, the glioma often is anterior to the chiasm, but in patients who do not have NF1, it more often is retrochiasmal. Additional intracranial manifestations of NF1, such as focal T2 hyperintensities and other central nervous system tumors, may aid in diagnosis. Chemotherapy represents the first-line treatment in most situations,

but there are also roles for molecular targeted therapies, radiotherapy, and surgical debulking.

Meningiomas of the optic nerve sheath account for 1% to 2% of all meningiomas and approximately one-third of primary optic nerve tumors. These lesions are more common in female patients, and typically present in the fourth or fifth decade with painless slowly progressive vision loss. An association exists with NF2. Fat-suppressed, gadolinium-enhanced magnetic resonance imaging is preferred to identify the lesion, which will appear as homogeneously enhancing thickening of the optic nerve sheath, and to determine the extent of disease. In the axial plane, the appearance of the enhancing tumor has been described as a "tram-track" configuration and as a "donut" appearance in the coronal plane. Calcifications are present in 20% to 50% of cases and best seen with CT.

The triad of vision loss, optociliary venous shunting, and optic disk atrophy, while associated with optic nerve sheath meningioma, also may be seen in a variety of other conditions including gliomas, central retinal vein occlusion, and glaucoma. In addition to optic nerve gliomas, differential considerations include optic neuritis, orbital sarcoid, and idiopathic orbital inflammatory disease. As such, the clinical history is essential.

Spectrum of Disease

The spectrum of disease is detailed in the preceding section.

Pearls

- An optic nerve glioma has the following features:
  - Arises from glial cells intrinsic to the optic nerve
  - Fusiform mass involves the optic nerve and/or chiasm
  - Smooth optic nerve enlargement; buckling or kinking may be seen
  - Variable enhancement pattern; cystic degeneration may be seen
- An optic nerve sheath meningioma has the following features:
  - Homogeneously enhancing optic nerve sheath thickening producing a "tram-track" configuration on axial images and a "donut" appearance on coronal images
  - Linear or punctate calcifications in up to half of cases
  - Optociliary venous shunting

Signs and Complications

Both optic pathway gliomas and optic nerve meningiomas may present with progressive painless visual field deficits, which often are unilateral, with associated proptosis. With optic nerve sheath meningiomas, edema of the optic disk often is seen initially, and the disk subsequently appears to be atrophic. Untreated lesions will cause progressive local mass effect based on their location. Both types of lesions may result in adjacent osseous scalloping or expansion of the bony canals. Differential considerations include sarcoidosis, demyelinating optic neuritis or perineuritis, orbital inflammatory disease of the optic nerve, orbital schwannoma, lymphoma, hemangiopericytoma, and optic nerve metastasis.

Suggested Readings

Avery RA, Fisher MJ, Liu GT: Optic pathway gliomas, *J Neuroophthalmol* 31(3):269–278, 2011.

Becker M, Masterson K, Delavelle J, et al: Imaging of the optic nerve, *Eur J Radiol* 74(2):299–313, 2010.

Ediriwickrema LS, Miller NR: Tumors of the optic nerve and its sheath, *Int Ophthalmol Clin* 58(2):237–260, 2018.

Farazdaghi MK, Katowitz WR, Avery RA: Current treatment of optic nerve gliomas, *Curr Opin Ophthalmol* 30(5):356–363, 2019.

Saeed P, Rootman J, Nugent RA, et al: Optic nerve sheath meningiomas, *Ophthalmology* 110:2019–2030, 2003.

Shapey J, Danesh-Meyer HV, Kaye AH: Diagnosis and management of optic nerve glioma, *J Clin Neurosci* 18(12):1585–1591, 2011.

Tailor TD, Gupta D, Dalley RW, et al: Orbital neoplasms in adults: clinical, radiologic, and pathologic review, *Radiographics* 33(6):1739–1758, 2013.

Turbin RE, Pokorny K: Diagnosis and treatment of orbital optic nerve sheath meningioma, *Cancer Control* 11(5):334–341, 2004.

74

Cavernous Sinus Masses

SWETHA ARIBINDI, BA, MD AND PAUL M. BUNCH, MD

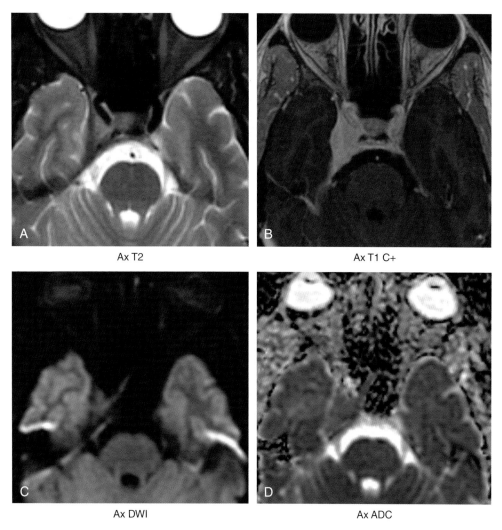

Ax T2

Ax T1 C+

Ax DWI

Ax ADC

CASE A: A 69-year-old female with headaches. *ADC*, Apparent diffusion coefficient; *Ax*, axial; *DWI*, diffusion-weighted imaging.

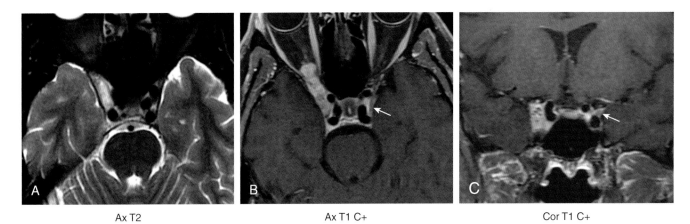

Ax T2   Ax T1 C+   Cor T1 C+

CASE B: A 56-year-old male with diplopia. *Ax*, Axial; *Cor*, coronal. The *arrows* mark a normal left-sided structure for comparison.

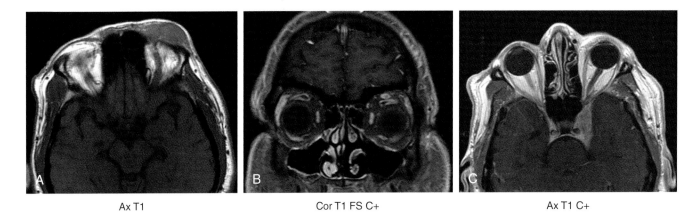

Ax T1   Cor T1 FS C+   Ax T1 C+

Case C: A 55-year-old male with left supraorbital melanoma. The patient also describes months of progressive left periorbital pain, as well as recent development of diplopia, ptosis, and numbness in a left V2 distribution. *Ax*, Axial; *Cor*, coronal; *FS*, fat saturated.

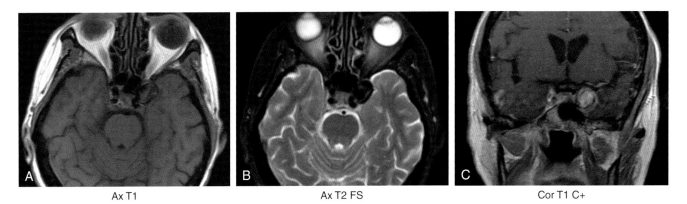

Ax T1   Ax T2 FS   Cor T1 C+

CASE D: An 85-year-old female with headaches. *Ax,* Axial; *Cor*, coronal; *FS*, fat saturated.

DESCRIPTION OF FINDINGS

- Case A: Homogeneously enhancing mass centered in the right cavernous sinus exhibiting T2 isointensity to gray matter and homogeneous low diffusivity suggestive of cellularity. The mass extends posteriorly along the right tentorial leaflet, where there is also an enhancing dural tail.
- Case B: Heterogeneously T2 hyperintense, heterogeneously enhancing mass involving the anterior aspect of the right cavernous sinus and extending anteriorly through and widening the right superior orbital fissure. On the postcontrast images, the mass is centered in the expected location of the right oculomotor nerve, and no normal right oculomotor nerve is identified. The normal left oculomotor nerve is marked with arrows for comparison.
- Case C: Mildly T1 hyperintense left supraorbital cutaneous mass consistent with the provided history of melanoma. Cord-like thickening of the ophthalmic division of the left trigeminal nerve along the superior aspect of the left superior muscle complex. This finding explains the patient's progressive left periorbital pain. Posterior extension of the left ophthalmic division abnormality reaches the left cavernous sinus, where a mildly enhancing mass is present. Left cavernous sinus involvement explains the additional cranial nerve deficits.
- Case D: Round T1, and T2 markedly hypointense, enhancing left cavernous sinus mass contiguous with the cavernous segment of the left internal carotid artery. Note the pulsation artifact on the coronal T1-weighted, gadolinium-enhanced image.

Diagnosis

Case A: Meningioma
Case B: Oculomotor schwannoma
Case C: Perineural tumor spread
Case D: Aneurysm

Summary

The cavernous sinuses are paired dural-lined venous structures located between the sphenoid wings and extending from the orbital apices anteriorly to the Meckel's caves posteriorly. Important structures associated with the cavernous sinuses include the cavernous segments of the internal carotid arteries; the oculomotor, trochlear, and abducens nerves; and the ophthalmic (V_1) and maxillary (V_2) divisions of the trigeminal nerves (Fig. 74.1). The normal cranial nerves traversing the cavernous sinuses can be identified as nonenhancing

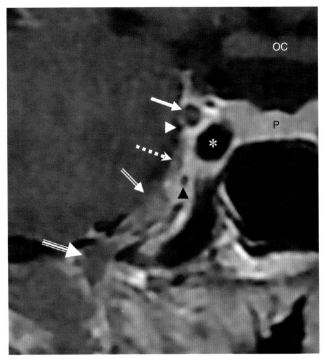

Cor T1 C+

• **Fig. 74.2** Coronal *(Cor)* T1-weighted, gadolinium-enhanced image demonstrates the normal anatomy of the cavernous sinus. The traversing cranial nerves are identifiable as nonenhancing structures within the enhancing cavernous sinus. The oculomotor *(solid arrow)*, trochlear *(white arrowhead)*, trigeminal nerve ophthalmic division *(dashed arrow)*, and trigeminal nerve maxillary division *(double line arrow)* course within the lateral aspect of the cavernous sinus. The abducens nerve *(black arrowhead)* passes more medially within the cavernous sinus and is surrounded by venous sinusoids. The cavernous segment of the right internal carotid artery is denoted by the *asterisk*. The mandibular division of the trigeminal nerve *(triple line arrow)* does not traverse the cavernous sinus and is shown passing through the right foramen ovale. The normal pituitary gland *(P)* and optic chiasm *(OC)* are labeled for reference.

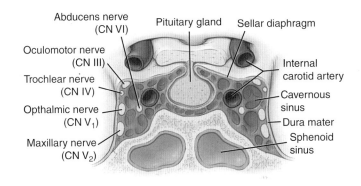

• **Fig. 74.1** Artist's rendering of the cavernous sinuses and associated anatomic structures.

structures on high-resolution, gadolinium-enhanced MR images (Fig. 74.2). Unlike the oculomotor nerves, trochlear nerves, and the ophthalmic and maxillary divisions of the trigeminal nerve, which course through the lateral walls of the cavernous sinuses, the abducens nerves are more medially located along the lateral margin of the internal carotid arteries and surrounded by venous sinusoids within the cavernous sinuses. The cavernous sinuses partially surround the pituitary gland and are located inferior and lateral to the optic chiasm.

Cavernous sinus masses may arise from adjacent (e.g., pituitary adenoma) and associated (e.g., schwannoma, aneurysm) structures or from the dural walls (e.g., meningioma). Additionally, infectious and inflammatory processes involving the cavernous sinuses may mimic a mass. Although the differential considerations for a cavernous sinus mass can be broad, clinical history and imaging characteristics are often sufficient to allow the radiologist to make a confident and informed imaging diagnosis.

Spectrum of Disease

Meningioma

Meningiomas are believed to arise from arachnoid cap cells, which form the outer layer of the arachnoid mater and arachnoid granulations. Typically attached to the dura, meningiomas may primarily involve the dural lining of the cavernous sinuses or secondarily invade the cavernous sinuses from an adjacent site of origin (e.g., Meckel's cave, tuberculum sellae, anterior clinoid process). Imaging features that favor meningioma include hyperostosis, intralesional mineralization (both best appreciated on CT; Fig. 74.3), T2 isointensity to gray matter, low diffusivity (due to cellularity), and homogenous enhancement on postcontrast images, often with an enhancing dural tail.

Meningiomas within the cavernous sinus may encase the cavernous segment of the internal carotid artery, in which case the tumor characteristically narrows the arterial lumen (Fig. 74.4).

Schwannoma

Schwannomas are benign neoplasms that arise from the Schwann cells surrounding the peripheral nerves, including cranial nerves III through XII. Although most schwannomas are sporadic, genetic conditions, including neurofibromatosis type 2 and schwannomatosis, predispose individuals to developing multiple schwannomas. Imaging features that favor

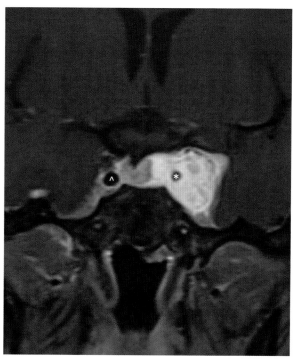

Cor T1 C+

• **Fig. 74.4** Coronal *(Cor)* T1-weighted, gadolinium-enhanced image demonstrates a left cavernous sinus meningioma encasing the left internal carotid artery. Note the associated narrowing of the left internal carotid artery flow void *(asterisk)* relative to the right *(carat)*.

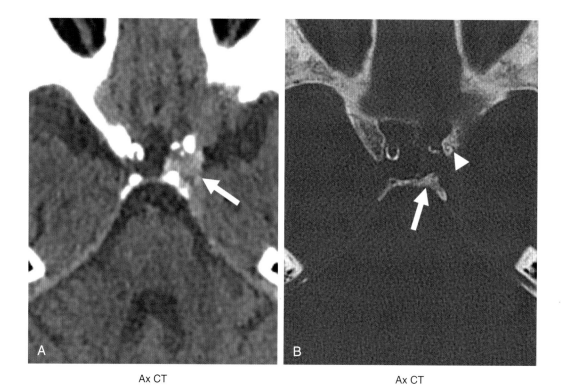

Ax CT   Ax CT

• **Fig. 74.3** Axial noncontrast CT images in (A) soft tissue and (B) bone windows demonstrate a mineralized mass *(arrow,* A) centered in the left cavernous sinus with associated focal hyperostosis involving the left aspect of the dorsum sellae *(arrow,* B) and the left anterior clinoid process *(arrowhead)*. These imaging features favor meningioma. *Ax,* Axial; *CT,* Computed tomography.

schwannoma include T2 hyperintensity and heterogeneous enhancement. Intralesional cystic spaces and intralesional blood products may also be seen. The long axis of the tumor is typically oriented along the path of the nerve. Although a schwannoma involving cranial nerves III through VI may be entirely located within the cavernous sinus, more commonly the lesion will extend proximally and/or distally along the course of the involved nerve, which can be a clue to the diagnosis. Because schwannomas are typically slow-growing tumors, widening of respective skull base foramina (e.g., superior orbital fissure for lesions involving cranial nerves III, IV, V_1, and VI; foramen rotundum for lesions involving V_2) may also be seen. Unlike with meningiomas, intralesional mineralization is not expected in schwannomas. Schwannomas involving the cavernous sinus most often arise from the trigeminal nerve.

Perineural Tumor Spread

Perineural tumor spread from a head and neck malignancy may result in a cavernous sinus mass, most commonly due to retrograde spread along branches of the trigeminal nerve. Perineural tumor spread is most commonly seen with squamous cell carcinoma and adenoid cystic carcinoma but also occurs in other malignancies, including mucoepidermoid carcinoma, melanoma, and lymphoma. Clinical symptoms of perineural tumor spread are referable to the nerve(s) involved, and multiple cranial neuropathies may occur with cavernous sinus involvement. However, up to 40% of patients with radiologic evidence of perineural tumor spread are asymptomatic. As such, a high index of suspicion is warranted in the presence of typical imaging findings even in the absence of clinically evident disease. The primary imaging findings of perineural tumor spread include abnormal thickening and enhancement of the involved nerve(s).

Loss of the normal fat surrounding the involved nerves, erosion or enlargement of the involved skull base foramina, and denervation changes (see Chapters 84 and 85) in the distribution of the involved nerve(s) may also be seen. Although both schwannoma and perineural tumor spread can produce enlargement and abnormal enhancement of cranial nerves within the cavernous sinus, schwannomas tend to be more focal, more T2 hyperintense, and more avidly enhancing as compared to perineural tumor spread, which tends to be more extensive, T2 intermediate, and mildly enhancing (the so-called "evil" gray). Perineural tumor spread, particularly disease reaching the cavernous sinus, is commonly treated with radiation therapy. Although some improvement in the pretreatment imaging findings may occur after therapy, persistent enlargement and enhancement is commonly observed after radiation and does not necessarily indicate persistent disease. However, progressive nerve enlargement or new areas of nerve enhancement should be viewed with suspicion.

Aneurysm

Aneurysms of the cavernous segment of the internal carotid artery and of its branches (i.e., meningohypophyseal trunk, inferolateral trunk) may manifest as a cavernous sinus mass. These aneurysms are usually asymptomatic and detected incidentally; however, large aneurysms may produce clinical symptoms secondary to mass effect on adjacent structures. Additionally, rupture (e.g., spontaneous, traumatic) of a cavernous segment aneurysm produces a cavernous-carotid fistula, as further discussed in Chapter 75. On noncontrast CT, a large, cavernous internal carotid aneurysm can be easily mistaken for neoplasm, such as meningioma. However, peripheral calcifications (Fig. 74.5) and smooth remodeling of the carotid canal

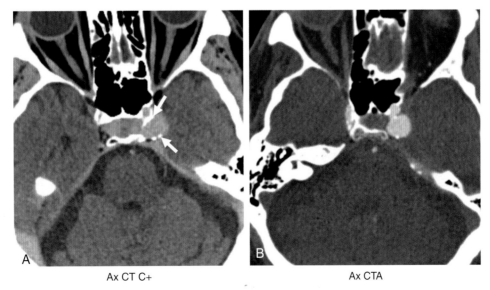

Ax CT C+   Ax CTA

• **Fig. 74.5** (A) The axial contrast-enhanced CT image demonstrates a round mass with peripheral calcifications (arrows) in the left cavernous sinus. The round morphology and peripheral calcifications were correctly interpreted as suspicious for aneurysm. (B) A head CTA was recommended for further evaluation and confirmed the suspected aneurysm. Ax, Axial; CT, Computed tomography; CTA, Computed tomography angiography.

can be clues to the presence of an aneurysm. The MR imaging appearance of cavernous internal carotid artery aneurysms is variable depending on the flow rate and presence or absence of thrombus. As such, a low threshold for vascular imaging (e.g., head CTA or MRA) is prudent before biopsy or attempted resection of a "mass" in this region, particularly if the "mass" exhibits a round morphology. A patent aneurysm with fast flow will exhibit a T2 hypointense "flow void." Partial thrombosis with slow flow in the aneurysm or complete aneurysm thrombosis will produce heterogeneous T2 hyperintensity with variable T1 signal depending on the age and composition of the thrombus. Finally, the presence of pulsation artifact propagating through the phase encode direction is an important clue that a "mass" is vascular in etiology and should prompt head CT angiogram (CTA) or magnetic resonance angiography (MRA) for further characterization.

Differential Diagnosis

1. The differential diagnosis for cavernous sinus masses is broad and includes numerous other conditions in addition to those previously discussed.
2. Cavernous sinus thrombosis can appear mass-like, particularly in the setting of infectious thrombophlebitis because the infected thrombus may enhance (Fig. 74.6). Cavernous sinus thrombosis warrants particular consideration in the clinical setting of an acute infection involving the paranasal sinuses, orbit, or face.
3. Cavernous sinus venous malformations (formerly known as cavernous sinus hemangiomas) are reported to account for up to 3% of all cavernous sinus lesions and exhibit a strong female predilection. These masses tend to be slow growing with insidious onset of clinical symptoms due to

local mass effect. Imaging features of cavernous sinus venous malformations include marked T2 hyperintensity, smooth osseous remodeling, small intralesional vessels, and progressive "filling in" with contrast on multiphase postcontrast imaging. If considering this diagnosis, a technetium-99m–tagged red blood cell scan can be useful, as these lesions typically exhibit photopenia during initial images with subsequent marked accumulation of radiotracer on delayed images. Although uncommon, the possibility of a cavernous sinus venous malformation is important for the radiologist to consider prior to biopsy or attempted resection because of the risk of catastrophic hemorrhage with intervention.

4. Pituitary macroadenomas do not arise in the cavernous sinus but can secondarily invade the cavernous sinus from the adjacent sella, thereby mimicking a cavernous sinus mass. The sella turcica is typically expanded by the macroadenoma (Fig. 74.7A). Most pituitary macroadenomas are nonfunctional and present with clinical symptoms related to mass effect (e.g., bitemporal hemianopia due to mass effect on the optic chiasm). Although the imaging appearance of pituitary macroadenomas may vary depending on the presence of cystic or hemorrhagic components, most lesions are hypoenhancing relative to the normal pituitary gland. As with meningiomas, pituitary macroadenomas that invade the cavernous sinus can encase the cavernous internal carotid arteries. However, unlike meningiomas, the relatively softer pituitary macroadenomas do not result in narrowing of the arterial lumen (Fig. 74.7B).

5. Tolosa-Hunt syndrome refers to an idiopathic steroid-responsive inflammation of the cavernous sinus and orbital apex manifesting clinically as painful ophthalmoplegia with

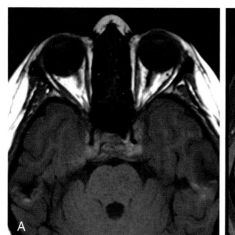 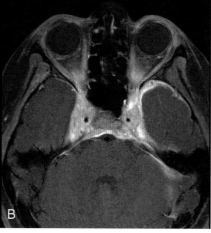 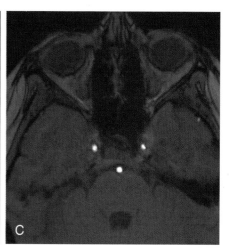

Ax T1   Ax T1 FS C+   Ax MRA

• **Fig. 74.6** An 11-year-old female with fusobacterium cavernous sinus thrombophlebitis after dental infection. (A) The axial T1-weighted image demonstrates-intrinsically T1 hyperintense material within the expanded cavernous sinuses. (B) The axial T1-weighted, fat-suppressed, gadolinium-enhanced image demonstrates heterogeneous enhancement of the expanded cavernous sinuses as well as dural thickening and enhancement along the dorsal clivus, the left greater than right sphenoid wings, and the left greater than right posterior petrous ridges. The axial head MRA image demonstrates associated narrowing of both internal carotid arteries. *Ax*, Axial; *FS*, fat saturated; *MRA*, magnetic resonance angiography.

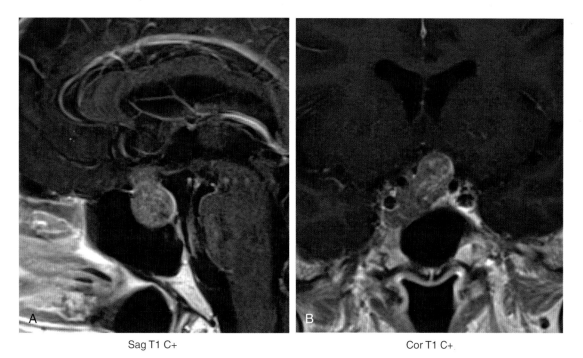

Sag T1 C+   Cor T1 C+

• **Fig. 74.7** Sagittal *(Sag)* T1-weighted, gadolinium-enhanced image demonstrates a heterogeneously hypoenhancing mass expanding the sella and exhibiting suprasellar extension. Coronal *(Cor)* T1-weighted, gadolinium-enhanced image demonstrates invasion of the right cavernous sinus by the mass with partial encasement of the right internal carotid artery. However, there is no associated luminal narrowing.

or without vision loss. Imaging features are nonspecific but typically include abnormal soft tissue and enhancement involving the orbital apex and cavernous sinus. This condition is typically considered a clinical diagnosis of exclusion, with a presumptive diagnosis often made if clinical symptoms and imaging findings resolve after corticosteroid therapy (Fig. 74.8).

Pearls

- Although the differential diagnosis for cavernous sinus masses is broad, clinical history and imaging characteristics are often sufficient to allow the radiologist to make a confident and informed imaging diagnosis.
- Cavernous sinus meningiomas exhibit T2 isointensity to gray matter, homogeneous enhancement, and often are associated with a dural tail. Hyperostosis, intralesional mineralization, and narrowing of the internal carotid artery are additional imaging clues.
- Schwannomas are typically T2 hyperintense with heterogeneous enhancement. Intralesional cystic spaces and intralesional blood products may also be seen, and the long axis of the tumor is typically oriented along the path of the nerve.
- Perineural tumor spread is most often the result of squamous cell carcinoma but also commonly occurs in salivary cancers (e.g., adenoid cystic carcinoma and mucoepidermoid carcinoma) and can be seen in the setting of melanoma and lymphoma. Because up to 40% of patients with radiologic evidence of perineural tumor spread are asymptomatic, the

typical imaging findings warrant a high index of suspicion even in the absence of clinically evident disease.
- Round morphology, T2 hypointense "flow voids," and pulsation artifacts are clues that a cavernous sinus "mass" is, in fact, an aneurysm. A low threshold for vascular imaging is prudent prior to biopsy or attempted resection.
- Marked T2 hyperintensity, intralesional vessels, and progressive contrast enhancement are characteristics of cavernous sinus venous malformations, an uncommon lesion with a strong female predilection. The possibility of a cavernous sinus venous malformation is important for the radiologist to consider prior to biopsy or attempted resection because of the risk of catastrophic hemorrhage with intervention.
- Pituitary macroadenomas invading the cavernous sinus are typically centered within an expanded sella turcica and exhibit hypoenhancement relative to the normal pituitary gland.

Signs and Complications

Clinical signs of the cavernous sinus lesions discussed in this chapter are similar and primarily related to mass effect, including headaches, cranial neuropathies, and visual field deficits.

Surgical access to the cavernous sinus carries substantial risk of bleeding and cranial nerve damage. As such, asymptomatic benign lesions are commonly observed. For symptomatic or enlarging cavernous sinus masses, a multidisciplinary approach is often most appropriate and commonly involves surgical debulking and/or radiotherapy.

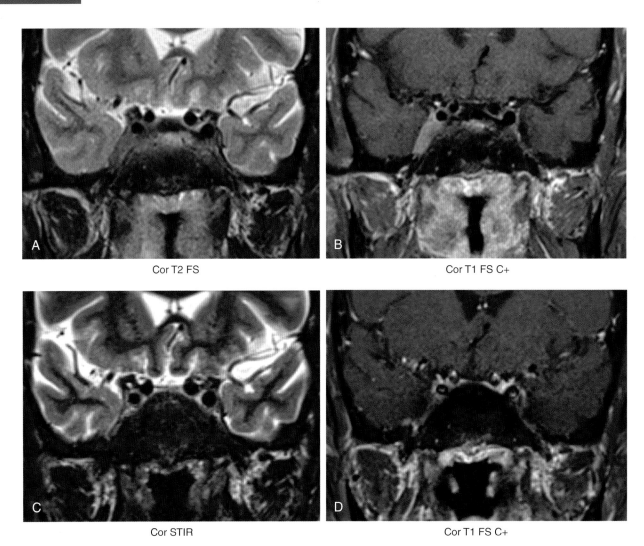

Cor T2 FS

Cor T1 FS C+

Cor STIR

Cor T1 FS C+

• **Fig. 74.8** A 65-year-old male with painful right ophthalmoplegia. (A, B) Coronal T2-weighted, fat-suppressed, and coronal T1-weighted, fat-suppressed, gadolinium-enhanced images demonstrate T2 hypointense, enhancing soft tissue involving the right cavernous sinus. Based on the clinical symptoms, a presumptive diagnosis of Tolosa-Hunt syndrome was made, and a trial of corticosteroids was initiated. The clinical symptoms resolved, and 6-month follow-up imaging (C, D) demonstrated resolution of the previous right cavernous sinus abnormality. *Cor,* Coronal; *FS,* fat saturated; *STIR,* short tau inversion recovery.

Suggested Readings

Agarwal M, Wangaryattawanich P, Rath TJ: Perineural tumor spread in head and neck malignancies, *Semin Roentgenol* 54(3):258–275, 2019.

Benson JC, Eschbacher KL, Raghunathan A, et al: Cavernous sinus vascular venous malformation, *AJNR Am J Neuroradiol* 43(1):19–23, 2022.

Eddleman CS, Hurley MC, Bendok BR, et al: Cavernous carotid aneurysms: to treat or not to treat? *Neurosurg Focus* 26(5):E4, 2009.

Hekmatpanah J: Evidence-based treatment of cavernous sinus meningioma, *Surg Neurol Int*, 10:228, 2019.

Klinger DR, Flores B, Lewis JJ, et al: The treatment of cavernous sinus meningiomas: evolution of a modern approach, *Neurosurg Focus* 35(6):E8, 2013.

Mahalingam HV, Mani SE, Patel B, et al: Imaging spectrum of cavernous sinus lesions with histopathologic correlation, *Radiographics* 39(3):795–819, 2019.

Paes FM, Singer AD, Checkver AN, et al: Perineural spread in head and neck malignancies: clinical significance and evaluation with 18F-FDG PET/CT, *Radiographics* 33(6):1717–1736, 2013.

Skolnik AD, Loevner LA, Sampathu DM, et al: Cranial nerve schwannomas: diagnostic imaging approach, *Radiographics* 36(5):1463–1477, 2016.

75

Dilated Superior Ophthalmic Vein/ Asymmetric Cavernous Sinus Enhancement

NICHOLAS A. TELISCHAK, MD, MS, PAUL M. BUNCH, MD, AND GUL MOONIS, MD

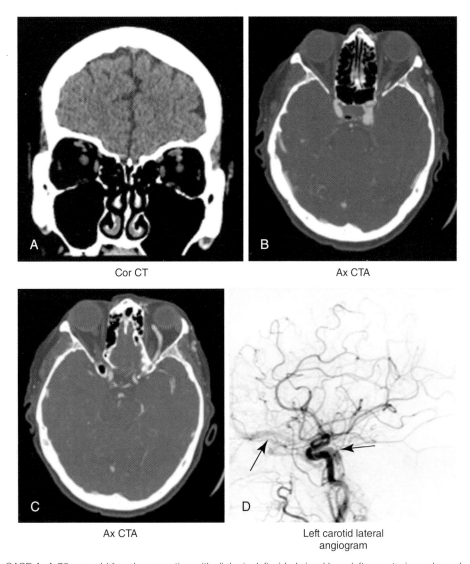

Cor CT

Ax CTA

Ax CTA

Left carotid lateral
angiogram

CASE A: A 76-year-old female presenting with diplopia, left-sided visual loss, left eye ptosis, and exophthalmos. *Ax,* Axial; *Cor,* coronal; *CT,* Computed tomography; *CTA,* CT angiography.

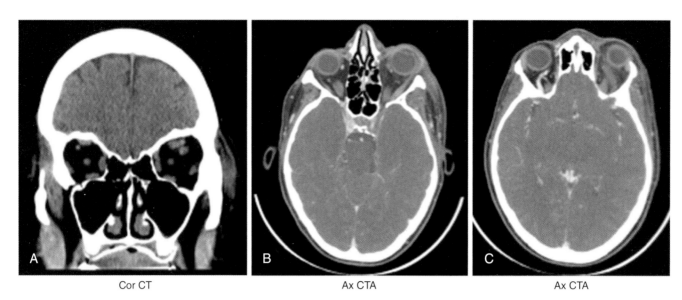

Cor CT · Ax CTA · Ax CTA

CASE B: A 51-year-old female presenting with headache and swelling of the left eye. *Ax,* Axial; *Cor,* coronal; *CT,* Computed tomography; *CTA,* CT angiography.

DESCRIPTION OF FINDINGS

- Case A: Noncontrast head CT in the coronal plane demonstrates enlargement of the left superior ophthalmic vein. Head CT angiography demonstrates arterial phase contrast filling of the cavernous sinus with filling of the enlarged left superior ophthalmic vein. A left common carotid angiogram demonstrates a fistulous connection between the cavernous segment of the internal carotid artery (ICA) with contrast filling and distending of the superior ophthalmic vein in a retrograde fashion.
- Case B: Noncontrast head CT in the coronal plane demonstrates enlargement of the left superior ophthalmic vein. Contrast-enhanced head CT demonstrates thrombus within the left cavernous sinus extending into the left superior ophthalmic vein.

Diagnosis

Case A: Carotid-cavernous fistula (CCF)
Case B: Cavernous sinus and superior ophthalmic vein thrombosis

Summary

The cavernous sinus, which is part of the anteroinferior group of dural venous sinuses, drains the insular cortex and parenchyma around the sylvian fissure via the sphenoparietal sinus. Each cavernous sinus communicates with the contralateral side, the pterygoid venous plexus, the inferior petrosal sinus, and the superior ophthalmic veins. Asymmetric contrast filling of the cavernous sinuses can be a normal finding on head CT angiography related to contrast bolus timing. However, when there is asymmetric enhancement and fullness of one cavernous sinus relative to the other, fistula, thrombosis, mass, inflammatory processes (e.g., sarcoid, Tolosa–Hunt syndrome), and infection should be considered. Enlargement of the ipsilateral superior ophthalmic vein may be seen in the setting of carotid-cavernous fistula and cavernous sinus thrombosis. However, superior ophthalmic vein enlargement can also be seen in intubated patients without associated intracranial or orbital pathology. When secondary to intubated status, this finding usually reverses following extubation.

CCFs are classified on the basis of etiology (traumatic or spontaneous), flow rate (high versus low), and angiographic architecture. The Barrow classification divides CCFs into four types based on arterial supply. Direct fistulas (type A) are usually traumatic and tend to affect young men. Up to 20% of direct fistulas may be spontaneous, resulting from aneurysmal rupture or rupture of a weakened cavernous ICA vessel wall. Predisposing factors to spontaneous rupture include fibromuscular dysplasia, Ehlers-Danlos syndrome, and pseudoxanthoma elasticum. The indirect types of CCFs comprise dural arteriovenous fistulas (DAVFs), either from dural branches of the ICA (type B), dural branches of the external carotid artery (type C), or meningeal branches of both the ICA and external carotid artery (type D, the most common type of indirect CCF). Indirect CCFs tend to occur in postmenopausal women, and sinus thrombosis, hypertension, and diabetes may be risk factors.

Clinically, direct or high-flow CCFs present as a triad of exophthalmos, bruit, and conjunctival chemosis. Associated

venous hypertension can result in ocular signs and symptoms of proptosis, chemosis, conjunctival injection, elevated intraocular pressure, cranial nerve palsies, and visual deficits. Bleeding can occur from the mouth, nose, or ears. Cerebral complications include intracranial hemorrhage, increased intracranial pressure, and vascular steal. Indirect CCFs (DAVFs) are low flow and tend to present with more subtle clinical symptoms, such as chronic red eyes.

Imaging demonstrates enlargement of the extraocular muscles, the superior (and/or inferior) ophthalmic vein, and the ipsilateral cavernous sinus. MRI also may show orbital edema and abnormal flow voids in the cavernous sinus, indicating arterialization of the cavernous sinus. Digital subtraction angiography is essential to confirm the diagnosis and classify the fistula and to identify sites of venous drainage. Endovascular treatment of high-flow CCFs can be accomplished with various methods, including stent-assisted coiling, detachable balloon occlusion, and more recently with the use of flow-diverting stents. Indirect CCFs are also commonly managed with endovascular approaches.

Cavernous sinus thrombosis (CST) presents most commonly with headache, often in a V1 and V2 distribution. Other common symptoms include orbital pain, periorbital edema, chemosis, ptosis, ophthalmoplegia, and vision loss. Cranial nerve signs and meningeal signs can occur. In persons with septic thrombosis, systemic signs of sepsis occur as a late finding. The most common organism responsible for septic CST (70%) is *Staphylococcus aureus*. Because the veins communicating with the cavernous sinus do not have valves, bacteria from facial, paranasal sinus, and odontogenic infections can pass into the cavernous sinus as a result of manipulation, for example, of a facial carbuncle. Contrast-enhanced MRI and contrast-enhanced CT imaging are equally suited to make the diagnosis, preferably with thin slices (e.g., 3 mm) through the cavernous sinus and orbits. Imaging findings include enlargement of the cavernous sinus with filling defects and enlargement and thrombosis of the superior and inferior ophthalmic veins. Treatment is with intravenous antibiotics, steroids, and supportive care.

Spectrum of Disease

The spectrum of disease is delineated in Figs. 75.1 and 75.2.

Differential Diagnosis

1. CST
2. Infected CST
3. Inflammation: sarcoid, Tolosa-Hunt syndrome, Wegener granulomatosis
4. Mass: meningioma, schwannoma, lymphoma
5. Vascular: CCF, aneurysm

Pearls

- Enlargement of the superior ophthalmic vein on noncontrast CT may be the only hint of serious pathology, such as CCF or CST. However, superior ophthalmic vein enlargement can

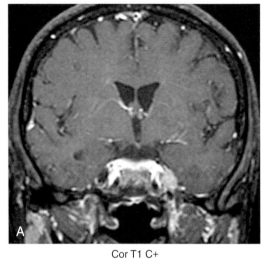

Cor T1 C+

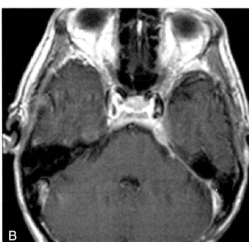

Ax T1 C+

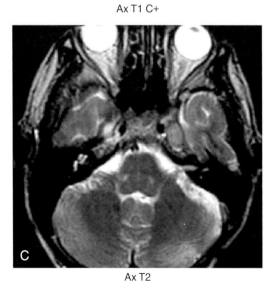

Ax T2

• **Fig. 75.1** A 40-year-old female with intermittent left trigeminal neuralgia. Coronal *(Cor)* T1 postcontrast image, axial *(Ax)* T1 postcontrast image, and axial T2-weighted image demonstrate a homogeneously enhancing, dural-based, extraaxial mass in the left cavernous sinus and left Meckel's cave with associated dural tail, consistent with meningioma.

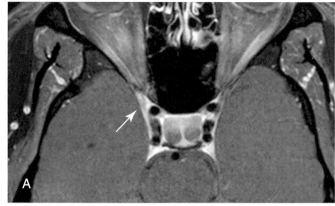

Ax T1 C+ FS

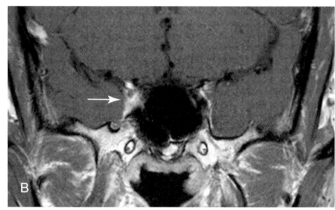

Cor T1 C+ FS

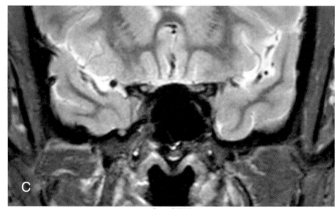

Cor STIR

• **Fig. 75.2** A 27-year-old male with limited movement of the right eye and pain. (A) Axial *(Ax)* gadolinium-enhanced, fat-suppressed, T1-weighted image (B) coronal *(Cor)* gadolinium-enhanced, fat-suppressed, T1-weighted image and (C) coronal short tau inversion recovery *(STIR)* image demonstrate asymmetric fullness and enhancement within the anterior aspect of the right cavernous sinus *(arrows, A and B)*, consistent with Tolosa–Hunt syndrome.

also occur in the setting of intubation and is therefore not necessarily pathologic.
- Veins communicating with the cavernous sinus do not have valves, predisposing to transmission of facial, odontogenic, and paranasal sinal infections.
- Direct CCFs are usually traumatic, although other predisposing conditions include Ehlers-Danlos syndrome, fibromuscular dysplasia, and pseudoxanthoma elasticum.

Signs and Complications

Signs and complications include intracranial hemorrhage in persons with CCF and propagation of a clot into deep veins and venous infarct in persons with CST.

Suggested Readings

Gemmette JJ, Ansari SA, Gandhi D: Endovascular treatment of carotid cavernous fistulas, *Neuroimaging Clin N Am* 19:241–255, 2009.

Grossman RI, Yousem DM: *Neuroradiology: the requisites*, ed 2, Philadelphia, 2003, Elsevier.

Mahalingam HV, Mani SE, Patel B, et al: Imaging spectrum of cavernous sinus lesions with histopathologic correlation, *Radiographics* 39: 795–819, 2019.

Munawar K, Nayak G, Fatterpekar GM, et al: Cavernous sinus lesions, *Clin Imaging* 68:71-89, 2020.

Nabavizadeh SA, Sundararajan SH, Schmitt JE, et al: Reversible dilation of the superior ophthalmic vein in intubated patients, *AJNR Am J Neuroradiol*, 39:1505–1508, 2018.

Rana RS, Moonis G: Head and neck infection and inflammation, *Radiol Clin North Am* 49(1):165–182, 2011.

76

Adult Globe Lesions

MARY D. MAHER, MD AND MARY E. CUNNANE, MD

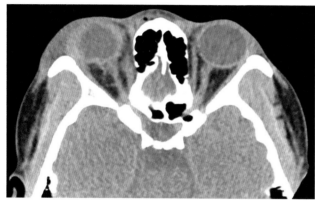

Ax CT

CASE A: A 23-year-old female presented with poor vision in the right eye after syncope and head strike. *Ax,* Axial; *CT,* Computed tomography.

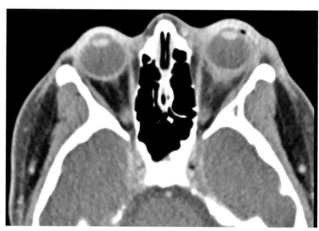

Ax CT

CASE B: A 36-year-old female presents with left eye swelling for 2 weeks and 1 day of eye pain, count fingers vision, headache, and nausea with vomiting. Ophthalmologic exam revealed elevated intraocular pressure and a "T sign" of choroidal thickening and extrascleral fluid. *Ax,* Axial; *CT,* Computed tomography.

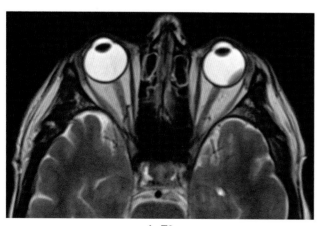

Ax T2

CASE C: A 69-year-old female presented with a nasal visual field defect in the left eye. *Ax,* Axial.

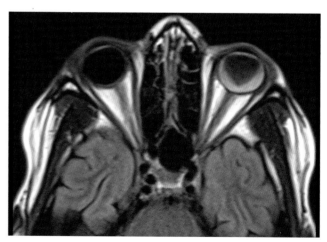

Ax FLAIR

CASE D: A 72-year-old male presented with hand motion vision in the left eye after seeing flashes of light. *Ax,* Axial; *FLAIR,* fluid attenuated inversion recovery.

DESCRIPTION OF FINDINGS

- Case A: Axial CT image demonstrates flattening and deformity of the right posterior globe.
- Case B: Axial CT image demonstrates severe thickening of the left globe scleral-uveal coat with retrobulbar stranding and a shallow anterior chamber related to acute angle closure glaucoma from posterior segment mass effect.
- Case C: Axial T2-weighted MR image demonstrates a T2 isointense lesion arising from the lateral aspect of the left posterior globe. There is no evidence of extrascleral extension.
- Case D: Axial FLAIR MR image demonstrates an abnormal "V" appearance of the left retina with hyperintense hemorrhage present posteriorly.

Diagnosis

Case A: Globe rupture
Case B: Scleritis
Case C: Choroidal melanoma
Case D: Retinal detachment

Summary

The globe can be understood anatomically and functionally in three layers. The outer layer is a strong, fibrous layer composed of the sclera and cornea. The middle layer is the vascular and muscular layer referred to as the uveal tract and composed of choroid, the ciliary body, and the iris. The inner layer is the sensorineural layer of the retina.

The globe is also divided by the lens into anterior and posterior segments. The anterior segment is located anterior to the lens and contains aqueous fluid, whereas the posterior segment is located posterior to the lens and contains vitreous fluid. The iris subdivides the anterior segment into anterior (i.e., anterior to the iris) and posterior (i.e., posterior to the iris) chambers. (Figs. 76.1, 76.2, and 76.3)

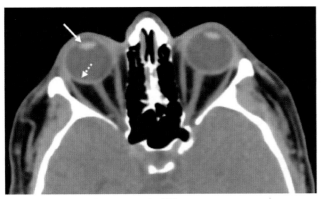

Ax CT

• **Fig. 76.1** On computed tomography (C- or C+) the walls of the globe are indistinguishable from each other *(serrated arrow)*. The native lens is hyperattenuating *(solid arrow)*. *Ax,* Axial.

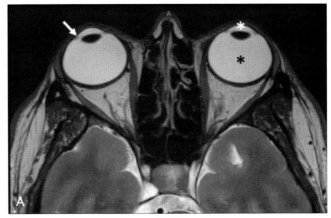

Ax T2

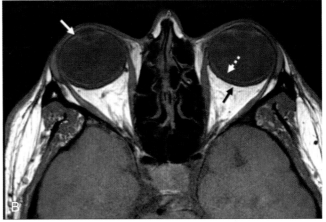

Ax T1

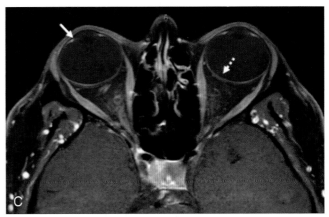

Ax T1 FS C+

• **Fig. 76.2** On magnetic resonance imaging T2-weighted images, the layers of the globe are indistinguishable from each other. On T1-weighted images, the middle uveal layer and the inner sensorineural layer are relatively hyperintense *(serrated arrow, B)* and enhance *(serrated arrow, C).* The normal sclera *(black arrow, B)* does not enhance on gadolinium-enhanced T1-weighted sequences. The ciliary body is T2 hypointense, T1 hyperintense, and enhances *(solid white arrows, A, B, C).* On T2-weighted images, the aqueous humor *(white asterisk, A)* and vitreous humor *(black asterisk, A)* are hyperintense. *Ax,* Axial; *FS,* fat saturated.

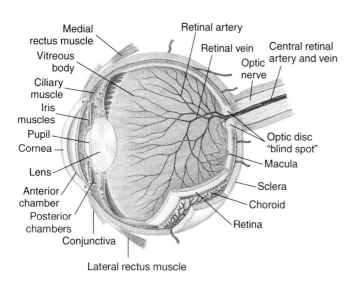

• **Fig. 76.3** Artist's rendering of the anatomy of the globe.

Spectrum of Disease

Open Globe Injury

For appropriate clinical management, traumatic ophthalmic injuries must be quickly and accurately triaged as either open versus closed globe. An open globe injury or globe rupture is defined as discontinuity of the outer layer (i.e., sclera and/or cornea) and requires emergent surgical repair. CT has a sensitivity of 75% and a specificity of 98% for globe rupture. The conspicuity of findings does not correlate with the severity of the injury, so inspection for globe rupture requires scrutiny of both primary and secondary findings.

The site of scleral discontinuity is described by zone. Zone one involves the cornea and limbus (i.e., the junction of the cornea and sclera). Zone two extends from the limbus to a 5 mm circumference of the sclera. Zone three involves the sclera beyond the 5 mm circumference and convey the poorest vision prognosis. Although an ophthalmologist can evaluate the entirety of zones one and two, intraocular hemorrhage and debris can obscure the ophthalmologist's fundoscopic view of zone three. In this setting, CT is critical for evaluating zone three's integrity (Tables 76.1 and 76.2).

Scleritis

Scleritis is rare but underdiagnosed. Clinically, scleritis is divided into anterior and posterior disease. Anterior disease is readily identified on ophthalmologic exam. Posterior disease is less common and traditionally diagnosed by history and ultrasound; however, ultrasound has a lower sensitivity for scleritis than CT and MRI. Histologically, immune-mediated scleritis causes necrosis of devitalized collagen, and severe cases or untreated cases can result in globe perforation and permanent vision loss.

TABLE 76.1	Open Globe Injury		
Finding	**Image and History**		**Description**
Flat tire sign: posterior globe deformity and ocular volume loss (Primary sign of globe rupture)	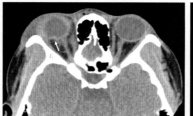 A 23-year-old female (same patient from Case A) presented with light perception vision in the right eye after syncope and head strike. The ophthalmologist was not able to see into the posterior segment due to hemorrhage in the anterior chamber. The patient was taken emergently to the operating room for repair of the posterior globe rupture.		Axial CT and sagittal CT images demonstrate zone three flattening and deformity *(arrows)* of the right globe, which confirmed the clinically suspected globe rupture.
Wall contour deformity (Primary sign of globe rupture)	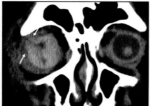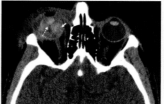 A 65-year-old male presented with no right eye light perception after a wood chip hit his eye while sawing. Subconjunctival hemorrhage, hyphema, and vitreous hemorrhage obscured the ophthalmologist's view into the posterior segment. Emergent surgery confirmed globe rupture involving zones two and three with uveal prolapse.		Coronal and axial CT images demonstrate contour irregularity in the supratemporal quadrant *(arrows, coronal CT)* concerning for globe rupture. There is also posterior lens displacement *(serrated arrow, axial CT)* and vitreous hemorrhage *(solid arrow, axial CT)*.

TABLE 76.1	Open Globe Injury—cont'd		
Finding	**Image and History**		**Description**
Intraocular air or foreign body (Secondary sign of globe rupture)	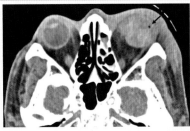 A 32-year-old male presented without left eye light perception after assault. Extensive vitreous hemorrhage can be present in an open or closed globe injury and limits the ophthalmologist's examination.		The focus of intraocular air *(black arrow)* on this axial CT image is diagnostic of globe rupture even though the globe contour is difficult to discern.
Anterior segment size (Secondary sign of globe rupture) Shallow anterior segment: corneal rupture with loss of aqueous humor Deep anterior segment: posterior segment rupture with decreased posterior pressure allowing the lens to drop posteriorly while remaining suspended.	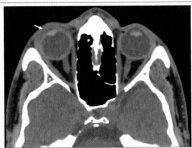 A 27-year-old male with a history of Steven Johnson Syndrome affecting his eyes 5 years ago presented with 2 weeks of right eye pain, redness, and light perception vision. An infected corneal ulcer was identified on ophthalmic exam.		Axial CT image demonstrates a shallow right anterior segment *(arrow)* corroborating corneal ulceration and perforation.

CT, Computed tomography.

TABLE 76.2	Additional Findings in Traumatic Globe Injury		
Finding	**Image and History**		**Description**
Hyphema: anterior chamber hemorrhage can be uniformly hyperattenuating or layer dependently. Once layered, hyperattenuating clot may only be seen on the inferior slices and may be more easily identified on reconstructed sagittal or coronal images.	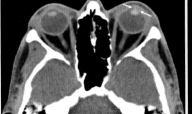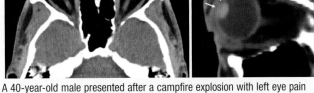 A 40-year-old male presented after a campfire explosion with left eye pain and hand motion vision. The patient was taken to the operating room for cleaning of a conjunctival laceration and hyphema washout.		Axial and sagittal CT images demonstrate high attenuation material layering superficial to the left lens, compatible with hyphema *(arrows)*.
Lens dislocation: blunt force compresses the globe, widening its transverse dimension and resulting in stretching and breaking of the zonular fibers, which suspend the lens from the ciliary body. Most lens dislocations are posterior because the iris blocks anterior dislocation. If the dislocated lens lies directly on the retina, communication of this finding to the ophthalmologist is important so that special care can be taken to minimize retinal injury during lens retrieval.	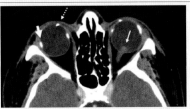 A 50-year-old male with a history of progressive high myopia, refractory glaucoma requiring shunts, retinal detachments requiring scleral bands, and a history of multiple posterior lens dislocations.		Axial CT image demonstrates the left lens laying upon the optic nerve insertion *(thin arrow)*. The elongated appearance of the globes relates to high myopia. Shunts *(serrated arrow)* have been placed to treat refractory glaucoma, and scleral bands *(thick arrow)* were placed to treat retinal detachment.

CT, Computed tomography.

The vast majority (~90%) of scleritis cases are noninfectious, among which systemic inflammatory diseases (e.g., rheumatoid arthritis, granulomatosis with polyangiitis, IgG4-related disease) and idiopathic processes (e.g., idiopathic orbital inflammatory disease) are most common. Infectious scleritis is rare but should be considered in the setting of immune suppression, after surgery, and after trauma.

When scleritis is suspected, MRI is the preferred imaging modality to evaluate the globe and surrounding soft tissues. In the setting of scleritis, the sclera will appear thickened and abnormally enhance. Surrounding cellulitis is commonly present. Findings of scleritis may be diffuse or focal and can appear mass-like. Enhancement may extend along the optic nerve sheath in the setting of optic perineuritis. Secondary findings may include retinal and choroidal detachments, choroidal effusions and uveitis, and complications including preseptal and postseptal cellulitis, myositis, and dacryoadenitis. Patients with extensive infectious and noninfectious disease can have both scleritis and uveitis (i.e., involvement of the middle layer of the globe) (Table 76.3).

Uveitis

Uveitis is inflammation of the uvea. As with scleritis, uveitis may be idiopathic or due to systemic disease, such as HLA-B27 spondyloarthropathy, rheumatoid arthritis, or sarcoidosis. Findings of uveitis include choroidal thickening, increased choroidal enhancement, increased signal intensity in the vitreous on FLAIR images, subretinal effusions with restricted diffusion, and inflammatory uveal nodules. Patients with Vogt–Koyanagi–Harada disease typically have bilateral findings, with posterior pole predominance of the choroidal enhancement.

Endophthalmitis

Bacterial or fungal infection of the globe is termed endophthalmitis. Endophthalmitis most commonly occurs as a complication of ocular surgery but may also result from hematogenous spread of bacteria or fungus in the setting of indwelling catheter, septicemia, or liver abscess. Findings in early endophthalmitis are similar to findings in noninfectious uveitis, with thickening and enhancement of the choroid. In advanced disease, there may be retinal or choroidal detachment, vitreal exudate, and peribulbar inflammation. Exudative retinal or choroidal effusions with decreased diffusivity may be present but are not specific for infection.

Intraocular Masses

An intraocular mass in an adult is a melanoma or a metastasis. The uveal tract is rich in melanocytes, and melanoma is the most common intraocular malignancy in adults. Ninety percent of uveal melanomas arise in the choroid with the remaining 10% occurring in the iris or ciliary body. Typically, the diagnosis of melanoma is made on fundoscopic

exam. MRI (local staging) and Positron emission tomography (PET)/CT (systemic staging) are adjuncts to ophthalmologic imaging modalities, including B scan ultrasound, fluorescein angiogram, autofluorescence and optical coherence tomography. MRI is particularly useful for the detection of extrascleral spread, which represents an adverse prognostic indicator of melanoma-related mortality. Imaging evaluation is especially helpful when vitreal hemorrhage or choroidal detachment obscures ophthalmologic visualization of the posterior segment.

The vascular lattice of the choroid makes it the most common site of metastasis within the globe. Choroidal metastases occur in the setting of widespread metastatic disease, most commonly from breast and lung cancer primaries (Table 76.4).

Choroidal Detachment

A choroidal effusion or detachment can occur in the setting of many ophthalmologic diseases. A detachment refers to the layer of choroid and retina lifted from the sclera, and an effusion refers to the fluid or hemorrhage that fills the potential space created by the detachment. In practice, the terms are interchangeable. A key point is that the retina remains adherent to the choroid. For this reason, a new choroidal detachment is a nonemergent finding, unlike a new retinal detachment in which retinal ischemia is a time-sensitive concern. The workup of choroidal effusion centers on determining the underlying cause. Notably, signal characteristics of intraocular hemorrhage cannot be used to determine age of hemorrhage.

Choroidal detachments have a broad base in the posterior globe. The choroid is anchored to the sclera by the short ciliary arteries, which pierce the sclera in a circle centered on the optic nerve. The choroid cannot be separated from the sclera posterior to these arterial insertions. Anteriorly, choroidal detachments can extend into the ciliary body as ciliochoroidal detachments. Adequate intraocular pressure is required to maintain apposition of the choroid to the sclera. In settings of low intraocular pressure or hypotony, the choroid falls away from the sclera. Hypotony can cause choroidal effusions after a complex ocular surgery. The term "kissing choroidal detachment" describes large effusions in which the convexities of the detached choroid approach each other in the center of the posterior segment.

The size and location of any enhancement or nodularity associated with the choroidal detachment should be described by the radiologist, as these findings raise suspicion for malignancy as the underlying cause.

Retinal Detachment

The retina is the neurosensory inner layer of the globe. A new retinal detachment is a semiemergent finding. Unlike choroidal detachments, the retina is no longer attached to the vascular choroid, leading to retinal ischemia and gradual cell death. Central vision in the fovea within the macula is entirely avascular in the absence of the choroid, so differentiation

TABLE 76.3 Scleritis

Finding	Image and History	Description
Diffuse scleral thickening and secondary acute angle glaucoma	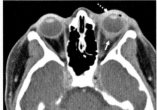 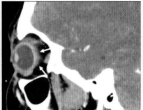 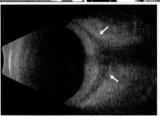 A 36-year-old female (same patient from Case B) presents with left eye swelling for 2 weeks and 1 day of left eye pain, decreased vision, headache, and nausea with vomiting. Ophthalmologic exam revealed elevated intraocular pressure.	Axial and sagittal CT images demonstrate severe left globe scleral and uveal thickening with retrobulbar stranding *(solid arrows)* and a shallow anterior segment *(serrated arrow)* related to acute angle closure glaucoma from posterior segment mass effect. B scan ultrasound demonstrates a "T sign" of scleral thickening and extrascleral fluid *(solid arrows)*.
Nodular scleral thickening	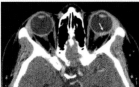 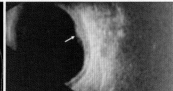 An 18-year-old female presented with left eye pain, blurry vision, and light sensitivity for 4 days.	Axial CT image demonstrates left posterior globe nodular thickening *(arrow)*. B scan ultrasound shows the same focus of nodular elevation of the macula *(arrow)* and diffuse thickening of the posterior pole.
Scleral enhancement and secondary choroidal effusion, lacrimal gland enlargement, and proptosis.	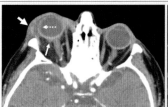 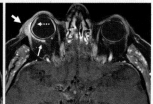 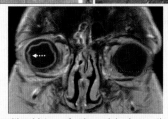 An 85-year-old male with a history of polymyalgia rheumatica and adrenal insufficiency presented with 3 days of progressive right eye pain and swelling.	Axial CT image demonstrates right globe uveoscleral thickening *(serrated arrow)*, retrobulbar soft tissue stranding *(solid thin arrow)*, lacrimal enlargement and edema *(solid thick arrow)*, and proptosis. Axial and coronal gadolinium-enhanced T1-weighted images demonstrate diffuse hyperenhancement of the right uvea with a ciliochoroidal detachment *(serrated arrows)*, episcleral enhancement *(solid thin arrow)*, and right lacrimal gland enlargement with hyperenhancement *(solid thick arrow)*.

CT, Computed tomography.

between a macula-sparing and macula-involving detachment determines the urgency of surgical repair. This differentiation is not possible on current MRI sequences. However, patients with altered mentation may not be able to communicate visual changes, and the radiologist may be the first to identify a critical retinal detachment.

In the posterior globe, the retina is anchored at the cribriform plate by the optic nerve. When a detachment involves the circumferential retina, the cribriform plate is the vertex of the classic, three-dimensional "V" detachment pattern. Anteriorly, the retina extends to the ora serrata at its junction with the ciliary body. The distinction between choroidal and retinal

TABLE 76.4	**Intraocular Masses**	
Finding	Image and History	Description
Intraocular mass (melanoma)	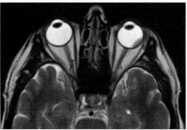 A 69-year-old female (same patient from Case C) presented with a snasal visual field defect in the left eye.	Axial T2-weighted image demonstrates a T2 isointense lesion arising from the lateral aspect of the left posterior globe. There is no evidence of extrascleral extension.
Intraocular mass (melanoma)	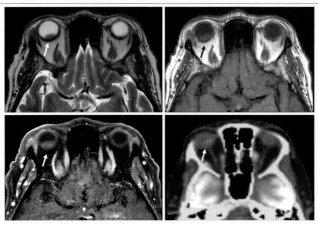 A 62-year-old female with a history of Lynch syndrome and rectal cancer presented with decreased vision in the right eye. Although metastasis is a differential consideration, fine needle aspiration revealed melanoma.	Axial T2-weighted, T1-weighted, and gadolinium-enhanced, fat-suppressed, T1-weighted images demonstrate a T2 isointense, T1 hypointense, enhancing lesion *(arrows)* in the right posterior globe. No extrascleral extension is present. Axial PET/CT image demonstrates FDG accumulation within the lesion. No distant metastases were identifed.

CT, Computed tomography; *FDG*, fluorodeoxyglucose; *PET*, positron emission tomography.

detachments may not always be clear, particularly in the setting of globe rupture or after a complex ocular surgery.

Retinal detachments are clinically classified as rhegmatogenous detachments from retinal tears, tractional detachments from scarring or diabetic neovascularization, and exudative detachments from trauma, inflammation, or malignancy. For this reason, patients with exudative retinal detachments are more likely to be imaged. The size and location of any enhancement or nodularity associated with the retinal detachment should be described by the radiologist because these findings raise suspicion for malignancy as the underlying cause (Table 76.5).

Differential Diagnosis

1. **Traumatic injury:**
   - Open globe injury
   - Closed globe injury
2. **Scleritis:**
   - Infectious
   - Inflammatory
3. **Uveitis**
4. **Endophthalmitis**
5. **Intraocular mass in an adult:**
   - Melanoma
   - Metastasis
6. **Detachment:**
   - Choroidal detachment
   - Retinal detachment

Pearls

- An open globe injury is an ophthalmologic emergency requiring immediate surgical repair.
- Scleritis is usually inflammatory rather than infectious.
- Endophthalmitis is most often a postsurgical complication.
- An ocular mass in an adult is either a melanoma or a metastasis.
- Choroidal detachments have a broad base.
- Retinal detachments have a narrow base and are centered on the optic nerve. A new retinal detachment is an urgent finding.
- Intraocular hemorrhage cannot be reliably dated on the basis of MR signal characteristics.

TABLE 76.5	Detachments		
Finding	**Image and History**		**Description**
Choroidal effusion from intraocular metastasis	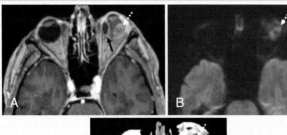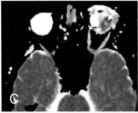A 66-year-old male with widely metastatic neuroendocrine tumor presents with new left eye vision loss.		Axial T1-weighted, gadolinium-enhanced, axial DWI, and axial ADC images demonstrate a heterogeneously enhancing intraocular lesion in the temporal aspect of the left globe (*serrated arrow*, A) with low diffusivity (*serrated arrow*, B and C). In the nasal aspect of the left globe, the nonenhancing T1 hypointense signal is a nonexudative choroidal effusion (*black arrow*, A), which does not restrict diffusion.
Kissing choroidal effusions	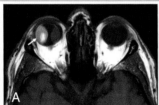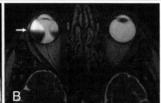A 68-year-old female presents with vision loss.		Axial T1-weighted and T2-weighted images demonstrate large right globe choroidal effusions, and the convexities of the choroidal detachments approach each other in the mid-globe. The intrinsic T1 hyperintense signal indicates a hemorrhagic effusion (*arrow*, A) with fluid-fluid level on the T2-weighted image (*arrow*, B). An exudative effusion could also have a layering effect similar to this hemorrhagic effusion.
Retinal detachment	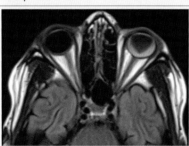A 72-year-old male (same patient from Case D) presented with hand motion vision in the left eye after seeing flashes of light.		Axial FLAIR image demonstrates the classic "V" pattern of a retinal detachment in the left globe. The "V" of the detachment is outlined posteriorly by a hyperintense hemorrhagic effusion.
Retinal detachment	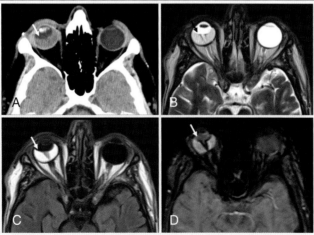A 66-year-old male presented with no light perception in the right eye.		Axial CT image demonstrates abnormal hyperattenuating material consistent with hemorrhage within the right posterior globe (*arrow*, A). On CT, the pattern of detachment is difficult to discern. Axial T2-weighted, T1-weighted, and GRE images demonstrate T2 iso- to hyperintense (*black arrow*, B), T1 hyperintense (*white arrow*, C) material with associated magnetic susceptibility (*white arrow*, D). The classic "V" pattern of retinal detachment is seen within the large hemorrhagic effusion.

Continued

TABLE 76.5 Detachments—cont'd

Finding	Image and History	Description
Retinal detachment from choroidal metastasis	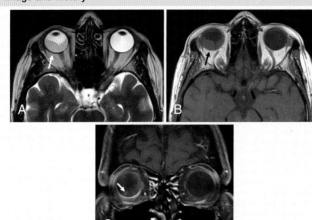 A 69-year-old female with a history of metastatic invasive ductal breast carcinoma presented with hand motion vision in the right eye.	Axial T2-weighted and axial T1-weighted images demonstrate a right globe subretinal effusion (*arrows,* A and B). Coronal T1-weighted, fat-suppressed, gadolinium-enhanced image demonstrates a small enhancing lesion (*arrow ,* C) representing a choroidal metastasis causing the retinal detachment.

ADC, Apparent diffusion coefficient; *CT,* Computed tomography; *DWI,* diffusion-weighted imaging; *FLAIR,* fluid attenuated inversion recovery.

Suggested Readings

Arepalli S, Kaliki S, Shields CL: Choroidal metastases: origin, features, and therapy, *Indian J Ophthalmol* 63(2):122–127, 2015.

Diogo MC, Jager MJ, Ferreira TA: CT and MR imaging in the diagnosis of scleritis, *AJNR Am J Neuroradiol* 37(12):2334–2339, 2016.

Ferreira TA, Saraiva P, Genders SW, et al: CT and MR imaging of orbital inflammation, *Neuroradiology* 60(12):1253–1266, 2018.

Fujikawa A, Mohamed YH, Kinoshita H, et al: Visual outcomes and prognostic factors in open-globe injuries, *BMC Ophthalmol;* 18(1):138, 2018.

Gragoudas ES. Proton beam irradiation of uveal melanomas: the first 30 years. The Weisenfeld lecture, *Invest Ophthalmol Vis Sci* 47(11): 4666–4673, 2006.

Hallinan JT, Pillay P, Koh LH, et al: Eye globe abnormalities on MR and CT in adults: an anatomical approach, *Korean J Radiol* 17(5): 664–673, 2016.

Hankins M, Margo CE: Histopathological evaluation of scleritis, *J Clin Pathol* 72(5):386–390, 2019.

Jager MJ, Shields CL, Cebula CM, et al: Uveal melanoma, *Nat Rev Dis Primers* 6(1):24, 2020.

Joseph DP, Pieramici DJ, Beauchamp NJ Jr: Computed tomography in the diagnosis and prognosis of open-globe injuries, *Ophthalmology* 107(10):1899–1906, 2000.

Karim F, de Hoog J, Paridaens D, et al: IgG4-related disease as an emerging cause of scleritis, *Acta Ophthalmol* 95(8):e795–e796, 2017.

Meng Y, Yan H: Prognostic factors for open globe injuries and correlation of Ocular Trauma Score in Tianjin, China, *J Ophthalmol* 2015:345764, 2015.

Shields CL, Welch RJ, Malik K, et al: Uveal metastasis: clinical features and survival outcome of 2214 tumors in 1111 patients based on primary tumor origin, *Middle East Afr J Ophthalmol* 25(2):81–90, 2018.

Wolff, E, Warwick R: *Anatomy of the eye and orbit: Including the central connections, development, and comparative anatomy of the visual apparatus,* Philadelphia, 1976, W.B. Saunders Company.

77

Orbital Masses

MARY D. MAHER, MD AND MARY E. CUNNANE, MD

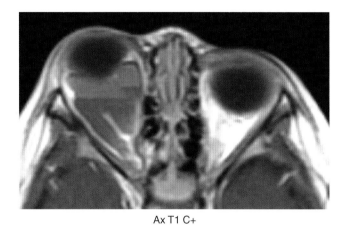

Ax T1 C+

CASE A: An 18-month-old male presents with sudden onset proptosis after a viral illness. *Ax*, Axial.

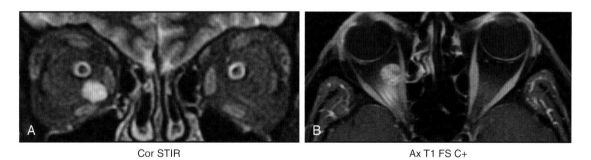

A

Cor STIR

B

Ax T1 FS C+

CASE B: A 36-year-old female undergoes magnetic resonance imaging (MRI) of the brain and orbits for evaluation of possible multiple sclerosis. *Ax*, Axial; *Cor*, coronal; *FS*, fat saturated; *STIR*, short tau inversion recovery.

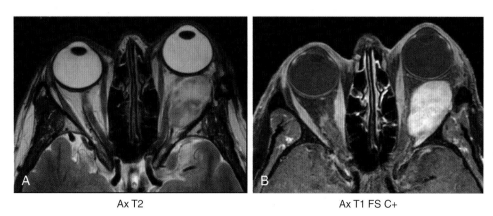

A

Ax T2

B

Ax T1 FS C+

CASE C: A 35-year-old male presented with left proptosis. *Ax*, Axial; *FS*, fat saturated.

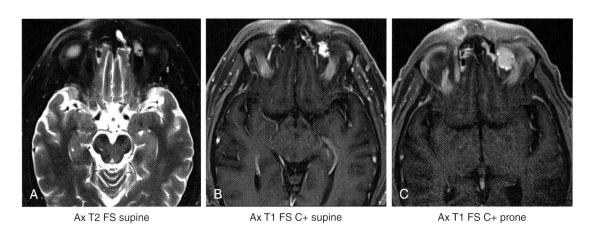

Ax T2 FS supine   Ax T1 FS C+ supine   Ax T1 FS C+ prone

CASE D: A 50-year-old male with left globe proptosis elicited by Valsalva. *Ax*, Axial; *FS*, fat saturated.

DESCRIPTION OF FINDINGS

- Case A: Axial T1-weighted, gadolinium-enhanced image demonstrates an expansile lesion in the right orbit with fluid-fluid levels and enhancing septae, but no focal nodularity.
- Case B: Coronal short TI inversion recovery (STIR) and axial T1-weighted, gadolinium-enhanced images of the orbit demonstrate a circumscribed, STIR hyperintense, heterogeneously enhancing right intraconal lesion. Review of multiple postcontrast phases showed the lesion to progressively fill in with contrast over time.
- Case C: Axial T2-weighted and axial T1-weighted, gadolinium-enhanced images of the orbit demonstrate an ovoid, T2 heterogeneous, avidly enhancing left intraconal mass resulting in left globe proptosis. This lesion was subsequently resected.
- Case D: The axial T2-weighted image demonstrates a T2 hyperintense lesion in the left superomedial orbit with a central round T2 hypointense focus suggestive of a phlebolith. Supine and prone axial T1-weighted, gadolinium-enhanced images demonstrate avid and homogeneous enhancement of the lesion, which substantially increases in size in the prone position.

Diagnosis

Case A: Venolymphatic malformation
Case B: Cavernous venous malformation
Case C: Schwannoma
Case D: Varix

Summary

Masses of the orbit can be broadly categorized by location as intraconal (i.e., within the "cone" defined by the extraocular muscles) or extraconal (i.e., outside this "cone"). Intraconal orbital lesions can be further subdivided into two groups based on the presence or absence of optic nerve involvement. This chapter focuses primarily on intraconal orbital masses without optic nerve involvement; however, select extraconal pathologies are also discussed. Optic nerve masses (Chapter 73) as well as globe lesions (Chapter 76), lacrimal gland lesions (Chapter 78), and extraocular muscle enlargement (Chapter 79) are discussed elsewhere in this book.

A brief discussion of vascular anomalies is relevant to the topic of intraconal orbital masses. The International Society for the Study of Vascular Anomalies 2018 classification differentiates vascular malformations (nonproliferative) from vascular neoplasms (proliferative), and both subtypes of vascular anomalies may occur in the orbit. Among children, both types of anomalies can grow. However, malformations will grow in proportion to the child, whereas neoplasms will grow faster than the child. Histologically distinct types of vascular malformations include lymphatic, capillary, venous, arteriovenous malformation, and arteriovenous fistula. Mixed lesions (e.g., venolymphatic malformation) also occur. Malformations may also be grouped into low-flow lesions (e.g., lymphatic, capillary, venous) or high-flow lesions (e.g., arteriovenous malformation, arteriovenous fistula) based on the absence or presence of an arterial component, respectively.

Spectrum of Disease

Vascular Anomalies

Lymphatic and Venolymphatic Malformations

Orbital lymphatic and venolymphatic malformations are both low-flow malformations, with the former originating entirely from lymphatic precursor cells and the latter arising from precursor cells, giving rise to both the venous and lymphatic systems. These malformations are usually identified during childhood as a result of slowly progressive proptosis and mass effect upon adjacent structures. Hemorrhage after minor trauma or infection can result in abrupt enlargement and sudden proptosis. Unlike orbital varices, these lesions do not increase in size with Valsalva because they are isolated from the normal orbital venous system. Lymphatic and venolymphatic malformations are notoriously difficult to resect due to their transspatial and "sticky" nature, and they frequently recur after surgery. If symptoms allow, observation is favored. If compressive symptoms require action, surgery, sclerosing agents, radiation, laser ablation, and steroids may be considered as treatment options. The absence of a capsule or pseudocapsule explains the transspatial nature of these lesions, which frequently insinuate between different anatomic structures and compartments. To aid appropriate treatment planning, radiologists should specifically assess for and report the presence or absence of an intracranial component.

On MR imaging, fluid-fluid levels are highly suggestive of a lymphatic or venolymphatic malformation (Fig. 77.1) with venolymphatic malformations exhibiting avidly enhancing components (Fig. 77.2) that pure lymphatic malformations lack. Notably, if osseous involvement is present, a telangiectatic osteosarcoma of the skull base should be included in the differential. The presence of T1 hyperintense signal indicates proteinaceous lymphatic components or subacute hemorrhage.

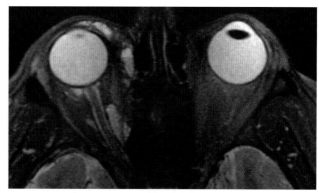

Ax T2 FS

• **Fig. 77.1** A 42-year-old female presents for imaging follow-up after multiple resections of a venolymphatic malformation. On the axial T2-weighted image, there are multifocal right orbital T2 hyperintense foci that are poorly defined, involving both preseptal and postseptal spaces. The close proximity to the right globe and the right optic nerve is clinically significant and should be reported by the radiologist. In the right medial extraconal fat, a fluid-fluid level is seen. *Ax*, Axial; *FS*, fat saturated.

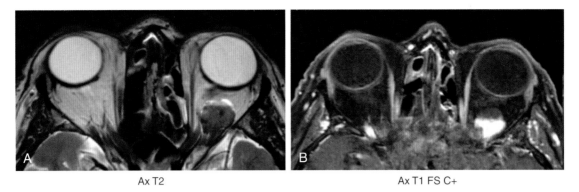

Ax T2   Ax T1 FS C+

• **Fig. 77.2** A 14-year-old female reports episodes of intermittent left visual field loss. (A) On the axial T2-weighted image, a left retrobulbar lesion with a fluid–fluid level encroaches upon the left orbital apex. (B) On the axial T1-weighted, gadolinium-enhanced image, contrast layers within the dependent venous component of this venolymphatic malformation. *Ax*, Axial; *FS*, fat saturated.

Phleboliths may be seen in venolymphatic malformations and confirm the low-flow state. On ultrasound, lymphatic and venolymphatic malformations appear cystic, and intralesional hemorrhage appears hyperechoic. Bone remodeling may be visualized on CT and indicates chronicity.

Cavernous Venous Malformation (Formerly Cavernous Hemangioma)

Orbital cavernous venous malformations are a common low-flow vascular malformation, representing the most common benign orbital mass in adults and frequently identified as an incidental finding. Cavernous venous malformations grow slowly and can result in progressive proptosis. The lesions are more common in women and can grow rapidly during pregnancy, suggesting hormonal responsiveness. These malformations are typically observed unless mass effect results in symptoms, which are largely determined by location within the orbit. For example, a small, cavernous venous malformation in the orbital apex may require surgical attention at a smaller size than one within the retrobulbar fat.

As a result of a pseudocapsule, these malformations appear on imaging as round or ovoid lesions exerting mass effect upon adjacent structures rather than conforming to the outline of the structures as occurs with lymphatic and venolymphatic malformations. Progressive central to peripheral enhancement on multiphase or delayed contrast-enhanced CT and MR images is characteristic (Fig. 77.3). On MRI, these malformations are T2 hyperintense and may have T2 hypointense

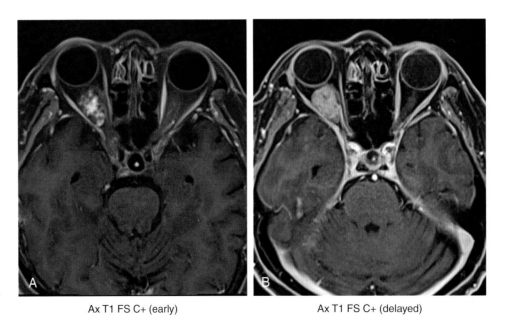

Ax T1 FS C+ (early)   Ax T1 FS C+ (delayed)

• **Fig. 77.3** An 85-year-old female with dizziness and an incidentally detected right orbital mass. (A) Early and (B) delayed T1-weighted, gadolinium-enhanced images demonstrate the typical progressive central to peripheral enhancement of cavernous venous malformations. *Ax*, Axial; *FS*, fat saturated.

septations. Intralesional phleboliths may be present as confirmation of their low-flow state. Smooth osseous remodeling may be seen and indicates chronicity.

Varix

A varix is a valveless venous low-flow malformation with a systemic connection which results in enlargement of the lesion with increased venous pressure. Clinically, patients may be able to induce proptosis by Valsalva, which can be captured on ultrasound or dynamic MRI sequences. On color Doppler ultrasound, there is reversal of flow toward the transducer with Valsalva. On CT or MR imaging, the lesion will increase during Valsalva or with the patient in prone position.

Varices are the most common cause of spontaneous orbital hemorrhage. They can enlarge suddenly and become painful with thrombosis. Treatment is often observation unless the patient is experiencing painful thrombosis.

Varices may exhibit different sizes and configurations, including fusiform, club-like, triangular and amorphous lesions. On MRI, varices are T2 hyperintense and variable on T1-weighted sequences. A varix avidly and homogeneously enhances. The presence of a phlebolith on CT or MRI (Fig. 77.4) confirms the low-flow state.

Arteriovenous Malformations and Arteriovenous Fistulae

Intraorbital arteriovenous malformations (AVMs) are rare lesions thought to be congenital in origin. These high-flow malformations exhibit a central nidus with multiple abnormal communications between arteries and veins, bypassing the normal capillary beds. Growth stimuli include menarche, pregnancy, and trauma with pain, proptosis, corkscrew conjunctival vessels, increased intraocular pressure, and bruit representing common clinical findings. Spontaneous hemorrhage is uncommon. Wyburn-Mason syndrome refers to a rare nonhereditary congenital phakomatosis characterized by multiple AVMs affecting the brain, eye, and facial structures, including the orbit.

Intraorbital arteriovenous fistulae (AVFs) are exceedingly rare acquired lesions (e.g., posttraumatic, iatrogenic) characterized by direct communications between arteries and veins without a central nidus. Unlike carotid cavernous fistulae, intraorbital AVFs lie purely within the orbit and do not connect to the cavernous sinus. Clinical manifestations are similar to those of intraorbital AVMs, and spontaneous resolution of intraorbital AVFs has been described.

Although CT and MR are useful for characterizing the extent of these high-flow lesions, catheter angiography is critical for treatment planning and best demonstrates the arterial supply and venous drainage. Management of these high-flow lesions depends on patient-specific features and may include observation, embolization, surgical excision, or a combination of embolization and surgery.

Infantile Hemangioma

An infantile hemangioma is a benign vascular *neoplasm* composed of capillary-sized spaces lined by proliferating endothelial cells representing the most common benign pediatric orbital tumor. These neoplasms are often small at birth and may go unnoticed initially. Subsequently, the typical course of these lesions is rapid growth for up to 1 year followed by slow involution over the course of childhood. Infantile hemangiomas can be isolated or part of PHACES, a syndrome characterized by a posterior fossa malformation, hemangiomas, arterial, cardiac, and eye abnormalities, and a sternal cleft. Because infantile hemangiomas are self-resolving lesions, observation is favored when possible. If vision threatening or otherwise symptomatic, an orbital infantile hemangioma can be treated with beta-blockers, steroids, interferon, or surgery.

While the natural history of infantile hemangiomas is distinct and adequate for diagnosis, imaging defines the depth of involvement and mass effect upon adjacent structures. Infantile hemangiomas are commonly extraconal (Fig. 77.5) and superficial, but can be intraconal or transspatial. Ultrasound allows for dynamic images, demonstrating compressible lesions that expand when the infant cries from increased venous pressure. A CT with contrast provides rapid acquisition of cross-sectional imaging and demonstrates a homogeneously enhancing lobulated lesion with irregular margins secondary to the absence of a capsule. MRI demonstrates an avidly enhancing lesion which is T2 iso- to hyperintense. Both T1- and T2-weighted sequences show intralesional and perilesional flow voids.

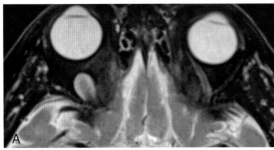
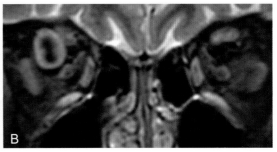

Ax T2 FS   Cor STIR

• **Fig. 77.4** A 70-year-old male presents with right retrobulbar pressure with Valsalva. (A) The axial T2-weighted and (B) coronal STIR images demonstrate a well-circumscribed, T2 and STIR hyperintense lesion in the right intraconal orbit along the expected course of the right superior ophthalmic vein. Centrally, there is T2 and STIR hypointensity suggestive of a phlebolith. *Ax,* Axial; *Cor,* coronal; *FS,* fat saturated; *STIR,* short tau inversion recovery.

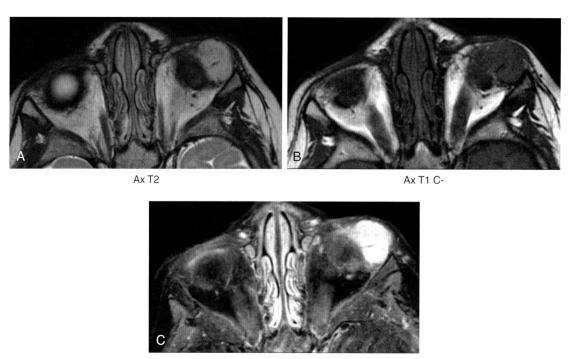

Ax T2

Ax T1 C-

Ax T1 FS C+

• **Fig. 77.5** A 3-month-old female presents with her parents because of an enlarging purple lesion overlying the left orbit, which has increased in size since her birth. Axial MR images demonstrate a T2 hyperintense, avidly enhancing lesion centered in the left periorbital soft tissues. (A) The linear T2 hypointensity within the lesion is consistent with a flow void. *Ax,* Axial; *FS,* fat saturated.

Benign Neoplasms

Schwannoma

Intraorbital schwannomas most commonly involve the ophthalmic division (V1) of the trigeminal nerve in the superior extraconal fat. However, schwannomas may also arise from peripheral branches of the oculomotor, trochlear, and abducens nerves, in which case they may be located in the intraconal fat. These lesions are well circumscribed and exhibit a nonaggressive appearance, but may produce compressive symptoms for which resection is the mainstay of treatment. Schwannomas are characteristically T2 hyperintense. As opposed to cavernous venous malformations, which initially enhance very focally within a portion of the lesion and then gradually fill in with contrast over time, schwannomas exhibit more diffuse early enhancement. Areas of cystic degeneration may also be seen.

Neurofibroma

Neurofibromas involving the orbit most commonly occur as plexiform neurofibromas in the setting of neurofibromatosis type I. Plexiform neurofibromas appear as rope-like lesions along the anterior-posterior course of the intraorbital nerves. The lesions are predominantly T2 hyperintense but may demonstrate a central T2 hypointense "target sign" (Fig. 77.6). Plexiform neurofibromas are infiltrative and can remodel the osseous orbit. Unfortunately, these lesions have a high rate of recurrence after resection. Nonsyndromic, solitary neurofibromas are possible but less common.

Solitary Fibrous Tumor

Solitary fibrous tumors (formerly hemangiopericytomas) are rare, hypervascular neoplasms that more commonly arise in the thoracic cavity but may occur in the head and neck, including within the orbit.

On MR imaging, T2 hypointensity is typical and reflects the fibrous nature of the lesion. Solitary fibrous tumors avidly enhance (Fig. 77.7), and washout is observed if delayed postcontrast images are acquired. Perilesional vessels and intralesional flow voids may also be present. Aggressive osseous erosion can also be seen and is best depicted by CT.

Malignant Neoplasms

Metastasis

Intraorbital metastases typically occur in the setting of a late-stage advanced malignancy. Breast carcinoma, melanoma, and lung cancer most commonly metastasize to the extraocular muscles due to their rich blood supply. Prostate carcinoma and neuroblastoma more commonly metastasize to the bony orbit with secondary soft tissue involvement resulting from extraosseous extension. Metastases to the intraconal fat may also occur. Imaging findings depend on the characteristics of the primary malignancy. Although orbital metastases frequently result in proptosis, scirrhous breast cancer can cause enophthalmos and restriction of extraocular muscle movement. Scirrhous breast cancer orbital metastases may appear T2 hypointense (Fig. 77.8) due to the desmoplastic response and associated fibrosis.

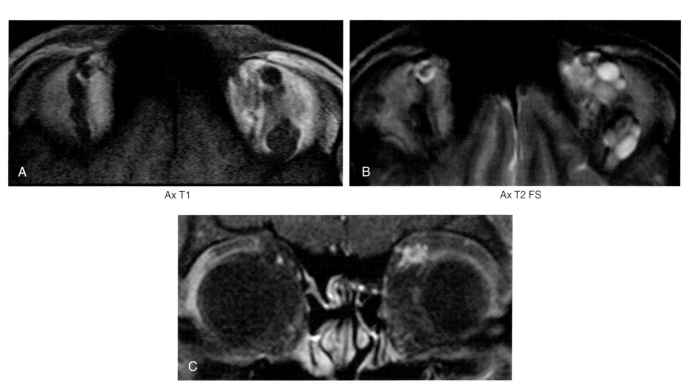

Ax T1

Ax T2 FS

Cor T1 FS C+

• **Fig. 77.6** A 19-year-old female with a history of neurofibromatosis type I presents for MRI of the orbits to assess for optic pathway glioma. No optic pathway glioma is identified; however, extraconal lesions extend along the expected course of the ophthalmic divisions of both trigeminal nerves. The lesions are T1 hypointense, T2 hyperintense, and demonstrate heterogeneous enhancement. Note the central T2 hypointense foci within some of the T2 hyperintense, rounded lesions representing the classical "target sign" of neurofibromas. *Ax,* Axial; *Cor,* coronal; *FS,* fat saturated.

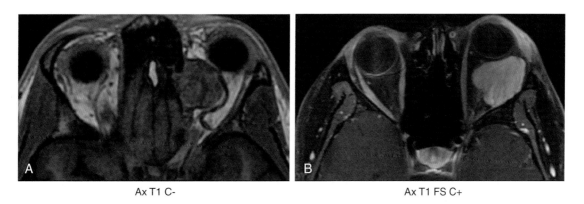

Ax T1 C-

Ax T1 FS C+

• **Fig. 77.7** A 32-year-old female presented with slowly progressive left proptosis. (A) Axial T1-weighted unenhanced and (B) gadolinium-enhanced, fat-suppressed images demonstrate an avidly enhancing T1 hypointense lesion in the left intraconal and extraconal space with erosion on the adjacent left lamina papyracea and a large flow void along the lateral aspect of the lesion. The combination of perilesional flow void and osseous erosion suggested solitary fibrous tumor, which was confirmed on biopsy. *Ax,* Axial; *FS,* fat saturated.

Lymphoma

Ocular adnexal lymphoma can arise in the conjunctiva, eyelids, lacrimal gland, and orbit and comprises 5% to 10% of all extranodal lymphomas. The vast majority of cases are B-cell lymphomas with marginal zone representing the most common subtype. These tumors exhibit a slight female predominance and occur most commonly in the 5th to 7th decades of life. Symptoms include proptosis, decreased visual acuity, and diplopia. Pain is uncommon. A palpable firm or rubbery mass may be encountered on physical examination. Homogeneous T2 hypointensity, homogeneous enhancement, and restricted diffusion are imaging features typical of

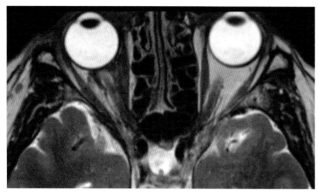

Ax T2

• **Fig. 77.8** A 56-year-old female with metastatic breast cancer presents with right enophthalmos and restricted eye movements. Axial T2-weighted image demonstrates an infiltrative, T2 hypointense lesion involving the right intraconal fat and right medial rectus muscle. The T2 hypointensity is characteristic of a scirrhous breast cancer metastasis. *Ax,* Axial.

lymphoma (Fig. 77.9), and this tumor has a tendency to mold to adjacent orbital structures.

Rhabdomyosarcoma

Rhabdomyosarcoma is a striated muscle sarcoma originating from primitive mesenchymal rhabdomyoblasts. Forty percent of rhabdomyosarcomas occur in the head and neck. The most common subtype is embryonal rhabdomyosarcoma, which predominantly affects infants and young children (Fig. 77.10). The alveolar subtype is seen in teens and young adults. A pleomorphic subtype affects adults typically greater than 60 years old. On imaging, these lesions commonly demonstrate diffuse enhancement, intermediate T2/STIR signal, and restricted diffusion. Management typically includes surgical resection followed by chemoradiation. Within the orbit, 5-year survival rates range from 75% to 95%.

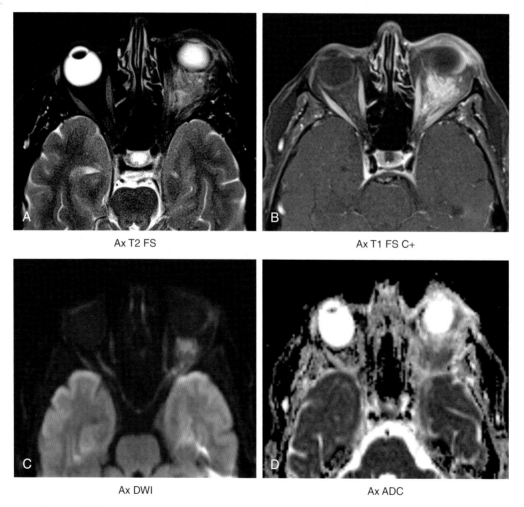

Ax T2 FS   Ax T1 FS C+

Ax DWI   Ax ADC

• **Fig. 77.9** A 77-year-old female with left proptosis. (A) Axial T2-weighted and (B) gadolinium-enhanced T1-weighted images demonstrate a T2 hypointense, homogeneously enhancing left intraconal mass that molds to the contour of the left posterior globe. (C) Axial DWI and (D) corresponding ADC images demonstrate restricted diffusion of the lesion consistent with hypercellularity. *ADC,* Apparent diffusion coefficient; *Ax,* axial; *DWI,* diffusion-weighted imaging; *FS,* fat saturated.

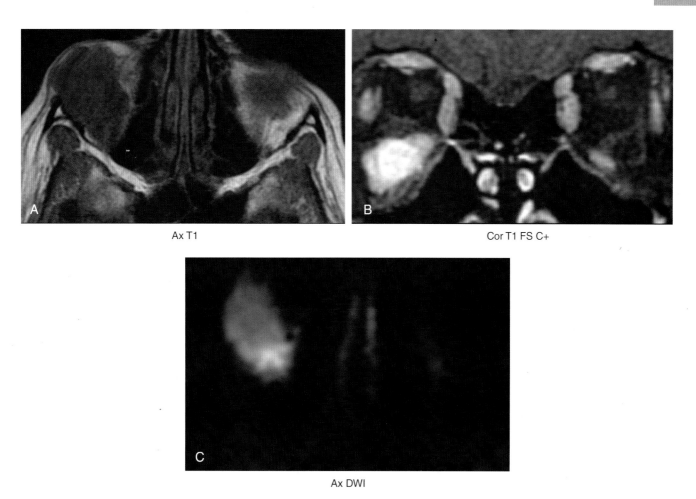

Ax T1

Cor T1 FS C+

Ax DWI

• **Fig. 77.10** A 9-year-old male presents with right proptosis and diplopia. (A) Axial T1-weighted and (B) coronal T1-weighted, gadolinium-enhanced, fat-suppressed images demonstrate an avidly enhancing soft tissue mass within the inferior right orbit inseparable from the right inferior rectus muscle. (C) Axial DWI image and corresponding ADC map (not shown) demonstrate low diffusivity consistent with hypercellularity. Rhabdomyosarcoma should always be considered as a differential diagnosis in a pediatric patient with an orbital soft tissue mass. *Ax*, Axial; *Cor*, coronal; *DWI*, diffusion-weighted imaging; *FS*, fat saturated.

Miscellaneous

Sarcoid

As one of the great mimickers, sarcoid is always a relevant differential consideration for enhancing soft tissue within the orbit. Sarcoid may appear as a discrete homogeneously enhancing soft tissue lesion (Fig. 77.11) or an infiltrative transspatial lesion. Secondary findings such as pachymeningeal, leptomeningeal, or intraparenchymal and intramedullary enhancement are clues to a systemic pathology.

Immunoglobulin G4-Related Disease

Immunoglobulin G4 (IgG4)-related disease can cause enlargement of discrete structures within the orbit or be transspatial. IgG4 warrants particular consideration in the setting of perineural soft tissue thickening and enhancement, particularly within the pterygopalatine fossa and along the infraorbital nerves (Fig. 77.12). Although nerve involvement in IgG4-related disease can mimic perineural spread of malignancy, in IgG4-related disease, the nerve function may be maintained, and the nerve involvement is usually painless.

Infection

Infection is an important differential consideration of an orbital mass, particularly in the emergency department. Patients often present with fever, pain, and proptosis. Imaging is important for determining the extent of infection to inform clinical decision-making. In the setting of preseptal cellulitis, oral antibiotics are sufficient. If orbital cellulitis is suspected, the patient will be admitted for intravenous antibiotics for disease control.

Sinus infection is the most common source of orbital cellulitis (Fig. 77.13). In the setting of sinus disease, the fat adjacent to the sinus will demonstrate infiltration. Hypoattenuation adjacent to the shared orbital/paranasal sinus wall may represent a periorbital abscess or phlegmon, which frequently lacks the classic enhancing rim of an abscess. The presence of an orbital abscess changes management because incision and drainage may be required for infection control. Abscesses may also be present in the lacrimal gland (Fig. 77.14) or the extraocular muscles in the setting of dacryocystitis or myositis. Both accidental and iatrogenic foreign bodies, such as a wood chip

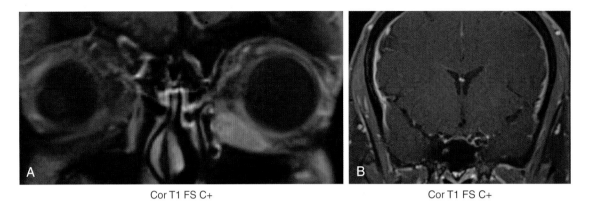

Cor T1 FS C+   Cor T1 FS C+

• **Fig. 77.11** A 32-year-old female presents with left hyperglobus and headache. (A) The coronal T1-weighted, gadolinium-enhanced image of the orbit demonstrates a focal homogeneously enhancing soft tissue mass along the inferomedial aspect of the left globe. Noncaseating granulomas were identified in this nodule at resection. Years later, the patient presented with new headaches, at which time (B) coronal T1-weighted, gadolinium-enhanced imaging of the brain demonstrated pachymeningeal thickening. These findings resolved with steroids and were considered to be consistent with neurosarcoid. *Cor,* coronal; *FS,* fat saturated.

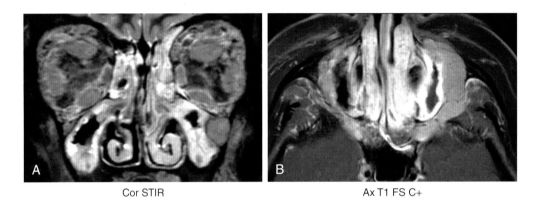

Cor STIR   Ax T1 FS C+

• **Fig. 77.12** A 35-year-old male presents after years of intermittent proptosis and diplopia. (A) The coronal STIR image demonstrates infiltrative soft tissue throughout the intraconal and extraconal fat, enlargement of the extraocular muscles, and enlargement of the left greater than right infraorbital nerves with expansion of the left infraorbital foramen. Pronounced paranasal sinus disease is also seen. (B) The axial T1-weighted, gadolinium-enhanced image demonstrates abnormal soft tissue extending along the course of the left greater than right infraorbital nerves, from the pterygopalatine fossae through the infraorbital canals to the level of the infraorbital foramina. *Ax,* Axial; *Cor,* coronal; *FS,* fat saturated; *STIR,* short tau inversion recovery.

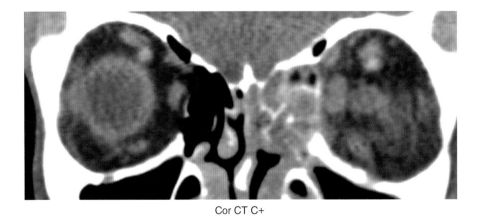

Cor CT C+

• **Fig. 77.13** An 18-year-old male presents to the emergency department with sinusitis failing to improve on antibiotics and new diplopia. The contrast-enhanced coronal CT image demonstrates opacification of the left ethmoid air cells, intraorbital fat stranding, and enlargement of the left medial rectus, consistent with ethmoid sinusitis complicated by orbital cellulitis. *CT,* Computed tomography; *Cor,* coronal.

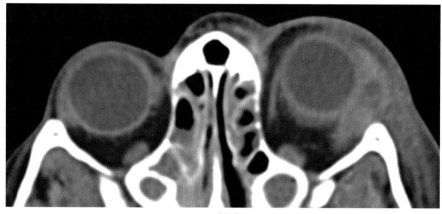

Ax CT C+

• **Fig. 77.14** A 72-year-old female presents to the emergency department with new left proptosis and hypoglobus after inadequate treatment of a left preseptal cellulitis. The contrast-enhanced axial CT image demonstrates a round focus of hypoattenuation within an enlarged left lacrimal gland, consistent with a lacrimal abscess secondary to dacryoadenitis. *Ax*, Axial; *CT*, Computed tomography.

after trauma or a glaucoma device should be noted, as they may need to be extracted for adequate control of the infection.

Differential Diagnosis

1. **Malformations**
   - Lymphatic
   - Venous
   - Venolymphatic
   - Arteriovenous
2. **Benign neoplasms**
   - Nerve sheath tumor
     - Schwannoma
     - Neurofibroma
   - Solitary fibrous tumor (hemangiopericytoma)
   - Infantile hemangioma (pediatric population)
3. **Malignant neoplasms**
   - Metastasis
   - Lymphoma
   - Sarcoma
4. **Miscellaneous processes**
   - Sarcoid
   - IgG4-related disease
   - Idiopathic Orbital Inflammation
   - Infection

Pearls

- Cavernous venous malformation (formerly cavernous hemangioma) represents the most common benign orbital mass in adults.
- Lymphatic and venolymphatic malformations may rapidly enlarge in the setting of recent infection or following trauma.
- Orbital varices connect with the systemic venous system and will therefore increase in size with increased venous pressure. As such, supine and prone imaging or imaging with and without Valsalva can be useful for diagnosis.
- Consider rhabdomyosarcoma in a pediatric patient with an enhancing orbital mass.

- Although most orbital metastases will produce proptosis due to mass effect, the desmoplastic reaction to scirrhous breast cancer orbital metastases may produce enophthalmos.
- A homogeneously enhancing, T2 hypointense orbital mass with restricted diffusion that molds to the contours of adjacent orbital structures is typical of lymphoma.
- Enlargement and enhancement of the infraorbital nerves is characteristic of IgG4-related disease; however, perineural spread of malignancy must also be considered.

Suggested Readings

Allen RC: Orbital metastases: when to suspect? when to biopsy?, *Middle East Afr J Ophthalmol* 25(2):60–64, 2018.

Leiner J, Le Loarer F: The current landscape of rhabdomyosarcomas: an updated, *Virchows Arch* 476(1):97–108, 2020.

Low CM, Stokken JK: Typical orbital pathologies: hemangioma, *J Neurol Surg B Skull Base* 82(1):20–26, 2021.

Olsen TG, Heegaard S: Orbital lymphoma, *Surv Ophthalmol* 64(1):45–66, 2019.

Priego G, Majos C, Climent F: Orbital lymphoma: imaging features and differential diagnosis. *Insights Imaging* 3(4):337–344, 2012.

Purohit BS, Vargas MI, Ailianou A, et al: Orbital tumours and tumour-like lesions: exploring the armamentarium of multiparametric imaging, *Insights Imaging* 7(1):43–68, 2016.

Smoker WRK, Gentry LR, Yee NK, et al: Vascular lesions of the orbit: more than meets the eye, *Radiographics* 28(1):185–204, 2008.

Tailor TD, Gupta D, Dalley RW, et al: Orbital neoplasms in adults: clinical, radiologic, and pathologic review, *Radiographics* 33(6):1739–1758, 2013.

Tiegs-Heiden CA, Eckel LJ, Hunt CH, et al: Immunoglobulin G4-related disease of the orbit: imaging features in 27 patients, *AJNR Am J Neuroradiol* 35(7):1393–1397, 2014.

Warrier S, Prabhakaran VK, Valenzuela A, et al: Orbital arteriovenous malformations, *Arch Ophthalmol* 126(12):1669–1675, 2008.

Wassef M, Blei F, Adams D, et al: Vascular anomalies classification: recommendations from the International Society for the Study of Vascular Anomalies, *Pediatrics* 136(1):e203–e214, 2015.

Yazc B, Yazc Z, Erdogan C, et al: Intraorbital arteriovenous fistula secondary to penetrating injury. *Ophthalmic Plast Reconstr Surg*, 23(4):275–278, 2007.

78

Lacrimal Gland Lesions

KATHARINE TANSAVATDI, MD

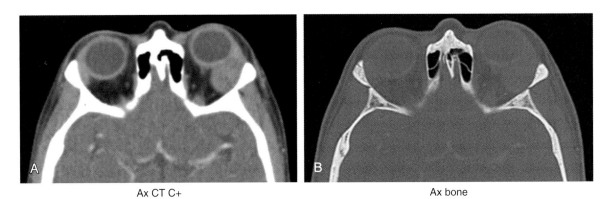

Ax CT C+

Ax bone

CASE A: A 37-year-old female presenting with blurred vision and a bulging left eye for the past 2 months. *Ax*, Axial; *CT*, Computed tomography.

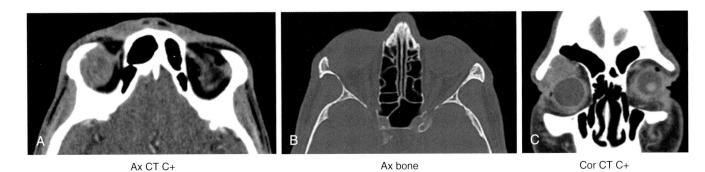

Ax CT C+

Ax bone

Cor CT C+

CASE B: A 59-year-old male presenting with ptosis of the right eye and an irregular superior orbital rim. *Ax*, Axial; *Cor*, coronal; *CT*, Computed tomography.

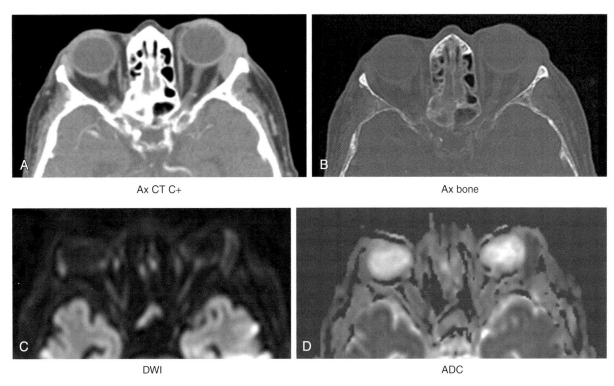

Ax CT C+

Ax bone

DWI

ADC

CASE C: A 76-year-old female presenting with a left superolateral orbit region lump. *ADC,* Apparent diffusion coefficient; *Ax,* Axial; *CT,* Computed tomography; *DWI,* diffusion-weighted imaging.

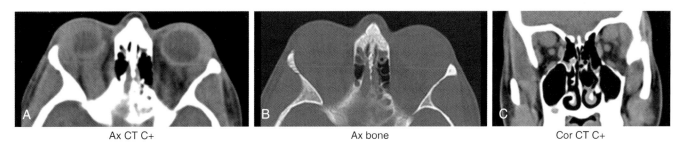

Ax CT C+

Ax bone

Cor CT C+

CASE D: A 23-year-old presenting with a 2-year history of bilateral eyelid swelling with proptosis. *Ax,* Axial; *Cor,* coronal; *CT,* Computed tomography.

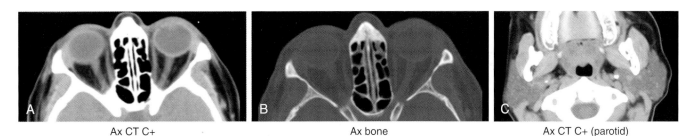

Ax CT C+

Ax bone

Ax CT C+ (parotid)

CASE E: A 54-year-old female presenting for evaluation after a motor vehicle crash. *Ax,* Axial; *CT,* Computed tomography.

DESCRIPTION OF FINDINGS

CT images demonstrate a variety of different lacrimal gland lesions with additional MR images provided for case C.

- Case A: Demonstrates a round mass involving the deep (i.e., orbital) lobe of the left lacrimal gland.
- Case B: Demonstrates a mass that appears to be similar to the mass shown in Case A; however, internal calcification and adjacent bony changes are present.
- Cases C, D, and E: Demonstrate a variety of entities diffusely involving the lacrimal glands.
- Case C: Lacks a discrete mass but instead demonstrates diffuse left lacrimal gland enlargement affecting both superficial and deep lobes with associated restricted diffusion (best appreciated on the ADC image).
- Case D: Demonstrates bilateral diffuse lacrimal gland involvement as well as enlargement of the bilateral superior recti muscles.
- Case E: Demonstrates mild bilateral lacrimal gland enlargement with fatty infiltration and small cystic spaces involving both parotid glands.

Diagnosis

Case A: Pleomorphic adenoma/benign mixed tumor
Case B: Adenoid cystic carcinoma
Case C: Lymphoma
Case D: Idiopathic orbital inflammation (IOI)
Case E: Sjögren syndrome

Summary

As with the radiographic analysis of all lesions, morphology and clinical presentation are the keys to arriving at the correct diagnosis or differential diagnosis. The lacrimal gland is divided into a deeper orbital lobe and a more superficial palpebral lobe that is one-third to half the size of the orbital lobe (Fig. 78.1). In general, neoplasms, particularly epithelial neoplasms, have a propensity to involve a single lobe of the lacrimal gland, whereas inflammatory, autoimmune, and lymphoproliferative processes tend to involve the entire gland.

Lacrimal lesions first should be evaluated for focal or diffuse involvement and can be divided into epithelial and nonepithelial lesions. Epithelial lesions, which make up 40% to 50% of lacrimal gland lesions, tend to involve the deeper orbital lobe and therefore have a greater propensity to grow posteriorly. Approximately half of all epithelial lesions are pleomorphic adenomas and present with a painless, slowly progressive mass, often over a period of more than 12 months. Pleomorphic adenomas occasionally present with internal calcifications and tend to scallop the adjacent bone. Malignant epithelial neoplasms have histologies similar to those seen in the salivary glands. Adenoid cystic carcinoma is the most common lacrimal malignant epithelial neoplasm. These tumors typically present with a short history of a painful, firm to hard mass with limited ocular motility because of their rapid growth and propensity for perineural and vascular invasion. Adenoid cystic carcinomas more commonly present with internal calcifications, can have an irregular edge as opposed to a more round to oval configuration of pleomorphic adenomas, can infiltrate orbital tissues, and can cause erosive changes of the adjacent bone.

Nonepithelial lesions often present with involvement of both lobes of the lacrimal gland and can be generalized into those typically having unilateral versus bilateral involvement. Inflammatory or infectious processes, namely acute dacryoadenitis and IOI, usually, but not always, present with unilateral diffuse (entire gland) lacrimal gland involvement. Acute dacryoadenitis often is related to a bacterial or viral infectious process commonly presenting in children and young adults with erythema, tenderness, and discharge. It is important to assess for orbital, cavernous, and intracranial extension to rule out venous sinus thrombosis. In IOI, also historically referred

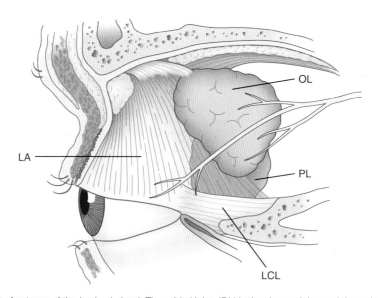

• **Fig. 78.1** Anatomy of the lacrimal gland. The orbital lobe *(OL)* is the deeper lobe and the palpebral lobe *(PL)* is the more superficial lobe. These lobes are separated by the lacrimal aponeurosis *(LA)*, which is attached to the orbital wall by the lateral canthal ligament *(LCL)*. When the upper eyelid is uplifted, a mass involving the PL can be seen as a bulging and enlarged gland. Lesions involving the orbital lobe may present with proptosis without a visible mass. (Modified from Levine MR, editor: *Manual of oculoplastic surgery*, ed 4, Thorofare, NJ, 2010, Slack.)

to as inflammatory pseudotumor, the lacrimal gland is the second most commonly involved intraorbital structure, and patients typically present with acute/subacute painful proptosis with symptoms over a period of less than 6 months. Extraocular muscle involvement, uveoscleral enhancement, and fluid in the Tenon capsule can be seen. The lacrimal gland typically is relatively T2 hypointense to muscle compared with other lacrimal lesions. Both dacryoadenitis and IOI can present with mild-to-moderate oblong enlargement of the lacrimal gland.

Lymphoproliferative, granulomatous, and autoimmune-related lesions tend to present with bilateral gland involvement. Lymphoproliferative lesions or lymphoid tumors include benign reactive lymphoid hyperplasia, atypical lymphoid hyperplasia, and lymphoma, and lymphoproliferative processes cannot be differentiated reliably from one another by imaging. These lesions can be associated with systemic involvement as part of primary or secondary disease, and they generally require further evaluation with systemic imaging. Lymphoproliferative lesions extend both anteriorly and posteriorly because of their diffuse involvement, often draping around rather than deforming the globe. These lesions do not cause destructive bony changes but can cause sclerosis and remodeling, demonstrate moderate-to-marked enhancement on MRI, and are T1 isointense to extraocular muscle and T2 hyperintense to the brain. In addition, restricted diffusion can be helpful in suggesting lymphoma rather than other lacrimal lesions.

Immunoglobulin G4 (IgG4)-related disease is an immune-mediated fibroinflammatory condition that was first recognized as a distinct disease in 2003 and is characterized by IgG4-positive plasma cell infiltration and sclerosing inflammation. Although the disease can involve virtually any organ, there is a strong predilection for the orbits and lacrimal glands. Lacrimal gland and extraocular muscle enlargement are commonly seen with the lateral recti representing the most commonly involved extraocular muscles. Many patients with IgG4-related orbital disease were previously diagnosed with IOI. There is overlap between the clinical and imaging features of both entities, and both are steroid-responsive. However, IgG4-related orbital disease (unlike IOI) is typically painless and bilateral. Infraorbital nerve enlargement can be a clue to diagnosis and is reported in approximately 30% of IgG4-related orbital disease cases. Notably, serum IgG4 levels cannot be used to reliably confirm or exclude this disease, and a low threshold to biopsy accessible sites is prudent because malignancy (e.g., lymphoma, metastasis) is often a differential consideration.

Lacrimal gland involvement in persons with sarcoidosis presents with diffuse, often bilateral enlargement and soft tissue characteristics similar to lymphoid tumors. The enlarged lacrimal gland typically has irregular margins, and patients often may present with dry eyes in the third to fifth decade of life. In persons with Sjögren syndrome, a bilateral change in lacrimal gland size is associated with accelerated fat deposition, showing a progression in appearance from normal-sized homogenous to hypertrophic homogenous to normal-sized heterogenous to small heterogenous to atrophic. The heterogenous appearance is the result of fat deposition within the lacrimal gland. A similar pattern of lacrimal gland involvement can be seen with granulomatosis with polyangiitis; however, the presence of nasal septal erosion and sinus involvement would favor granulomatosis with polyangiitis, whereas the presence of salivary gland involvement would favor Sjögren syndrome. Additional features favoring granulomatosis with polyangiitis include renal, upper airway, and pulmonary disease.

Spectrum of Disease

Developmental cysts (e.g., dermoid cysts, epidermoid cysts, and teratoma) can occur within the orbit. They arise from the inclusion of ectodermal elements during neural tube closure and often become trapped within suture lines. These cysts often are found adjacent to the zygomaticofrontal or frontoethmoidal sutures, with most demonstrating adjacent nonaggressive bony changes (Fig. 78.2). Because these developmental cysts are more commonly located laterally in the extraconal orbit, they can mimic a lacrimal gland mass, but the cysts usually demonstrate areas of low density or have a density that is greater than fat but less than vitreous. Calcification and fluid levels are uncommon. The bone margins adjacent to the cyst are typically smooth, but the developmental cyst can extend into and even through the bone.

Differential Diagnosis

1. Pleomorphic adenoma/benign mixed tumor
2. Adenoid cystic carcinoma
3. Lymphoproliferative disorders
4. Dacryoadenitis
5. Idiopathic orbital inflammation
6. IgG4-related orbital disease
7. Sarcoidosis
8. Sjögren syndrome
9. Granulomatosis with polyangiitis

Pearls

- Laterality: Bilateral disease favors lymphoproliferative disease, IgG4-related disease, sarcoid, and Sjögren syndrome, whereas unilateral disease favors epithelial neoplasms, infection, and IOI.
- Focal versus diffuse: Focal disease involving a particular lobe is more typically the presentation of epithelial neoplasms, whereas infectious, inflammatory, and autoimmune diseases tend to involve the entire gland.
- Morphology: Among epithelial neoplasms, pleomorphic adenoma tends to scallop the adjacent bone with smooth contours, whereas adenoid cystic carcinoma can have irregular margins, infiltrate adjacent orbital tissue, and cause erosion of the adjacent bone.
- DWI/ADC: Statistically significant lower ADC values and ADC ratios (lesion to thalamus) have been demonstrated when differentiating between lymphoid lesions, IOI, and orbital cellulitis.

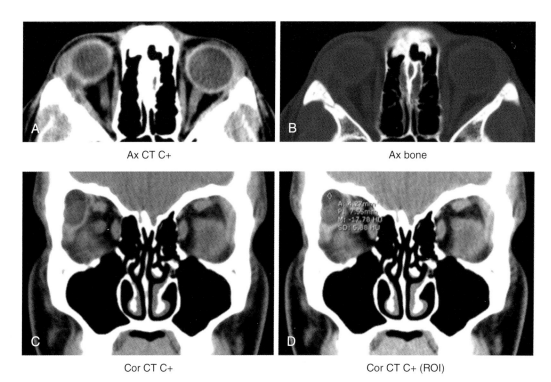

Ax CT C+   Ax bone

Cor CT C+   Cor CT C+ (ROI)

• **Fig. 78.2** Orbital dermoid cyst. (A) An axial *(Ax),* computed tomography *(CT),* contrast-enhanced image, (B) an axial CT bone window image, and (C) a coronal *(Cor),* CT postcontrast image demonstrate a heterogeneous, smooth-contoured, oval-shaped mass in the upper outer quadrant of the right orbit. The mass is located in close proximity to the right zygomaticofrontal suture (B), and a region of interest *(ROI)* in D clearly demonstrates fat attenuation (−17.78 HU [Hounsfield units]); these findings are consistent with a dermoid cyst. *ST,* Soft tissue.

Signs and Complications

Proptosis is a common sign of an underlying lacrimal gland lesion.

Suggested Readings

Gündüz AK, Yeşiltaş YS, Shields CL: Overview of benign and malignant lacrimal gland tumors, *Curr Opin Ophthalmol* 29(5):458–468, 2018.

Huang S, Juniat V, Satchi K, et al: Bilateral lacrimal gland disease: clinical features and outcomes, *Eye (Lond)* 36(11):2163–2171, 2022.

Hughes GK, Miszkiel KA: Imaging of the lacrimal gland, *Semin Ultrasound CT MRI* 27:476–491, 2006.

Jung WS, Kook JA, Park MR, et al: The radiological spectrum of orbital pathologies that involve the lacrimal gland and the lacrimal fossa, *Korean J Radiol* 8:336–342, 2007.

Kapur R, Sepahdari AR, Mafee MF, et al: MR imaging of orbital inflammatory syndrome, orbital cellulitis, and orbital lymphoid lesions: the role of diffusion-weighted imaging, *AJNR Am J Neuroradiol* 30:64–70, 2009.

Obata H: Anatomy and histopathology of the human lacrimal gland, *Cornea* 25(suppl):S82–S89, 2006.

Sullivan TJ, Valenzuela AA: Imaging features of ocular adnexal lymphoproliferative disease, *Eye* 20:1189–1195, 2006.

Tan TT, Davagnanam I, Isa H, et al: Clinical and imaging features of lacrimal gland involvement in granulomatosis with polyangiitis, *Ophthalmology* 122(10):2125–2129, 2015.

Tiegs-Heiden CA, Eckel LJ, Hunt CH, et al: Immunoglobulin G4-related disease of the orbit: imaging features in 27 patients, *AJNR Am J Neuroradiol* 35(7):1393–1397, 2014.

Tonami H, Matoba M, Yokota H, et al: CT and MR findings of bilateral lacrimal gland enlargement in Sjögren syndrome, *J Clin Imaging* 26:392–396, 2002.

Vaidhyanath R, Kirke R: Lacrimal fossa lesions: pictorial review and CT and MR features, *Orbit* 27:410–418, 2008.

Valmaggia C, Neuweiler J: Orbital involvement as the first manifestation in classic Wegener's granulomatosis, *Orbit* 20:231–237, 2001.

Wallace ZS, Naden RP, Chari S, et al: The 2019 American College of Rheumatology/European League Against Rheumatism classification criteria for IgG4-related disease, *Arthritis Rheumatol* 72(1):7–19, 2020.

79

Extraocular Muscle Enlargement

JEFFREY R. SACHS, MD

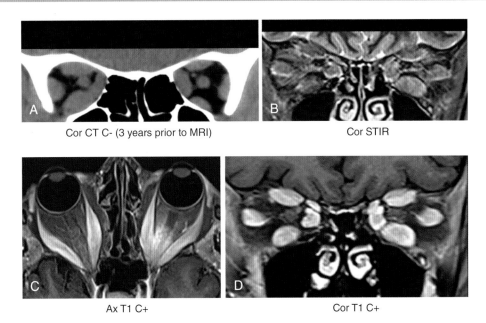

Cor CT C- (3 years prior to MRI)

Cor STIR

Ax T1 C+

Cor T1 C+

CASE A: A 57-year-old female with a history of thyroid dysfunction. *Ax,* Axial; *Cor,* coronal; *CT,* Computed tomography; *MRI,* magnetic resonance imaging; *STIR,* short tau inversion recovery.

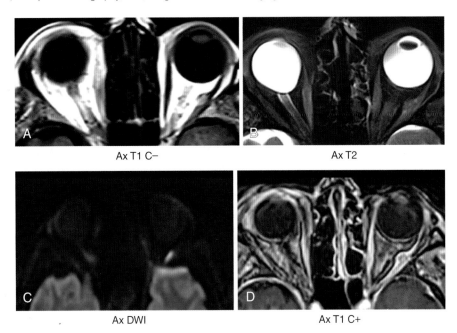

Ax T1 C−

Ax T2

Ax DWI

Ax T1 C+

CASE B: A 72-year-old male with malignant melanoma presents for a staging MRI of the brain. *Ax,* Axial; *DWI,* diffusion-weighted imaging; *MRI,* magnetic resonance imaging.

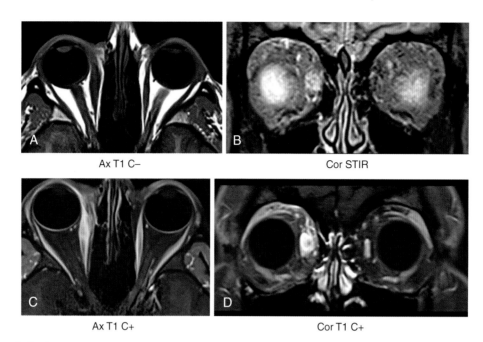

Ax T1 C–

Cor STIR

Ax T1 C+

Cor T1 C+

CASE C: A 27-year-old male presents with right eye pain. *Ax,* Axial; *Cor,* coronal; *STIR,* short tau inversion recovery.

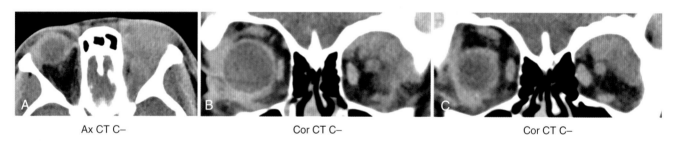

Ax CT C–

Cor CT C–

Cor CT C–

CASE D: A 25-year-old female presents with 1-year history of left eye swelling with occasional diplopia and pressure sensation. *Ax,* Axial; *Cor,* coronal; *CT,* Computed tomography.

DESCRIPTION OF FINDINGS

- Case A: Marked enlargement of the mid-muscle bellies of the extraocular muscles with sparing of the tendinous insertions. There has been progression of muscle enlargement on the left since the CT was performed 3 years prior. Crowding of the right optic nerve near the orbital apex is noted.
- Case B: A focal round mass in the mid-muscle belly of the left lateral rectus muscle is noted. The lesion is hyperintense to muscle on T1, isointense to muscle on T2 with minimal surrounding edema, restricts diffusion (confirmed on ADC map, not shown), and enhances.
- Case C: Asymmetric and focal nonmass–like enlargement of the anterior and mid-portions of the right medial rectus muscle is seen with involvement of the tendinous insertion. The muscle as well as the surrounding fat are inflamed, as evidenced by T2 hyperintensity and enhancement. The other extraocular muscles (EOMs) appear normal.
- Case D: Mass-like soft tissue is centered in the left superotemporal orbit involving both the intraconal and extraconal fat, inseparable from both the superior and lateral rectus muscles as well as the lacrimal gland. The remainder of the orbital fat is unremarkable, and the right orbit is normal.

Diagnosis

Case A: Thyroid eye disease (TED)
Case B: Metastasis
Case C: Idiopathic orbital inflammation (IOI)
Case D: IgG4-related orbital disease

Summary

The presentation of EOM enlargement can be a diagnostic dilemma. A broad differential diagnosis for this finding can include TED, metastasis, IOI, immunoglobulin G4 (IgG4)-related orbital disease, sarcoidosis, and lymphoproliferative disorders. Features that may help a radiologist narrow the differential include the presence or absence of involvement of the tendinous insertions, the pattern of EOM enlargement (i.e., which muscles are enlarged?), and ancillary findings elsewhere in the head and neck, in addition to characteristic clinical and laboratory features.

Spectrum of Disease

Thyroid Eye Disease

TED, also referred to as thyroid orbitopathy or Graves dysthyroid ophthalmopathy, represents an autoimmune orbital inflammation in the setting of autoimmune thyroid dysfunction, such as Graves disease. The most common clinical presentations include eyelid retraction, periorbital swelling, and proptosis, but pain and restricted gaze also occur. There is a female predilection, and most cases occur in young and middle-aged adults, increasing in severity with age and uncommon in children. While TED is primarily a clinical diagnosis, imaging is helpful for confirmation and to exclude other etiologies of proptosis in atypical cases, most notably a mass. At imaging, even in the early acute stages of the disease, there is usually enlargement of the EOM bellies with relative sparing of the tendinous insertions (though they can rarely be

involved), an important differentiating feature. Imaging in the coronal plane is generally most helpful for assessing the extent and severity of EOM enlargement with the exception of the lateral rectus muscle, which is better assessed in the axial plane due to its oblique orientation within the orbit. Additionally, the orbital apex and any degree of associated optic nerve compression are well seen in the coronal plane. Areas of hypoattenuation within the enlarged muscle bellies are a helpful clue to the diagnosis (Fig. 79.1), thought to be due to glycosaminoglycan or fat deposition. On MRI, the enlarged muscle bellies will be T1 isointense, with T2 signal dependent on the stage of disease. Acutely, the affected EOM may demonstrate T2 hyperintensity reflecting edema and inflammation. As a chronic fibrotic phase develops, the EOMs lose their elasticity, and the patient develops restricted eye movement. This phase will appear on imaging as thin, string-like EOMs that may show fatty replacement or potentially T2 hypointensity due to fibrosis. Affected muscles may demonstrate decreased enhancement relative to unaffected muscles. Secondary signs of TED include increased orbital fat, proptosis, eyelid edema, anterior displacement of the orbital septum, a straightened or stretched-appearing optic nerve, lacrimal gland enlargement/prolapse, and stranding of the orbital fat, especially in the acute phase.

The muscles which are typically involved by TED can be remembered by the mnemonic IM SLO, which represents the **I**nferior rectus, **M**edial rectus, **S**uperior rectus, **L**ateral rectus, and superior **O**blique muscles in decreasing order of frequency of involvement. However, exceptions to this rule occur and are under-recognized. For instance, there may be isolated involvement of the levator palpebrae superioris/superior rectus muscle complex (Fig. 79.2). This finding can be very subtle, but should be specifically sought for in the clinical setting of upper eyelid retraction. If found, this finding should prompt the radiologist to suggest the possibility of TED and trigger laboratory investigation for thyroid-stimulating immunoglobulin or thyrotropin receptor antibodies if not previously performed. Such patients are likely to develop the more typical pattern of EOM involvement in TED when encountered at future imaging.

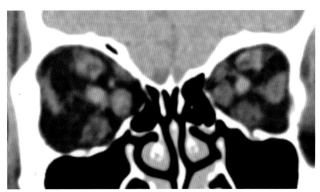

Cor CT C–

• **Fig. 79.1** Coronal CT image obtained in a 60-year-old male with Graves disease demonstrates hypoattenuation within the enlarged muscle bellies secondary to deposition of glycosaminoglycan or fat. *Cor,* Coronal; *CT,* Computed tomography.

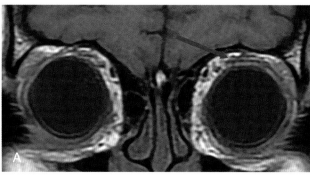 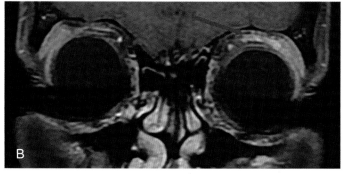

Cor T1 C–   Cor T1 C+

• **Fig. 79.2** Isolated involvement of the left levator palpebrae superioris/superior rectus muscle complex in a 50-year-old female presenting with left facial weakness and upper lid retraction. Pre- and postcontrast coronal T1-weighted images demonstrate asymmetric thickening of the left superior muscle complex *(arrows)*. Findings were more conspicuous on postcontrast imaging. All other EOMs appeared normal. Graves disease was subsequently confirmed by laboratory analysis. *Cor,* Coronal; *EOMs,* extraocular muscles.

Metastasis

Metastasis to the EOMs is rare. The most common primary malignancies that metastasize to the EOMs are breast, melanoma, and carcinoid. The lateral rectus has been implicated as the most common EOM involved. It has been speculated that this is a result of the differing blood supply to the lateral rectus via the lacrimal artery, whereas the other EOMs take their blood supply via muscular branches of the ophthalmic artery. Rather than diffuse EOM swelling, a metastasis is more likely to be focal (discrete borders), round, and expansile without involvement of the tendinous insertion. Generally, the T1 and T2 signal are heterogeneous with variable heterogeneous postcontrast enhancement.

Idiopathic Orbital Inflammation

IOI, commonly referred to as orbital pseudotumor, is the most common cause of a painful orbital mass in adults and the third most common orbital disease after thyroid orbitopathy and lymphoproliferative disease. In general, IOI refers to a nongranulomatous inflammation with no known cause, but that is responsive to steroids. Pain is an important distinguishing feature from other orbital processes (but may be absent in the chronic phase), and other symptoms may include diplopia, proptosis, restricted eye movement, and impaired vision. There are protean manifestations of this disease, and there are several different anatomical patterns of orbital pseudotumor that are recognized, which include myositis, dacryoadenitis, apical, anterior, and diffuse disease. When EOMs are involved, 90% to 95% of cases are unilateral. The medial rectus is the most frequently involved muscle, followed by the superior rectus, lateral rectus, and inferior rectus. Tendon involvement is expected, which, when coupled with the muscle belly involvement produces a tubular-like configuration of the abnormality. This pattern helps to distinguish IOI from TED. Fat stranding is often seen, but unlike TED, increased volume of orbital fat

is not expected. Additionally, TED is more frequently bilateral, affects an older population, and has a more insidious, typically painless clinical onset. When IOI is clinically suspected, a trial of therapeutic steroids is often initiated. A presumptive diagnosis of IOI is supported if symptoms improve. If symptoms persist or if there is clinical or imaging evidence of disease progression, biopsy is indicated.

Immunoglobulin G4-Related Disease

IgG4-related disease is characterized by infiltration of tissues by IgG4 plasma cells and sclerosing inflammation. It is a systemic disorder of unknown etiology and was recognized as a distinct disease entity in 2003. Many patients previously diagnosed with IOI are now recognized to actually have IgG4-related disease. When IgG4-related disease affects the orbit, EOM enlargement is the most common finding. The lateral rectus muscle is most frequently affected, and often to the greatest degree and bilaterally. In contrast to TED, where lateral rectus involvement is a late finding in IgG4-related disease, the lateral rectus is prominently affected early in the disease course. Unlike IOI, the tendinous insertion sites are usually spared in IgG4-related disease. IOI is also most commonly unilateral, whereas the bilateral orbital involvement more often seen with TED and IgG4-related disease reflects the systemic nature of the pathology. Orbital pain is a clinical feature that would support IOI over IgG4-related disease or TED. There are a number of secondary features that the head and neck imager can use to support the diagnosis of IgG4-related disease. These include lacrimal gland enlargement, paranasal sinus mucosal thickening, and evidence of perineural involvement, often the infraorbital nerve. Occasionally there is abnormal soft tissue in the orbital apex, cavernous sinus, or Meckel's cave. Because IgG4-related disease represents a systemic, multiorgan pathology, the radiologist should review available imaging outside of the head and neck to assess for findings attributable to IgG4-related disease, most notably the classic sausage-shaped pancreas or infrarenal periaortic soft tissue infiltration. The American College of Rheumatology/European League Against Rheumatism has developed a validated set of classification criteria for IgG4-related disease (see Suggested Readings). It is important to maintain a low threshold to biopsy accessible sites when there is concern for malignancy or infection, as it is only a minority of patients that will have classic clinical, radiologic, and supportive laboratory evidence that allow for diagnosis of IgG4-related disease in the absence of biopsy. Importantly, normal serum IgG4 levels do not exclude IgG4-related disease, and elevated serum IgG4 levels are not diagnostic.

Lymphoproliferative Disease

A discussion of orbital mass lesions affecting the EOMs would be incomplete without the inclusion of lymphoproliferative lesions. Lymphoma can involve any part of the orbit but has a predilection for the lacrimal gland. There are many case reports of orbital lymphoma mimicking TED. Moreover, a history of TED predisposes to orbital lymphoma. However, isolated involvement of the EOMs by lymphoma is rare. Features favoring lymphoma include presence of a soft tissue mass focally expanding the EOM or lacrimal gland, extension of abnormal soft tissue to involve the tendinous insertion, or abnormal soft tissue adjacent to the muscle. Lymphoma tends to appear as a soft, pliable tumor that encases rather than destroys or

displaces adjacent structures. T2 intermediate or low signal and restricted diffusion are present due to the highly cellular nature of this tumor that has a high nuclear/cytoplasmic ratio. IgG4-related orbital disease can also restrict diffusion, but the mean diffusivity in lymphoma is typically lower than in IgG4-related disease.

Sarcoidosis

Orbital involvement by sarcoidosis is rarely characterized by EOM enlargement. When present, multifocal, asymmetric EOM infiltration will be seen. The most common location for orbital involvement in sarcoidosis is the lacrimal gland (~60%). One may also see thickening of the optic nerve sheath, preseptal soft tissue thickening/infiltration, uveitis, intraorbital soft tissue masses, or involvement of the nasolacrimal apparatus. Involved tissues will appear isoattenuating on CT relative to the EOMs, hypointense on T1WI, variably hyperintense on T2, and demonstrate homogeneous postcontrast enhancement.

Differential Diagnosis

Characteristic features of disorders resulting in extraocular muscle enlargement are summarized in the Table below: Note that exceptions to these typical or classic features occur. Biopsy may be required to differentiate neoplasm from inflammatory/granulomatous processes.

	Most Common EOM(s) Involved	Unilateral or Bilateral	Tendinous Insertion Involvement	Ancillary Imaging Findings	Clinical Features
Thyroid eye disease, typical	IM SLO (inferior rectus, medial rectus, superior rectus, lateral rectus, and superior oblique in decreasing order of frequency)	Bilateral	No	Increased orbital fat, proptosis, straightened or stretched-appearing optic nerve, lacrimal gland enlargement, orbital fat stranding	Eyelid retraction, periorbital swelling, proptosis
Idiopathic orbital inflammation	Medial rectus most common	Unilateral	Yes	Fat stranding, dacryoadenitis, optic perineuritis, episcleritis, orbital mass, fullness in region of orbital apex/superior orbital fissure/cavernous sinus (combination of these findings may be present)	Pain
IgG4-related disease	Lateral rectus involvement early in disease course, often pronounced	Bilateral	No	lacrimal gland enlargement, paranasal sinus mucosal thickening, perineural disease spread	Often indolent course; painless periorbital swelling, proptosis, diplopia; serum IgG4 levels may be normal
Metastasis	Lateral rectus most common; can be any EOM	Unilateral	No	Mass-like morphology, may extend out of EOM to affect orbital fat or bone	Known history of malignancy

	Most Common EOM(s) Involved	Unilateral or Bilateral	Tendinous Insertion Involvement	Ancillary Imaging Findings	Clinical Features
Lymphoma	Any	Unilateral or bilateral	Possible	Protean imaging manifestations; predilection for lacrimal gland involvement	Up to 50% have systemic lymphoma at time of diagnosis; insidious onset of eyelid or anterior orbital swelling
Sarcoidosis	Any	Bilateral, asymmetric	Possible	Lacrimal gland infiltration, optic nerve sheath thickening and enhancement, intraorbital soft tissue mass, periorbital preseptal infiltration, uveitis, obstruction of nasolacrimal apparatus	Uveitis, diplopia, lacrimal mass, dacryoadenitis

IgG4, Immunoglobulin G4.

Additional rare differential considerations for EOM enlargement include inflammatory bowel disease–related myositis and granulomatosis with polyangiitis (formerly Wegener's granulomatosis). The EOM imaging findings can overlap with the other more common pathologies discussed in this chapter. However, a clinical history of Crohn's disease or ulcerative colitis should prompt consideration of inflammatory bowel disease–related myositis, and destructive sinonasal changes should prompt consideration of granulomatosis with polyangiitis.

Pearls

Careful attention to the pattern and morphology of muscle enlargement, presence or absence of involvement of the tendinous insertion sites, and appropriate integration of clinical symptoms, laboratory data, and ancillary orbital or extraorbital imaging findings is key to narrowing the differential diagnosis when the radiologist is presented with extraocular muscle enlargement.

Signs and Complications

A notable complication of TED is dysthyroid optic neuropathy (DON) due to compression of the optic nerve at the orbital apex by enlarged extraocular muscles (Fig. 79.3).

Suggested Readings

Cunnane MB, Sepahadari AR, Gardiner M, et al: Chapter 9: Pathology of the eye and orbit. In Som PM, Curtin HD, editors: *Head and neck imaging*, ed 5, St. Louis, MO 591–756, 2011, Elsevier/Mosby.

Ding ZX, Lip G, Chong V: Idiopathic orbital pseudotumor, *Clin Radiol* 66(9):886–892, 2011.

Leung V, Wei M, Roberts TV: Metastasis to the extraocular muscles: a case report, literature review and pooled data analysis, *Clin Exp Ophthalmol* 46:687–694, 2018.

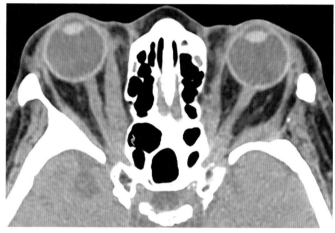

Ax CT C–

• **Fig. 79.3** Axial CT image obtained in a 71-year-old male with Graves disease demonstrates compression and flattening of the right optic nerve at the orbital apex due to a markedly enlarged right medial rectus muscle. The patient had previously undergone left orbital decompression for compressive left optic neuropathy. *Ax*, Axial; *CT*, Computed tomography.

Neto AM, Denardi FC, Delamain MT, et al: Orbital lymphoma mimicking ophthalmopathy in a patient with Graves', *Am J Med Sci* 344(5):418–421, 2012.

Tiegs-Heiden CA, Eckel LJ, Hunt CH, et al: Immunoglobulin G4-related disease of the orbit: imaging features in 27 patients, *AJNR Am J Neuroradiol* 35(7):1393–1397, 2014.

Wallace ZS, Naden RP, Chari S, et al: The 2019 American College of Rheumatology/European League against Rheumatism Classification Criteria for IgG4-related disease, *Arthritis Rheumatol* 72(1):7–19, 2020.

Wang Y, Mettu P, Broadbent T, et al: Thyroid eye disease presenting with superior rectus/levator complex enlargement, *Orbit* 39(1):5–12, 2020.

80

Nasal Cavity Masses

JOHN M. FAGNOU, MD AND PAUL M. BUNCH, MD

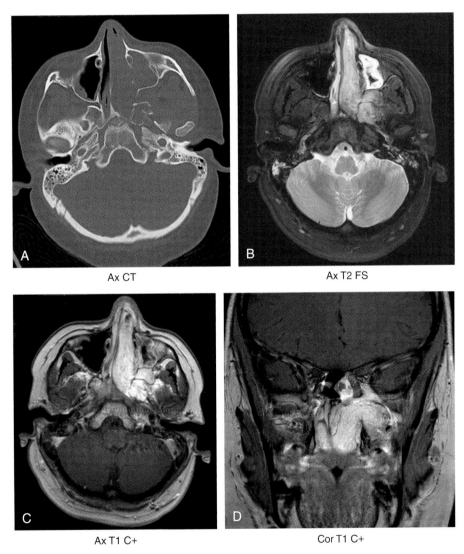

Ax CT

Ax T2 FS

Ax T1 C+

Cor T1 C+

CASE A: A 13-year-old male presenting with epistaxis. *Ax*, Axial; *Cor*, coronal; *CT*, Computed tomography; *FS*, fat saturated.

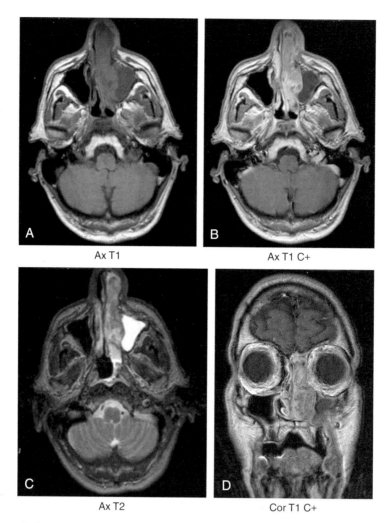

A — Ax T1

B — Ax T1 C+

C — Ax T2

D — Cor T1 C+

CASE B: A 62-year-old male presenting with epistaxis. *Ax*, Axial; *Cor*, coronal.

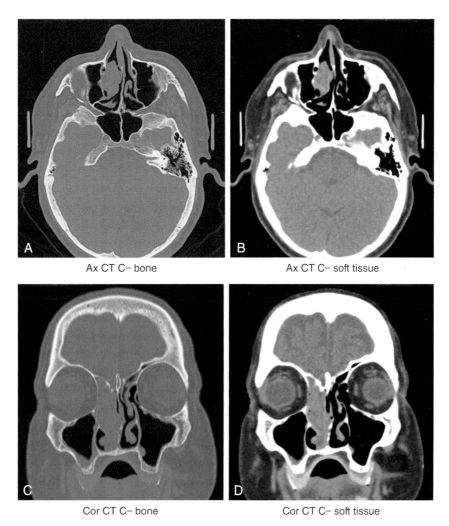

Ax CT C− bone

Ax CT C− soft tissue

Cor CT C− bone

Cor CT C− soft tissue

CASE C: A 73-year-old male presenting with chronic sinusitis. *Ax*, Axial; *Cor*, coronal; *CT,* Computed tomography.

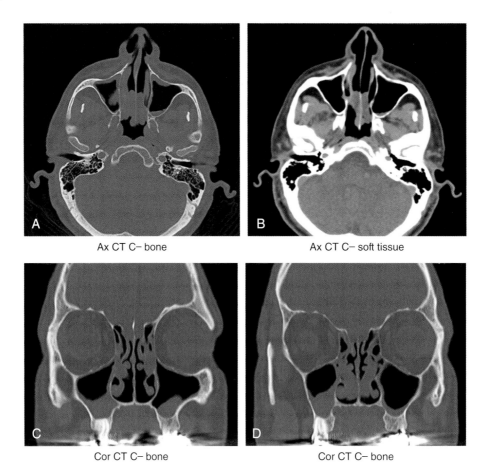

Ax CT C− bone

Ax CT C− soft tissue

Cor CT C− bone

Cor CT C− bone

CASE D: A 51-year-old male presenting with persistent nasal congestion. *Ax*, Axial; *Cor*, coronal; *CT,* Computed tomography.

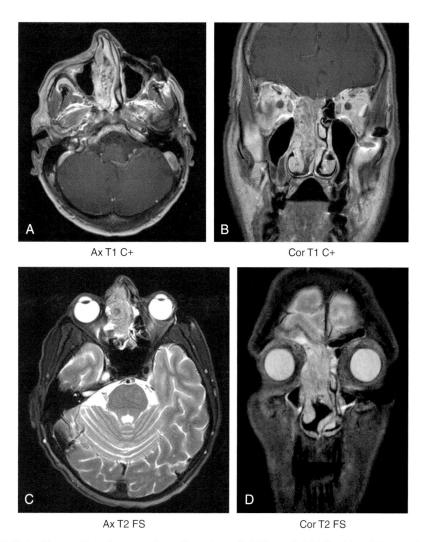

Ax T1 C+

Cor T1 C+

Ax T2 FS

Cor T2 FS

CASE E: A 47-year-old male presenting with a 1-month history of right frontal and temporal pain. *Ax*, Axial; *Cor*, coronal; *FS,* fat saturated.

DESCRIPTION OF FINDINGS

- Case A: An avidly enhancing, expansile mass is centered at the left sphenopalatine foramen with extension into the left nasal cavity, pterygopalatine fossa, pterygomaxillary fissure, and inferior orbital fissure.
- Case B: An avidly enhancing left nasal cavity mass extends anteriorly into the nasal vestibule. On the axial T1-weighted image, there are areas of intrinsic mild T1 hyperintensity within the mass.
- Case C: A nonspecific right nasal cavity mass.
- Case D: Bilateral low-density polypoid nasal cavity lesions with associated paranasal sinus mucosal thickening.
- Case E: A heterogeneous mass involving the right greater than left nasal cavities and extending into the ethmoid air cells.

Diagnosis

Case A: Juvenile angiofibroma
Case B: Melanoma
Case C: Inverted papilloma
Case D: Sinonasal polyposis
Case E: Squamous cell carcinoma (SCC) ex inverted papilloma

Summary

Because most disease in the nasal cavity relates to inflammatory mucosal thickening or polyp formation, the radiologist must be attuned to subtle findings that might suggest a different diagnostic possibility. More broadly, nasal cavity lesions may include neoplastic, inflammatory, or infectious etiologies. Often a nasal cavity mass has nonspecific imaging characteristics, and accurate prediction of the histologic diagnosis using imaging features is not possible. Fortunately, nasal cavity masses are typically amenable to endoscopic tissue sampling. On pretreatment imaging of a known, suspected, or possible nasal cavity malignancy, the role of the radiologist is to determine the anatomic extent of the lesion, to evaluate for metastatic lymph nodes, and to assess for perineural tumor spread.

When faced with an unknown nasal cavity lesion, it is useful to evaluate for aggressive imaging features, such as bone destruction on CT, which might suggest a more sinister diagnosis compared with remodeling, which is suggestive of a slow-growing lesion. However, even malignant lesions can be slow-growing and produce a pushing margin with remodeling. In addition, "evil gray" at MRI (i.e., intermediate T2 signal and intermediate enhancement on postcontrast T1-weighted images) is strongly suggestive of tumor, in contradistinction to typically T2 bright and peripherally enhancing inflammatory change.

Benign nasal cavity lesions include polyps/polyposis, papilloma, hamartoma, and juvenile angiofibroma. Malignant nasal cavity lesions include sinonasal carcinoma (including squamous cell carcinoma (SCC), sinonasal undifferentiated carcinoma, and adenocarcinoma), esthesioneuroblastoma, lymphoma, sarcoma, and melanoma. Neither of these lists is exhaustive.

Nasal septal perforation constitutes a unique and somewhat specific differential diagnosis. This condition is also discussed in the following sections.

Spectrum of Disease

Nasal Polyp

The benign inflammatory nasal polyp is the most common nasal cavity mass. These lesions are often multiple and occur in the setting of inflammatory paranasal sinus disease. A nasal polyp is typically well defined, low density, T2 hyperintense, and T1 hypointense, although both CT and MRI characteristics may vary depending on protein content. On noncontrast CT, polyps may be indistinguishable from malignant neoplasm, such that recommending correlation with direct inspection is prudent. On contrast-enhanced MR imaging, enhancement is usually thin and peripheral. Nodular enhancement should raise concern for neoplasm. Inflammatory polyps may arise in the nasal cavity primarily or extend into the nasal cavity from an origin in a paranasal sinus. A nasal polyp extending from the maxillary antrum into the nasal cavity is referred to as a "nasoantral" polyp, and a polyp extending from the maxillary antrum posteriorly to reach the nasopharynx is known as an "antrochoanal" polyp.

Juvenile Angiofibroma

Juvenile angiofibroma is a benign but locally aggressive neoplasm that occurs in adolescent males. Nasal obstruction and epistaxis are common presenting symptoms. These tumors typically arise in the lateral nasal cavity near the sphenopalatine foramen, with typical early spread to the pterygopalatine fossa and variably into the nasopharynx, masticator space, skull base, inferior orbital fissure, and paranasal sinuses. These lesions are highly vascular and therefore commonly demonstrate multiple flow voids with intense enhancement. Common feeding vessels at angiography include the internal maxillary artery and ascending pharyngeal artery, with variable internal carotid artery supply (e.g., the Vidian artery). Preoperative embolization prior to resection has been shown to reduce blood loss and operative duration. Caution is warranted if considering biopsy because of the high risk of hemorrhage.

Inverted Papilloma

Nasal papillomas are benign neoplasms accounting for up to 5% of sinonasal tumors. The inverted papilloma represents the most common subtype and typically occurs in middle-aged to elderly men. Most inverted papillomas arise from the lateral wall of the nasal cavity in the region of the middle meatus, though they also commonly occur in the maxillary sinus. These lesions may calcify and commonly exhibit a "convoluted cerebriform" appearance on T2-weighted and T1-weighted, gadolinium-enhanced MR images (Fig. 80.1). A focal area of hyperostosis is frequently seen (Fig. 80.1) and has been shown to correlate with the site of tumor attachment, which is useful information for surgical planning. Importantly, 5% to 15% undergo malignant degeneration into SCC or harbor SCC at diagnosis (i.e., an SCC ex inverted papilloma). As such, these lesions are typically surgically removed.

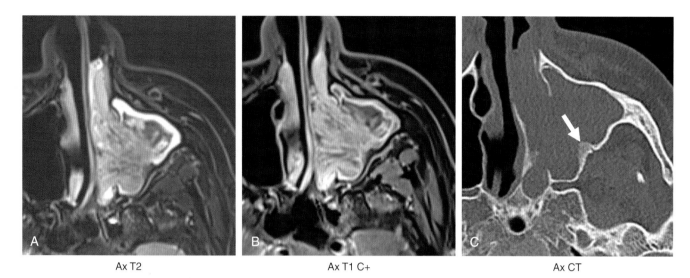

Ax T2   Ax T1 C+   Ax CT

• **Fig. 80.1** (A) Axial T2-weighted and (B) axial T1-weighted, gadolinium-enhanced images demonstrate a left maxillary sinus and left nasal cavity mass exhibiting the "convoluted cerebriform" pattern typical of inverted papilloma. (C) On the axial CT image, note the focal hyperostosis *(arrow)* along the posterior wall of the left maxillary sinus, which also favors inverted papilloma as the diagnosis and has been shown to correlate with the site of attachment. *Ax,* Axial; *CT,* Computed tomography.

Hamartoma

Sinonasal epithelial hamartomas are benign lesions that contain normal ciliated respiratory epithelium. Subtypes include seromucinous hamartoma (SH) and respiratory epithelial adenomatoid hamartoma (REAH). These hamartomas are observed in adults with a strong male predilection. Rhinorrhea, nasal congestion, and loss of smell are common presenting symptoms. These lesions manifest on imaging as well-defined, homogenous soft tissue filling the bilateral superior nasal cavities and commonly resulting in expansion or smooth remodeling (Fig. 80.2). Erosion and other aggressive osseous changes should be absent. On sagittal images, a characteristic discoid or half-moon appearance has been described.

Squamous Cell Carcinoma

SCC typically affects older male smokers with refractory sinonasal symptoms. SCCs most commonly arise from the maxillary sinus rather than the nasal cavity. Although frequently indistinguishable from other sinonasal malignancies by imaging, these tumors have been described as relatively

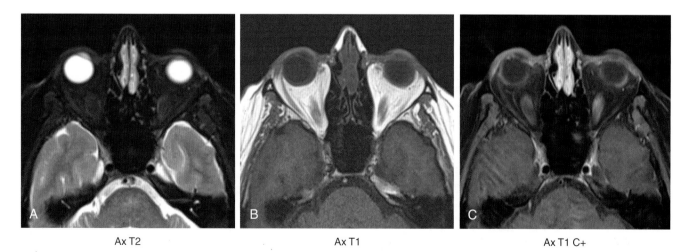

Ax T2   Ax T1   Ax T1 C+

• **Fig. 80.2** Axial *(Ax)* magnetic resonance images demonstrate mildly expansile, homogeneously enhancing lesions involving the bilateral olfactory clefts. Although tissue sampling is necessary for definitive diagnosis, the imaging appearance favors sinonasal epithelial hamartomas, of which the subtypes include respiratory epithelial adenomatoid hamartoma and seromucinous hamartoma.

hypoenhancing after gadolinium contrast administration compared to other sinonasal malignancies (e.g., esthesioneuroblastoma, melanoma) and are commonly associated with aggressive osseous changes.

Esthesioneuroblastoma (Olfactory Neuroblastoma)

Esthesioneuroblastoma appears in persons with a broad age range, including bimodal peaks in the second and sixth decades. Esthesioneuroblastoma arises from the basal stem cells of the olfactory neuroepithelium, which is typically confined to the superior nasal cavity; however, rare cases of "ectopic" esthesioneuroblastoma have been described in the nasopharynx, maxillary sinus, and sella turcica. The classically described imaging appearance is a dumbbell-shaped or bilobed mass with intracranial and superior nasal cavity components and a "waist" at the cribriform plate. Marginal cysts (Fig. 80.3) within the intracranial component have been described as pathognomonic of this diagnosis but are rarely seen. This tumor may calcify; however, calcification is also seen in other nasal cavity tumors, including inverted papilloma and chondrosarcoma.

Melanoma

Sinonasal melanoma is a rare, aggressive malignancy that most commonly arises from the nasal septum. Nasal obstruction and epistaxis are the most commonly reported symptoms. Most CT and MR imaging features overlap with those of other sinonasal malignancies; however, the presence of intrinsic T1

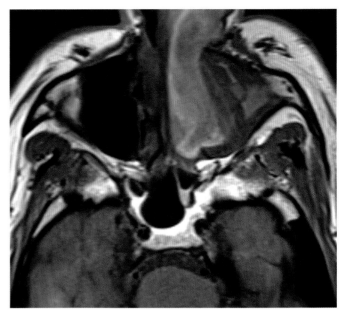

Ax T1

• **Fig. 80.4** Axial *(Ax)* T1-weighted image demonstrates an intrinsically T1 hyperintense left nasal cavity melanoma.

hyperintensity (Fig. 80.4) would favor melanoma over other sinonasal neoplasms.

Lymphoma

Sinonasal lymphoma may occur in isolation or in conjunction with systemic disease. B-cell lymphomas account for most cases and are associated with a more favorable prognosis. Extranodal natural killer/T-cell lymphoma is associated with rapid progression and death. Imaging features favoring sinonasal lymphoma (Fig. 80.5) include restricted diffusion, homogeneously intermediate signal on T1- and T2-weighted images, homogeneous enhancement, and transosseous extension with relatively little osseous destruction.

Sarcoma

Sarcomas are rare in the head and neck; however, among head and neck subsites, the sinonasal tract is relatively commonly involved. Rhabdomyosarcoma represents the most common subtype of sinonasal sarcoma and warrants particular consideration in a pediatric patient. Less common subtypes of sinonasal sarcoma with more characteristic, although not necessarily diagnostic, imaging features include chondrosarcoma and osteosarcoma. Chondrosarcoma may occur at the cartilaginous junctions of the facial bones or within the cartilaginous nasal septum and exhibits "ring and arc" mineralization. Osteosarcoma is associated with the formation of osteoid and "sunburst" periosteal reaction.

Nasal Septal Perforation

Causes of nasal septal perforation include ischemic necrosis relating to trauma (including surgery), cocaine use, overuse of

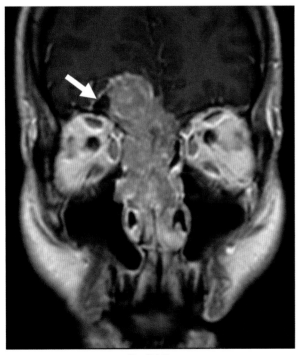

Cor T1 C+

• **Fig. 80.3** Coronal *(Cor)* T1-weighted, gadolinium-enhanced image demonstrates a marginal cyst *(arrow)* along the right lateral aspect of the intracranial component of this esthesioneuroblastoma.

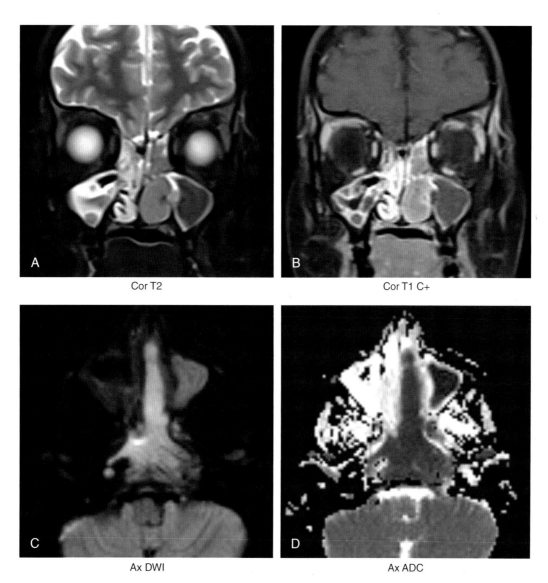

Cor T2

Cor T1 C+

Ax DWI

Ax ADC

• **Fig. 80.5** (A) Coronal T2-weighted and (B) coronal T1-weighted, gadolinium-enhanced images demonstrate a homogeneously T2 hypointense, homogeneously enhancing left nasal cavity mass. (C) Axial DWI image and (D) corresponding ADC map show marked restricted diffusion in the mass, which also involves the left nasopharynx and left prevertebral musculature. The mass obstructs the left maxillary sinus drainage, and the left maxillary sinus is filled with proteinaceous material. This mass represents biopsy-proven lymphoma. *ADC,* Apparent diffusion coefficient; *Ax,* axial; *Cor,* coronal; *DWI,* diffusion-weighted imaging.

vasoconstrictive nasal medications, sarcoidosis, granulomatosis with polyangiitis (formerly Wegener granulomatosis), and malignancy (SCC, lymphoma, and melanoma). A soft tissue mass should raise suspicion for malignancy. Chest imaging may be useful in the setting of granulomatous disease.

Differential Diagnosis

1. Nasal polyp
2. Juvenile angiofibroma
3. Inverted papilloma
4. Hamartoma
5. Squamous cell carcinoma
6. Esthesioneuroblastoma (olfactory neuroblastoma)
7. Melanoma
8. Lymphoma
9. Sarcoma
10. Nasal septal perforation

Pearls

• Nasal polyp: An extremely common, nonaggressive, low-density, polypoid nasal cavity mass, often multiple and occurring in the setting of paranasal sinus mucosal thickening and fluid
• Juvenile angiofibroma: A multispatial hypervascular mass centered at the sphenopalatine foramen in an adolescent male with epistaxis
• Inverted papilloma: A lateral nasal cavity or maxillary sinus mass with a convoluted cerebriform pattern on MRI and focal hyperostosis corresponding to the site of attachment

- Hamartoma: Well-defined soft tissue filling both superior nasal cavities with no aggressive osseous changes and exhibiting a discoid or half-moon appearance on sagittal images
- SCC: An aggressive maxillary sinus mass in an elderly male smoker
- Esthesioneuroblastoma: A dumbbell-shaped lesion with intracranial and superior nasal cavity components; the intracranial component may demonstrate marginal cysts
- Melanoma: An avidly enhancing, intrinsically T1 hyperintense mass associated with the nasal septum
- Lymphoma: A homogeneous mass with restricted diffusion
- Sarcoma: Imaging features depend on sarcoma subtype; consider rhabdomyosarcoma in a pediatric patient, chondrosarcoma when there is "ring and arc" mineralization, and osteosarcoma when there is "sunburst" periosteal reaction and osteoid formation
- Nasal septal perforation: The clinical history is critical but beware of malignant etiologies

Signs and Complications

Craniofacial, orbital, and skull base involvement is common with nasal cavity malignancy, and accurate anatomic delineation is important for staging and to facilitate treatment planning.

Suggested Readings

Agarwal M, Policeni B: Sinonasal Neoplasms. *Semin Roentgenol* 54(3): 244–257, 2019.

Curtin HD: The "evil gray": cancer and cartilage, *Radiology* 249(2): 410–412, 2008.

Bunch PM, Kelly HR: Esthesioneuroblastoma. In: Small JE, Noujaim DL, Ginat DT, Kelly HR, Schaefer PW, editors: *Neuroradiology: spectrum and evolution of disease*, ed 1, 346–356, 2018, Philadelphia, PA, Elsevier.

Dammann F, Pereira P, Laniado M, et al: Inverted papilloma of the nasal cavity and the paranasal sinuses: using CT for primary diagnosis and follow-up, *AJR Am J Roentgenol* 172(2):543–548, 1999.

Dean KE, Shatzkes D, Phillips CD: Imaging review of new and emerging sinonasal tumors and tumor-like entities from the fourth edition of the World Health Organization Classification of Head and Neck Tumors. *AJNR Am J Neuroradiol* 40(4):584–590, 2019.

Jeon TY, Kim H-J, Chung S-K, et al: Sinonasal inverted papilloma: value of convoluted cerebriform pattern on MR imaging, *AJNR Am J Neuroradiol* 29(8):1556–1560, 2008.

Kim Y-K, Choi JW, Kim H-J, et al: Melanoma of the sinonasal tract: value of a septate pattern on precontrast T1-weighted MR imaging, *AJNR Am J Neuroradiol* 39(4):762–767, 2018.

Lee DK, Chung SK, Dhong H-J, et al: Focal hyperostosis on CT of sinonasal inverted papilloma as a predictor of tumor origin, *AJNR Am J Neuroradiol* 28(4):618–621, 2007.

Lopez F, Triantafyllou A, Snyderman CH, et al: Nasal juvenile angiofibroma: current perspectives with emphasis on management, *Head Neck* 39(5):1033–1045, 2017.

Shirazi N, Bist SS, Puri N, et al: Primary sinonasal lymphoma in immunocompetent patients: a 10 years retrospective clinicopathological study, *J Oral Maxillofac Pathol* 22(2):280–281, 2018.

Som PM, Lidov M, Brandwein M, et al: Sinonasal esthesioneuroblastoma with intracranial extension: marginal tumor cysts as a diagnostic MR finding, *AJNR Am J Neuroradiol* 15(7):1259–1262, 1994.

Yu T, Xu YK, Li L, et al: Esthesioneuroblastoma methods of intracranial extension: CT and MR imaging findings, *Neuroradiology* 51(12): 841–850, 2009.

81

Solitary Parotid Masses

MICHAEL T. PREECE, MD AND PAUL M. BUNCH, MD

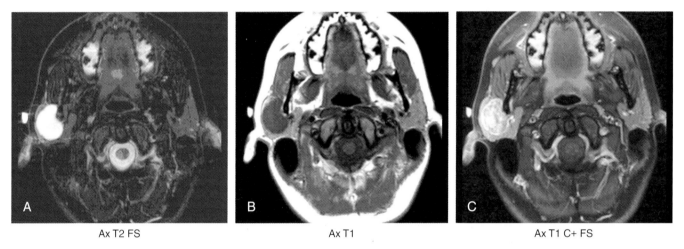

Ax T2 FS | Ax T1 | Ax T1 C+ FS

CASE A: A 20-year-old female with a gradually enlarging right parotid mass. *Ax*, Axial; *FS*, fat saturated.

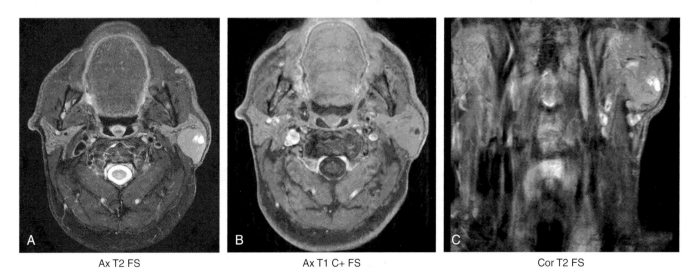

Ax T2 FS | Ax T1 C+ FS | Cor T2 FS

CASE B: A 74-year-old male with a history of smoking presenting with a nontender left parotid mass. *Ax*, Axial; *Cor*, coronal; *FS*, fat saturated.

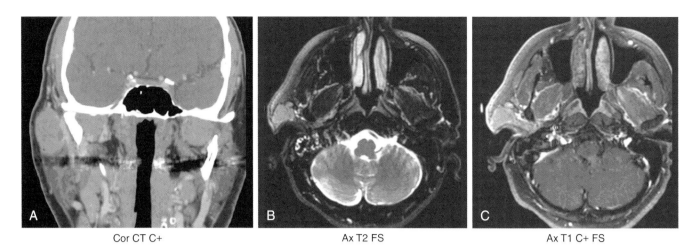

Cor CT C+ | Ax T2 FS | Ax T1 C+ FS

CASE C: A 67-year-old male presenting with an enlarging right preauricular mass. *Ax*, Axial; *Cor*, coronal; *CT*, Computed tomography; *FS*, fat saturated.

DESCRIPTION OF FINDINGS

MRIs from three patients demonstrate well-defined unilateral parotid masses.
- Case A: Features a well-defined, T2 hyperintense, T1 hypointense enhancing mass centered within the right parotid gland with slightly lobulated (bosselated) margins. Early postcontrast images demonstrate heterogeneous enhancement.
- Case B: A well-circumscribed enhancing mass is seen centered within the left parotid tail with predominantly T2 isointense signal when compared with the remainder of the parotid gland. Note the small, internal, T2 hyperintense, nonenhancing cystic foci.
- Case C: Features a homogenously enhancing mass within the right parotid gland with the same signal intensity as a small adjacent intraparotid lymph node on T2 and T1 postcontrast images.

Diagnosis

Case A: Pleomorphic adenoma
Case B: Warthin tumor
Case C: Primary lymphoma of the parotid gland

Summary

The parotid gland is the largest of the salivary glands and can be divided into superficial and deep lobes along the plane of the facial nerve. Lesions affecting the gland often arise from salivary, lymphoid, or neural tissue within the gland.

Most parotid tumors are benign (approximately 85%). Pleomorphic adenomas, also known as benign mixed tumors, are the most common neoplasms of the parotid, accounting for approximately 70% of lesions. These lesions are twice as common in women and occur most commonly in the superficial lobe of the parotid gland. Pleomorphic adenomas are composed of solid, glandular, or ductal elements and often have a hyperintense signal on T2-weighted images as a result of an internal myxoid matrix. The margin is well defined and not infiltrative. The border can have a slightly undulating margin, which has been referred to as "bosselated." Surgical removal is warranted because of the risk of malignant transformation to carcinoma ex pleomorphic adenoma, which is reported to occur eventually in approximately 10% to 25% of nonresected lesions. Care must be taken during surgical removal because inadvertent tumor spillage from a tear of the pseudocapsule can result in a multinodular recurrence.

Tissue sampling or resection of parotid masses is generally recommended because the imaging features of benign and malignant lesions can overlap. However, an irregular margin increases suspicion of malignancy. Perineural tumor spread (most commonly across the facial and auriculotemporal nerves) indicates malignancy regardless of the primary tumor appearance. Facial weakness on clinical examination should also be viewed with suspicion. Of note, a smoothly marginated solitary mass is not necessarily reassuring, as malignancies such as low-grade mucoepidermoid carcinoma can have this imaging appearance.

Warthin tumors are the second most common benign parotid tumor, representing 10% to 25% of lesions. Masses arise more commonly in male patients (3:1) and are highly associated with cigarette smoking. The diagnosis should not be suggested in patients younger than 40 years. Lesions often arise in the lower portion of the superficial lobe (tail) of the parotid gland and are multiple and bilateral in 15% to 20% of cases. T2 hypointense soft tissue components are suggestive, and approximately one-third of masses demonstrate T2 hyperintense cyst formation.

Lesions appear heterogeneous because of cystic and hemorrhagic change. Growth is slow, and malignant transformation is uncommon. Oncocytomas may also exhibit T2 hypointense soft tissue components and have been termed "the vanishing parotid mass" because, although they are easily visible on T1-weighted images without fat suppression, they are commonly isointense to the normal parotid gland on fat-suppressed T2-weighted images and on fat-suppressed, gadolinium-enhanced T1-weighted images.

Lymphoma affecting the parotid gland can be primary or secondary. Primary lymphoma of the parotid gland is uncommon. Lymphoma may arise in intraglandular lymph nodes or from the parenchyma (mucosa-associated lymphoid tissue). Prospective diagnosis of parotid lymphoma can be difficult based on imaging alone. Features that raise the possibility of parotid lymphoma include a known history of lymphoma, an autoimmune disorder such as Sjögren syndrome or rheumatoid arthritis, a history of human immunodeficiency virus, or a parotid mass in the setting of bilateral cervical lymphadenopathy.

A solitary parotid mass may also represent an intraparotid lymph node metastasis, most commonly from a cutaneous malignancy involving the face, external ear, or scalp. A pathology report describing "squamous cell carcinoma" of the parotid gland should be viewed with particular suspicion for nodal metastatic disease, and careful skin examination for an occult cutaneous primary malignancy should be performed.

Spectrum of Disease

The spectrum of disease is delineated in Fig. 81.1.

Differential Diagnosis

1. Pleomorphic adenoma
2. Warthin tumor
3. Oncocytoma
4. Mucoepidermoid carcinoma
5. Adenoid cystic carcinoma
6. Acinic cell carcinoma
7. Lymphoma
8. Metastasis
9. First branchial cleft cyst
10. Neurogenic tumor (e.g., schwannoma)
11. Lymphatic malformation
12. Venous malformation

Pearls

- Larger salivary glands (i.e., the parotid gland) are associated with a higher percentage of benign lesions, whereas smaller

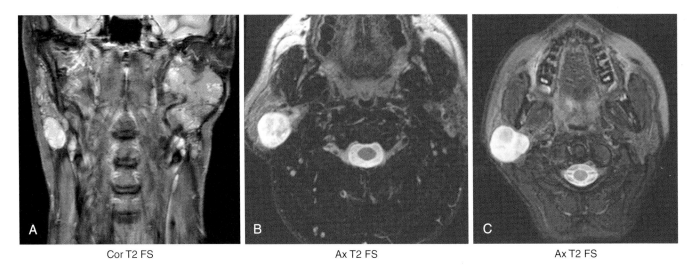

Cor T2 FS · Ax T2 FS · Ax T2 FS

• **Fig. 81.1** (A) Bilateral oncocytomas. (B) Acinic cell carcinoma (pleomorphic adenoma mimic). (C) Schwannoma (pleomorphic adenoma mimic). *Ax*, Axial; *Cor*, coronal; *FS*, fat saturated.

salivary glands (i.e., the submandibular and sublingual glands) have a higher association with malignant lesions. Eighty-five percent of parotid neoplasms are benign.

• Low-grade malignant neoplasms such as mucoepidermoid tumors or acinic cell carcinomas can have the appearance of well-circumscribed benign tumors.

• The diagnosis of Warthin tumor should be considered in a solid mass with a cystic component.

• Warthin tumors, oncocytomas, and lymphoma often present as bilateral solid parotid masses.

• Warthin tumors have a strong association with smoking and typically are seen in persons older than 40 years.

• Primary differential considerations for a T2 hypointense parotid mass include Warthin tumor and oncocytoma.

• Pleomorphic adenoma is favored in the case of a T2 hyperintense, homogenously enhancing lesion with a smooth, sharp, slightly undulating margin (bosselation).

• Consider lymphoma or metastatic disease in the setting of concomitant bilateral cervical adenopathy.

• Metastases to the parotid gland typically arise from primary malignancies of the face, external ear, and scalp.

• An irregular margin and facial paralysis are strong indicators of malignancy.

Signs and Complications

Pleomorphic adenomas can recur as multinodular T2 hyperintense lesions years after resection as a result of inadvertent tumor spillage.

The most significant common surgical complication in parotid surgery is facial nerve injury. On imaging, the retromandibular vein serves as a landmark for the intraparotid facial nerve. Most commonly, the facial nerve passes just superficially to the retromandibular vein.

Suggested Readings

Baert AL, Brady LW, Heilmann HP: *Medical radiology: diagnostic imaging and radiation oncology series.* Berlin, 219–241, 2008.

Hamilton BE, Salzman KL, Wiggins RH, et al: Earring lesions of the parotid tail, *AJNR Am J Neuroradiol* 24(9):1757–1764, 2003.

Moonis G, Patel P, Koshkareva Y, et al: Imaging characteristics of recurrent pleomorphic adenoma of the parotid gland, *AJNR Am J Neuroradiol* 28(8):1532–1536, 2007.

Myers LL, Ahn C: Cutaneous squamous cell carcinoma metastasis to the parotid region lymph nodes, *Laryngoscope* 129(7):1579–1586, 2019.

Patel ND, van Zante A, Eisele DW, et al: Oncocytoma: the vanishing parotid mass, *AJNR Am J Neuroradiol* 32(9):1703–1706, 2011.

Shellenberger TD, Williams MD, Clayman GL, et al: Parotid gland oncocytosis: CT findings with histopathologic correlation, *AJNR Am J Neuroradiol* 29(4):734–736, 2008.

82
Bilateral Parotid Lesions

KATHARINE TANSAVATDI, MD

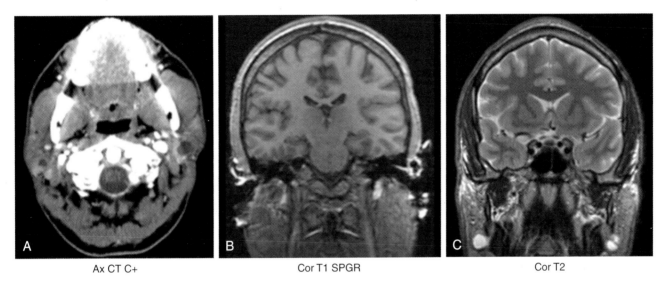

| Ax CT C+ | Cor T1 SPGR | Cor T2 |

CASE A: Images of a 39-year-old male (A, computed tomography [CT]) and a 30-year-old male (B and C, magnetic resonance imaging) with incidental parotid lesions. *Ax,* Axial; *Cor,* coronal; *SPGR,* spoiled gradient.

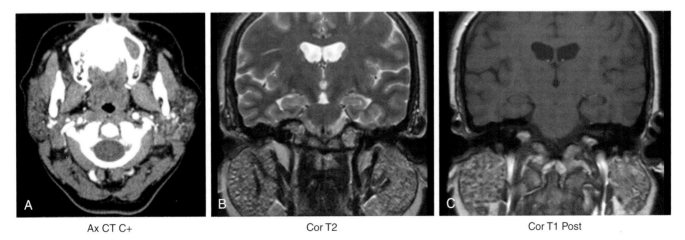

| Ax CT C+ | Cor T2 | Cor T1 Post |

CASE B: A 54-year-old female (A, computed tomography [CT]) and a 39-year-old female (B and C, magnetic resonance imaging) with chronic dry eyes and mouth. *Ax,* Axial; *Cor,* coronal.

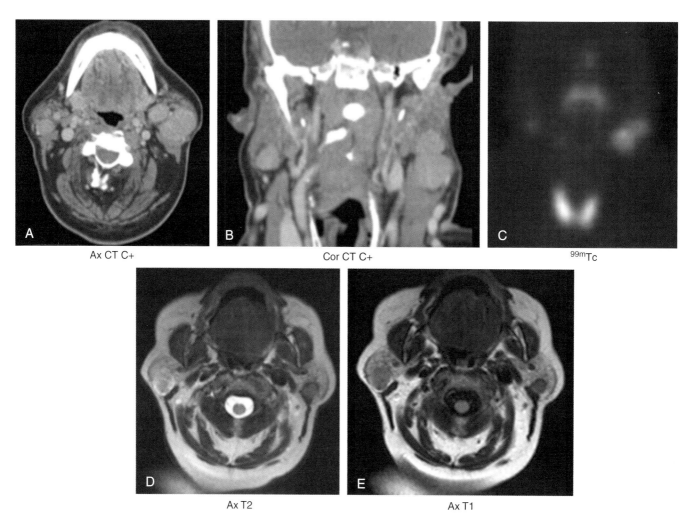

Ax CT C+

Cor CT C+

^{99m}Tc

Ax T2

Ax T1

CASE C: A 66-year-old male (A to C, computed tomography [CT]) and a 68-year-old female (D and E, magnetic resonance imaging) presenting with palpable parotid masses. *Ax,* Axial; *Cor,* coronal; *Tc,* technetium.

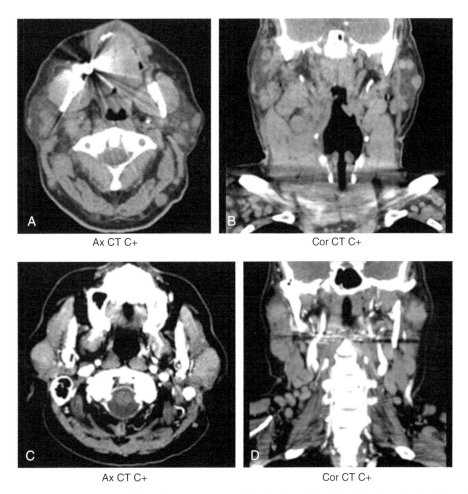

Ax CT C+   Cor CT C+

Ax CT C+   Cor CT C+

CASE D: A 59-year-old male (A and B) and a 71-year-old male (C and D) with multilevel, enlarging, bilateral neck masses. *Ax,* Axial; *Cor,* coronal; *CT,* Computed tomography.

DESCRIPTION OF FINDINGS

- Cases A and B demonstrate entities that commonly present with cystic lesions.
- Case A demonstrates several bilateral, fluid-attenuated, large (>10 mm), cystic-appearing parotid lesions following fluid signal by MRI.
- Case B demonstrates innumerable small (1 to 3 mm), fluid-attenuated cysts present diffusely throughout the bilateral parotid glands.
- Cases C and D demonstrate entities that commonly present solid-appearing lesions.
- Case C demonstrates large, bilateral, solid, enhancing lesions, many of which are found in the parotid tail. A technetium-pertechnetate study shows prompt uptake of radiotracer by these masses.
- Case D demonstrates numerous bilateral parotid masses with marked multilevel cervical chain lymphadenopathy.

Diagnosis

Case A: Lymphoepithelial cysts
Case B: Sjögren syndrome
Case C: Warthin tumor
Case D: Lymphoma

Summary

A simple approach toward identifying bilateral parotid gland lesions begins by dividing processes into those that predominantly present with cysts versus those that present with solid lesions. Although some degree of overlap exists and some combination of the two appearances can be seen, this approach, when combined with a thorough history, often will lead to a clinically relevant differential diagnosis.

In general, benign lymphoepithelial cysts in persons with HIV and Sjögren syndrome can be thought of as processes presenting with cysts. The development of cysts in these processes, although they differ in their pathophysiology, can result in a similar picture in end-stage disease because ductal obstruction and periductal epimyoepithelial islands can occur.

The lymphoepithelial cysts seen in persons with HIV are macroscopic cysts presenting as a result of cystification of lymph nodes and periductal obstruction. However, epimyoepithelial islands, which are seen in persons with benign lymphoepithelial lesions of Sjögren syndrome and typically are solid, also can be seen in persons with HIV. When this is the case, the presence of cervical lymphadenopathy and the prominence of lymphoid tissue within the nasopharynx can help suggest HIV as the leading diagnosis. More recently, with effective treatment of HIV, the cysts have been seen in isolation without adenoid prominence or lymphadenopathy. Cysts follow fluid signal on both CT and MRI sequences.

Sjögren syndrome is characterized by immune-mediated infiltration of periductal lymphocyte aggregates, proliferation of the ductal epithelium obstructing the ducts, and production of epithelial islands. The parotid gland usually is diffusely involved with more localized areas of involvement, simulating a mass otherwise known as benign lymphoepithelial lesions. These lesions are few in number but necessary for the diagnosis of Sjögren syndrome. Early in the disease process, Sjögren syndrome manifests on CT as enlarged glands of increased density that are nonspecific and can be seen with chronic sialadenitis or sialosis. As the disease progresses, obstruction of the ducts leads to increasing microscopic cyst size that may be difficult to identify with CT imaging but are easily seen with MRI as discrete T1 hypointense/T2 hyperintense fluid collections (1 to 2 mm). At later stages, the gland has a honeycomb appearance on CT scans. In end-stage disease, increased glandular destruction occurs, resulting in progressive fatty infiltration or replacement. Less commonly, macroscopic cysts can be seen mimicking the lymphoepithelial cysts seen in persons with HIV, but, unlike in HIV, diffuse cervical lymphadenopathy is not seen in Sjögren syndrome.

Lymphoma and Warthin tumors can present as bilateral and/or multiple solid masses in the parotid glands. Warthin tumors commonly present with cystic components because of cystic fluid related to the heterotopic incorporation of salivary tissue into preexisting intraparotid or periparotid lymph nodes.

Non-Hodgkin lymphoma involving the parotid glands typically is a diffuse large B-cell lymphoma and can be seen as part of systemic involvement or, less commonly, as the primary site of involvement. The incidence of lymphoma in the parotid glands is increased with immunosuppression and autoimmune disorders, including Sjögren syndrome. Patients present with solitary or multiple intraparotid masses, typically with homogenous enhancement, and these masses often are accompanied by periparotid and cervical lymphadenopathy. The masses usually appear as intraparotid lymph nodes that are mildly hyperdense to parotid parenchyma, are intermediate in T1 and T2 signal intensity, and exhibit mild-to-moderate homogenous enhancement. Occasionally they may exhibit central areas of necrosis. Restricted diffusion is a feature of lymphoma; however, normal intraparotid lymph nodes also exhibit low diffusivity.

Warthin tumor, also termed *papillary cystadenoma lymphomatosum*, is the second most common benign parotid tumor and is the most common tumor to present with multifocal lesions, with up to 14% presenting with bilateral masses. Positive associations with smoking and radiation exposure have been described, and the incidence appears to be increasing. It has been postulated that Warthin tumors arise as a result of heterotopic salivary gland tissue in preexisting intraparotid and periparotid lymph nodes. As a result, these lesions can be found at the margin of the parotid. They frequently are found in the lower parotid or as a parotid tail mass. Because of the inclusion of salivary tissue, they commonly are partially cystic. The solid components enhance poorly and often exhibit relative T2 hypointensity. The cystic components are typically T1 hypointense but can contain proteinaceous contents and may be T1 hyperintense. Technetium pertechnetate is avidly taken up by mitochondrial-rich oncocytes in Warthin tumors and demonstrates delayed washout when compared with other lesions or a normal parotid gland. This study can be helpful in suggesting the diagnosis of Warthin tumors, with a reported sensitivity and specificity ranging from 78% to 95% and 91% to 92%, respectively.

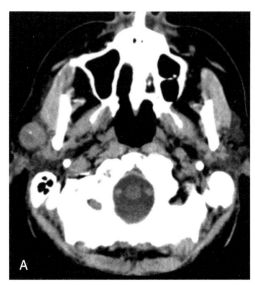 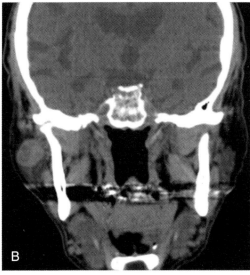

• **Fig. 82.1** (A) Axial and (B) coronal noncontrast computed tomography images of an 88-year-old male with a large squamous cell carcinoma on the right side of the forehead presenting with an enlarging right parotid mass. A solid lesion with central areas of hypoattenuation is seen.

Spectrum of Disease

Metastatic disease to the parotid glands can occur. Metastatic disease typically is the result of nodal spread of disease from local skin malignancies of the skin of the face, external ear, and scalp and also should be considered in the differential diagnosis when multiple solid or mixed cystic-solid masses are seen. Parotid metastases are more commonly seen as unilateral disease but can be bilateral. The nodes typically have a round morphology and can have central necrosis with a central cystic appearance (Fig. 82.1).

Differential Diagnosis

1. Benign lymphoepithelial cysts (HIV)
2. Sjögren syndrome
3. Warthin tumor
4. Lymphoma
5. Metastatic lymphadenopathy
6. Sarcoidosis
7. Oncocytoma

Pearls

• Cystic versus solid: Sjögren syndrome, sarcoidosis, and HIV typically present with cysts, whereas Warthin tumors, metastatic lymphadenopathy, and lymphoma are more commonly solid but can be found with cystic components.
• Lymphadenopathy: Cervical lymphadenopathy can be helpful in favoring lymphoepithelial cysts of HIV over Sjögren syndrome in the case of cystic lesions of the parotid gland and can be helpful in favoring lymphoma in the case of multiple solid lesions.
• Technetium pertechnetate: Avid radiotracer uptake and delayed washout can suggest Warthin tumors or oncocytomas because of the presence of mitochondrial-rich oncocytes.

Signs and Complications

Patients with parotid involvement in Sjögren syndrome have a 44 times greater risk of developing mucosa-associated lymphoid tissue lymphoma. An enlarging solid mass or cervical lymphadenopathy should raise concern.

Suggested Readings

Chen S, Paul BC, Myssiorek D: An algorithm approach to diagnosing bilateral parotid enlargement, *Otolaryngol Head Neck Surg* 148:732–739, 2013.

Iida E, Wiggins RH 3rd, Anzai Y: Bilateral parotid oncocytoma with spontaneous intratumoral hemorrhage: a rare hypervascular parotid tumor with ASL perfusion, *Clin Imaging* 40:357–360, 2016.

Ikeda M, Motoori K, Ito H, et al: Warthin tumor of the parotid gland: diagnostic value of MR imaging with histopathologic correlation, *AJNR Am J Neuroradiol* 25:1256–1262, 2004.

Ko KWS, Bhatia KS, Ai QYH, et al: Imaging of head and neck mucosa-associated lymphoid tissue lymphoma (MALToma), *Cancer Imaging* 21(1):10, 2021.

Kremp AN, Nelson BL: Bilateral Warthin tumors of the parotid gland, *Head Neck Pathol* 2:175–176, 2008.

Myers LL, Ahn C: Cutaneous squamous cell carcinoma metastasis to the parotid region lymph nodes, *Laryngoscope* 129:1579–1586, 2019.

Nikitakis NG, Rivera H, Sauk JJ, et al: Primary Sjögren syndrome in childhood: report of a case and review of the literature, *Oral Surg Oral Med Oral Pathol Oral Radiol Endod* 96:42–47, 2003.

Som PM, Curtin HD: *Head and neck imaging*, ed 5, St Louis, 2011, Mosby.

Sujatha D, Bibtha K, Prasad RS, et al: Parotid lymphoepithelial cysts in human immunodeficiency virus: a review, *J Laryngol Otol* 127:1046–1049, 2013.

Sun Z, Zhang Z, Fu K, et al: Diagnostic accuracy of parotid CT for identifying Sjögren's syndrome, *Eur J Radiol* 81:2702–2709, 2012.

Takita H, Takeshita T, Shimono T, et al: Cystic lesions of the parotid gland: radiologic-pathologic correlation according to the latest World Health Organization 2017 Classification of Head and Neck Tumours, *Jpn J Radiol* 35:629–647, 2017.

83
Retropharyngeal Space Abnormalities

HUI J. JENNY CHEN, MD AND PAUL M. BUNCH, MD

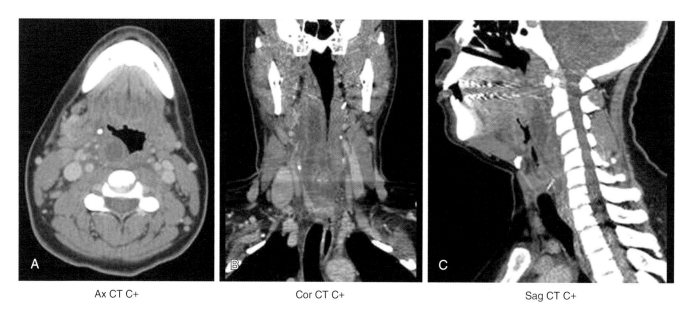

Ax CT C+   Cor CT C+   Sag CT C+

CASE A: A 42-year-old female with a sore swollen throat, dysphagia, fever, and chills for 2 days presented to the emergency department, saying, "It feels like I have a baseball in my throat." *Ax,* Axial; *Cor,* coronal; *CT,* Computed tomography; *Sag,* sagittal.

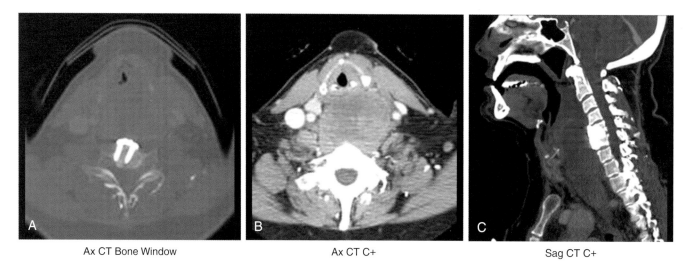

Ax CT Bone Window   Ax CT C+   Sag CT C+

CASE B: A 52-year-old female who recently underwent anterior spinal fusion at C5–C6 complicated by deep venous thrombosis, now receiving anticoagulation therapy. *Ax,* Axial; *CT,* Computed tomography; *Sag,* sagittal.

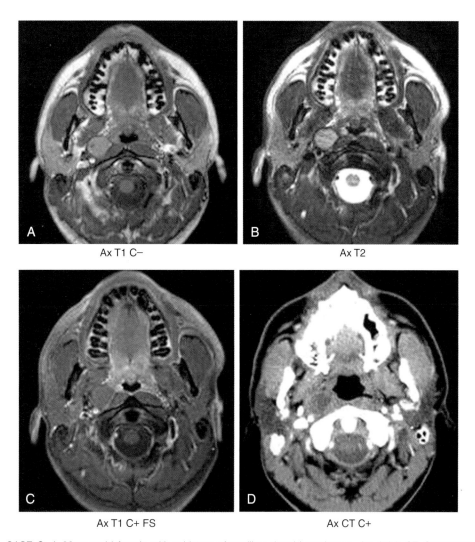

Ax T1 C−

Ax T2

Ax T1 C+ FS

Ax CT C+

CASE C: A 38-year-old female with a history of papillary thyroid carcinoma. *Ax*, Axial; *CT*, Computed tomography; *FS*, fat saturated.

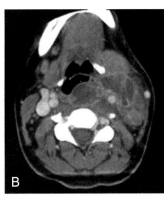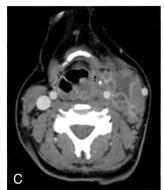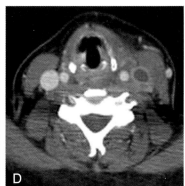

Ax CT C+

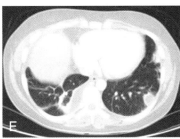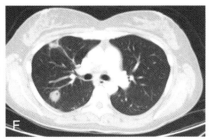

Ax CT Lung Window

CASE D: A 31-year-old previously healthy female presenting with cough, fever, a sore throat, and thrombosis of the left internal jugular vein, as revealed by ultrasound. *Ax*, Axial; *CT*, Computed tomography.

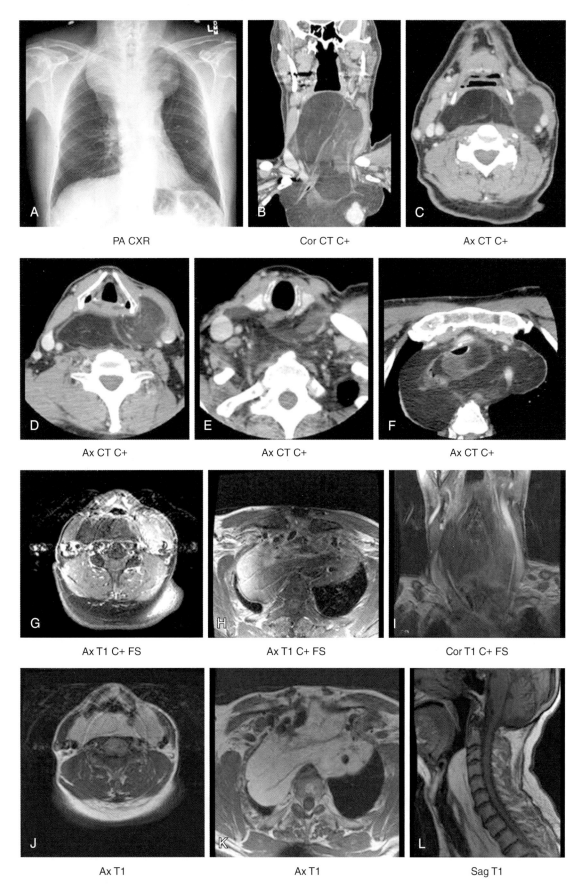

PA CXR

Cor CT C+

Ax CT C+

Ax CT C+

Ax CT C+

Ax CT C+

Ax T1 C+ FS

Ax T1 C+ FS

Cor T1 C+ FS

Ax T1

Ax T1

Sag T1

CASE E: A 70-year-old male presenting with increased swelling in the neck and shortness of breath during the past 7 to 8 months. *Ax,* Axial; *Cor,* coronal; *CT,* Computed tomography; *CXR,* chest x-ray; *FS,* fat saturated; *PA,* posteroanterior; *Sag,* sagittal.

- Case A: CT images demonstrate a large, oblong fluid collection with an enhancing rim in the retropharyngeal space (RPS) (bilateral but predominantly on the right) extending from the level of the tonsillar pillar to the level of the thyroid cartilage, which is most consistent with a retropharyngeal abscess. This fluid collection began as a peritonsillar abscess (the round area on the axial image) and extended secondarily into the RPS.
- Case B: CT images demonstrate a large prevertebral hematoma from C4 through T3 with a patent airway. Edema or phlegmon in the retropharyngeal region of the hematoma also is noted on the sagittal image, without frank abscess.
- Case C: A necrotic lateral retropharyngeal lymph node is seen in the right RPS.
- Case D: CT images demonstrate left internal jugular vein thrombosis with a heterogeneous, rim-enhancing, septated fluid collection deep to the left sternocleidomastoid muscle and extending into the RPS. Asymmetric enlarged and necrotic left level II lymph nodes also are present. Multiple pulmonary septic emboli also are seen on the chest CT.
- Case E: A frontal chest radiograph demonstrates widening of the mediastinum. CT of the neck and chest demonstrates a very large heterogeneous fatty mass that extends from the level of the hypopharynx to the carina and displaces the trachea and esophagus. MRI shows a large, septated, slightly heterogeneous lipomatous mass extending from the angle of the mandible down through the RPS and into the lower neck behind the right thyroid gland. From the thoracic inlet, the mass extends into the mediastinum, enveloping the trachea and displacing it anteriorly.

Diagnosis

Case A: Retropharyngeal and right peritonsillar abscesses

Case B: Prevertebral hematoma resulting from anticoagulation in a patient who recently underwent anterior spinal fusion surgery

Case C: Thyroid cancer metastasis to a lateral retropharyngeal lymph node

Case D: Thrombophlebitis of the left jugular vein with abscess formation extending into the RPS in a patient with Lemierre syndrome

Case E: Well-differentiated retropharyngeal liposarcoma

Summary

Anatomy

The RPS is a small space that contains mainly fat and lymph nodes. The RPS typically is defined by the following borders (Fig. 83.1):
- Anteriorly, the border is the buccopharyngeal fascia surrounding the viscera.
- Posteriorly, the alar fascia separates the RPS from the danger space. The danger space extends from the skull base to the level of the diaphragm and can serve as a conduit for the spread of infection. The danger space (usually defined as the posterior compartment of the RPS) is separated from the prevertebral space by the prevertebral fascia.
- The cloison sagittale (sagittal partition) separates the RPS from the carotid space (or alternatively the poststyloid compartment of the parapharyngeal space) on each side, as the *lateral* borders of the RPS.
- The skull base forms the *superior* border of the RPS.
- The buccopharyngeal and alar fasciae fuse between the T2 and T6 spinal levels to form the *inferior* border for the RPS.

The RPS contains two main groups of lymph nodes in the suprahyoid neck, the lateral (nodes of Rouvière) and medial retropharyngeal nodes. The medial lymph nodes are seldom seen in adults.

It is difficult to talk about the RPS without also mentioning prevertebral space lesions, which may mimic a retropharyngeal location because of proximity. Accurate localization of lesions to their respective deep cervical spaces is important because this characterization will significantly affect the differential diagnosis.

Imaging Strategies

On radiography (lateral view), the average thickness of the retropharyngeal soft tissue is 3.4 mm (range, 1–7 mm) at the level of the second cervical vertebra and 14 mm (range, 9–22 mm)

Fascial Spaces of the Neck

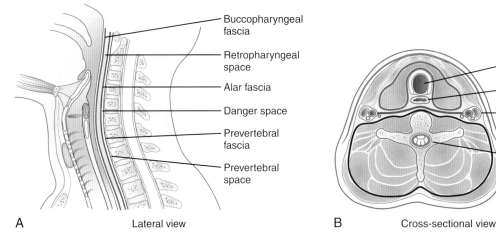

A   Lateral view   B   Cross-sectional view

- **Fig. 83.1** Fascial layers and soft tissue compartments of the neck.

at the level of the sixth cervical vertebra. However, CT and MRI with intravenous contrast are the primary modalities for imaging the retropharyngeal and prevertebral spaces. CT is preferred for evaluating bony lesions or air in soft tissues. MRI allows for excellent characterization of the soft tissues of the neck, but MRI can be difficult to perform in patients with significant neck and airway disease. A neck coil often is used to optimally evaluate the entire neck for nodal disease. Under optimal conditions, head motion and pharyngeal motion (e.g., swallowing and snoring) are minimized. The typical MRI protocol includes the following sequences, with coverage including at least the palate to the hyoid bone and a slice thickness of 3 to 4 mm for T1 images and not greater than 5 mm for T2 images:

- Axial T1 precontrast images for fat/muscle and fat/tumor contrast
- Axial T1 postcontrast (preferably with fat saturation) for visualization of tumor enhancement
- Axial T2-weighted images (preferably with fat saturation) for good muscle/lymphoid tissue contrast
- Coronal T1 images, especially for lesions near the skull base and submandibular and sublingual spaces
- Sagittal T1 images for midline lesions

Pathology

A variety of pathologies can occur in the retropharyngeal and prevertebral spaces (Box 83.1) that often are hidden from direct endoscopic visualization.

A tortuous carotid artery can push into the area behind the pharynx, which may raise clinical concern for a retropharyngeal mass lesion. However, the artery technically is not in the true RPS. This less typical course of the cervical internal carotid artery occurs unilaterally in 31% of cases and bilaterally in 67% of cases (Fig. 83.2).

Primary lesions in the RPS are rare, but a lipoma or liposarcoma can occur. An RPS lipoma often is elliptical and homogeneous in density, conforming to the configuration of a distended RPS, and it has a relatively slow growth rate. In contrast, a liposarcoma often demonstrates heterogeneous density and enhancing soft tissue components with a more rapidly progressive clinical course. Lipomas tend to occur in subcutaneous tissues, and liposarcomas tend to occur more frequently in the deep soft tissues, such as the RPS, the retroperitoneum, and the mediastinum. Transformation of a lipoma to a liposarcoma is extremely rare. A well-differentiated liposarcoma tends to have predominantly adipose tissue (>75% according to the literature) with irregularly thickened linear or nodular septa, whereas a myxoid liposarcoma will exhibit high signal intensity on T2-weighted images (due to high water content) and a dedifferentiated liposarcoma will exhibit predominantly soft tissue (i.e., rather than fatty) components.

The majority of retropharyngeal and prevertebral pathologies are secondary and most commonly are neoplastic, infectious, or inflammatory in etiology. The retropharyngeal and prevertebral regions are frequently affected by direct invasion

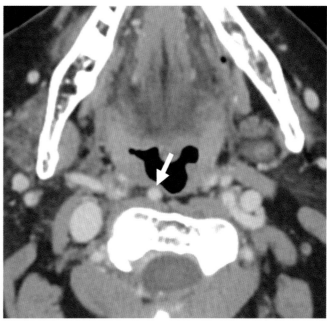

Ax CT

• **Fig. 83.2** Axial CT image demonstrates a medial course of the right internal carotid artery *(arrow)*, which bulges toward the right retropharyngeal space (i.e., so-called "retropharyngeal course"). *Ax,* Axial; *CT,* Computed tomography.

of neoplasms (Fig. 83.3), osseous metastases (Fig. 83.4), and metastases to the retropharyngeal lymph nodes (Case C). Superior extension of malignancy is limited by the attachment of the fascial layers defining the RPS to the skull base, which may lead to bony (clival) erosion.

Retropharyngeal infection can be a consequence of spread of microorganisms (typically in pediatric patients) to the retropharyngeal lymph nodes, or it can result from direct extension of an infectious process involving the cervical spine. However, the incidence of frank retropharyngeal abscess formation has decreased as a result of the timely administration of antibiotics. A concerning aspect of RPS infection is the potential spread of infection along the danger space into the posterior mediastinum and pleural spaces, which can be life threatening. Patients also can have spasm and even rupture of the adjacent carotid artery.

Spectrum of Disease

A disease that often mimics retropharyngeal abscess or infection is acute calcific tendonitis of the longus colli muscles. Clinically, the patient may present with acute onset of a stiff neck, limited neck motion, odynophagia, dysphagia, neck pain, low-grade fever, and even leukocytosis. Acute calcific tendonitis of the longus colli is an inflammatory process caused by calcium hydroxyapatite crystal deposition in the superior oblique tendon fibers of the longus colli muscle of the prevertebral space (Fig. 83.5). Occasionally this deposition can occur at lower levels, that is, at C5–C6 at the inferior oblique tendon fibers of the longus colli. The crystal deposits can rupture and may provoke a painful inflammatory response. Typically, amorphous calcification is present anterior to

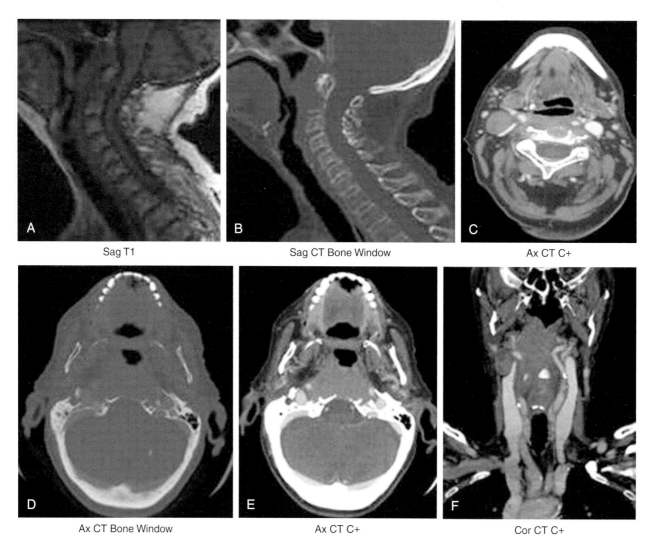

• **Fig. 83.3** Direct extension of metastatic nasopharyngeal squamous cell carcinoma to the retropharyngeal and prevertebral spaces with adjacent bony destruction and vessel encasement at the C2 vertebral level. A metastatic right jugulodigastric lymph node also is seen. *Ax,* Axial; *Cor,* coronal; *CT,* Computed tomography; *Sag,* sagittal.

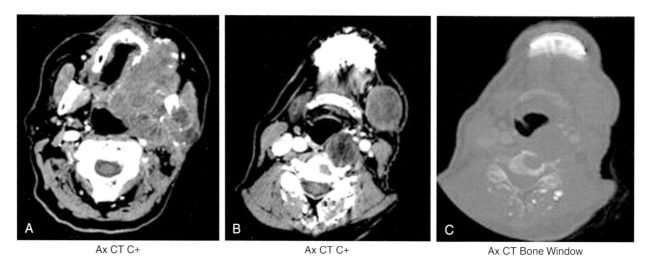

• **Fig. 83.4** A patient with a history of recurrent left parotid adenocarcinoma. (A) Recurrent adenocarcinoma of the left parotid involves multiple spaces of the neck. (B and C) Adenocarcinoma metastasis to a cervical vertebral body with extension into the prevertebral space, mimicking a lateral retropharyngeal nodal metastasis. *Ax,* Axial; *CT,* Computed tomography.

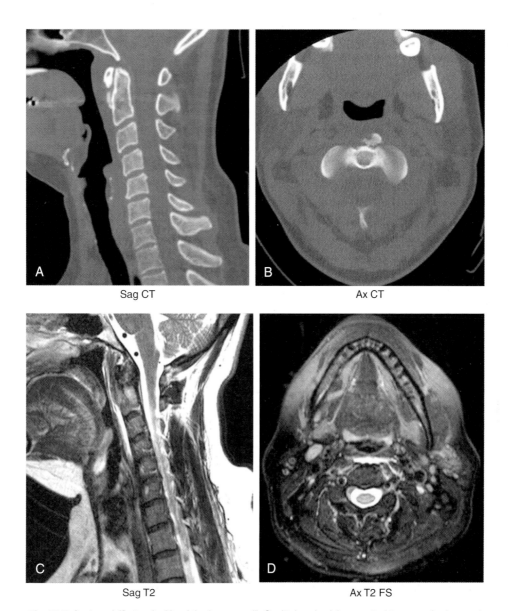

• **Fig. 83.5** Acute calcific tendonitis of the longus colli. Sagittal and axial computed tomography images in bone window demonstrate amorphous calcification along the anterior aspect of the C2 vertebral body associated with the superior oblique tendon fibers of the longus colli muscles. A simple-appearing, nonenhancing (post-contrast T1-weighted images not shown) small retropharyngeal fluid collection is seen on both sagittal and axial T2-weighted images. *Ax,* Axial; *CT,* Computed tomography; *FS,* fat saturated; *Sag,* sagittal.

C1–C3. Typically, amorphous calcification is present anterior to C1-C3, and a small associated RPS fluid collection is also seen, most often without rim enhancement.

Differential Diagnosis

The differential diagnosis is outlined in Box 83.1.

Pearls

• Confusing retropharyngeal air with lipomatous lesions (especially lipoma) on CT is a potential pitfall related to the RPS. Using the correct window and level settings and measuring the attenuation of the hypoattenuating abnormality are essential steps to avoid this pitfall.

• Edema within the RPS is commonly seen after radiotherapy for head and neck cancer. Unlike retropharyngeal abscess, postradiotherapy edema will not demonstrate rim-enhancement, and will not appear as a space-occupying collection or exert mass effect on adjacent structures.

• Suppurative lymphadenitis of lateral retropharyngeal lymph nodes (i.e., intranodal abscess) can occur after pharyngitis and tonsillitis, most commonly in the pediatric population. Extension of the lateral retropharyngeal intranodal abscess into the RPS is a common mechanism for retropharyngeal abscess development. Whereas true retropharyngeal abscess often requires surgical drainage, a suppurative retropharyngeal lymph node (i.e., intranodal abscess) can often be adequately treated with antibiotics, As such, differentiation of suppurative lymphadenitis from true retropharyngeal

• BOX 83.1 Differential Diagnosis of Pathology Involving the Retropharyngeal and Prevertebral Regions

Vascular
- Tortuous internal carotid artery
- Hematoma from thoracic aortic dissection

Infectious/Inflammatory/Autoimmune
- Abscess/cellulitis (Cases A and D)
- Reactive adenopathy
- Suppurative adenopathy (intranodal abscess)
- Vertebral body osteomyelitis (prevertebral)
- Angioedema
- Castleman disease
- Acute calcific tendonitis of longus colli (Fig. 83.5)

Neoplasm
- Liposarcoma/lipoma (Case E)
- Nodal metastasis from head and neck cancers (most commonly nasopharyngeal squamous cell carcinoma and thyroid carcinoma) (Case C)
- Lymphoma
- Direct invasion from primary squamous cell carcinoma
- Chordoma from vertebral bodies

Degenerative
- Anterior vertebral body osteophyte/anterior disk herniation

Iatrogenic
- Instrumentation, endotracheal intubation
- Postradiation fluid collection
- Anticoagulation (hematoma) (Case B)

Congenital
- Venous malformation
- Lymphatic malformation

Acquired
- Edema or lymph spilling into the retropharyngeal space as a result of venous or lymphatic obstruction

Trauma
- Hematoma
- Penetrating wound to the neck

Environmental/endocrine/metabolic
- Hemorrhage from a parathyroid adenoma
- Goiter or thyroid tumor

---

abscess is important for determining appropriate clinical management.

- Imaging findings that favor acute calcific tendonitis of the longus colli include amorphous calcification in the superior oblique tendon of the longus colli, the presence of a nonenhancing retropharyngeal fluid collection, and the lack of lymphadenopathy, abscess, or bony destruction.

Signs and Complications

- Liposarcoma can grow to a large size without pain and produce symptoms (such as obstructive sleep apnea and dyspnea) that are most often related to compression of adjacent structures. Patients with well-differentiated liposarcoma have a better prognosis. However, RPS liposarcomas have a high frequency of recurrence because of their challenging location for clean margin resection.
- A retropharyngeal/prevertebral region hematoma (both traumatic and spontaneous) can cause rapid, life-threatening airway obstruction from compression of the trachea and larynx. Even minor trauma (such as hyperextension) can result in an RPS hematoma, typically in an elderly patient undergoing anticoagulation treatment. The most commonly reported nontraumatic cause of hematoma in the retropharyngeal region is hemorrhage from a parathyroid adenoma.
- A retropharyngeal course of the internal carotid artery can increase the risk of life-threatening hemorrhage with certain head and neck surgical procedures (e.g., tonsillectomy), particularly if the surgeon is not alerted to the presence of this anatomic variant preoperatively.
- Necrotic or cystic metastatic retropharyngeal lymph nodes (most commonly from squamous cell carcinoma and

thyroid carcinoma) often maintain a distinct nodal margin with no signs of surrounding inflammation. In addition, patients with retropharyngeal nodal metastases will not typically exhibit infectious signs or symptoms.

- Spread of retropharyngeal infection into the posterior mediastinum and pleural spaces along the danger space can result in mediastinitis, pleural empyema, and pericarditis.
- Although acute calcific tendonitis of the longus colli can be treated conservatively with nonsteroidal antiinflammatory drugs, an otolaryngology evaluation and short interval follow-up should be considered, especially in the setting of fever and leukocytosis, even when the characteristic radiological findings are present, to exclude a potential alternative diagnosis such as early retropharyngeal abscess.

Suggested Readings

Bhatt AA: Non-traumatic causes of fluid in the retropharyngeal space, *Emerg Radiol* 25:547–551, 2018.

Debnam JM, Guha-Thakurta N: Retropharyngeal and prevertebral spaces: anatomic imaging and diagnosis, *Otolaryngol Clin North Am* 45(6):1293–1310, 2012.

Gavid M, Dumollard JM, Habougit C, et al: Anatomical and histological study of the deep neck fasciae: does the alar fascia exist? *Surg Radiol Anat* 40:917–922, 2018.

Gundelach R, Ullah R, Coman S, et al: Liposarcoma of the retropharyngeal space, *J Laryngol Otol* 119:651–654, 2005.

Hoang JK, Branstetter BF 4th, Eastwood JD, et al: Multiplanar CT and MRI of collections in the retropharyngeal space: is it an abscess? *AJR Am J Roentgenol* 196(4):W426–W432, 2011.

Kochilas X, Ali A, Montague ML, et al: Retropharyngeal space swelling secondary to minor blunt head and neck trauma, *J Laryngol Otol* 118:465–467, 2004.

Newton AI: Spontaneous retropharyngeal hematoma: an unusual presentation of thoracic aortic dissection, *J Emerg Med* 31(1):45–48, 2006.

Offiah CE, Hall E: Acute calcific tendinitis of the longus colli muscle: spectrum of CT appearances and anatomical correlation, *Br J Radiol* 82(978):e117–e121, 2009.

Palacios E, Kirsch D: Anomalous course of the carotid arteries in the retropharyngeal space poses a surgical risk, *Ear Nose Throat J* 84(6):336–337, 2005.

Park SY, Jin W, Lee SH, et al: Acute retropharyngeal calcific tendinitis: a case report with unusual location of calcification, *Skeletal Radiol* 39:817–820, 2010.

Pinto A, Scaglione M, Scuderi MG, et al: Infections of the neck leading to descending necrotizing mediastinitis: role of multi-detector row computed tomography, *Eur J Radiol* 65:389–394, 2008.

Scali F, Nash LG, Pontl ME: Defining the morphology and distribution of the alar fascia: a sheet plastination investigation, *Ann Otol Rhinol Laryngol* 124:814–819, 2015.

Shefelbine SE, Mancuso AA, Gajewski BJ, et al: Pediatric retropharyngeal lymphadenitis: differentiation from retropharyngeal abscess and treatment implications, *Otolaryngol Head Neck Surg* 136(2):182–188, 2007.

Snosek M, Macchi V, Stecco C, et al: Anatomical and histological study of the alar fascia, *Clin Anat* 34:609–616, 2021.

Som PM, Curtin HD: Fascia and spaces of the neck. In Som PM, Curtin HD, editors: *Head and neck imaging*, ed 5, St Louis, 2011, Mosby.

Som PM, Smoker WRK, Reidenberg SJ: Embryology and anatomy of the neck. In Som PM, Curtin HD, editors: *Head and neck imaging*, ed 5, St Louis, 2011, Mosby.

Tomita H, Yamashiro T, Ikeda H, et al: Fluid collection in the retropharyngeal space: a wide spectrum of various emergency diseases, *Eur J Radiol* 85(7):1247–1256, 2016.

Wang YP, Lee KS: Extraosseous chordoma of the retropharyngeal space, *Otolaryngol Head Neck Surg* 30(3):383–385, 2004.

Wu K, Ahmed A: Penetrating injury to the soft palate causing retropharyngeal air collection, *Emerg Med J* 22:148–149, 2005.

84

Cranial Nerve Denervation Patterns Part 1: III–VI

THOMAS G. WEST, MD, ADAM SWEENEY, MD, AND PAUL M. BUNCH, MD

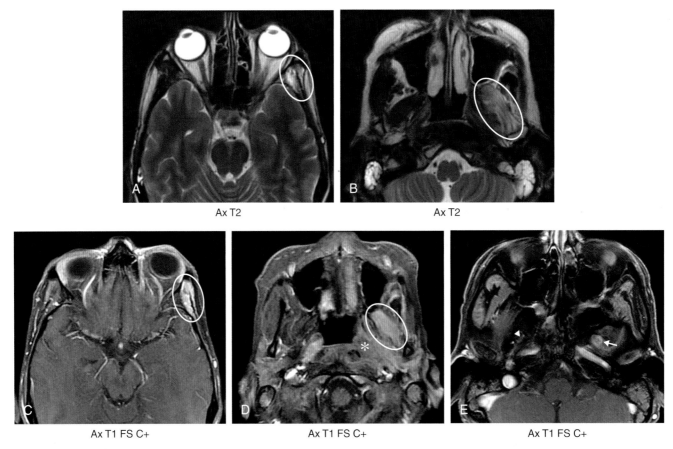

Ax T2

Ax T2

Ax T1 FS C+

Ax T1 FS C+

Ax T1 FS C+

CASE A: A 38-year-old female with left-sided headaches and difficulty opening her mouth. *Ax*, Axial; *FS*, fat saturated.

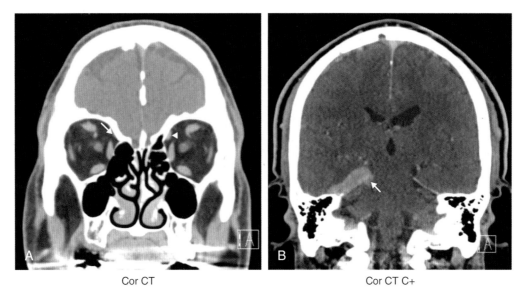

Cor CT   Cor CT C+

CASE B: A 55-year-old female with headaches, blurred vision, and generalized fatigue. *Cor*, Coronal; *CT*, Computed tomography.

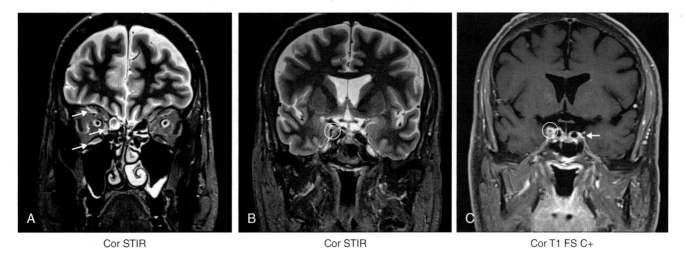

Cor STIR   Cor STIR   Cor T1 FS C+

CASE C: A 47-year-old male with history of renal cell carcinoma now experiencing diplopia and inability to hold the right eye open. *Cor*, Coronal; *FS*, fat saturated; *STIR*, short tau inversion recovery.

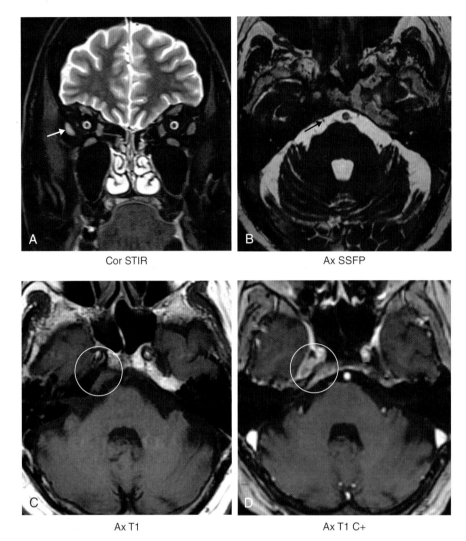

Cor STIR

Ax SSFP

Ax T1

Ax T1 C+

CASE D: A 62-year-old male with metastatic prostate cancer and new onset diplopia. *Ax*, Axial; *Cor*, coronal; *SSFP*, steady-state free precession; *STIR*, short tau inversion recovery.

DESCRIPTION OF FINDINGS

- Case A: Large, infiltrative mass centered in the left nasopharynx (*asterisk*, D) with abnormal enhancement and enlargement of the mandibular division (V3) of the left trigeminal nerve at the level of the left foramen ovale (*arrow*, E). For comparison, the normal right foramen ovale is marked with an arrowhead. Edema and enhancement within the asymmetrically enlarged left temporalis (*ovals*, A and C) and left lateral pterygoid muscles (*ovals*, B and D).
- Case B: Marked atrophy of the right superior oblique muscle (*arrow*, A) compared to the normal left superior oblique muscle (*arrowhead*, A). Enhancing extraaxial lesion centered on the right tentorial leaflet, including involvement along the expected course of the right trochlear nerve (*arrow*, B).
- Case C: Abnormal STIR hyperintensity involving the right superior, medial, and inferior rectus muscles (*arrows*, A). Abnormal soft tissue effaces the right oculomotor cistern (*circle*, B) and surrounds the right oculomotor nerve within the right cavernous sinus (*circle*, C). The normal nonenhancing left oculomotor nerve (*arrow*, C) is seen within the normal enhancing left cavernous sinus.
- Case D: Abnormal STIR hyperintensity involving the right lateral rectus muscle (*arrow*, A). Loss of the normal marrow signal within the right petrous apex with extraosseous extension of soft tissue into the right Meckel cave and right inferior petrosal sinus (*circles*, C and D) along the course of the right abducens nerve (*arrow*, B).

Diagnosis

Case A: Left nasopharyngeal carcinoma with perineural tumor spread along the mandibular division (V3) of the left trigeminal nerve producing acute denervation changes within the left muscles of mastication.

Case B: Sarcoidosis resulting in right trochlear nerve palsy with denervation atrophy of the right superior oblique muscle.

Case C: Renal cell carcinoma metastasis to the right cavernous sinus and right oculomotor cistern producing denervation changes of the extraocular muscles innervated by the right oculomotor nerve.

Case D: Prostate carcinoma skull base metastasis resulting in right abducens palsy.

Summary

This chapter and the next chapter (Chapter 85) discuss cranial nerve denervation patterns. The current chapter focuses on cranial nerves III through VI, whereas the following chapter discusses cranial nerves VII through XII. Cranial nerves I, II, and VIII are purely sensory (as opposed to the other cranial nerves, each with motor components) and are therefore excluded from the discussion. Denervation involving a single cranial nerve is classified as "simple," while involvement of multiple cranial nerves is considered "complex." Denervation can also be divided into proximal and distal patterns, depending on the site of the causative lesion. Importantly, if the inciting lesion is accurately identified and appropriately treated early in the course of disease, denervation changes can be reversible.

Denervation can be broadly divided into acute (0 to 1 month), subacute (1 to 20 months) and chronic phases (>20 months) (Fig. 84.1); however, this represents a continuum, and the time course can vary for different cranial nerves (e.g., fatty atrophy may occur as early as 2 weeks following hypoglossal denervation but often takes at least 3 months to become apparent after trigeminal denervation), individuals, and causative etiologies. During the acute phase of denervation, T2 hyperintensity and enhancement are often evident with increased muscle volume. These findings can simulate a mass, but careful inspection reveals that the striations of the muscle belly are maintained. Edema related to radiation therapy can mimic acute denervation as well, such that knowledge of the treatment history is relevant to accurate interpretation. In the subacute phase of denervation, enhancement and T2 hyperintensity decrease and eventually resolve with gradual transition to fatty replacement and volume loss characteristic of the chronic phase (Fig. 84.2).

When faced with cranial nerve denervation, it is critically important for the radiologist to accurately localize and characterize the causative lesion. Familiarity with the underlying anatomy, expected appearance of stages of denervation, common etiologies of denervation, and typical pathways of tumor spread are prerequisites for the consistent execution of this important task. In addition to assessing the central and cisternal portions of the relevant cranial nerve(s), search patterns should also include identification of normal fat surrounding the cranial nerves and their major branches (e.g., immediately inferior to the relevant skull base foramina, within the

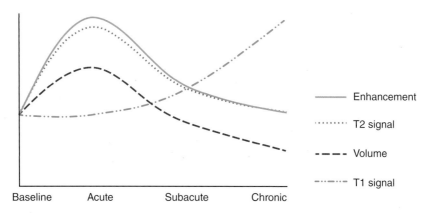

Temporal evolution of denervated musculature

- **Fig. 84.1** Changes in denervated muscle enhancement, T2 (edema) signal, volume, and T1 (fat) signal as a function of time.

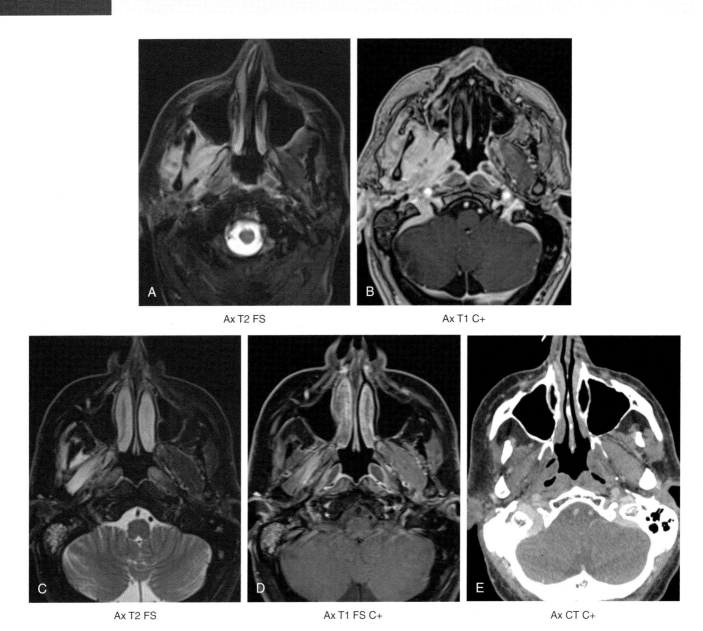

Ax T2 FS   Ax T1 C+

Ax T2 FS   Ax T1 FS C+   Ax CT C+

• **Fig. 84.2** Muscle denervation changes over time as illustrated in a 65-year-old male patient with perineural tumor spread involving the right mandibular nerve. At the time of diagnosis (A, B), there is enlargement, marked T2 hyperintensity, and avid enhancement of the right masseter and pterygoid musculature that could potentially be mistaken for a mass. However, the normal muscle striations are preserved. At imaging follow-up performed 7 months later (C, D), the muscles have decreased in size; however, some T2 hyperintensity and enhancement persist. The axial CT image (E) acquired 27 months after initial imaging demonstrates marked atrophy and fatty infiltration of the right masseter and pterygoid musculature. *Ax,* Axial; *CT,* Computed tomography; *FS,* fat saturated.

infraorbital and mandibular foramina, and within the pterygopalatine fossa). This expected fat is typically best appreciated on noncontrast T1-weighted images (Fig. 84.3) but can also be identified on CT.

Understanding the different denervation patterns of the cranial nerves will inform appropriate imaging protocol selection and assist in localization of inciting lesions. High-quality imaging maximizes the radiologist's chances of detecting the often-subtle causative lesions, and imaging protocols must cover the entire extent of the nerve(s) in question (i.e., from the brainstem nuclei to the innervated tissues). Homogenous

fat suppression on postcontrast images is very helpful in identifying abnormal enhancement, especially in the bone marrow and the fat pads along the skull base. Failure of fat suppression risks obscuring pathology and commonly occurs at the skull base and adjacent to the paranasal sinuses with spectral fat suppression techniques due to susceptibility artifacts at the bone-air interfaces. Newer fat suppression techniques based on chemical shift, such as the Dixon method, have gained popularity in head and neck imaging due to their ability to generate images with near uniform fat suppression. The Dixon sequence can be T1- or T2-weighted and provides images without and

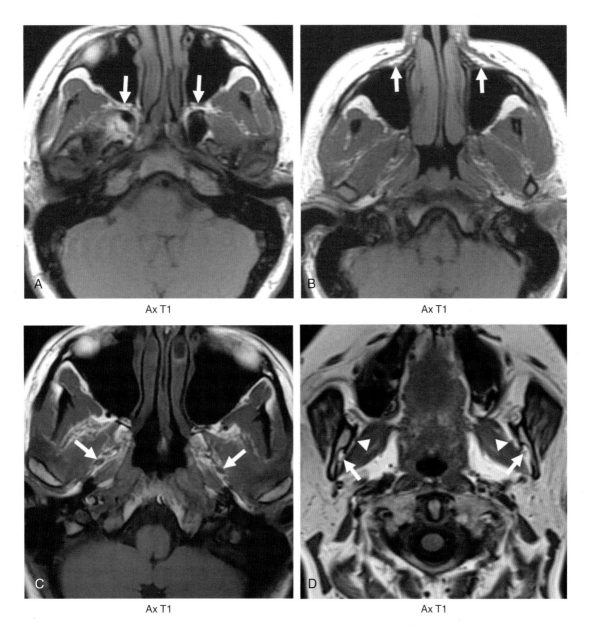

• **Fig. 84.3** Normal fat (A) within the pterygopalatine fossae *(arrows)*, (B) surrounding the infraorbital nerves *(arrows)* at the level of the infraorbital foramina, (C) surrounding the mandibular divisions *(arrows)* of the trigeminal nerve at a level just inferior to the foramina ovale, and (D) surrounding the inferior alveolar nerves *(arrows)* at the mandibular foramina. Note the normal lingual nerves *(arrowheads)* located anteromedial to the mandibular foramina at this level. *Ax*, Axial.

with fat suppression in a single acquisition. To minimize the risk of fat suppression failure (Fig. 84.4A) on T2-weighted images, fluid-sensitive inversion recovery sequences such as STIR (Fig. 84.4B) and the T2-weighted Dixon sequence are both useful with the inversion recovery method benefitting from additive T1 and T2 contrast.

Spectrum of Disease

Oculomotor Nerve

The oculomotor nerve innervates the superior, medial, and inferior rectus muscles, the inferior oblique muscle, the levator palpebrae superioris muscle, and the pupillary constrictor and ciliary muscles. The oculomotor nuclei reside within the midbrain in a paramidline location immediately ventrolateral to the cerebral aqueduct at the level of the superior colliculi. There are multiple subnuclei for each of the innervated extraocular muscles.

The oculomotor nerves exit the ventral midbrain at the interpeduncular cistern, course anteriorly between the posterior cerebral and superior cerebellar arteries, and pass through the oculomotor cisterns before entering the superolateral aspect of the cavernous sinuses (Fig. 84.5). Fibers from the sympathetic carotid plexus join the oculomotor fibers within the cavernous sinuses.

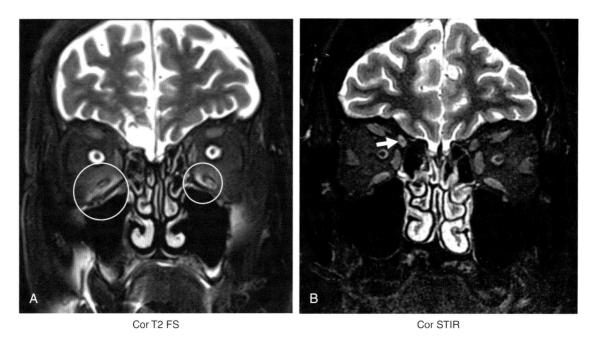

Cor T2 FS   Cor STIR

• **Fig. 84.4** Comparing (A) spectral fat suppression to (B) inversion recovery fat suppression. The coronal T2-weighted image with spectral fat suppression (A) demonstrates multifocal failure of fat suppression along the margins of the maxillary sinuses, including within the inferior orbits *(circles)* where the failed fat suppression could potentially be mistaken for pathology involving the inferior rectus muscles. In contrast, the coronal STIR image (B) obtained in a 77-year-old female with right trochlear nerve palsy exhibits homogeneous fat suppression enabling confident identification of abnormally increased fluid signal within the right superior oblique muscle *(arrow)*. *Cor,* Coronal; *FS,* fat saturated; *STIR,* short tau inversion recovery.

The oculomotor nerves then pass through the superior orbital fissures into the orbits, dividing into superior and inferior divisions. The superior division innervates the superior rectus and levator palpebrae superioris muscles. The inferior division innervates the medial rectus, inferior rectus, and inferior oblique muscles. A complete oculomotor palsy will cause a "down and out" eye due to unopposed action of the lateral rectus and superior oblique muscles, ptosis due to paralysis of the levator palpebrae superioris, as well as dilated pupil and loss of accommodation due to absent parasympathetic function.

Trochlear Nerve

The trochlear nerve innervates the superior oblique muscle and represents the smallest cranial nerve with the longest intracranial course. The trochlear nuclei reside within the dorsal midbrain in a paramidline location immediately ventrolateral to the cerebral aqueduct at the level of the inferior colliculi. The fibers decussate through the superior medullary velum before exiting the dorsal midbrain. The nerves then course anteriorly through the ambient cisterns between the posterior cerebral and superior cerebellar arteries at a level lateral to the oculomotor nerves and closely approximating the free edges of the tentorial leaflets within small depressions referred to as the trochlear grooves (Fig. 84.6A). The trochlear nerves then pass through the trochlear cisterns (Fig. 84.6B) immediately inferolateral to the oculomotor cisterns before entering the cavernous sinuses. The trochlear nerves enter the orbits through the superior orbital fissures and then pass anteromedially to reach the superior oblique muscles.

Because of their small size, the trochlear nerves are difficult to discretely identify with routine clinical imaging; however, knowledge of their location along the inferior aspect of the tentorial free edge and within the superolateral aspect of the cavernous sinus allows the radiologist to suspect nerve compression by pathology in these regions even if the nerve cannot be confidently identified (Fig. 84.7). Furthermore, the trochlear nerves' long cisternal course and close proximity to the tentorium render them particularly susceptible to traumatic injury.

Trigeminal Nerve

The trigeminal nerve comprises three divisions—the ophthalmic (V1), maxillary (V2), and mandibular (V3). The ophthalmic and maxillary divisions have no motor function, such that pathologic involvement manifests as sensory dysfunction (e.g., pain, numbness). The mandibular division provides motor function to the muscles of mastication as well as to the tensor veli palatini and tensor tympani muscles.

Immediately after passing through the foramen ovale, the motor roots of the mandibular division provide branches to the tensor veli palatini, tensor tympani, and medial pterygoid muscles before subsequently dividing into anterior and posterior divisions. Denervation proximal to the tensor veli palatini nerve branch can result in middle ear and mastoid effusion because the tensor veli palatini muscle functions to open the nasopharyngeal orifice of the Eustachian tube.

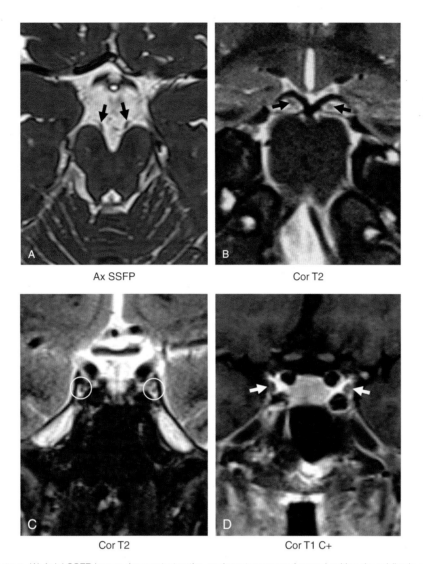

Ax SSFP

Cor T2

Cor T2

Cor T1 C+

• **Fig. 84.5** (A) Axial SSFP image demonstrates the oculomotor nerves *(arrows)* exiting the midbrain along the lateral aspects of the interpeduncular cistern. (B, C) Coronal T2-weighted images demonstrate the oculomotor nerves *(arrows,* B) coursing between the posterior cerebral and superior cerebellar arteries to reach the oculomotor cisterns *(circles,* C). (D) Coronal T1-weighted, gadolinium-enhanced image demonstrates the oculomotor nerves *(arrows)* as nonenhancing structures within the superolateral aspects of the contrast-filled cavernous sinuses. *Ax,* Axial; *Cor,* coronal; *SSFP,* steady-state free precession.

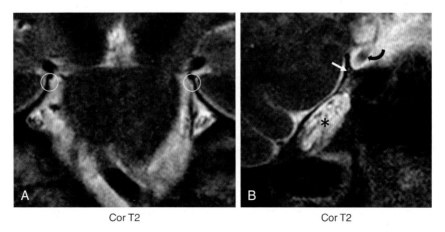

Cor T2

Cor T2

• **Fig. 84.6** Coronal *(Cor)* T2-weighted images demonstrate the trochlear nerves within the trochlear grooves *(circles,* A) along the inferior aspect of the free tentorial edges and the right trochlear nerve within the right trochlear cistern *(arrow,* B) located inferolateral to the right oculomotor nerve *(curved arrow,* B) entering the right oculomotor cistern and superomedial to the right Meckel cave *(asterisk,* B).

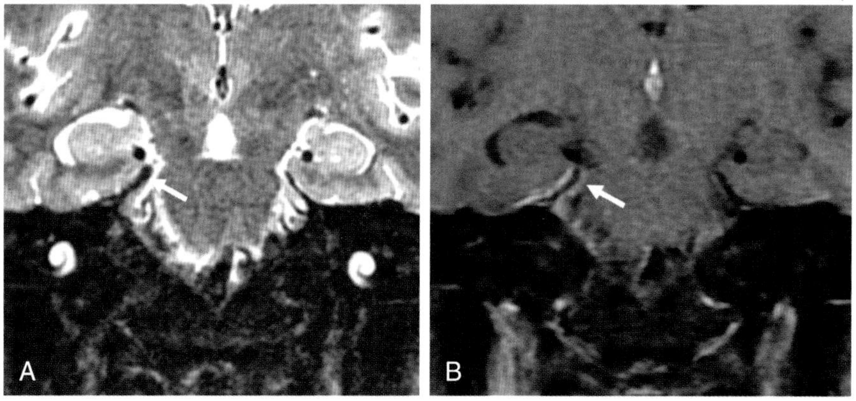

• **Fig. 84.7** (A) Coronal T2-weighted and (B) coronal T1-weighted, gadolinium-enhanced images obtained in the 77-year-old female with right trochlear nerve palsy shown in Fig. 84.4B demonstrate abnormal thickening and enhancement of the right tentorial leaflet including involvement of the expected location of the right trochlear groove *(arrows)*. Although the right trochlear nerve cannot be directly visualized on these images, knowledge of its course within the right trochlear groove allows the radiologist to infer that the cranial nerve deficit is caused by the right tentorial presumed meningioma. *Cor,* Coronal; *FS,* fat saturated.

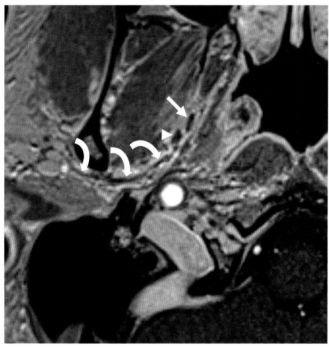

Ax T1 C+

• **Fig. 84.8** Axial *(Ax)* T1-weighted, gadolinium-enhanced image demonstrates the posterior division branches of V3—the lingual *(straight arrow)*, inferior alveolar *(arrowhead)*, and auriculotemporal *(curved arrows)* nerves.

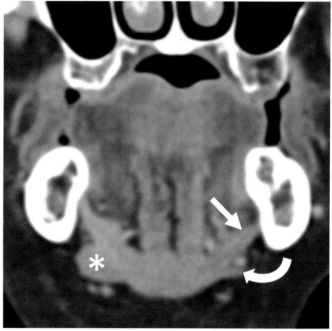

Cor CT C+

• **Fig. 84.9** Coronal CT image obtained in a 65-year-old female with perineural tumor spread involving the left inferior alveolar nerve demonstrates atrophy of the left mylohyoid muscle *(straight arrow)* and of the anterior belly of the left digastric muscle *(curved arrow)*. The normal right digastric muscle anterior belly is marked by the *asterisk*. *Cor,* Coronal; *CT,* computed tomography.

The anterior division gives rise to the masseteric, deep temporal, buccal, and lateral pterygoid branches. The deep temporal branch innervates the temporalis muscle, and the buccal branch provides sensory innervation to the buccal mucosa. The posterior division divides into the auriculotemporal, lingual, and inferior alveolar nerves (Fig. 84.8). The inferior alveolar nerve gives off the mental nerve (sensory) and nerve to the mylohyoid, which provides motor innervation to the mylohyoid muscle and to the anterior belly of the digastric muscle.

A lesion proximal to the branching of the anterior and posterior divisions will result in atrophy involving the muscles of mastication and the musculature innervated by the nerve to mylohyoid (i.e., mylohyoid and digastric anterior belly). A distal lesion involving the inferior alveolar nerve will result in atrophy of the mylohyoid and anterior belly of the digastric muscles (Fig. 84.9) but will spare the muscles of mastication. Careful inspection of fat within the mandibular foramen aids detection of lesions involving the inferior alveolar nerve. A

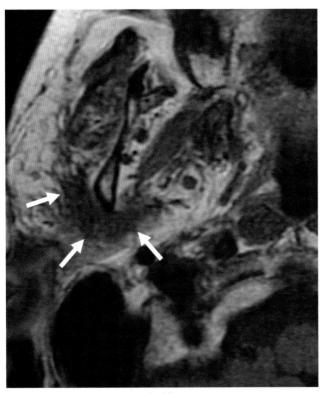

Ax T1

• **Fig. 84.10** Axial *(Ax)* T1-weighted imaged obtained in a 71-year-old male with prior history of right cheek squamous cell carcinoma now presenting with two months of right face pain and two days of right facial droop demonstrates abnormal soft tissue *(arrows)* along the course of the right auriculotemporal nerve and accounting for clinical symptoms referable to both the right trigeminal and right facial nerves.

distal lesion involving the anterior division but sparing the posterior division will produce denervation of the muscles of mastication with sparing of the mylohyoid and anterior belly of the digastric muscles. This pattern of denervation has also been reported following radiation therapy for palatine tonsil cancer.

After arising from the posterior division of V3, the auriculotemporal nerve splits to encircle the middle meningeal artery before rejoining laterally to travel along the posterior aspect of the mandibular condylar neck to reach the parotid gland. Within the parotid gland, the auriculotemporal nerve arborizes with the facial nerve. The auriculotemporal nerve provides sensory innervation to the ear, external auditory canal, temporal scalp, and temporomandibular joint. Additionally, secretomotor parasympathetic fibers from cranial nerve IX course with the auriculotemporal nerve to reach the parotid gland. Of greatest clinical relevance, the auriculotemporal nerve represents an access route for malignancy involving the trigeminal nerve to reach the facial nerve and vice versa (Fig. 84.10).

Abducens Nerve

The abducens nerve innervates the lateral rectus muscle. The abducens nuclei reside within the pontine tegmentum immediately anterior to the facial colliculi, which are eminences on the floor of the fourth ventricle created by the facial nerve fibers looping around the abducens nuclei (Fig. 84.11).

The abducens fibers extend anteriorly to exit the brainstem along the ventral pontomedullary junction. The abducens nerves then course through the prepontine cistern (Fig. 84.12A) and the basilar venous plexus (Fig. 84.12B) to reach the

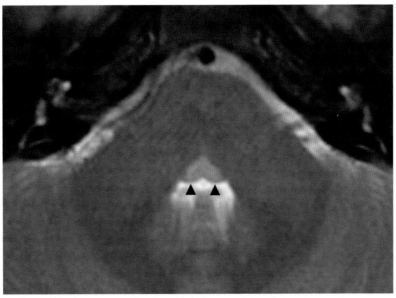

Ax T2 FS

• **Fig. 84.11** Axial T2-weighted image obtained in a 22-year-old female with bilateral lateral gaze palsy occurring in the setting of multiple sclerosis demonstrates a demyelinating lesion involving both abducens nuclei. The facial colliculi are denoted by the *arrowheads*. *Ax,* Axial; *FS,* fat saturated.

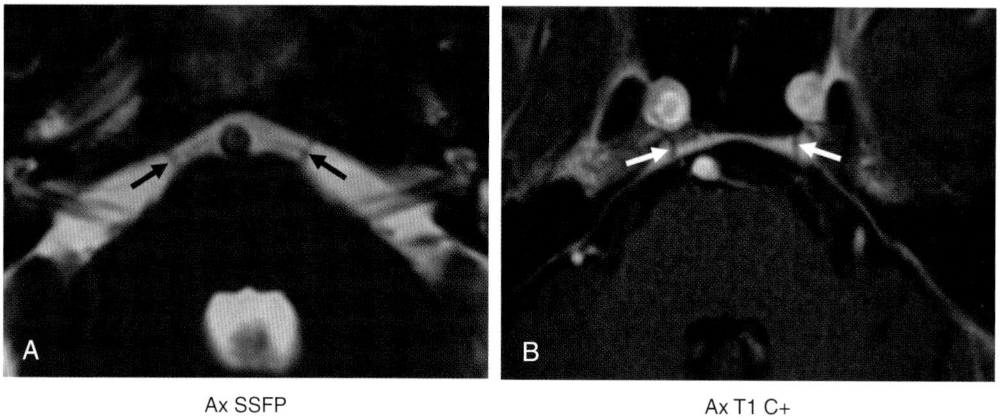

Ax SSFP   Ax T1 C+

• **Fig. 84.12** (A) Axial SSFP image demonstrates the normal abducens nerves *(arrows)* traversing the prepontine cistern. (B) Axial T1-weighted, gadolinium-enhanced image demonstrates the normal nonenhancing abducens nerves *(arrows)* traversing the contrast-filled basilar venous plexus. *Ax,* Axial; *SSFP,* steady-state free precession.

Dorello canals. The abducens nerves then turn anteriorly to pass through the medial aspects of the cavernous sinuses along the lateral margin of the internal carotid artery cavernous segments. Unlike the oculomotor nerves, trochlear nerves, and the ophthalmic and maxillary divisions of the trigeminal nerve, which course through the lateral walls of the cavernous sinuses, the abducens nerves are more medially located and surrounded by venous sinusoids within the cavernous sinuses.

After exiting the cavernous sinuses, the abducens nerves enter the orbit through the superior orbital fissures before turning anterolaterally to reach the lateral rectus muscles. The lateral rectus muscles function to abduct the globes. As such, denervation results in lateral gaze palsy with medial deviation of the affected globe in forward gaze (esotropia).

Additional Considerations

By recognizing complex patterns of denervation, (e.g., muscles innervated by the trigeminal and facial nerves), radiologists can narrow the region of interest requiring an intensive targeted search for subtle pathology. Although the ophthalmic and maxillary divisions of the trigeminal nerves have no motor function, knowledge of sensory deficits in this distribution is also useful for image interpretation. For example, facial numbness involving the ophthalmic and maxillary trigeminal nerve divisions in a patient with diplopia should prompt the radiologist to scrutinize the region of the cavernous sinus (Table 84.1).

Differential Diagnosis

Intracranially, all cranial nerves and their nuclei can be affected by infarction, hemorrhage, trauma, neoplasm, demyelination, inflammatory and autoimmune disorders (e.g., sarcoid, IgG4-related disease), and vascular lesions. Myriad extracranial pathology can also involve the cranial nerves with perineural spread of head and neck malignancy representing

TABLE 84.1	Summary of the Component Muscles and Innervation of Commonly Referenced Muscle Groups Related to Cranial Nerves III–VI		
Muscle Group	**Component Muscles**		**Innervation**
Extraocular muscles	Superior rectus, inferior rectus, medial rectus, inferior oblique		III
	Superior oblique		IV
	Lateral rectus		VI
Muscles of mastication	Temporalis, masseter, medial pterygoid, lateral pterygoid		V

an important consideration. Cranial nerve III palsy should direct the radiologist to assess for a posterior communicating artery aneurysm due to the close proximity of the oculomotor cistern to the posterior communicating artery origin. Bilateral abducens nerve palsy should prompt consideration of an abnormality of intracranial pressure (i.e., intracranial hypertension or intracranial hypotension). Finally, Duane syndrome refers to a rare form of strabismus in which the abducens nerve is commonly hypoplastic or absent (Fig. 84.13).

Pearls

- Minimize the risk of fat suppression failures by utilizing Dixon and inversion recovery techniques rather than spectral fat suppression.
- An enlarged, edematous, acutely denervated muscle may mimic a mass. However, the normal striations of the muscle belly are maintained.
- Volume loss and fatty infiltration within a chronically denervated muscle may cause the radiologist to mistake the contralateral normal muscle for pathology. Correlate with the side of the clinical deficit to differentiate.

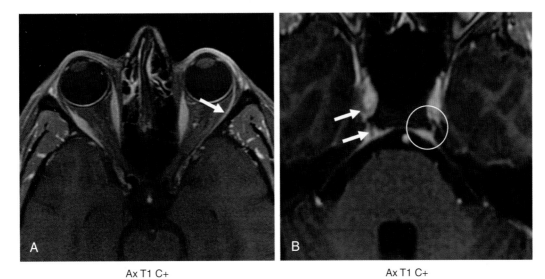

Ax T1 C+   Ax T1 C+

• **Fig. 84.13** Axial T1-weighted, gadolinium-enhanced images of (A) the orbits and of (B) the central skull base obtained in a 54-year-old female with Duane syndrome demonstrate marked atrophy of the left lateral rectus muscle (*arrow*, A) and absence of the expected nonenhancing abducens nerve within the left basilar venous plexus, left Dorello canal, and left cavernous sinus (*circle*, B). Note the expected nonenhancing right abducens nerve (*arrows*, B) within the right basilar venous plexus, right Dorello canal, and posterior aspect of the right cavernous sinus along the lateral margin of the right internal carotid artery.

- Careful inspection of fat (e.g., on T1-weighted MR or CT images) along the courses of the cranial nerves facilitates detection of subtle pathology.
- Although the trochlear nerves are often difficult to depict with routine clinical imaging, the trochlear grooves and trochlear cisterns are useful landmarks for identifying the tentorial segments.
- A mastoid effusion may occur in the setting of V3 disease due to dysfunction of the tensor veli palatini muscle.
- By recognizing complex patterns of denervation and understanding the relevant anatomy (e.g., muscles of mastication and facial expression → auriculotemporal nerve, face numbness and diplopia → cavernous sinus), radiologists can narrow the region of interest requiring an intensive targeted search for subtle pathology.

Suggested Readings

Borges A: Imaging of denervation in the head and neck, *Eur J Radiol* 72(2):323–340, 2010.

Bunch PM, Kelly HR, Zander DA, et al: Trochlear groove and trochlear cistern: useful anatomic landmarks for identifying the tentorial segment of cranial nerve IV on MRI, *AJNR Am J Neuroradiol* 38(5):1026–1030, 2017.

Connor SE, Chaudhary N, Fareedi S, et al: Imaging of muscular denervation secondary to motor cranial nerve dysfunction, *Clin Radiol* 61(8):659–669, 2006.

Ferreira T, Verbist B, van Buchem M, et al: Imaging the ocular motor nerves, *Eur J Radiol* 74(2):314–322, 2010.

Harnsberger HR, Dillon WP: Major motor atrophic patterns in the face and neck: CT evaluation, *Radiology* 155(3):665–670, 1985.

Vanderah TW, Gould DJ: *Nolte's the human brain: an introduction to its functional anatomy.* Philadelphia, 2021, Elsevier.

Patel VA, Zacharia TT, Goldenberg D, et al: End-organ radiographic manifestations of cranial neuropathies: a concise review, *Clin Imaging* 44:5–11, 2017.

Russo CP, Smoker WR, Weissman JL: MR appearance of trigeminal and hypoglossal motor denervation, *AJNR Am J Neuroradiol* 18(7):1375–1383, 1997.

Smoker WR, Reede DL: Denervation atrophy of motor cranial nerves, *Neuroimaging Clin N Am* 18(2):387–411, 2008.

Thatcher J, Chang Y, Chapman MN, et al: Clinical-radiologic correlation of extraocular eye movement disorders: seeing beneath the surface, *Radiographics* 36(7):2123–2139, 2016.

85

Cranial Nerve Denervation Patterns Part 2: VII–XII

THOMAS G. WEST, MD, ADAM SWEENEY, MD, AND PAUL M. BUNCH, MD

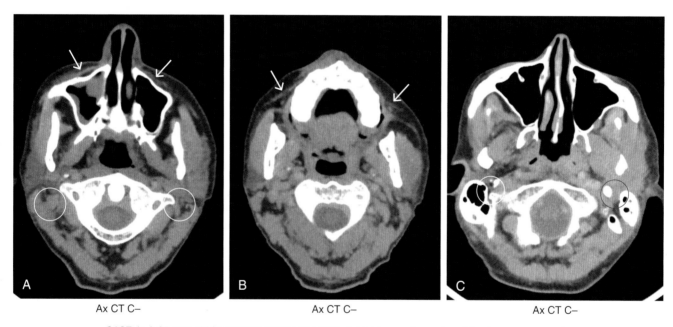

| Ax CT C– | Ax CT C– | Ax CT C– |

CASE A: A 65-year-old female with history of multiple cutaneous malignancies of the face now presents with progressive left facial weakness. *Ax*, Axial; *CT*, Computed tomography.

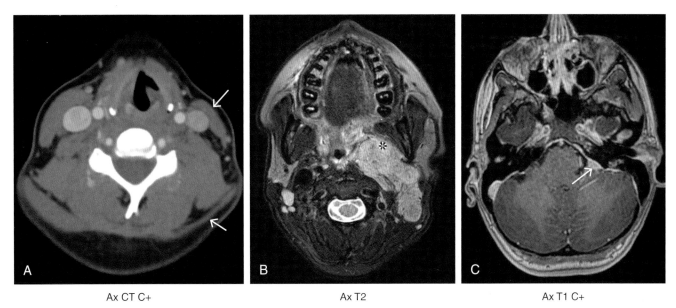

Ax CT C+   Ax T2   Ax T1 C+

CASE B: A 29-year-old female with hoarseness. *Ax*, Axial; *CT*, Computed tomography.

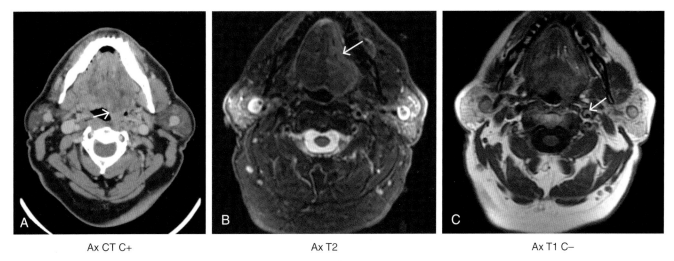

Ax CT C+   Ax T2   Ax T1 C–

CASE C: A 55-year-old male with sudden onset dysphagia and dysarthria who was found to have left tongue base fullness on office endoscopic examination. *Ax*, Axial; *CT*, Computed tomography.

DESCRIPTION OF FINDINGS

- Case A: Atrophy of the left levator labii superioris muscle (*arrows*, A), the posterior belly of the left digastric muscle (*circles*, A), and of the left zygomaticus major muscle (*arrow*, B) with abnormal soft tissue within the left parotid gland with effacement of the normal fat at the left stylomastoid foramen (*red circle*, C) compared to the normal right stylomastoid foramen (*white circle*, C).
- Case B: Asymmetric enlargement of the left laryngeal ventricle with atrophy (*arrows*, A) of the left sternocleidomastoid and left trapezius muscles. A large left poststyloid parapharyngeal (carotid) space mass anteriorly displaces the left internal carotid artery (*asterisk*, B), and a smaller intracranial extra-axial component of the mass with associated dural tail lies along the left posterior petrous ridge (*arrow*, C).
- Case C: Posterior prolapse of the left tongue base (*arrow*, A) without discrete mass lesion. Diffuse left tongue T2 hyperintensity (*arrow*, B), which respects the midline. Crescentic T1 hyperintensity along the anterior aspect of the left internal carotid artery (*arrow*, C).

Diagnosis

Case A: Recurrent malignancy involving the left parotid gland, resulting in a left facial nerve denervation pattern secondary to perineural tumor spread.

Case B: Left poststyloid pharyngeal (carotid) space meningioma resulting in denervation changes in the left vagus and spinal accessory nerves.

Case C: Left internal carotid artery dissection resulting in left hypoglossal nerve palsy.

Summary

This chapter represents the second of a two-part discussion of cranial nerve denervation and focuses on cranial nerves VII through XII. A comprehensive overview of cranial nerve denervation, associated imaging findings, and strategies for obtaining high-quality images are provided in Part 1

(Chapter 84). Whereas cranial nerves VII, IX, X, XI, and XII all have motor components, cranial nerve VIII is purely sensory and will therefore not be discussed.

Pharyngeal arch embryology provides a framework for intuitively understanding denervation patterns of cranial nerves V (discussed in further detail in Part 1), VII, IX, and X. Each of the pharyngeal arches has a mesenchymal core consisting of mesoderm and neural crest from which blood vessels, nerve, muscle, and cartilage develop. The muscles arising from the mesoderm of a given pharyngeal arch are innervated by the cranial nerve associated with that same pharyngeal arch (Table 85.1).

Cranial nerve XI derives from the basal plate of the embryonic spinal segments of C1 to C6 with the sternocleidomastoid and trapezius muscles forming from the third through seventh somites. Cranial nerve XII derives from the first pair of occipital somites, and the innervated musculature develops from the myotomes of the first four pairs of occipital somites.

Spectrum of Disease

Facial Nerve

The facial nerve is predominantly a motor nerve supplying the muscles of facial expression with minor sensory and parasympathetic components. The facial motor nucleus in the pons receives contralateral supranuclear motor input for the inferior muscles of facial expression but bilateral motor input for the more superior muscles of facial expression (periorbital, forehead). As such, a supranuclear lesion (Fig. 85.1) spares the superior muscles of facial expression and involves only the contralateral lower musculature. The intratemporal facial nerve provides motor innervation to the stapedius muscle. Just after exiting the skull base at the stylomastoid foramen, the facial

TABLE 85.1 Summary of the Pharyngeal Arches and Their Key Mesenchymal Core Derivatives

Pharyngeal Arch	Cranial Nerve	Muscles	Artery	Cartilage
1	V[a]	Tensor tympani, tensor veli palatini, muscles of mastication, anterior belly of the digastric, mylohyoid	Maxillary	Meckel: incus, malleus, maxilla, mandible
2	VII	Stapedius, Stylohyoid, posterior belly of digastric, muscles of facial expression	Stapedial, caroticotympanic	Reichert: stapes, styloid process, stylohyoid ligament, lesser cornu, and upper body of hyoid
3 (Contributes to pharyngeal plexus)	IX	Stylopharyngeus	Common carotid, internal carotid	Greater cornu and lower body of hyoid
4 (Fuses with 6)	X (superior laryngeal)	Soft palate, pharynx (except tensor veli palatine and stylopharyngeus)	Proximal right subclavian	Thyroid, cricoid, arytenoid, corniculate, cuneiform
5 (Regresses)	None	None	None	None
6 (Fuses with 4)	X (recurrent laryngeal)	Intrinsic laryngeal muscles (except cricothyroid), skeletal esophageal	Ductus arteriosus, proximal pulmonary	Thyroid, cricoid, arytenoid, corniculate, cuneiform

[a]Although cranial nerve V is discussed in detail in the previous chapter, it is included here for completeness.

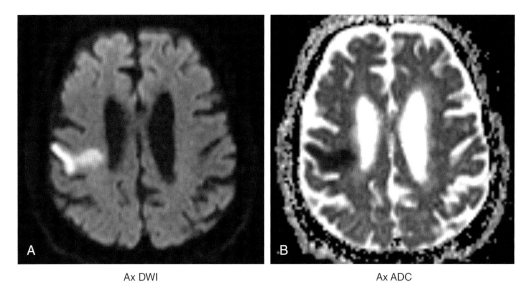

Ax DWI

Ax ADC

• **Fig. 85.1** In this 80-year-old male with acute onset left facial droop, axial DWI image and corresponding ADC map demonstrate restricted diffusion consistent with acute to early subacute ischemic infarction in the lateral aspect of the right precentral gyrus in the expected location of motor function to the left face. *ADC,* Apparent diffusion coefficient; *Ax,* axial; *DWI,* diffusion-weighted imaging.

nerve gives off branches to the posterior belly of the digastric and stylohyoid muscles, subsequently dividing into the temporofacial and cervicofacial branches. The temporofacial branch further divides into the temporal and zygomatic branches, and the cervicofacial branch divides into the mandibular and cervical branches. The buccal branch can arise from either the temporofacial or cervicofacial branches. Multiple connections are frequently present between the five terminal branches of the facial nerve, and these five terminal branches innervate the muscles of facial expression.

Lesions proximal to the stylomastoid foramen (e.g., temporal bone fracture) will result in denervation atrophy of the posterior belly of the digastric and muscles of facial expression, while lesions within the parotid gland will spare the posterior belly of the digastric. Cross-connections between motor branches of the facial nerves exist that preclude selective motor denervation of individual muscles unless the lesion is extremely peripheral. Atrophy of the larger muscles of facial expression can be seen in the subacute and chronic phase but is more difficult to appreciate in the acute phase due to the relatively small size of these muscles.

Glossopharyngeal Nerve

Cranial nerve IX exits the skull base through the medial aspect of the jugular foramen and courses in the poststyloid parapharyngeal (carotid) space along the posterior aspect of the internal carotid artery before terminating in the posterior aspect of the sublingual space. The glossopharyngeal nerve is a mixed motor-sensory nerve with motor innervation to a single muscle—the stylopharyngeus. Atrophy of the small stylopharyngeus muscle is difficult to appreciate directly with imaging. The normal gag reflex relies on intact glossopharyngeal

and vagus nerve function, such that an absent gag reflex should prompt the radiologist to assess for pathology affecting these lower cranial nerves.

Vagus Nerve

Cranial nerve X also exits the skull base through the medial aspect of the jugular foramen to subsequently course in the poststyloid parapharyngeal (carotid) space between the internal carotid artery and internal jugular vein. The vagus nerve gives off three motor branches to muscles in the neck: the pharyngeal nerve, the superior laryngeal nerve, and the recurrent laryngeal nerve. Through the pharyngeal plexus, the pharyngeal nerve supplies all the muscles of the pharynx except the stylopharyngeus (IX) and all the muscles of the soft palate except the tensor veli palatini (V3). Denervation of the muscles innervated by the pharyngeal nerve can result in atrophy of the superior constrictor muscle and fatty infiltration of the soft palate. The superior laryngeal nerve innervates the cricothyroid muscle, and the recurrent laryngeal nerve innervates the remaining intrinsic laryngeal musculature.

A distal pattern of vagal denervation spares muscles innervated by the pharyngeal plexus but results in involvement of the superior laryngeal or recurrent laryngeal nerves. Recurrent laryngeal nerve palsy is much more common, resulting in atrophy of the intrinsic laryngeal musculature (except the cricothyroid) with vocal cord paralysis. Findings of vocal cord paralysis include atrophy of the thyroarytenoid and posterior cricoarytenoid muscles with anteromedial displacement of the ipsilateral arytenoid cartilage, medialization of the ipsilateral vocal fold, and thickening of the ipsilateral aryepiglottic fold along with associated enlargement of the vallecula, laryngeal ventricle, and pyriform sinus. When a distal cranial nerve X

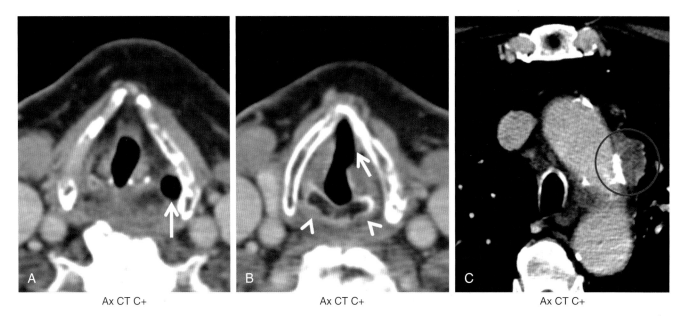

• **Fig. 85.2** Axial contrast-enhanced CT images obtained in an 80-year-old male with progressive hoarseness demonstrate asymmetric enlargement of the left pyriform sinus (*arrow*, A) and left laryngeal ventricle (*arrow*, B). There is atrophy of the left posterior cricoarytenoid muscle relative to the right (*arrowheads*, B). The causative lesion compressing the left recurrent laryngeal nerve lies along the left lateral aspect of the aortic arch (*red circle*, C) in this patient subsequently diagnosed with metastatic lung cancer. *Ax*, Axial; *CT*, Computed tomography.

denervation pattern is identified, imaging must extend through the aortopulmonary window to assess the inferior extent of the left recurrent laryngeal nerve extending inferior to the aortic arch and the right recurrent laryngeal nerve extending inferior to the right subclavian artery (Fig. 85.2). A nonrecurrent right laryngeal nerve occurs in the presence of an aberrant right subclavian artery, and the nonrecurrent laryngeal nerve is at increased risk for iatrogenic injury (e.g., thyroidectomy, parathyroidectomy, and carotid endarterectomy) because of this nerve's variable and unpredictable course.

Spinal Accessory Nerve

Cranial nerve XI also exits the skull base through the medial aspect of the jugular foramen into the poststyloid parapharyngeal (carotid) space. Cranial nerve XI can be injured by trauma or resected as part of a neck dissection, resulting in atrophy of the trapezius and sternocleidomastoid muscles. Less commonly, cranial nerve XI denervation may result from nerve sheath tumor or metastasis. Thus, in the absence of prior surgery or known trauma, a careful search for a lesion along the course of cranial nerve XI, including within the jugular foramen and along the sternocleidomastoid muscle, should be performed to exclude an underlying lesion. In the setting of cranial nerve XI denervation, compensatory hypertrophy of the ipsilateral levator scapulae commonly occurs (Fig. 85.3) and can simulate a mass.

Hypoglossal Nerve

The hypoglossal nerve is purely a motor nerve innervating all of the intrinsic and extrinsic muscles of the tongue except for

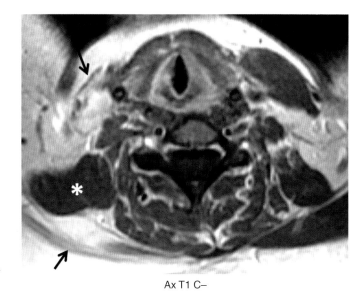

Ax T1 C–

• **Fig. 85.3** Axial T1-weighted image in a 37-year-old female with right cranial nerve XI paralysis demonstrates atrophy of the right sternocleidomastoid and trapezius muscles *(arrows)* with compensatory hypertrophy of the right levator scapulae muscle *(asterisk)*. *Ax*, Axial.

the palatoglossus muscle, which is innervated by the vagus nerve. The tongue also has embryologic contributions from the first four pharyngeal arches, including innervation from the associated cranial nerves: the lingual nerve (somatosensory) from V, the chorda tympani (taste to the anterior two-thirds) from VII, as well as contributions from IX (taste to the posterior one-third) and X (the palatoglossus). The hypoglossal nerve exits the skull base through the hypoglossal canal into the poststyloid parapharyngeal (carotid) space lateral to the jugular vein. The nerve exits the poststyloid parapharyngeal space along the inferior margin of the digastric muscle posterior belly and courses anteroinferiorly to the tongue between the hyoglossus and mylohyoid muscles.

The strap musculature is innervated by fibers from C1 and C2, which travel with the hypoglossal nerve and ansa cervicalis. Lesions of the hypoglossal nerve proximal to the contributions from C1 and C2 will result in a proximal pattern of denervation sparing the strap musculature, whereas lesions distal to this contribution will result in atrophy of the strap musculature as well (Fig. 85.4).

Additional Considerations

Recognition of complex patterns of denervation can narrow the region of intensive search for pathology. For example, cranial nerves IX to XII are in close proximity immediately inferior to the skull base, such that denervation of multiple lower cranial nerves should prompt a careful search of the suprahyoid poststyloid parapharyngeal (carotid) space. The combination of loss of gag reflex, hoarseness, and atrophy of the sternocleidomastoid muscle should be a clue to a lesion involving the jugular foramen, and jugular foramen pathology is further discussed in Chapter 74. Finally, a denervation pattern affecting the muscles of mastication (V3) and facial expression (VII) should prompt a search for pathology along the auriculo-temporal nerve (Table 85.2).

Differential Diagnosis

Intracranially, all cranial nerves and their nuclei can be affected by infarction, hemorrhage, trauma, neoplasm, demyelination, and vascular lesions. Lyme disease may produce facial paralysis secondary to facial nerve involvement.

Diverse extracranial pathology can also produce cranial nerve denervation and varies with the specific nerve involved. Specific extracranial etiologies for each of the cranial nerves discussed in this chapter include:

VII: Perineural tumor spread, iatrogenic (e.g., parotidectomy), trauma, viral infection, venous malformation (formerly facial nerve hemangioma), schwannoma

IX: Meningioma, paraganglioma, metastasis, internal carotid artery dissection

X: Meningioma, paraganglioma, metastasis, iatrogenic (e.g., thyroidectomy, parathyroidectomy), trauma, viral infection, internal carotid artery dissection

XI: Iatrogenic (e.g., radical neck dissection), trauma, nerve sheath tumor, metastasis

XII: Perineural tumor spread, metastasis, invasive nasopharyngeal carcinoma, meningioma, paraganglioma, internal carotid artery dissection, craniocervical junction degenerative disease

Bell palsy is a clinical diagnosis that warrants special mention. Long considered idiopathic, evidence now implicates reactivation of a latent viral infection. Although imaging is commonly not performed if the clinical features are classic, when imaging is performed and abnormal facial nerve thickening or enhancement is present (Fig. 85.5), continued clinical follow-up to complete resolution is prudent to avoid a delayed or missed diagnosis of perineural tumor spread from occult (often cutaneous) malignancy.

Pearls

- Careful inspection of fat (e.g., on T1-weighted MR or CT images) along the courses of the cranial nerves facilitates detection of subtle pathology.

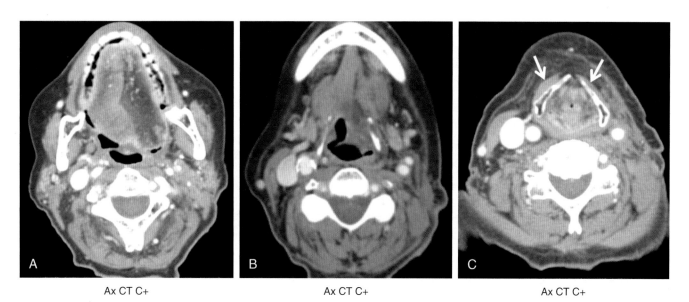

Ax CT C+   Ax CT C+   Ax CT C+

• **Fig. 85.4** Axial contrast-enhanced CT images demonstrate atrophy of the left (A) intrinsic and (B) extrinsic tongue musculature as well as of the left strap musculature (*arrows*, C) in this patient with a left hypoglossal nerve distal denervation pattern. *Ax*, Axial.

TABLE 85.2 **Summary of the Component Muscles and Innervation of Commonly Referenced Muscle Groups Related to Cranial Nerves VII–XII**

Muscle Group	Component Muscles	Innervation
Muscles of facial expression	Depressor anguli oris, levator anguli oris, levator labii superioris, levator labii superioris alaeque nasi, zygomaticus major, zygomaticus minor, orbicularis oris, risorius, depressor labii inferioris, levator anguli, buccinator, mentalis, platysma procerus, nasalis, depressor septi nasi, orbicularis oculi, corrugator supercilia, depressor supercilia, auricular	VII
Intrinsic tongue musculature (no bony attachment)	Superior longitudinal, inferior longitudinal, vertical, transverse	XII
Extrinsic tongue musculature (bony attachment)	Genioglossus, hyoglossus, styloglossus Palatoglossus	XII X
Infrahyoid strap muscles	Thyrohyoid Sternothyroid, sternohyoid, omohyoid	C1 via XII Ansa cervicalis
Suprahyoid muscles	Geniohyoid Stylohyoid, digastric (posterior belly) Mylohyoid, digastric (anterior belly)	C1 via XII VII Mylohyoid nerve (V)
Intrinsic laryngeal muscles	Cricothyroid Thyroarytenoid, posterior cricoarytenoid, lateral cricoarytenoid, transverse arytenoid, oblique arytenoid	External branch of superior laryngeal nerve (X) Recurrent laryngeal (X)
Extrinsic laryngeal muscles	Sternothyroid, omohyoid, sternohyoid (depress) Thyrohyoid, geniohyoid (elevate) Anterior belly of digastric, mylohyoid Posterior belly of digastric, stylohyoid Hyoglossus, genioglossus Inferior constrictor	Ansa cervicalis C1 Mylohyoid nerve (V) VII XII X

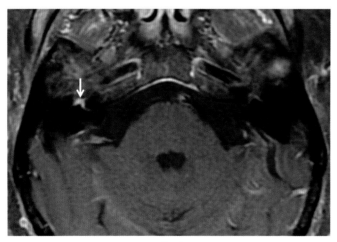

Ax T1 C+

• **Fig. 85.5** Axial T1-weighted, gadolinium-enhanced image demonstrates abnormal, asymmetric enhancement of the labyrinthine segment, geniculate ganglion *(arrow)*, and proximal tympanic segment of the right facial nerve in a patient with sudden onset right facial weakness. Although these imaging findings may be seen in the clinical setting of Bell palsy, suspicion of possible perineural tumor spread should remain until complete clinical resolution of symptoms. *Ax,* Axial.

- An enlarged, edematous, acutely denervated muscle may mimic a mass while volume loss and fatty infiltration within a chronically denervated muscle may result in contralateral normal tissue erroneously being suspected as pathologic. More specifically, loss of normal tongue tone from hypoglossal palsy will produce posterior prolapse of the ipsilateral tongue base in the supine position (e.g., during CT or MR imaging) that may be mistaken for tongue base fullness or mass.

- Infranuclear lesions of the facial nerve pathway involve both the superior (forehead, periorbital) and inferior muscles of facial expression, whereas supranuclear lesions spare the superior muscles secondary to bilateral supranuclear motor pathways.

- Distal denervation pattern of X spares the superior constrictor musculature and involves the laryngeal musculature, which should prompt a search for pathology along the course of the recurrent laryngeal nerve, requiring imaging extending inferiorly to the aortopulmonary window.

- Involvement of the musculature innervated by the pharyngeal plexus differentiates a proximal X denervation pattern from a distal X pattern, which affects only the laryngeal muscles.

- Compensatory hypertrophy of the ipsilateral levator scapulae may mimic a mass in the setting of cranial nerve XI denervation.

- Proximal denervation pattern of cranial nerve XII spares the strap musculature (sternothyroid, geniohyoid), as these muscles are innervated by C1 nerve roots which travel with the hypoglossal nerve and ansa cervicalis.

- Loss of gag reflex, hoarseness, and atrophy of the sternocleidomastoid muscle are clues to a lesion involving the jugular foramen.

Signs and Complications

Sail sign: Appearance of atrophic thyroarytenoid muscle with enlarged ipsilateral laryngeal ventricle in the setting of vocal cord paralysis.

Suggested Readings

Alves P: Imaging the hypoglossal nerve, *Eur J Radiol* 74(2):368–377, 2010.

Borges A: Imaging of denervation in the head and neck, *Eur J Radiol* 72(2):323–340, 2010.

Chhabra A, Bajaj G, Wadhwa V, et al: MR neurographic evaluation of facial and neck pain: normal and abnormal craniospinal nerves below the skull base, *Radiographics* 38(5):1498–1513, 2018.

Harnsberger HR, Dillon WP: Major motor atrophic patterns in the face and neck: CT evaluation, *Radiology* 155(3):665070, 1985.

Pascual PM, Maranillo E, Vazques T: Extracranial course of the facial nerve revisited, *Anat Rec* 302:599–608, 2019.

Patel VA, Zacharia TT, Godenberg D, et al: End-organ radiographic manifestations of cranial neuropathies: A concise review, *Clinical Imaging* 44:5–11, 2017.

Russo CP, Smoker WR, Weismman JL: MR appearance of trigeminal and hypoglossal motor denervation, *AJNR Am J Neuroradiol*: 18(7):1375–1383, 1997.

Smoker WR, Reede DL: Denervation atrophy of motor cranial nerves, *Neuroimagin Clin N Am* 18(2):387–411, 2008.

Thompson EO, Smoker WRK: Hypoglossal nerve palsy: a segmental approach, *Radiographics* 14:939–958, 1994.

Weindling SM, Goff RD, Wood CP, et al: Is hypoglossal nerve palsy caused by craniocervical junction degenerative disease an underrecognized entity?, *AJNR Am J Neuroradiol* 37(11):2138–2143, 2016.

86

Intraventricular Posterior Fossa Tumors

JENNIFER HUANG, MD, MED AND ASHA SARMA, MD

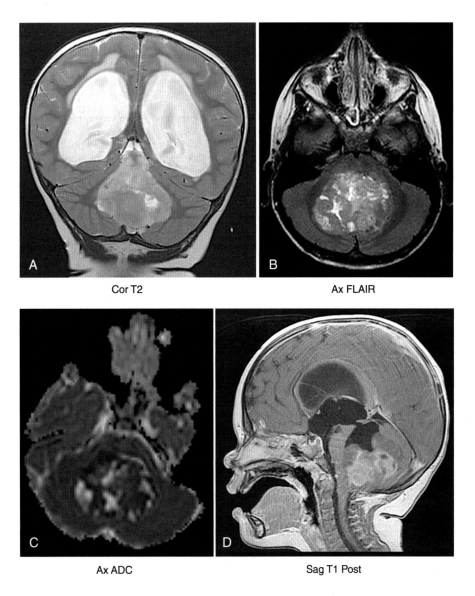

| Cor T2 | Ax FLAIR |
| Ax ADC | Sag T1 Post |

CASE A: A 2-year-old child with vomiting and inability to walk or hold her head up. *ADC*, Apparent diffusion coefficient; *Ax*, axial; *Cor*, coronal; *FLAIR*, fluid attenuated inversion recovery; *Sag*, sagittal.

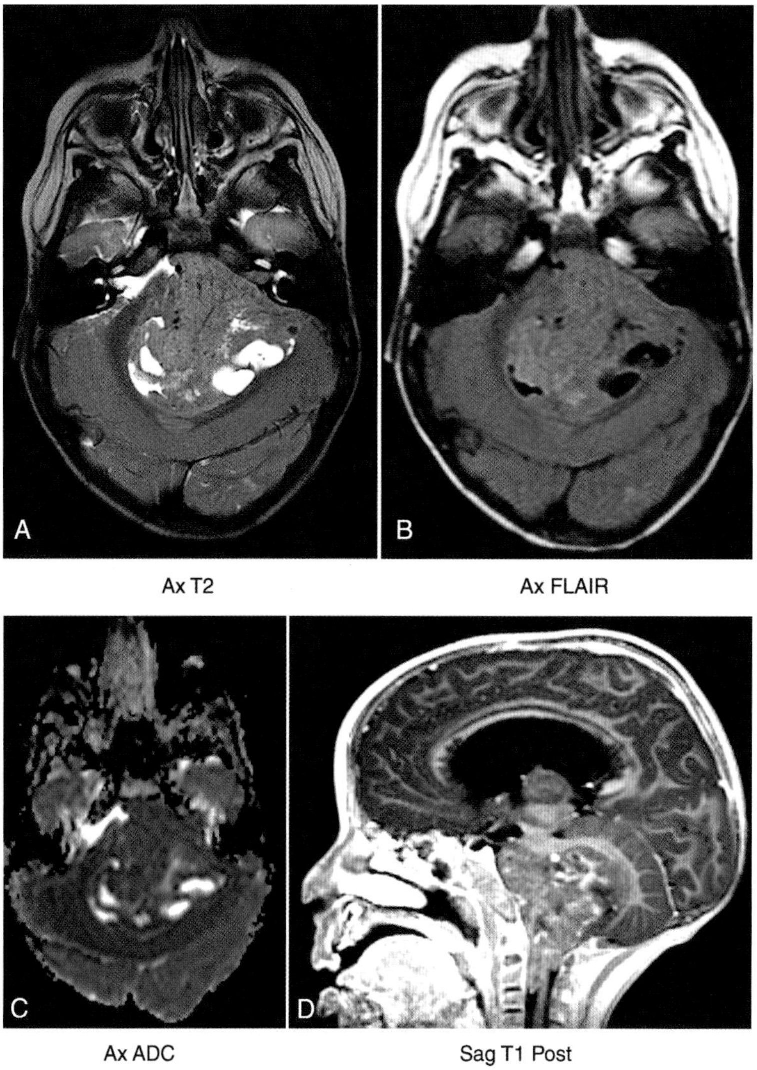

A Ax T2

B Ax FLAIR

C Ax ADC

D Sag T1 Post

CASE B: A 1-year-old child with irritability, difficulty walking, head tilt, and poor appetite. *ADC*, Apparent diffusion coefficient; *Ax*, axial; *FLAIR*, fluid attenuated inversion recovery; *Sag*, sagittal.

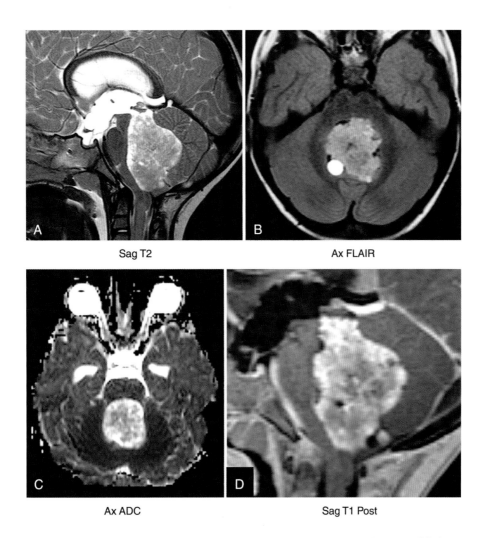

Sag T2

Ax FLAIR

Ax ADC

Sag T1 Post

CASE C: A 3-year-old child with one month of progressive intermittent headaches and emesis. *ADC*, Apparent diffusion coefficient; *Ax*, axial; *FLAIR*, fluid attenuated inversion recovery; *Sag*, sagittal.

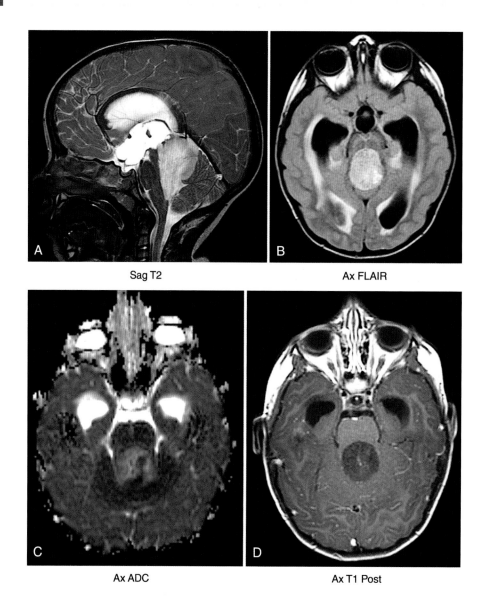

Sag T2

Ax FLAIR

Ax ADC

Ax T1 Post

CASE D: A 3-year-old child with headaches. *ADC*, Apparent diffusion coefficient; *Ax*, axial; *FLAIR*, fluid attenuated inversion recovery; *Sag*, sagittal.

DESCRIPTION OF FINDINGS

- Case A: Heterogeneously enhancing mass located at the inferior aspect of the fourth ventricle along the ventral aspect of the vermis. Marked low diffusivity and heterogeneous enhancement.
- Case B: Heterogeneous fourth ventricular mass with areas of internal cystic change and hemorrhage. Intermediate diffusivity. Characteristic extension through the left foramen of Luschka.
- Case C: Fourth ventricular mass with "frondlike" or "papillary" architecture. Increased diffusivity.
- Case D: Mass with enhancement arising from superior medullary velum with heterogeneous low diffusivity and little enhancement.

Diagnosis

Case A: Medulloblastoma
Case B: Ependymoma
Case C: Choroid plexus tumor
Case D: Atypical teratoid/rhabdoid tumor

Summary

Medulloblastoma and ependymoma are the most common pediatric intraventricular posterior fossa tumors, with ependymomas, atypical teratoid/rhabdoid tumors (ATRTs), and choroid plexus tumors as additional considerations. Other tumor types, including metastases, are more unusual (Fig. 86.1).

Medulloblastoma

Medulloblastoma is a highly cellular "small round blue cell" embryonal tumor. Although it classically arises in the fourth ventricle, there has been significant progress in radiogenomic subtyping in recent years, which is discussed in greater detail in Chapter 87. The group III/IV subtypes of medulloblastoma are typically found within the fourth ventricle. On magnetic resonance imaging (MRI), the mass tends to be relatively homogeneous, exhibiting features of high cellularity such as hyperdensity on unenhanced computed tomography (CT), relatively low signal on T2-weighted MRI, and low diffusivity. While the majority of medulloblastomas enhance, the enhancement pattern is highly variable. Calcifications can be seen in up to 20% of cases, and hemorrhage is rare. Due to the tumor's propensity to demonstrate microscopic or nodular seeding of the subarachnoid space, MRI of the total spine is recommended at diagnosis to evaluate for disseminated disease. Medulloblastoma is associated with several familial cancer syndromes, including Gorlin syndrome, Li–Fraumeni syndrome, Turcot syndrome, Gardner syndrome, and Cowden syndrome.

Ependymoma

The majority of intracranial ependymomas are infratentorial, making ependymoma the third most common posterior fossa

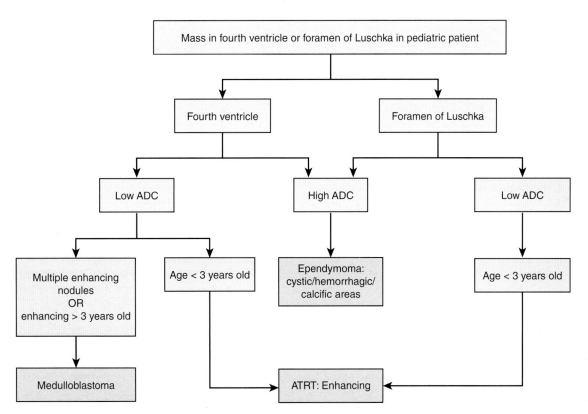

• **Fig. 86.1** A diagnostic algorithm for diagnosis of intraventricular posterior fossa tumors. *ADC*, Apparent diffusion coefficient; *ATRT*, atypical teratoid/rhabdoid tumor. (Adapted from Alves CAPF, Löbel U, Martin-Saavedra JS, et al: A diagnostic algorithm for posterior fossa tumors in children: a validation study, *AJNR Am J Neuroradiol* 42(5):961–968, 2021.)

tumor in children after pilocytic astrocytoma and medulloblastoma. Ependymomas classically arise from the ventrally located "floor" of the fourth ventricle, which can help differentiate them from medulloblastomas (which typically arise from the dorsally located "roof"). Calcifications and hemorrhage are common, and enhancement tends to be heterogeneous. Tumoral cysts are common. Although not pathognomonic, a helpful clue to the diagnosis of ependymoma is the plastic-like extension of tumor through the foramina of Luschka or Magendie (hence the useful moniker, "toothpaste" tumor). Because of the tumor's tendency to insinuate around neurovascular structures, complete resection is often difficult, and therefore radiation and/or chemotherapy are often considered as adjuvant treatments.

Choroid Plexus Tumors

Compared to medulloblastoma and ependymoma, choroid plexus tumors are less common. The majority (70% to 80%) is found in young children, particularly within the first year of life. Choroid plexus papillomas (CPPs) arise from the epithelial cells lining the choroid plexus and therefore occur within the ventricular system. The most common location in children is the atrium of the lateral ventricle, followed by the fourth ventricle and then the third ventricle. The fourth ventricle is the most common location in adult patients. Rarely, choroid plexus tumors may occur at the cerebellopontine angle or arise from the brain parenchyma (postulated to arise from embryonic remnants of the choroid plexus). The "papillary" or "frondlike" lobulated architecture of the intraventricular mass helps to differentiate choroid plexus tumor from other intraventricular neoplasms. Calcification, hemorrhage, and large flow voids are common. Due to propensity for CSF dissemination, craniospinal MRI is recommended for diagnosis and follow-up. Choroid plexus tumors often cause hydrocephalus, which is thought to result from a combination of obstruction, increased CSF production, and decreased CSF reabsorption from the arachnoid granulations. The degree of hydrocephalus may appear disproportionate to the degree of obstruction of the CSF circulation pathway. More aggressive variants (atypical choroid plexus papilloma and choroid plexus carcinoma) are rare. Active investigation of findings that help to differentiate among the variants is ongoing. A large amount of parenchymal edema or other signs suggestive of frank parenchymal invasion may raise suspicion for carcinoma.

Atypical Teratoid/Rhabdoid Tumor

ATRT is a more rarely seen infratentorial embryonal tumor in children and is most common in infants and children under the age of 3 years. ATRT may be indistinguishable from medulloblastoma on imaging, and recent development of specific immunohistochemical markers and discovery of characteristic gene mutations (most commonly *SMARCB1/INI1*) have aided in distinguishing between these two entities. ATRT often contains cysts, hemorrhage, and calcifications, with a hyperattenuating appearance on noncontrast CT and a heterogeneous appearance on T1- and T2-weighted MRI. Reduced diffusivity is often seen, and there is a tendency toward minimal enhancement. An off-midline location, at the foramen of Luschka or in the cerebellopontine angle, is suggestive. In summary, it is appropriate to put ATRT in the differential diagnosis along with medulloblastoma for a hypercellular fourth ventricular tumor in a child under age 3 years.

Spectrum of Disease

The spectrum of disease is detailed in the preceding section.

Pearls

- Medulloblastoma is a highly cellular tumor with reduced diffusivity and variable enhancement.
- Ependymoma often arises from the floor of the fourth ventricle with "plastic" extension through the fourth ventricular outlet foramina.
- Choroid plexus tumors have a "frondlike" or "papillary" architecture. The lateral ventricular trigone is a more common location than the fourth ventricle in children.
- ATRT is a highly aggressive tumor in the differential diagnosis for a hypercellular posterior fossa mass in a child under the age of 3 years.

Signs and Complications

- Obstructive hydrocephalus and increased intracranial pressure are common complications of intraventricular posterior fossa masses.

Suggested Readings

Alves CAPF, Lobel U, Martin-Saavedra JS, et al: A diagnostic algorithm for posterior fossa tumors in children: a validation study, *AJNR Am J Neuroradiol* 42(5):961–968, 2021.

D'Arco F, Khan F, Mankad K, et al: Differential diagnosis of posterior fossa tumours in children: new insights, *Pediatr Radiol* 48(13): 1955–1963, 2018.

Plaza MJ, Borja MJ, Altman N, et al: Conventional and advanced MRI features of pediatric intracranial tumors: posterior fossa and suprasellar tumors, *AJR Am J Roentgenol* 200(5):1115–1124, 2013.

Smith AB, Smirniotopoulos JG, Horkanyne-Szakaly I: From the radiologic pathology archives: intraventricular neoplasms: radiologic-pathologic correlation, *Radiographics* 33(1):21–43, 2013.

87

Pediatric Cerebellar Tumors

JENNIFER HUANG, MD, MED AND ASHA SARMA, MD

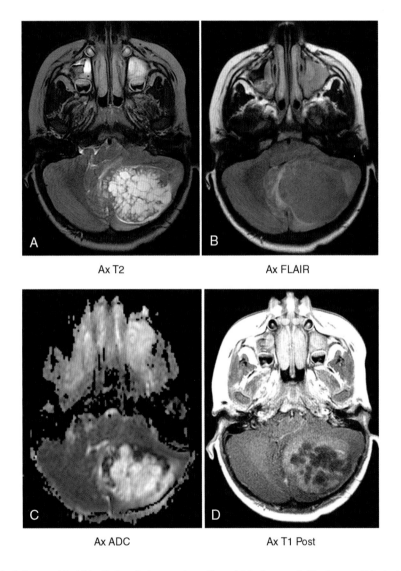

Ax T2

Ax FLAIR

Ax ADC

Ax T1 Post

CASE A: A 6-year-old child with headaches and vomiting. *ADC*, Apparent diffusion coefficient; *Ax*, axial; *FLAIR*, fluid attenuated inversion recovery.

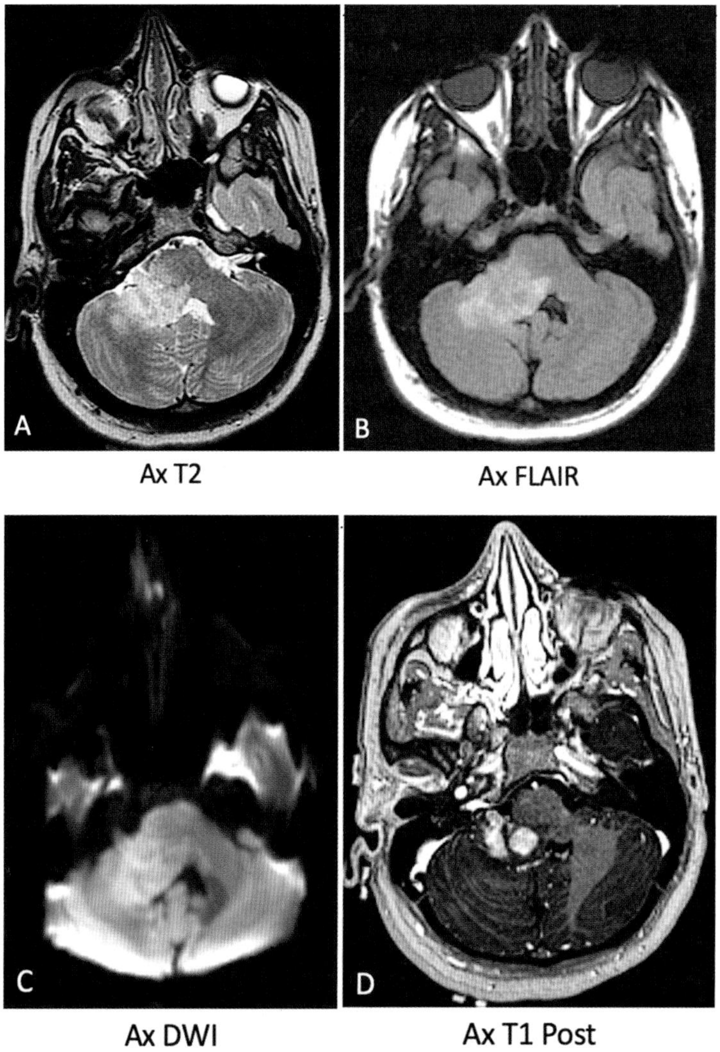

Ax T2

Ax FLAIR

Ax DWI

Ax T1 Post

CASE B: A 15-year-old child with one month of severe headaches and vomiting. *Ax*, Axial; *DWI*, diffusion-weighted imaging; *FLAIR*, fluid attenuated inversion recovery.

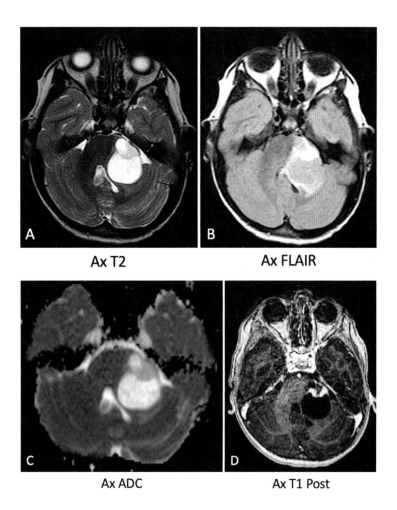

CASE C: A 6-year-old child with torticollis. *ADC*, Apparent diffusion coefficient; *Ax*, axial; *FLAIR*, fluid attenuated inversion recovery.

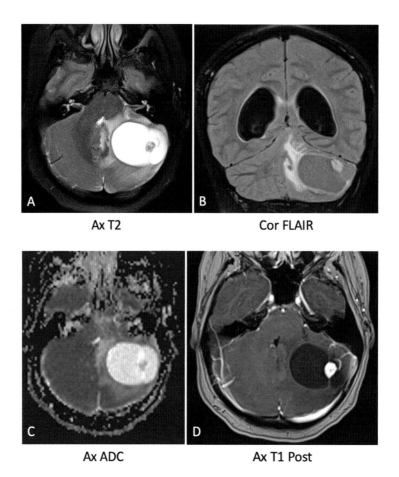

Ax T2   Cor FLAIR

Ax ADC   Ax T1 Post

CASE D: An 18-year-old with headaches. *ADC*, Apparent diffusion coefficient; *Ax*, axial; *Cor*, coronal; *FLAIR*, fluid attenuated inversion recovery.

DESCRIPTION OF FINDINGS

- Case A: Large partially solid and multicystic mass centered in the left cerebellar hemisphere, with mild enhancement and reduced diffusivity in the solid portions and mild hyperintensity on fluid attenuated inversion recovery (FLAIR) imaging. Severe local mass effect with tonsillar herniation, brainstem compression, and severe hydrocephalus.
- Case B: Mildly T2 and FLAIR hyperintense mass centered in the right cerebellar peduncle with extension into the adjacent right cerebellar hemisphere. The mass demonstrates multifocal areas of enhancement and moderate effacement of the fourth ventricle.
- Case C: Mass in the left cerebellar hemisphere with cystic-appearing T2 hyperintense component that does not suppress on FLAIR and small nodular enhancing component. No associated reduced diffusivity or hemorrhage. Mass effect and rightward deviation of midbrain and pons.
- Case D: Large T2 hyperintense cystic mass with a solid enhancing nodule and incomplete suppression on FLAIR in the left cerebellar hemisphere. No associated reduced diffusivity and a small amount of surrounding edema.

Diagnosis

Case A: Desmoplastic medulloblastoma
Case B: Ganglioglioma
Case C: Pilocytic astrocytoma
Case D: Hemangioblastoma

Summary

Posterior fossa tumors are much more common in pediatric patients compared to adults, comprising up to 60% of childhood brain tumors. Due to limited space within the posterior fossa and proximity to vital brainstem structures, tumors in this area are often associated with findings warranting rapid surgical intervention, including hydrocephalus and tonsillar herniation. The presenting symptoms depend on the site of origin and involvement of regional anatomic structures: common clinical manifestations include headache, neck pain, and vomiting. Compared to adults, there is a very different differential diagnosis for infratentorial tumors in children. Common pediatric posterior fossa tumors include juvenile pilocytic astrocytoma (JPA), medulloblastoma, and ependymoma. Less commonly seen are atypical teratoid/rhabdoid tumor, hemangioblastoma, and high-grade glioma. Although some of these tumors demonstrate overlapping imaging characteristics, there are several key imaging features to aid the interpreting radiologist in coming to an accurate diagnosis. The most important sequences to evaluate are T2, FLAIR, diffusion-weighted imaging (DWI), and postcontrast T1-weighted imaging, which can be used to evaluate the degree of cellularity and vascularity of the lesion.

Differential Diagnosis

Juvenile Pilocytic Astrocytoma

JPA is one of the most common pediatric posterior fossa brain tumors. There is overall increased risk for JPA in patients with neurofibromatosis type 1 (NF1), although the more common location for JPA in NF1 patients is the optic pathway. On imaging, cerebellar JPA is classically described as having a "cyst with enhancing nodule" appearance. However, JPA may also present as a predominantly solid mass. JPA is a low-grade neoplasm (WHO grade 1) with less associated vasogenic edema than that which is seen in high-grade tumors. Solid components are typically T2 hyperintense with increased diffusivity due to low cellularity and avid enhancement due to high vascularity. Importantly, these tumors may show increased perfusion and elevated lactate on MR spectroscopy, which could lead to a false impression of high-tumor grade.

In comparison to JPA, ganglioglioma is much less common and tends to have more solid and nodular enhancement. Hemangioblastoma, which can also present as a cystic mass with an enhancing mural nodule, is also less common than JPA. The nodule tends to be located peripherally, along the pia. Enlarged regional flow voids may be seen. The patient may also have additional brain, spine, or retinal hemangioblastomas, other tumors, and lesions such as cysts in kidneys, pancreas, and genital tract in the context of associated von Hippel–Lindau (VHL) syndrome.

Medulloblastoma

Medulloblastoma accounts for approximately 35% to 40% of infratentorial tumors in children. There are known molecular groups of medulloblastoma (e.g., group III, group IV, and WNT- and SHH-activated tumors), which demonstrate different clinical and imaging manifestations, as well as clinical outcomes. Recently, subgroups have been identified within group III, group IV, and SHH groups in the WHO 2021 brain tumor classification. There are four main histologic subtypes: classic, desmoplastic/nodular, extensive nodularity, and large cell/anaplastic. Although somewhat variable in appearance depending on genetic subgroup, medulloblastoma most commonly arises in midline from the roof of the fourth ventricle and thus must be distinguished from intraventricular tumors such as ependymoma and choroid plexus tumor. However, it is important to recognize that in pediatric patients, desmoplastic medulloblastoma can present off midline in the cerebellar hemisphere as a minimally enhancing mass. Medulloblastoma is a highly cellular "small round blue cell" tumor, characterized by hyperattenuation on CT and marked reduced diffusivity. It tends to be relatively lower in signal intensity on T2-weighted imaging in comparison with JPA. The degree and pattern of enhancement are highly variable and can be associated with the subgroup. Calcifications can be seen in up to 20% of cases, and hemorrhage is rare. Due to its propensity to demonstrate microscopic or nodular seeding of the subarachnoid space, MRI of the total spine is recommended at diagnosis to evaluate for disseminated disease. Medulloblastoma is associated with several familial cancer syndromes, including Gorlin, Li-Fraumeni, Turcot, Gardner, and Cowden syndromes.

Ganglioglioma

Ganglioglioma is a well-differentiated tumor that most commonly involves the temporal cerebral cortex; however, it can rarely be seen as an infratentorial lesion. The peak age of incidence is between 10 and 20 years, and the clinical presentation depends on the structures involved. Imaging characteristics of posterior fossa ganglioglioma are variable. These tumors are often hyperintense on T2-weighted images and can be cystic, solid, or mixed. When ganglioglioma presents as a cystic and solid mass, it can be difficult to differentiate from JPA, although JPA is much more common. Enhancement is seen in approximately 44% of cases. Surrounding vasogenic edema is uncommon due to the tumor's slow-growing nature. Complete surgical resection is the recommended treatment of choice, although this is often not possible with involvement of vital brain structures such as the brainstem.

Hemangioblastoma

Hemangioblastomas are more common in adults than children, but in children, they are often seen in the setting of von Hippel–Lindau (VHL) disease. An estimated 25% to 40% of hemangioblastomas are associated with VHL syndrome. Hemangioblastomas are highly vascular and, with equal frequency, can present as a cystic mass with a mural nodule or a solid tumor. They frequently demonstrate a growth phase (characterized by enlargement) followed by a quiescent phase (a period of stabilization and arrested growth).

Spectrum of Disease

The spectrum of disease is detailed in the preceding section.

Pearls

- Posterior fossa tumors are common in children, with different differential considerations compared to adults.

- Cerebellar JPA most often presents as a cystic mass with enhancing mural nodule.
- Medulloblastoma is a highly cellular tumor with reduced diffusivity and variable enhancement. There are multiple subtypes with differing genetic signatures, imaging appearances, and clinical outcomes.
- Ganglioglioma is a rare infratentorial mass with variable imaging appearance.
- Hemangioblastoma is a cystic mass with enhancing mural nodule or purely solid enhancing mass that is seen in greater frequency in VHL syndrome. The enhancing nodule tends to be peripheral, along the pial surface.

Signs and Complications

- The limited space within the posterior fossa often leads to tumor presentation with hydrocephalus or herniation. Alternatively, patients may present with ataxia.

Suggested Readings

Camacho AC, Chaljub G, Uribe T, et al: MR imaging of pediatric posterior fossa tumors, *Contemp Diagn Radiol* 30(14):1–6, 2007.
D'Arco F, Khan F, Mankad K, et al: Differential diagnosis of posterior fossa tumours in children: new insights, *Pediatr Radiol* 48(13): 1955–1963, 2018.
Plaza MJ, Borja MJ, Altman N, et al: Conventional and advanced MRI features of pediatric intracranial tumors: posterior fossa and suprasellar tumors, *AJR Am J Roentgenol* 200(5):1115–1124, 2013.
Shin JH, Lee HK, Khang SK, et al: Neuronal tumors of the central nervous system: radiologic findings and pathologic correlation, *Radiographics* 22(5):1177–1189, 2002.
WHO Classification of Tumours Editorial Board. World Health Organization classification of tumours of the central nervous system. ed 5: Lyon: International Agency for Research on Cancer; 2021.

88
Pediatric Extraaxial Posterior Fossa Tumors

JENNIFER HUANG, MD, MED AND ASHA SARMA, MD

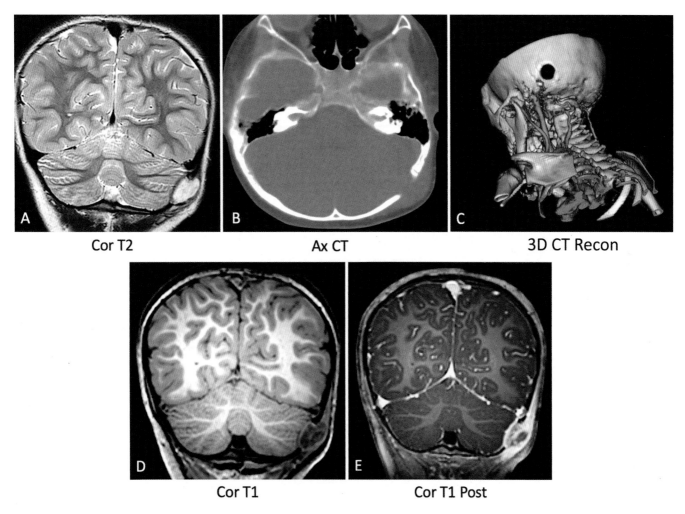

CASE A: A 4-year-old child presenting with lump over left occiput. *Ax*, Axial; *Cor*, coronal; *CT*, Computed tomography; *Recon*, Reconstruction.

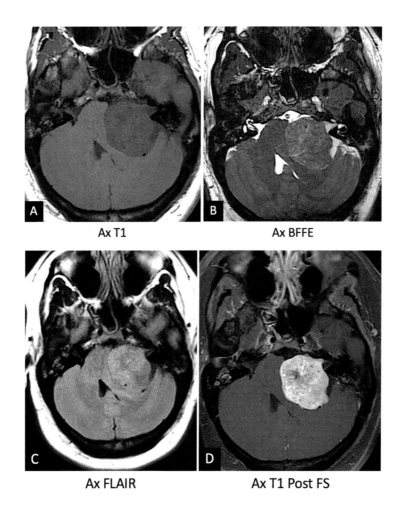

Ax T1

Ax BFFE

Ax FLAIR

Ax T1 Post FS

CASE B: An 18-year-old with headache. *Ax*, Axial; *BFFE*, balanced fast field echo; *FLAIR*, fluid attenuated inversion recovery; *FS*, fat saturated.

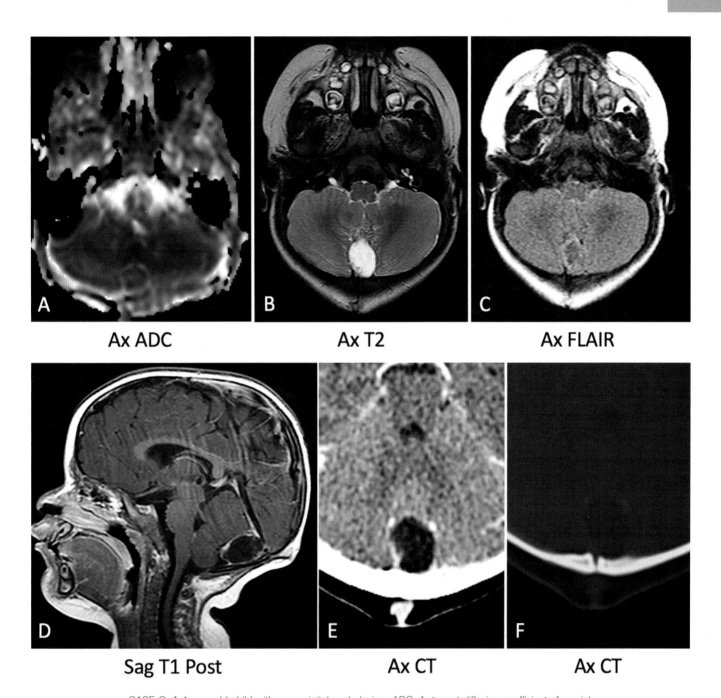

Ax ADC   **Ax T2**   **Ax FLAIR**

Sag T1 Post   **Ax CT**   **Ax CT**

CASE C: A 1-year-old child with an occipital scalp lesion. *ADC*, Apparent diffusion coefficient; *Ax*, axial; *CT*, Computed tomography; *FLAIR*, fluid attenuated inversion recovery; *Sag*, sagittal.

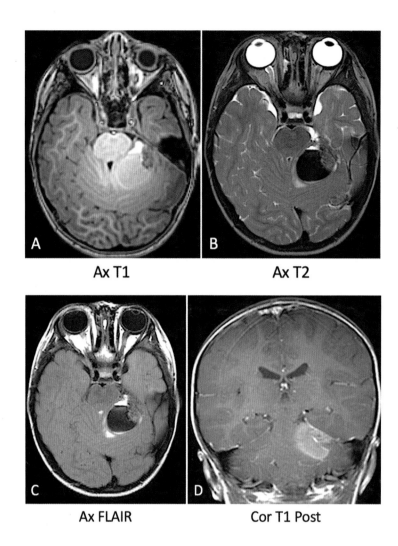

Ax T1

Ax T2

Ax FLAIR

Cor T1 Post

CASE D: A 2-year-old child with history of neuroblastoma who presents for follow-up magnetic resonance imaging (MRI). *Ax,* Axial; *Cor,* coronal; *FLAIR,* fluid attenuated inversion recovery.

DESCRIPTION OF FINDINGS

- Case A: Heterogeneously enhancing extraaxial mass involving the left occipital bone and scalp, with associated "punched-out" lytic appearance of bone lesion. Mild mass effect on the left cerebellar hemisphere and mild smooth dural enhancement of the underlying left cerebellar convexity dura.
- Case B: Relatively homogeneously enhancing mass in the region of the left cerebellopontine angle cistern, with a small portion extending into the left internal auditory canal. Moderate mass effect on the fourth ventricle and brainstem.
- Case C: Ovoid mass located inferior to and slightly to the left of the torcular herophili. Near-fluid isoattenuation on CT and isointensity on T2-weighted MRI, with incomplete suppression of signal on fluid-attenuated inversion recovery (FLAIR) images and reduced diffusivity. Small amount of patchy enhancement along the margins, likely normal veins, with no internal enhancement. CT more clearly depicts a corticated bony tract between the midline subcutaneous nodule and the subjacent posterior fossa cystic structure.
- Case D: Cystic and solid dural-based mass in the cerebellopontine angle. Hematocrit level within the cystic portion of the mass and mildly enhancing solid portion. Mild dural thickening and enhancement, along the tentorium with moderate mass effect on the pons, midbrain, and fourth ventricle. Minimal edema in the adjacent brain parenchyma.

Diagnosis

Case A: Langerhans cell histiocytosis (LCH)
Case B: Schwannoma
Case C: Epidermoid cyst in posterior fossa communicating with a scalp dermoid cyst
Case D: Metastatic neuroblastoma

Summary

Extraaxial posterior fossa masses in the pediatric population include LCH, epidermoid or dermoid inclusion cysts, arachnoid cysts, schwannomas, and metastases. Associated findings, including the nature of bone involvement and other intracranial and extracranial abnormalities as detailed below, are key in narrowing the differential diagnosis. CT and MRI may play complementary roles in lesions involving bone.

Langerhans Cell Histiocytosis

LCH is a common dendritic cell disorder in the pediatric population, with a wide range of possible organ involvement. Classic findings in the skull include "punched-out" lytic lesions with beveled edges, which result from asymmetric destruction of the inner and outer cortex, although a more permeative pattern is sometimes encountered. A solitary calvarial lesion is the most common manifestation. The bone lesion is often best characterized with CT. Curettage, steroid injections, or radiation therapy may be used to treat single skull lesions, although multiple skull lesions often warrant chemotherapy. Intracranial abnormalities, including absence of the posterior pituitary bright spot and enhancing infundibular thickening, may clinically manifest with diabetes insipidus and should be assessed for in affected patients with craniofacial lesions. Rarely, neurodegenerative brain parenchymal disease may be found, with characteristic abnormal T2 prolongation in the globi pallidi, pontine tegmentum, and cerebellar dentate nuclei. Another rare intracranial manifestation is a mass with enhancement, which may involve the meninges, choroid plexus, or basal ganglia. Outside the central nervous system (CNS), there may be additional involvement of bone, marrow, liver, lymph nodes, and/or spleen.

Schwannoma

Schwannomas are well-defined, enhancing tumors arising from Schwann cells. They are the most common tumor of peripheral nerves, including the cranial nerves (most commonly CN VIII—"vestibular schwannoma"). Although more common in adults, Children with neurofibromatosis type 2 may present with multiple schwannomas, although this is more commonly seen in adults. Vestibular schwannomas often present with smooth bone remodeling with enlargement of the porus acousticus and marginal bony sclerosis, indicating chronicity and benignity. Larger masses often show internal heterogeneity due to cystic degeneration or hemorrhage. Compared to meningiomas, calcification is rare in schwannomas. Schwannoma may be difficult to distinguish from neurofibroma when small, although an encapsulated mass that is eccentric relative to the affected nerve favors schwannoma. Although the "target" sign (describing the appearance on T2-weighted imaging of centrally low and peripherally high signal intensity) is classically associated with plexiform neurofibromas, it can also be seen in schwannoma. Clinical symptoms depend on the location of the tumor and are due to local mass effect or dysfunction of the nerve from which they arise. Malignant transformation is rare.

Dermoid/Epidermoid Inclusion Cyst

Intracranial epidermoid cysts can be congenital or acquired. Unlike epidermoid cysts, dermoid cysts contain dermal elements such as hair follicles and sweat glands. Both are lined by stratified squamous epithelium, but epidermoid cysts show reduced diffusivity, and dermoid cysts may follow attenuation or signal of fat CT or MR. Epidermoid cysts also demonstrate incomplete suppression on FLAIR imaging, aiding in distinction from arachnoid cyst. These lesions are characteristically nonenhancing, which differentiates them from neoplasm. The cerebellopontine angle is the most common location for intracranial epidermoid cysts, while dermoid cysts often arise at or near midline. Epidermoid cysts often insinuate between structures, encasing adjacent vessels and nerves, without causing vascular stenosis or occlusion. As in the case presented, sinus tracts connecting the intra- and extracranial tissues may be revealed by identification of defects traversing bone, which may be better seen on CT and/or fat-suppressed MRI sequences. Lesions with sinus tracts may present due to complicating meningitis.

Metastases

Extraaxial metastatic lesions are rare in the pediatric population. The most common associated pediatric malignancies are neuroblastoma, Ewing sarcoma, and rhabdomyosarcoma. In particular, neuroblastoma has a predilection for metastasis to the dura, with very rare involvement of the brain parenchyma. Involvement of the posterior fossa extraaxial space by metastatic sarcoma is rare and is most often due to osseous or dural involvement. A history of primary malignancy should raise concern for metastatic disease when an extraaxial posterior fossa mass is discovered.

Spectrum of Disease

The spectrum of disease is detailed in the preceding section.

Pearls

- LCH is a common multi-organ disorder in the pediatric population, with classic "punched-out" lytic calvarial lesions with beveled edges.
- Schwannoma is a slow-growing enhancing tumor that is often multiple in neurofibromatosis type 2.
- Epidermoid cysts demonstrate reduced diffusivity and incomplete suppression on FLAIR imaging. CT and fat-suppressed MRI may be helpful in identifying intracranial and extracranial communication via an associated sinus tract.

- A history of primary malignancy in a patient with extraaxial posterior fossa lesions should raise concern for metastatic disease.

Signs and Complications

- Lesions in the posterior fossa are at high risk for causing brainstem compression, hydrocephalus, or herniation due to limited space.

Suggested Readings

Beaman FD, Kransdorf MJ, Menke DM: Schwannoma: radiologic-pathologic correlation, *Radiographics* 24(5):1477–1481, 2004.

D'Ambrosio N, Lyo JK, Young RJ, et al: Imaging of metastatic CNS neuroblastoma, *AJR Am J Roentgenol* 194(5):1223–1229, 2010.

Poretti A, Meoded A, Huisman TAGM: Neuroimaging of pediatric posterior fossa tumors including review of the literature, *J Magn Reson Imaging* 35(1):32–47, 2012.

Smith AB, Smirniotopoulos JG, Horkanyne-Szakaly I: From the radiologic pathology archives: intraventricular neoplasms: radiologic-pathologic correlation, *Radiographics* 33(1):21–43, 2013.

Zaveri J, La Q, Yarmish G, et al: More than just Langerhans cell histiocytosis: a radiologic review of histiocytic disorders, *Radiographics* 34(7):2008–2024, 2014.

89

Midline Posterior Fossa Extraaxial Cystic Lesions

JUAN E. SMALL, MD, MSC, EMILY HAAS, MD, AND ASHA SARMA, MD

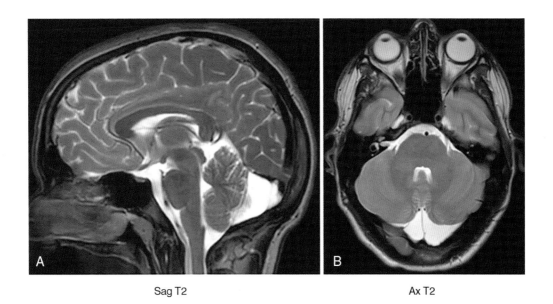

Sag T2   Ax T2

CASE A: A 17-year-old male presenting with an incidental finding on head CT after a motor vehicle accident. *Ax*, Axial; *Sag,* sagittal.

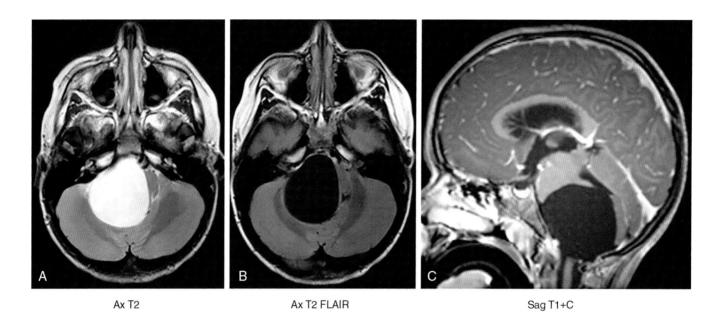

Ax T2   Ax T2 FLAIR   Sag T1+C

CASE B: A 4-year-old male presenting with headaches and vomiting for several weeks. *Ax,* Axial; *FLAIR,* fluid attenuated inversion recovery; *Sag,* sagittal; +*C,* postcontrast.

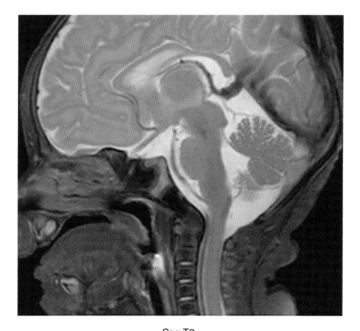

Sag T2

CASE C: A 3-week-old female presenting with short stature. *Sag,* sagittal.

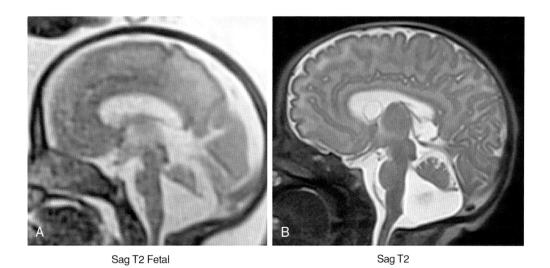

Sag T2 Fetal   Sag T2

CASE D: A newborn male with congenital abnormality diagnosed prenatally. *Sag,* sagittal.

DESCRIPTION OF FINDINGS

- Case A: Prominent retrocerebellar cerebrospinal fluid (CSF) space without mass effect or hydrocephalus. Normal vermis and posterior fossa.
- Case B: Large, round CSF isointense, nonenhancing cyst centered in the right cerebellopontine angle. Significant mass effect on the brainstem with effacement of the fourth ventricle and obstructive hydrocephalus. Structurally normal cerebellum.
- Case C: Prominent posterior fossa CSF space continuous with the mildly enlarged fourth ventricle. Dorsal rotation of the normally formed vermis.
- Case D: Marked vermian hypoplasia with dorsal rotation. Flattened fastigium. Absence of normal vermian fissural landmarks.

Diagnosis

Case A: Mega cisterna magna
Case B: Arachnoid cyst
Case C: Blake pouch cyst
Case D: Dandy–Walker malformation

Summary

When normally developed, the posterior fossa is predominantly filled by the brainstem and cerebellum, with only a small CSF-filled space (the *vallecula*) located inferior and posterior to the vermis and between the cerebellar hemispheres. When the CSF space is enlarged, the radiologist must be able to differentiate among various congenital variants and pathologies, as there is substantial variation in prognosis among entities.

Special attention to the appearance of the vermis and choroid plexus, as well as identification of any mass effect, helps to narrow the differential diagnosis. Key entities that will be discussed include mega cisterna magna, arachnoid cyst, Blake pouch cyst, and Dandy–Walker malformation. A key factor determining prognosis in affected patients is whether the cerebellum, particularly the cerebellar vermis, is normally formed.

Mega Cisterna Magna

The term *mega cisterna magna* refers to a prominent infra- or retrocerebellar CSF space with a normal vermis and fourth ventricle. The posterior fossa is either normal in size or enlarged, and there may be scalloping of the occipital bone. Mega cisterna magna is thought to result from delayed fenestration of Blake pouch during embryonic development, which is described in more detail below in the section covering Blake pouch cyst. Unlike Blake pouch cyst, mega cisterna magna is not continuous with an enlarged fourth ventricle and the vermis is not dorsally rotated. Unlike in arachnoid cyst, there is no mass effect. Mega cisterna magna can vary considerably in size but is typically of no clinical consequence, as the vast majority of affected patients develop normally.

Arachnoid Cyst

Arachnoid cyst is often the most easily diagnosed posterior fossa cyst based on characteristic mass effect. It is important

to note that there is no communication with the fourth ventricle, and the choroid plexus is normally in position with respect to the fourth ventricle. An arachnoid cyst appears as a CSF isointense, nonenhancing, space-occupying cyst with imperceptibly thin walls. If the cyst is large, there may be mass effect on the adjacent cerebellar hemisphere, vermis, or other posterior fossa or supratentorial structures. When the arachnoid cyst is inferior to the vermis, it may compress the inferior vermis and lead to diagnostic uncertainty; however, normal vermian fissural anatomy and relative proportions of the superior, posterior, and inferior vermian lobes may be recognizable and allow exclusion of inferior vermian hypoplasia.

Blake Pouch Cyst

Blake pouch is an embryologic structure formed from a midline evagination of the fourth ventricular roof and lined by ependyma, glia, and choroid plexus. In normal early fetal development, this fluid-filled structure along the inferior surface of the vermis ruptures and forms the median aperture (foramen of Magendie) that opens into the subarachnoid space. If this fenestration does not occur, the pouch continues to expand and eventually forms a midline posterior fossa cyst termed "Blake pouch cyst." This cyst can sometimes be difficult to differentiate from mega cisterna magna, arachnoid cyst, and Dandy–Walker malformation. The characteristic appearance is enlarged posterior fossa CSF space *in continuity* with an enlarged fourth ventricle (differentiating it from mega cisterna magna and arachnoid cyst) with a *dorsally rotated but structurally normal appearing vermis* (differentiating it from Dandy–Walker malformation). Although it has been stated that hydrocephalus is more common in Blake pouch cyst, it is not invariably present. Furthermore, hydrocephalus can also be associated with arachnoid cyst with mass effect or Dandy–Walker malformation. In addition, the choroid plexus in a Blake pouch cyst may sometimes be displaced into the cyst inferior and posterior to the vermis, whereas choroid plexus will be normally positioned in mega cisterna magna and arachnoid cyst (although this finding may not be visible unless thin-section high-resolution T2-weighted imaging is acquired). Because of frequent difficulty in distinguishing among mega cisterna magna, arachnoid cyst, and Blake pouch cyst, many investigators suggest that when the histologic identity of a posterior fossa cyst is unknown, descriptive language should be utilized in lieu of suggestion of a specific diagnosis. Regarding the clinical prognosis of a Blake pouch cyst, outcomes are typically favorable. Unfortunately, in some cases, it is difficult to differentiate Blake pouch cyst from Dandy–Walker malformation, especially on fetal imaging, due to distortion of the vermis.

Dandy–Walker Malformation

Dandy–Walker and related malformations are primarily characterized by abnormal development of the vermis, which is associated with developmental abnormalities. The spectrum of imaging findings is produced by dysgenetic development of the rhombencephalic roof. Classically, a Dandy–Walker malformation consists of an enlarged posterior fossa, an absent or marked hypoplastic vermis, and prominent cystic dilatation of the fourth ventricle. Newer research from the internation Dandy–Walker consortium has indicated that the diagnostic features are (1) the degree of vermian hypogenesis including the caudal severity gradient, (2) obtuse fastigial recess angle, (3) large tegmentovermian angle, (4) inferolateral displacement of tela choroidea and choroid plexus (when visible), and (5) "tail sign" (T2 hypointense line located along the inferior vermis). This group asserts that posterior fossa size should be eliminated from the diagnostic criteria, particularly on fetal imaging. It is crucial to note that the identification of a normal choroid plexus within the fourth ventricle/inferior medullary velum excludes Dandy–Walker malformation as a diagnostic consideration. Associated malformations that may be identified include callosal dysgenesis/agenesis, encephalocele, and migrational abnormalities. The term "Dandy–Walker variant" has been used in the past to label findings that do not meet criteria for Dandy–Walker malformation; however, it has been noted to cause confusion; therefore, interpreters are encouraged to use the umbrella term "Dandy–Walker complex" or (better yet) specifically describe the findings in this heterogeneous group of malformations. Recognizing that inferior vermian hypoplasia may exist without a cystic posterior fossa lesion is also important.

Spectrum of Disease

The spectrum of disease is detailed in the preceding section.

Differential Diagnosis

The differential diagnosis is detailed in the preceding section.

Pearls

The most important determinations to make in evaluating a prominent posterior fossa CSF space are:

- Is the posterior fossa normal or mildly enlarged, with no abnormality apart from the enlarged retrocerebellar CSF space? If so, consider mega cisterna magna.
- Is there a cyst with mass effect on an otherwise normal appearing fourth ventricle, with normal formation of the cerebellum? If so, consider arachnoid cyst.
- Is there a cyst in continuity with the fourth ventricle with dorsal rotation of a normal appearing vermis (sometimes associated with hydrocephalus)? If so, consider Blake pouch cyst.
- Is the cerebellum (especially the vermis) abnormal, is the choroid plexus displaced, and/or is "tail sign" present? If so, consider Dandy–Walker malformation (see Table 89.1).

Signs and Complications

Signs and complications are generally related to mass effect and associated malformations.

TABLE 89.1 Diagnostic Differentiating Features of Posterior Fossa Cystic Lesions

	Vermis	Fourth Ventricle	Associated Central Nervous System Malformations	Fourth Ventricle Choroid Plexus	Posterior Fossa Size	Hydrocephalus
Dandy–Walker complex	Agenetic or hypoplastic (especially the inferior vermis)	Cystic dilation, communicates with cyst	70% of the time	Inferolaterally displaced	Not considered important to diagnosis, but commonly enlarged	Often present at the time of diagnosis
Arachnoid cyst	Normal or compressed	Typically normal, may be compressed	Rarely	Normal	Normal or enlarged	Typically absent, unless the cyst is large and effaces the fourth ventricle
Blake pouch cyst	Normal	Enlarged	Rarely	Displaced (inferiorly and/or posteriorly)	Usually normal, although may be enlarged	Variable
Mega cisterna magna	Normal	Normal	None	Normal	Usually normal, although may be enlarged	Absent

Suggested Readings

Barkovich AJ, Raybaud C: *Pediatric neuroimaging*, ed 6, Philadelphia, 2018, Lippincott Williams & Wilkins.

Bosemani T, Orman G, Boltshauser E, et al: Congenital abnormalities of the posterior fossa, *Radiographics* 35(1):200–220, 2015.

Cornips EM, Overvliet GM, Weber JW, et al: The clinical spectrum of Blake's pouch cyst: report of six illustrative cases, *Childs Nerv Syst* 26(8):1057–1064, 2010.

De Nardi S, Porcu C, di Paolo PL, et al: Cystic lesion of posterior cranial fossa: is it Dandy-Walker?, *J Pediatr Neonat Individual Med* 7(1):e070104, 2018.

Kau T, Birnbacher R, Schwärzler P, et al: Delayed fenestration of Blake's pouch with or without vermian hypoplasia: fetal MRI at 3 tesla versus 1.5 tesla, *Cerebellum Ataxias* 6:4, 2019.

Kau T, Marterer R, Kottke R, et al: Blake's pouch cysts and differential diagnoses in prenatal and postnatal MRI: a pictorial review, *Clin Neuroradiol* 30(3):435–445, 2020.

Robinson AJ, Ederies MA: Diagnostic imaging of posterior fossa anomalies in the fetus, *Semin Fetal Neonatal Med* 21(5):312–320, 2016.

Schlatterer SD, Sanapo L, du Plessis AJ, et al: The role of fetal MRI for suspected anomalies of the posterior fossa, *Pediatr Neurol* 117:10–18, 2021.

Venkatesan C, Kline-Fath B, Horn PS, et al: Short- and long-term outcomes of prenatally diagnosed Dandy-Walker malformation, vermian hypoplasia, and Blake Pouch cyst, *J Child Neurol* 36(12):1111–1119, 2021.

Whitehead MT, Vezina G, Schlatterer SD, et al: Taenia-tela choroidea complex and choroid plexus location help distinguish Dandy-Walker malformation and Blake pouch cysts, *Pediatr Radiol* 51(8):1457–1470, 2021.

90

Pediatric Supratentorial Intraaxial Malignancies

ALEXANDRA M. FOUST, DO AND ASHA SARMA, MD

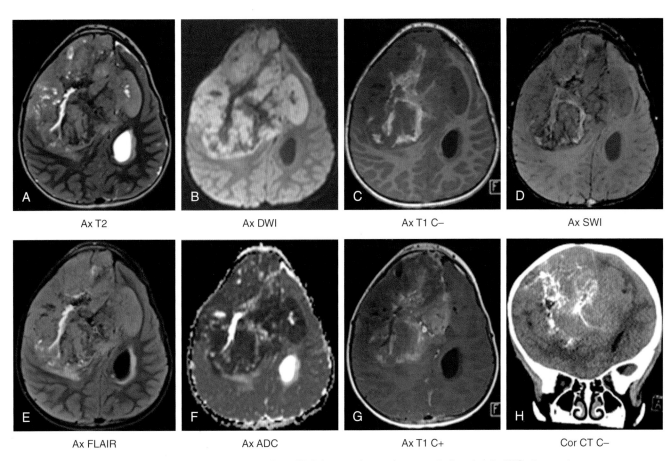

Ax T2   Ax DWI   Ax T1 C−   Ax SWI

Ax FLAIR   Ax ADC   Ax T1 C+   Cor CT C−

CASE A: A 4-year-old male presenting with left extremity weakness and altered gait. *ADC*, Apparent diffusion coefficient; *Ax*, axial; *Cor*, coronal; *CT*, Computed tomography; *DWI*, diffusion-weighted imaging; *FLAIR*, fluid attenuated inversion recovery; *SWI*, susceptibility-weighted imaging.

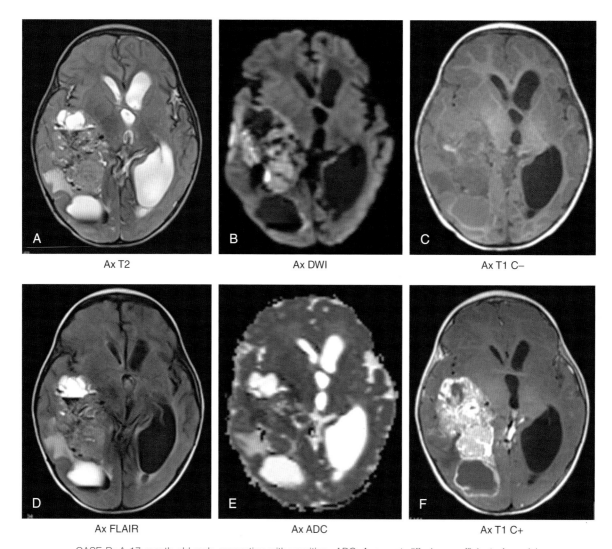

CASE B: A 17-month-old male presenting with vomiting. *ADC,* Apparent diffusion coefficient; *Ax,* axial; *DWI,* diffusion-weighted imaging; *FLAIR,* fluid attenuated inversion recovery.

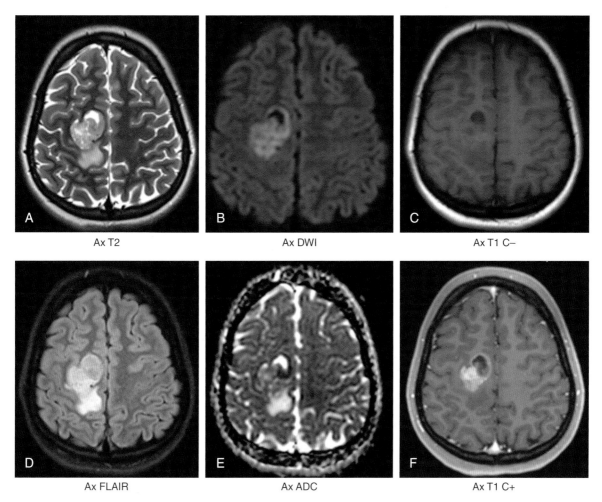

Ax T2

Ax DWI

Ax T1 C–

Ax FLAIR

Ax ADC

Ax T1 C+

CASE C: A 14-year-old female with left arm paresthesias and weakness. *ADC*, Apparent diffusion coefficient; *Ax*, axial; *DWI*, diffusion-weighted imaging; *FLAIR*, fluid attenuated inversion recovery.

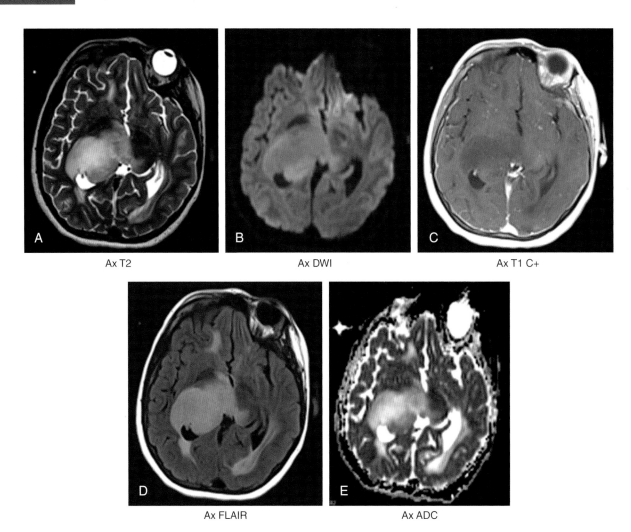

Ax T2

Ax DWI

Ax T1 C+

Ax FLAIR

Ax ADC

CASE D: A 12-year-old female presenting with left-sided weakness and personality change. *ADC*, Apparent diffusion coefficient; *Ax*, axial; *DWI*, diffusion-weighted imaging; *FLAIR*, fluid attenuated inversion recovery.

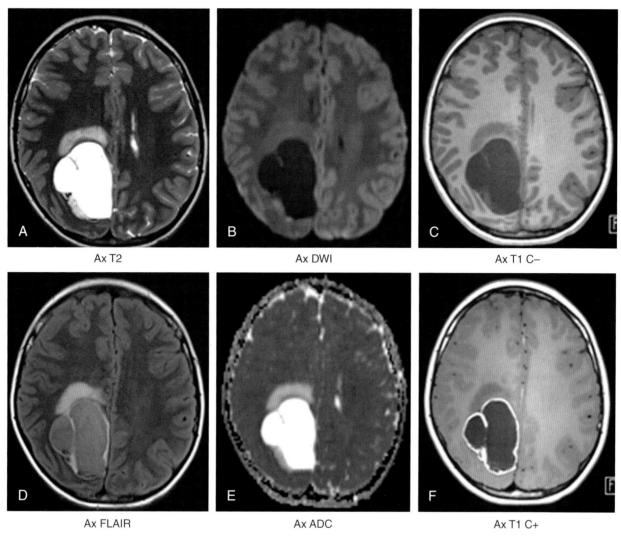

Ax T2   Ax DWI   Ax T1 C−

Ax FLAIR   Ax ADC   Ax T1 C+

CASE E: A 10-year-old male with worsening headaches associated with blurry vision. *ADC*, Apparent diffusion coefficient; *Ax*, axial; *DWI*, diffusion-weighted imaging; *FLAIR*, fluid attenuated inversion recovery.

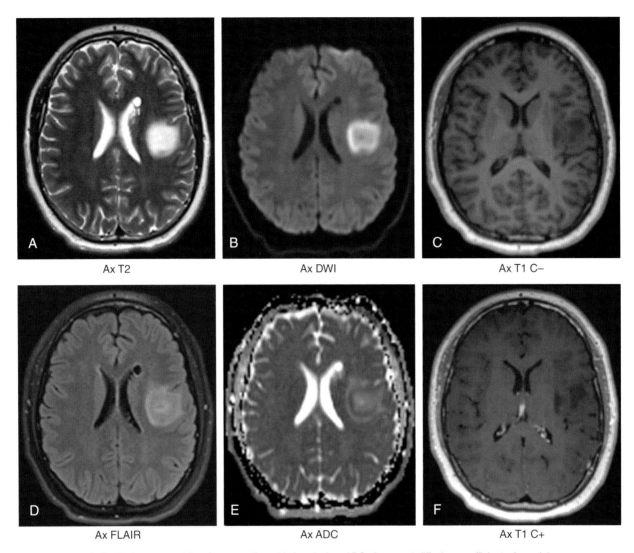

Ax T2

Ax DWI

Ax T1 C−

Ax FLAIR

Ax ADC

Ax T1 C+

CASE F: A 15-year-old male presenting with headache. *ADC,* Apparent diffusion coefficient; *Ax,* axial; *DWI,* diffusion-weighted imaging; *FLAIR,* fluid attenuated inversion recovery.

DESCRIPTION OF FINDINGS

- Case A: Large, heterogeneous intraaxial right frontal lobe mass with T1 shortening (C), mild enhancement (G), and internal hyperattenuation (H)/ magnetic susceptibility artifact (D) consistent with extensive calcification. Relatively low signal on T2 WI (A, E) and reduced diffusivity (B, F), connoting hypercellularity. Small area of central necrosis (A).
- Case B: Large heterogeneous intraaxial mass centered in the right temporoparietal region, with solid and cystic components. The solid component demonstrates marked reduced diffusivity (B, E) and avid enhancement on postcontrast imaging (F). Incomplete suppression on FLAIR and hematocrit levels are seen in the cystic components (A, D, E). Axial T2 fluid-attenuated inversion recovery (FLAIR) weighted image (D) demonstrates peritumoral edema.
- Case C: Right frontal solid and cystic intraaxial mass that demonstrates avid enhancement on postcontrast imaging (F). The cystic focus is peripherally located (A, D) and there is marked peritumoral edema (D). The solid portion of the tumor demonstrates marked reduced diffusivity (B, E), while the area of surrounding vasogenic edema shows facilitated diffusivity.
- Case D: Large, infiltrative-appearing intraaxial mass centered in the right thalamus, extending into the left thalamus and right periventricular white matter. Mixed hypointense and hyperintense appearance on T2 WI (A, D), and mixed reduced and facilitated diffusivity (B, E). Minimal adjacent edema (D). No intralesional enhancement (C).
- Case E: Right parietal intraaxial tumor with cystic and nodular appearance. Incomplete suppression of the "cyst" contents on FLAIR (A, D), with avid enhancement of the rim (F). Avid enhancement (F) and reduced diffusivity (B, E) of the solid nodular portion of the tumor located posterolaterally. Small amount of adjacent vasogenic edema (D).
- Case F: Nonenhancing (C, F), T2 hyperintense (A, D) intraaxial left temporal mass with peripheral reduced diffusivity and central facilitated diffusivity (B, E). Minimal peritumoral edema (D). Small unrelated periventricular cysts are noted adjacent to the left frontal horn (A, D).

Diagnosis

Case A: Embryonal tumor with multilayered rosettes
Case B: Atypical teratoid/rhabdoid tumor
Case C: Supratentorial ependymoma (*ST-EPN-C11orf95*)
Case D: Diffuse midline glioma (*H3 K27-altered*)
Case E: Pediatric-type high-grade glioma (*H3-wildtype; IDH-wildtype*)
Case F: Oligodendroglioma (*1p19q co-deleted, IDH2-mutant*)

Summary

Large, aggressive-appearing intraaxial supratentorial neoplasms tend to be difficult to differentiate from one another by MRI. Many exhibit characteristics such as findings of hypercellularity (hyperattenuation on CT, relatively hypointense signal on T2-weighted imaging, and low apparent diffusion coefficient (*ADC*), necrosis, hemorrhage or calcification, perilesional edema, and propensity for leptomeningeal dissemination. This summary focuses on selected distinctive features, acknowledging that histopathologic and genetic evaluation of tissue is essentially always needed for definitive diagnosis in current practice. Although a specific diagnosis cannot often not be determined by imaging alone, a cogent neuroradiological differential diagnosis is helpful.

The discovery of specific gene mutations associated with pediatric brain tumors has led to development of new molecular targeted therapies. In response, the 2021 World Health Organization (WHO) classification of central nervous system (CNS) neoplasms update focuses on an integrated classification of pediatric brain tumors, which includes molecular profile, histologic features, and tumor grade. It is important for neuroradiologists to be aware of both imaging features and molecular profile when approaching pediatric supratentorial intraaxial malignancies, as these findings often have bearing on important clinical factors such as treatment decision-making and risk of recurrence and metastasis.

Embryonal tumors with multilayered rosettes (ETMRs) are rare embryonal tumors that are associated with amplification or gain of the C19MC region of chromosome 19, or alterations in *DICER1*. These aggressive tumors are most frequently reported as large intraaxial supratentorial masses, though they can also occur in the posterior fossa and spinal canal. On CT and MRI, these tumors often exhibit features of hypercellularity and calcification. Different from many high-grade tumors, there is a tendency toward minimal peritumoral edema and minimal or no postcontrast enhancement. Intratumoral veins connected to cortical veins have been described.

Atypical teratoid/rhabdoid tumors (ATRTs) are aggressive embryonal neoplasms most frequently occurring in infants and young children. These tumors are generally intraaxial, arising in the supra- or infratentorial compartments, or rarely, the spinal canal. Leptomeningeal tumor dissemination may be present at diagnosis. At the molecular level, biallelic mutations in *SMARCB1*, or rarely *SMARCA4*, are identified. Generally, ATRTs tend to appear heterogeneous, with features of hypercellularity, intratumoral hemorrhage, peripheral cysts, variable calcification, and heterogeneous band-like enhancement. More recently, radiogenomic description of three molecular subgroups has been published, based on DNA methylation profiles and gene expression patterns: ATRT-MYC (myelocytomatosis oncogene), ATRT-TYR (tyrosine), and ATRT-SHH (sonic hedgehog).

Supratentorial ependymomas are neuroepithelial tumors characterized by gene fusions on chromosome 11. These are subdivided into those involving ZFTA (zinc finger translocation associated gene, formerly *CR11orf95*) fusions and those involving YAP1 (yes-associated protein 1). Although these two subgroups are not reliably differentiated by imaging, they have important prognostic implications, with YAP1 fusions having a better prognosis than ZFTA fusions. Supratentorial ependymomas are most often intraaxial hemispheric tumors, though they can also be periventricular or intraventricular in location. They tend to be cystic and solid masses, with variable proteinaceous content within peripheral tumoral cysts that sometimes leads to areas of T1 hyperintensity. Calcifications, hemorrhage, and necrosis are not uncommon, and peritumoral edema is typically present. Enhancement of solid components tends to be avid, though heterogeneous.

Pediatric supratentorial high-grade gliomas are members of the newly defined *pediatric-type diffuse high-grade glioma* group in WHO 2021 CNS tumors, which is comprised of four tumor types: *diffuse midline glioma, H3 K27-altered; diffuse hemispheric glioma, H3 G34-mutant; diffuse pediatric-type high-grade glioma, H3-wildtype and IDH-wildtype; and infant-type hemispheric glioma.* MRI reveals a hypercellular-appearing tumor, often with internal necrosis, peritumoral edema, and variable hemorrhage. Solid components often demonstrate moderate to strong enhancement, although the degree of enhancement does not correlate with tumor grade.

Diffuse midline gliomas, H3 K27-altered are members of the new tumor group of *pediatric-type diffuse high-grade gliomas* in the WHO 2021 CNS neoplasm update. This tumor type includes diffuse intrinsic pontine gliomas and midline non-brainstem high-grade gliomas that are characterized genetically by H3 K27 alteration (histone mutation). Supratentorial histone-mutant gliomas often present as large midline thalamic or bithalamic masses that may extend into the brainstem. Tumors tend to be hyperintense on T2/FLAIR MRI and are often well defined, with little or no perilesional edema. Contrast enhancement is variable, and areas of necrosis and hemorrhage may be observed. Mass effect is common and aqueductal compression may result in obstructive hydrocephalus.

Pediatric oligodendrogliomas (pODGs) are rare intraaxial CNS neoplasms in the pediatric population, accounting for approximately 1% of pediatric brain tumors. Genetic mutations in pediatric tumors are more variable compared to those in adult tumors (1p19q co-deletion and isocitrate dehydrogenase 1 [IDH1] mutations). pODGs are generally low-grade hemispheric tumors arising in temporal lobes or frontal lobes, although 19% of cases are extracortical in location. On imaging, pODGs often contain calcifications and exhibit variable enhancement. Diffusion-weighted imaging characteristics vary according to tumor grade.

Spectrum of Disease

Although less common than posterior fossa tumors, supratentorial intraaxial neoplasms do occur in the pediatric population, including several of the high-grade lesions discussed in this chapter. As with other pediatric tumors, age and location can be helpful in narrowing the differential diagnosis. For example, a large supratentorial mass in an infant would be concerning for an ATRT, ETMR, or some other form of embryonal tumor, while an expansile midline mass would be suspicious for a histone-mutant diffuse glioma. Additional features, such as the presence or absence of peritumoral edema, calcification, and/or contrast enhancement, can also be helpful.

Differential Diagnosis

1. ETMRs
2. ATRT
3. Supratentorial ependymoma
4. Diffuse midline glioma, H3 K27-altered
5. Other pediatric-type diffuse high-grade gliomas
6. Oligodendroglioma

Pearls

- Embryonal tumors such as ETMR and ATRT are highest on the differential diagnosis for large, aggressive-appearing supratentorial masses in infants and young children.
- Unlike posterior fossa ependymomas, pediatric supratentorial ependymomas are more likely to be hemispheric and extraventricular in location.
- H3 K27 alteration is the key molecular feature of diffuse midline gliomas, which include thalamic gliomas and diffuse intrinsic pontine gliomas.

Signs and Complications

Supratentorial intraaxial malignancies have a variable clinical presentation largely dictated by location and degree of related mass effect. Many of the high-grade intraaxial supratentorial neoplasms have a propensity for leptomeningeal dissemination; thus, MRI of the entire neural axis should be performed when one of these tumors is encountered.

Suggested Readings

Aboian MS, Solomon DA, Felton E, et al: Imaging characteristics of pediatric diffuse midline gliomas with histone H3 K27M mutation, *AJNR Am J Neuroradiol* 38(4):795–800, 2017.

AlRayahi J, Zapotocky M, Ramaswamy V, et al: Pediatric brain tumor genetics: what radiologists need to know, *Radiographics* 38(7):2102–2122, 2018.

Braunstein S, Raleigh D, Bindra R, et al: Pediatric high-grade glioma: current molecular landscape and therapeutic approaches, *J Neurooncol* 134(3):541–549, 2017.

Dangouloff-Ros V, Tauziede-Espariat A, Roux CJ, et al: CT and multimodal MR imaging features of embryonal tumors with multilayered rosettes in children, *AJNR Am J Neuroradiol* 40(4):732–736, 2019.

Goel NJ, Abdullah G, Lang S: Outcomes and prognostic factors in pediatric oligodendroglioma: a population-based study, *Pediatr Neurosurg* 53(1):24–35, 2018.

Gutierrez DR, Jones C, Varlet P, et al: Radiological evaluation of newly diagnosed non-brainstem pediatric high-grade glioma in the HERBY phase II trial, *Clin Cancer Res* 26(8):1856–1865, 2020.

Li YX, Aibaidula A, Shi Z, et al: Oligodendrogliomas in pediatric and teenage patients only rarely exhibit molecular markers and patients have excellent survivals, *J Neurooncol* 139(2):307–322, 2018.

Louis DN, Perry A, Wesseling P, et al: The 2021 WHO classification of tumors of the central nervous system: a summary, *Neuro Oncol* 23(8):1231–1251, 2021.

Meyers SP, Khademian ZP, Biegel JA, et al: Primary intracranial atypical teratoid/rhabdoid tumors of infancy and childhood: MRI features and patient outcomes, *AJNR Am J Neuroradiol* 27(5):962–971, 2006.

Nowak J, Junger ST, Huflage H, et al: MRI phenotype of RELA-fused pediatric supratentorial ependymoma, *Clin Neuroradiol* 29(4):595–604, 2019.

Nowak J, Nemes K, Hohm A, et al: Magnetic resonance imaging surrogates of molecular subgroups in atypical teratoid/rhabdoid tumor, *Neuro Oncol* 20(12):1672–1679, 2018.

Wagner MW, Poretti A, Huisman TAGM, et al: Conventional and advanced (DTI/SWI) neuroimaging findings in pediatric oligodendroglioma. *Childs Nerv Syst* 31(6):885–891, 2015.

Wang B, Gogia B, Fuller GN, et al: Embryonal tumor with multilayered rosettes, C19MC-altered: clinical, pathological, and neuroimaging findings, *J Neuroimaging* 28(5):483–489, 2018.

WHO Classification of Tumours Editorial Board: World Health Organization Classification of Tumours of the Central Nervous System, ed 5, Lyon, 2021, International Agency for Research on Cancer.

91
Occipital Cephalocele

JUAN E. SMALL, MD, MSC, EMILY HAAS, MD, AND ASHA SARMA, MD

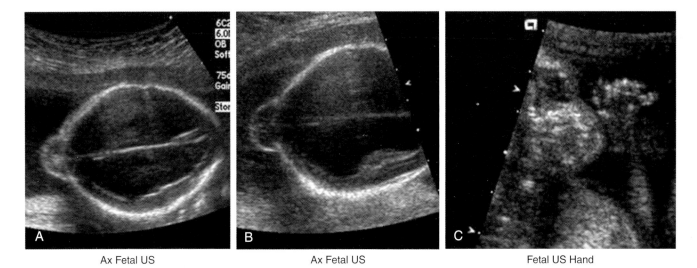

| Ax Fetal US | Ax Fetal US | Fetal US Hand |

CASE A: A 25-week-old gestational age fetus with cystic enlargement of the kidneys (not shown). *Ax*, Axial; *US*, ultrasound.

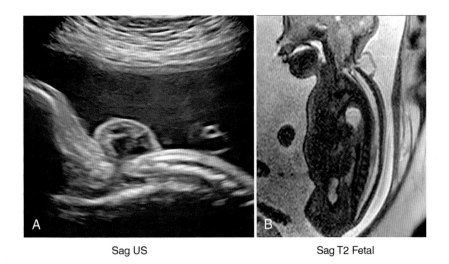

| Sag US | Sag T2 Fetal |

CASE B: A 34-week-old gestational age fetus with craniocervical abnormalities on early prenatal ultrasound. *Sag*, sagittal; *US*, ultrasound.

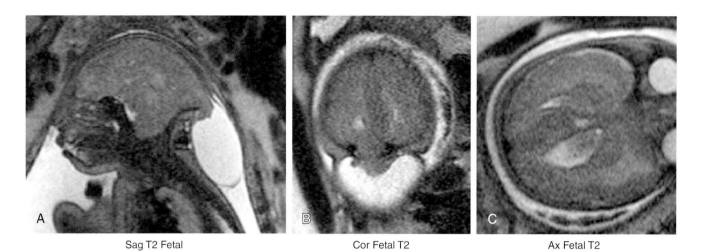

Sag T2 Fetal   Cor Fetal T2   Ax Fetal T2

CASE C: A 35-week-old gestational age fetus with ocular abnormalities. *Ax,* Axial; *Cor,* coronal; *Sag,* sagittal.

DESCRIPTION OF FINDINGS

- Case A: Occipital encephalocele, postaxial polydactyly. The history of cystic renal enlargement in conjunction with postaxial polydactyly and an occipital encephalocele is diagnostic.
- Case B: High cervical encephalocele containing herniated cervical spinal cord tissue. Small posterior fossa with hindbrain herniation.
- Case C: Occipital meningoencephalocele with a large cephalocele sac extending inferiorly. Cobblestone malformation, including a thickened, smooth cortex with only minimal shallow sulci and irregularity of the gray-white matter junction. The brainstem is dysmorphic.

Diagnosis

Case A: Meckel–Gruber syndrome
Case B: Chiari III malformation
Case C: Walker–Warburg syndrome

Summary

A cephalocele is defined as a skull defect with extracranial protrusion of intracranial contents. Cephalocele represents a form of neural tube defect and may be further classified by the intracranial contents it contains. A meningocele includes meninges and cerebrospinal fluid (CSF), while an encephalocele contains meninges, CSF, and brain parenchyma. An atretic cephalocele is a midline scalp nodule containing meninges, dysplastic brain tissue, and fibrous tissue (Fig. 91.1). In general, cephaloceles may be primary/congenital or secondary (i.e., posttraumatic or postsurgical). Congenital cephaloceles are typically midline abnormalities and most commonly occur in the occipital region (70% to 80% of cases). Less common locations include frontoethmoidal, cranial vault, and skull base. Most occipital cephaloceles are readily detected on prenatal ultrasound or are identified as occipital masses at birth.

Many patients with occipital cephaloceles present with associated anomalies or syndromes; however, cephaloceles can exist in isolation as well. The primary differential diagnosis for an occipital cephalocele includes simple occipital encephalocele, Meckel–Gruber syndrome, Chiari III malformation, and Walker–Warburg syndrome, among other rare syndromes. The primary consideration upon discovery of an occipital cephalocele in the fetal or neonatal setting is the identification of associated abnormalities, which can guide prognostication and assist in narrowing the differential diagnosis. Microcephaly is commonly seen with larger cephaloceles (Fig. 91.2). Associated malformations of cortical development, midline anomalies, and venous sinus anomalies are very common.

Meckel–Gruber Syndrome

Meckel–Gruber syndrome is an autosomal recessive syndrome characterized by renal, extremity, and brain abnormalities. Specifically, cystic dysplastic kidneys, postaxial polydactyly, and occipital encephalocele are considered the classic triad on imaging. In addition, microcephaly, cleft lip and palate, cardiac anomalies, hepatic fibrosis, and oligohydramnios are associated with Meckel–Gruber syndrome. Identification of the cephalocele late in pregnancy may be difficult in the presence of severe associated oligohydramnios. Prognosis is very poor, and the disease is typically fatal at birth due to pulmonary hypoplasia and renal failure.

Chiari III Malformation

The Chiari III malformation is extremely rare and is the most severe of the Chiari malformations. High cervical/occipital cephalocele in conjunction with hindbrain herniation is the imaging hallmark of this condition. Only cases that involve the upper cervical spinal canal should be classified as Chiari III malformations. Accordingly, some investigators believe that this condition should be considered a high cervical myelocystocele. The cerebellum (and sometimes the brainstem) herniates

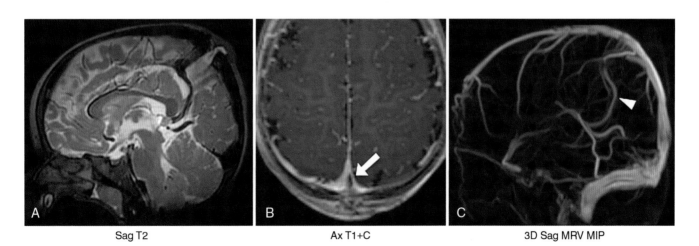

Sag T2   Ax T1+C   3D Sag MRV MIP

• **Fig. 91.1** Small CSF-containing midline parietal scalp lesion consistent with an atretic cephalocele. There is associated fenestration of the superior sagittal sinus (*arrow*) with a persistent falcine sinus (*arrowhead*). *Ax*, Axial; *MIP*, Maximum Intensity Projection; *MRV*, magnetic resonance venography; *Sag*, sagittal.

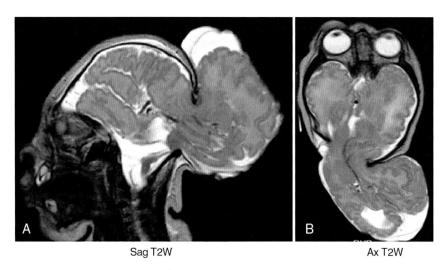

Sag T2W   Ax T2W

• **Fig. 91.2** Large occipital encephalocele with significant microcephaly and flattening of the forehead. There is marked architectural distortion of the brain parenchyma. Flow voids are also seen traversing the occipital defect. MRA/MRV should be performed in cases such as this to evaluate the positions of the major intracranial vessels, which is a vital step in surgical treatment planning. *Ax,* Axial; *MRA,* magnetic resonance angiography; *MRV,* magnetic resonance venography.

into the cephalocele sac. Dysgenesis/hypogenesis of the corpus callosum is often also seen.

Walker–Warburg Syndrome

Walker–Warburg syndrome is a rare multisystem form of congenital muscular dystrophy (in the category of alpha-dystroglycanopathies) characterized by muscle disease as well as brain and eye abnormalities. The typical brain abnormalities seen in this syndrome are cobblestone cortical malformation, occipital cephalocele, and cerebellar hypoplasia and dysplasia with associated small cysts. Multiple other associated brain abnormalities have been reported, including callosal dysgenesis/hypoplasia and Dandy–Walker malformation. The major diagnostic criteria (of Dobyns) include (1) lissencephaly, (2) cerebellar malformation, (3) retinal dysplasia, and (4) congenital muscular dystrophy. Prognosis is extremely poor, as death usually occurs within the first months of life. Correspondingly, the imaging diagnosis occurs in the fetal or neonatal period. It is noteworthy that the normal developing fetal brain remains relatively agyric and smooth until approximately 16 weeks of gestation. It is only after this stage in development that the absence of developing sulci and gyri should raise the suspicion of cobblestone malformation, which is described in the chapter covering malformations of cortical development (Chapter 101). In addition, a characteristic brainstem "kink" is usually observed in the dorsal pons and ventral cervicomedullary junction ("Z-shaped brainstem"; Fig. 91.3).

Spectrum of Disease

The spectrum of disease is detailed in the preceding section.

Differential Diagnosis

Care should be taken not to confuse a cervical lymphatic malformation (formerly known as cystic hygroma) with a cephalocele sac. Assessment of continuity of intracranial and/or cervical spinal canal contents and detection of a bone defect are key findings.

Pearls

- The primary consideration when presented with an occipital cephalocele in the fetal or neonatal setting is the exclusion of associated abnormalities.
- When the cephalocele is the only abnormality, a simple occipital cephalocele is diagnosed.
- The presence of cystic dysplastic kidneys, postaxial polydactyly, and an occipital cephalocele suggests the diagnosis of Meckel–Gruber syndrome.
- Hindbrain herniation with an associated high cervical/occipital cephalocele suggests a Chiari III malformation.
- The presence of ocular abnormalities and cobblestone lissencephaly in conjunction with an occipital cephalocele or cerebellar hypoplasia suggests the diagnosis of Walker–Warburg syndrome.

Signs and Complications

Evaluation of an occipital cephalocele should include evaluation of the adjacent venous sinuses, because the superior sagittal sinus and torcula may be found within the cephalocele sac (Fig. 91.4). Ventricular herniation into the cephalocele may result in a trapped ventricle or hydrocephalus.

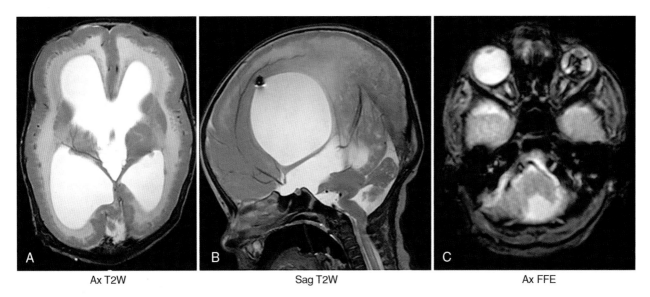

| Ax T2W | Sag T2W | Ax FFE |

• **Fig. 91.3** Severe hydrocephalus with cobblestone malformation in a patient with Walker-Warburg syndrome. Sagittal T2W image shows cerebellar hypoplasia and characteristic "kinking" of the brainstem Note small cerebellar cysts in B. Axial FFE image demonstrates left-sided microphthalmia with intravitreal hemorrhage. *Ax*, Axial; *FFE*, fast field echo; *Sag*, sagittal.

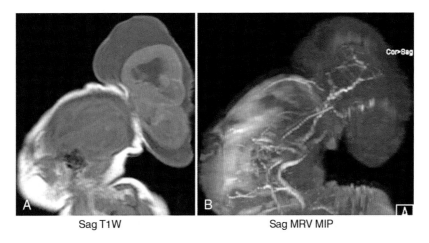

| Sag T1W | Sag MRV MIP |

• **Fig. 91.4** Large occipital encephalocele containing a large amount of brain parenchyma. MR venography *(MRV)* maximum intensity projection *(MIP)* image shows the encephalocele containing portions of the transverse, straight, and superior sagittal sinuses. *Sag*, sagittal.

Suggested Readings

Atlas SW: *Magnetic resonance imaging of the brain and spine*, ed 5, Philadelphia, 2016, Lippincott Williams & Wilkins.

Barkovich AJ, Raybaud C: *Pediatric neuroimaging*, ed 6, Philadelphia, 2018, Lippincott Williams & Wilkins.

Chen CP: Meckel syndrome: genetics, perinatal findings, and differential diagnosis, *Taiwan J Obstet Gynecol* 46(1):9–14, 2007.

Khurana S, Saini V, Wadhwa V, et al: Meckel-Gruber syndrome: ultrasonographic and fetal autopsy correlation, *J Ultrasound* 20(2):167–170, 2017.

Lacalm A, Nadaud B, Massoud M, et al: Prenatal diagnosis of cobblestone lissencephaly associated with Walker-Warburg syndrome based on a specific sonographic pattern, *Ultrasound Obstet Gynecol* 47(1):117–122, 2016.

Low AS, Lee SL, Tan AS, et al: Difficulties with prenatal diagnosis of the Walker-Warburg syndrome, *Acta Radiol* 46(6):645–651, 2005.

Markovic I, Bosnjakovic P, Milenkovic Z: Occipital encephalocele: cause, incidence, neuroimaging and surgical management, *Curr Pediatr Rev* 16(3):200–205, 2019.

Pejic M, Luecke K, Meoded A, et al: Pediatric cephaloceles: a multimodality review, *Appl Radiol* 49(5):26–32, 2020.

92

Congenital Brainstem Abnormalities

ALEXANDRA M. FOUST, DO AND ASHA SARMA, MD

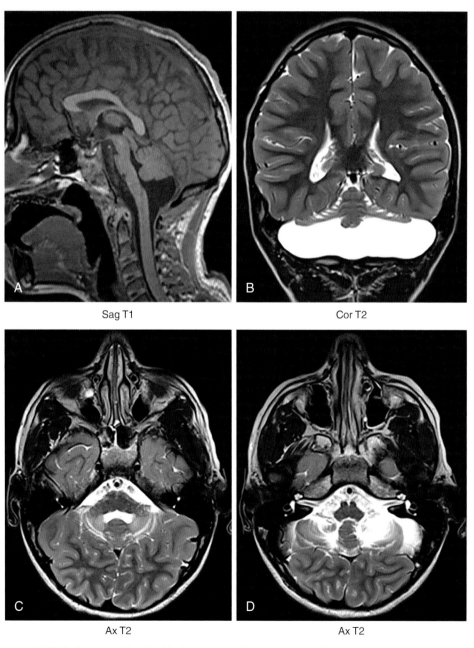

Sag T1

Cor T2

Ax T2

Ax T2

CASE A: A 6-year-old male with developmental delay. *Ax*, Axial; *Cor*, coronal; *Sag*, sagittal.

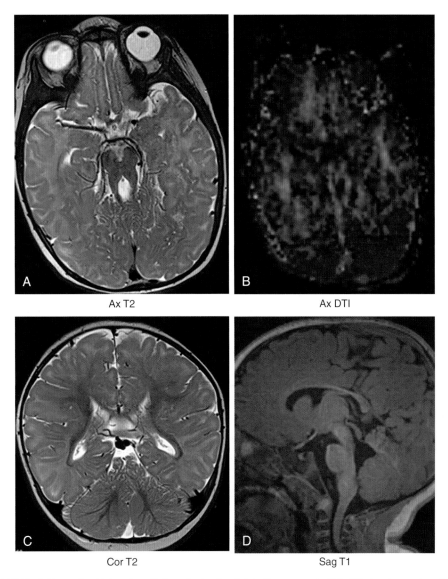

CASE B: A 5-month-old female with hypotonia. *Ax*, Axial; *Cor*, coronal; *DTI*, diffusion tensor imaging; *Sag*, sagittal.

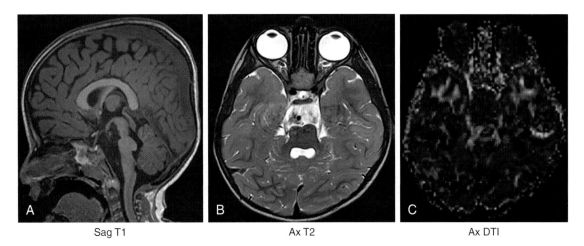

CASE C: A 2-year-old female with developmental delay, unilateral facial palsy, abnormal eye movements, and failure to thrive. *Ax*, Axial; *DTI*, diffusion tensor imaging; *Sag*, sagittal.

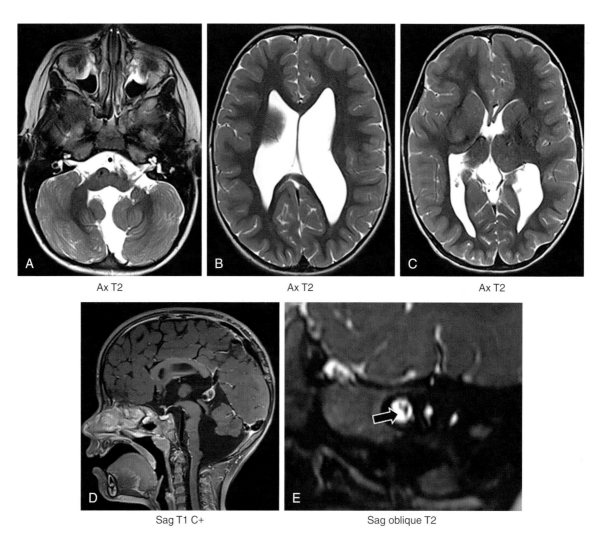

Ax T2   Ax T2   Ax T2

Sag T1 C+   Sag oblique T2

CASE D: A 2-year-old female with developmental delay. *Ax*, Axial; *Sag*, sagittal.

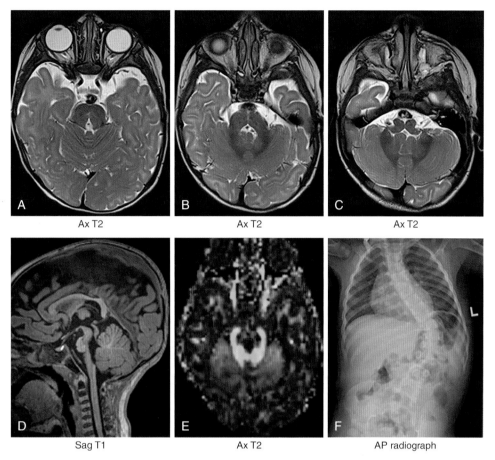

Ax T2 Ax T2 Ax T2

Sag T1 Ax T2 AP radiograph

CASE E: A 7-month-old male with left-sided weakness and horizontal nystagmus. *Ax*, Axial; *Sag*, sagittal.

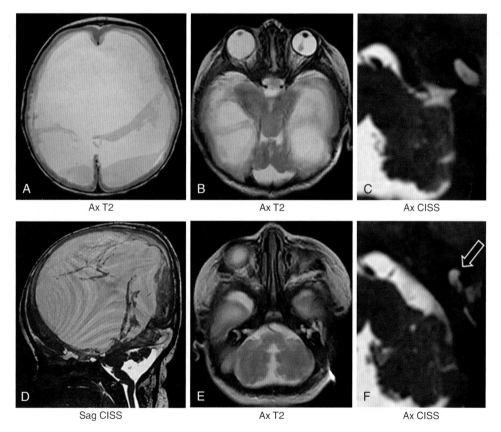

Ax T2 Ax T2 Ax CISS

Sag CISS Ax T2 Ax CISS

CASE F: A 3-month-old male with fever and history of congenital hydrocephalus. *Ax*, Axial; *CISS*, constructive interference in steady state; *Sag*, sagittal.

DESCRIPTION OF FINDINGS

- Case A: Marked hypoplasia of the pons (A), with shortening of both length and width. Severe cerebellar hypoplasia disproportionately involving the cerebellar hemispheres relative to the vermis (B, C, D) resulting in a "dragonfly" appearance. Prominent cerebrospinal fluid (CSF) collection inferior to the cerebellum.
- Case B: Deep interpeduncular cistern (A, D) and thick, elongated, and horizontally orientated superior cerebellar peduncles giving rise to a "molar tooth" appearance of the midbrain (A). Absence of the normal "red-dot" corresponding to the superior cerebellar decussation in the midbrain (B) on diffusion tensor color fractional anisotropy map. Dysplastic vermis, which is deficient inferiorly with dysplastic nodular appearance superiorly (C, D). Dysmorphic cerebellar hemispheres (C).
- Case C: Hypoplastic midbrain and ventral pons with a dorsal "cap"-like protrusion of the dorsal pons (A). Splayed superior cerebellar peduncles (B), which are not as elongated or horizontally oriented as in Joubert syndrome. Abnormally positioned "red line" of transverse pontine fibers crossing through the dorsal cap (C) on the diffusion tensor imaging color fractional anisotropy map, rather than through the mid-pontine tegmentum.
- Case D: Hypoplastic pons with crossed asymmetry (right side larger than left) and a ventral cleft (A). Small medulla and mild inferior vermian hypoplasia with an uplifted cerebellar vermis (D). Supratentorially, bilateral perisylvian malformations of cortical development (B), dysmorphic lateral ventricles (B, C) and enlarged, dysmorphic appearing basal ganglia with poor demarcation between structures (C). Absent right cochlear nerve (*black arrow*, E).
- Case E: Hypoplasia of the pons (A, B, D) and medulla (C, D) with a deep sagittal cleft of the dorsal pons extending from the fourth ventricle (A) and resulting in a split appearance of the mid-pons (B). The "red-dot" of the superior cerebellar decussation is absent and the transverse pontine fibers are ventrally displaced (E). The medullary pyramids have a splayed appearance resulting in a butterfly-like appearance of the medulla (C). There is moderate-to-severe levoscoliotic curvature of the thoracolumbar spine (F).
- Case F: Severe dilatation of the lateral ventricles (A, B, D) with intraventricular debris related to ventriculitis (unrelated to congenital malformation). "Cobblestone lissencephaly" cortical malformation with agyria (A, B). Dysmorphic midbrain with fusion of the colliculi and tectum (B, D), resulting in an absent cerebral aqueduct. Combined with a kinked pontomesencephalic junction, this results in a "Z-shaped" configuration of the brainstem (D). Hypoplastic inferior vermis and dorsally rotated small, dysmorphic cerebellar hemispheres (D, E) with tiny cysts (C, F). Normal cochlear basal turns (C), but with small and offset middle and apical turns (*black arrow*, F). Persistent hyperplastic primary vitreous is noted in the left globe (B).

Diagnosis

Case A: Pontocerebellar hypoplasia
Case B: Joubert syndrome ("molar tooth" malformation), pathogenic mutation in *AHI1*
Case C: Pontine tegmental cap dysplasia
Case D: Tubulinopathy, *TUBB3* mutation
Case E: Horizontal gaze palsy and progressive scoliosis, *ROBO3* mutation
Case F: Walker–Warburg Syndrome, mutation in *ISPD* gene

Summary

Congenital brainstem malformations are relatively uncommon. They are often accompanied by additional supratentorial and infratentorial abnormalities, most commonly of the cerebellum, given its common embryologic origin with the brainstem. Although there is some imaging overlap among these disorders, some characteristic brainstem appearances (i.e., "molar tooth" midbrain, dorsal pontine "cap", crossed asymmetry, and "Z-shape") can aid in narrowing the differential diagnosis.

Pontocerebellar Hypoplasia

The term pontocerebellar hypoplasia refers to a rare group of inherited autosomal recessive disorders characterized by volume loss of the brainstem and cerebellum with a prenatal onset. Imaging reveals hypoplasia, often with superimposed atrophy, of the brainstem and cerebellum, although the pattern and potential for progression of volume loss depend upon the underlying genetic mutation and disease subtype. Some of the subtypes demonstrate disproportionate atrophy of the cerebellar hemispheres relative to the vermis, resulting in a "dragonfly" appearance (Case A, image B). Absence of the expected cerebellar vermis lobulation is another potential finding. Associated supratentorial abnormalities may include agenesis of the corpus callosum, a simplified gyral pattern, and hypomyelination. Ultimately, diagnosis requires correlation with clinical and genetic evaluation as the imaging findings are not specific and can occur with other genetic (e.g., *CASK* mutation and disorders of congenital glycosylation) and acquired etiologies (e.g., sequelae of prenatal parenchymal injury/infection).

Molar Tooth Malformation

Joubert syndrome is an autosomal recessive disorder caused by several different genetic mutations (resulting in the term "Joubert syndrome–related disorders") that result in dysfunction of the primary cilium during embryogenesis. Consequently, there is impaired neuronal proliferation and axonal migration. The underlying ciliary dysfunction also results in additional systemic abnormalities involving the renal, hepatic, ocular, and skeletal systems. MRI of the brain demonstrates elongated, thick, horizontally oriented superior cerebellar peduncles and a deep interpeduncular cistern, resulting in the classic "molar tooth" appearance of the midbrain on axial images. The midbrain itself may also demonstrate elongation and thickening in association with a small pons. The underlying abnormality in axonal migration can be appreciated on diffusion tensor color fractional anisotropy maps by the absence of the normal "red-dot" of the superior cerebellar decussation in the center of the midbrain. The cerebellar vermis is generally hypoplastic and/or dysplastic (often with a coronal cleft) and, in some cases, completely absent. Supratentorial abnormalities occur in up to 30% of cases and include dysgenesis of the corpus callosum, ventriculomegaly, cephaloceles, migrational disorders, and hippocampal malrotation.

Pontine Tegmental Cap Dysplasia

Pontine tegmental cap dysplasia is a rare sporadic brainstem malformation with a characteristic imaging appearance of a small and flattened ventral pons and prominent vaulted dorsal tegmentum along the floor of the fourth ventricle ("pontine tegmental cap"). Diffusion tensor imaging reveals ectopic transverse pontine fibers centered within the "pontine tegmental cap." The superior cerebellar peduncles may be splayed and/or elongated and the middle and inferior cerebellar peduncles are generally small or, in some cases, completely absent. Cerebellar vermian hypoplasia is generally present and the inferior olivary nuclei are often hypoplastic or absent. Temporal bone abnormalities are common and include duplication of the internal auditory canals, vestibulocochlear or cochlear nerve aplasia, and aberrant course of the facial nerve. Associated systemic manifestations include vertebral segmentation anomalies and congenital heart defects.

Tubulinopathy

The term "tubulinopathy" describes a spectrum of brain malformations caused by mutations in the tubulin genes, resulting in altered microtubule structure and function. This results in abnormal neuronal migration and organization. Variable brainstem abnormalities are frequently present, including asymmetry (either homolateral or crossed), clefts, and pontine hypoplasia. Brainstem abnormalities on diffusion tensor imaging are also frequent, including a small superior cerebellar peduncle decussation, fusion of the corticospinal tracts and medial lemnisci, and thinned/altered transverse pontine fibers. The cerebellar vermis is usually hypoplastic, and dysplasia of the cerebellar hemispheres is common. Supratentorial abnormalities include variable commissural dysgenesis/agenesis and malformations of cortical development. Dysmorphic, incompletely separated striatal nuclei and absence of the internal capsule anterior limb are helpful distinctive features.

Horizontal Gaze Palsy and Progressive Scoliosis

Horizontal gaze palsy and progressive scoliosis are a rare autosomal recessive disorder caused by mutation of the *ROBO3* gene, which encodes a protein required for normal axonal guidance. MRI of the brain reveals hypoplasia of the pons and medulla. The medulla has a characteristic "butterfly"-shaped appearance on axial images, secondary to absent gracile and cuneate nuclear prominences and prominence of the inferior olivary nuclei relative to the medullary pyramids. Additionally, a dorsal midline cleft in the pons with absent facial nuclear prominences results in a "split pons" appearance. On diffusion tensor imaging, the expected decussations of the corticospinal tracts, pontine sensory tracts, and superior cerebellar peduncles are frequently absent. Spine imaging demonstrates progressive childhood scoliosis.

Dystroglycanopathies

Walker–Warburg syndrome is the most severe form of congenital muscular dystrophy, a group of autosomal recessive disorders affecting the brain, muscles, and eyes. These disorders are caused by mutations in genes responsible for glycosylation of α-dystroglycan (hence the collective term "dystroglycanopathies"). Fukuyama congenital muscular dystrophy and muscle-eye-brain disease are

the less severe forms. Imaging reveals a dysmorphic brainstem with fused colliculi, a small pons with or without a ventral cleft, and typical "Z-shape" of the brainstem caused by kinking of the pontomesencephalic and pontomedullary junctions. The cerebellar vermis is hypoplastic and the cerebellar hemispheres are often small and dysmorphic, containing tiny subcortical cysts. Supratentorial abnormalities include cobblestone malformation of the cerebral cortex, hypomyelination of the cerebral white matter, and hydrocephalus. In the orbit, buphthalmos and microphthalmia are the most common manifestations, although persistent hyperplastic primary vitreous, retinal detachment, vitreous hemorrhage, and colobomas have also been observed. Temporal bone imaging frequently demonstrates bilateral cochlear hypoplasia type 4, characterized by a small cochlea with a normal basal turn and hypoplastic, anteriorly offset middle and apical turns.

Spectrum of Disease

The spectrum of disease is detailed in the preceding sections.

Differential Diagnosis

1. In utero vascular insult or infection
2. Pontocerebellar hypoplasia
3. Joubert syndrome–related disorders
4. Pontine tegmental cap dysplasia
5. Tubulinopathies
6. Horizontal gaze palsy and progressive scoliosis
7. Dystroglycanopathies—Walker–Warburg syndrome
8. CHARGE syndrome

Pearls

- Congenital brainstem malformations frequently occur in conjunction with additional anomalies of the cerebellum and supratentorial brain, and thus should prompt a careful search for additional abnormalities.
- Thick horizontally oriented superior cerebellar peduncles and a deep interpeduncular cistern result in the classic "molar tooth" appearance of the midbrain in Joubert syndrome–related disorders.
- A small, flattened ventral pons and prominent dorsal tegmental cap along the floor of the fourth ventricle are characteristic of pontine tegmental cap dysplasia.
- Brainstem asymmetry with or without a brainstem cleft, in addition to dysmorphic striatal nuclei, absent anterior limb of internal capsule, and cortical malformations, is suggestive of a tubulinopathy.
- A "Z-shaped" brainstem, cobblestone cortical malformation, dysplastic cerebellum with subcortical cysts, and ocular abnormalities are common imaging features of Walker–Warburg syndrome and other dystroglycanopathies.

Signs and Complications

The signs and complications are detailed in the preceding sections.

Suggested Readings

Alharbi S, Alhashem A, Alkuraya F, et al: Neuroimaging manifestations and genetic heterogeneity of Walker-Warburg syndrome in Saudi patients, *Brain Dev* 43(3):380–388, 2021.

Arrigoni F, Romaniello R, Peruzzo D, et al: The spectrum of brainstem malformations associated to mutations of the tubulin genes family: MRI and DTI analysis, *Eur Radiol* 29:770–782, 2019.

Bosemani T, Orman G, Boltshauser E, et al: Congenital abnormalities of the posterior fossa, *Radiographics* 35(1):200–220, 2015.

Nixon JN, Dempsey JC, Doherty D, et al: Temporal bone and cranial nerve findings in pontine tegmental cap dysplasia, *Neuroradiology* 58:179–187, 2016.

Poretti A, Boltshauser E, Huisman TAGM: Cerebellar and brainstem malformations, *Neuroimaging Clin N Am* 26:341–357, 2016.

Rüsch CT, Bolsterli BK, Kottke R, et al: Pontocerebellar hypoplasia: a pattern recognition approach, *Cerebellum* 19:569–582, 2020.

Sarma A, Heck JM, Ndolo J, et al: Magnetic resonance imaging of the brainstem in children, part 1: imaging techniques, embryology, anatomy and review of congenital conditions, *Pediatr Radiol* 51:172–188, 2021.

Talenti G, Robson C, Severino MS, et al: Characteristic cochlear hypoplasia in patients with Walker-Warburg syndrome: A radiologic study of the inner ear in α-dystroglycan-related muscular disorders, *AJNR Am J* 42(1):167–172, 2021.

93

Congenital Cerebellar Abnormalities

ALEXANDRA M. FOUST, DO AND ASHA SARMA, MD

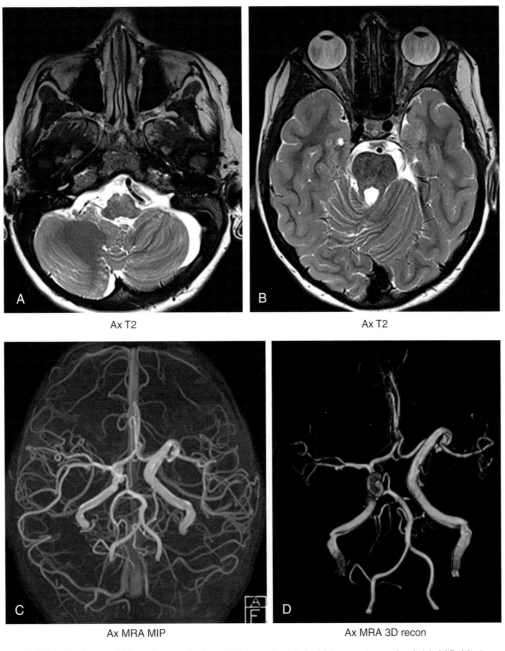

Ax T2

Ax T2

Ax MRA MIP

Ax MRA 3D recon

CASE A: An 8-year-old female with ataxia and history of a left facial hemangioma. *Ax*, Axial; *MIP*, Maximum Intensity Projection; *MRA*, magnetic resonance angiography; *Recon*, reconstruction.

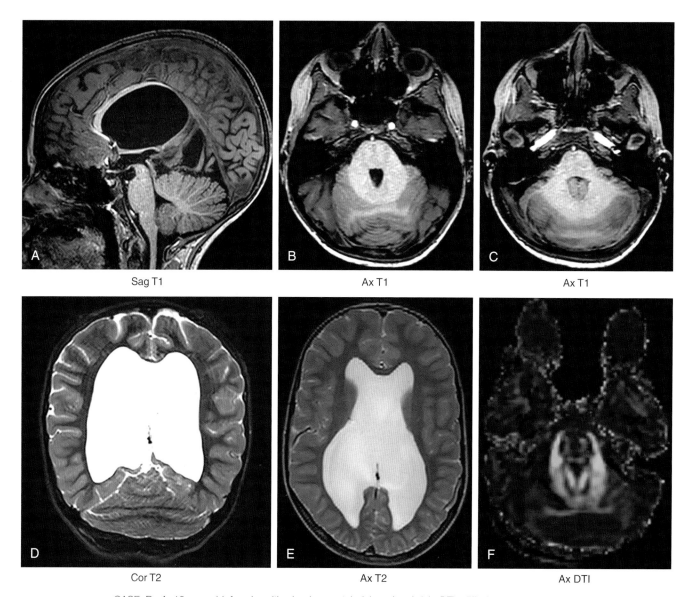

Sag T1   Ax T1   Ax T1

Cor T2   Ax T2   Ax DTI

CASE B: A 10-year-old female with developmental delay. *Ax*, Axial; *DTI*, diffusion tensor imaging; *Sag*, sagittal.

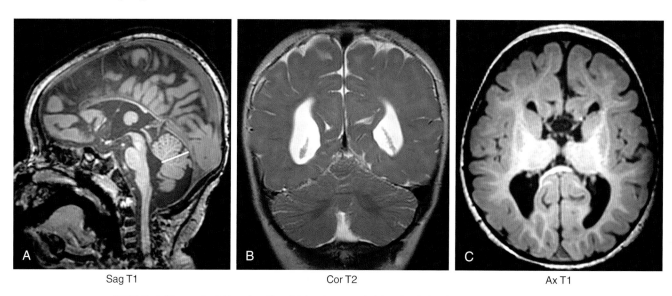

Sag T1   Cor T2   Ax T1

CASE C: A 22-month-old female with mild developmental delay. *Ax*, Axial; *Cor*, coronal; *Sag*, sagittal.

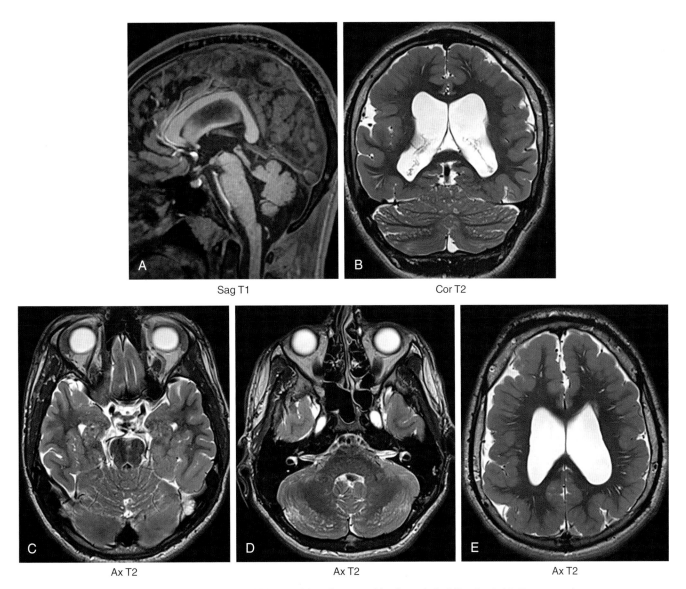

Sag T1

Cor T2

Ax T2

Ax T2

Ax T2

CASE D: A 14-year-old male with intractable epilepsy and intellectual disability. *Ax*, Axial; *Cor*, coronal; *Sag*, sagittal.

DESCRIPTION OF FINDINGS

- Case A: Hypoplasia and distortion of the left cerebellar hemisphere and asymmetric prominent left preauricular fatty tissue with a few small flow voids at site of involuted hemangioma (A, B). Dilated tortuous internal carotid arteries (ICAs) with an unusual course of the left ICA.
- Case B: Complete absence of normal vermian structures (A, B, C), thinned callosal body with absent splenium (A), aqueductal stenosis (A), and ventriculomegaly (A, D, E). Absent septum pellucidum (E). Continuity of the cerebellar folia (D) and white matter tracts (B, C, F) across the midline and "keyhole"-shaped fourth ventricle (B).
- Case C: Mildly dorsally rotated cerebellar vermis with smaller inferior half (A, B; line drawn from fastigial point through declive in (A) and mild blunting of the fastigial recess (A). Hypogenesis of the corpus callosum with absent rostrum and genu and thinned body and splenium (A, C). Simplified gyral pattern (C).
- Case D: Dysmorphic superior cerebellar vermis, mild flattening of the ventral pons, and vertical dysmorphic appearing splenium of the corpus callosum (A). Symmetric thickened cortex with extensive symmetric thickened cobblestone cortex of the frontal and parietal lobes (B, E), with relative sparing of the temporal lobes (C). Diffuse cerebellar dysplasia with nodular, abnormal appearing cerebellar folia with small interspersed cerebellar cysts, most pronounced superiorly (B, C, D).

Diagnosis

Case A: PHACE syndrome
Case B: Rhombencephalosynapsis
Case C: Vermian hypoplasia and additional anomalies in a patient with *1q43q44* deletion.
Case D: Cerebellar dysplasia and cortical malformation in a patient with pathologic *GPR56* mutation

Summary

Although the cerebellum is best known for its role in motor coordination, congenital cerebellar malformations are associated with a much broader range of neurodevelopmental disabilities, including deficits in cognition, social behavior, and language. Furthermore, while congenital cerebellar anomalies can occur in isolation, they are frequently associated with other anomalies of the cerebrum, corpus callosum, and brainstem. Thus, neuroradiologists must carefully scrutinize other brain regions when a cerebellar malformation is encountered. Finally, although not covered in this chapter, it is important to remember that in utero cerebellar injuries (e.g., related to germinal matrix hemorrhage or vascular insults) are an important differential consideration when evaluating an abnormal appearing cerebellum in a pediatric patient. When present, encephalomalacia, gliosis, and peripheral cerebellar magnetic susceptibility artifact can help differentiate in utero injury from genetic causes of hypoplasia. However, accurate distinction is not always possible. Many congenital and acquired cerebellar disorders involve both the brainstem and the cerebellum due to shared embryologic origin and intertwined white matter pathways. Pontocerebellar hypoplasia and Joubert syndrome and related disorders are two such conditions that are discussed in Chapter 92.

PHACE Syndrome

PHACE is a neurocutaneous syndrome that stands for *Posterior* fossa brain malformations, *H*emangioma, *A*rterial anomalies, *C*ardiac defects, and *E*ye anomalies. Occasionally, *S*ternal cleft/*S*upraumbilical raphe is also included in descriptions of this association (PHACES). Neuroimaging studies are often requested in children with segmental facial hemangiomas in order to assess for concurrent intracranial vascular, orbital, and brain parenchymal malformations that may occur with PHACE. The most frequent structural brain abnormality is unilateral cerebellar hypoplasia, sometimes with vermian hypoplasia. Frequently, the cerebellar hemisphere ipsilateral to the facial hemangioma is hypoplastic. Dandy–Walker malformations are less commonly associated. Selected key findings on MRI/MRA include intracranial arterial anomalies, such as vascular aplasia/hypoplasia or progressive steno-occlusive disease, tortuous ectatic or anomalous vascularity, aneurysms, and persistent embryonic vascular connections.

Rhombencephalosynapsis

Rhombencephalosynapsis is defined by continuity of the cerebellar hemispheres across the midline and can be further classified depending on the degree of associated vermian hypoplasia (partial) or aplasia (complete). Cases are generally sporadic and frequently co-occur with other midline abnormalities, including absence of the septum pellucidum, holoprosencephaly, callosal dysgenesis, thalamic fusion, or fusion of the midbrain colliculi. Commonly associated aqueductal stenosis often results in hydrocephalus. MRI reveals partial or complete absence of the cerebellar vermis. On midline sagittal images, landmarks of normal vermian architecture, such as the primary fissure, cannot be identified. The cerebellar folia and fissures continue without interruption across the midline on axial and coronal images. The fourth ventricle has a dysmorphic "keyhole" appearance in the axial plane, and the dentate nuclei are often fused.

Vermian Hypoplasia and Related Disorders

Inferior vermian hypoplasia, defined as a small, underdeveloped vermis, can occur in conjunction with other cerebral and cerebellar malformations or in isolation; the latter scenario is associated with better neurodevelopmental outcomes. Although the term "inferior vermian hypoplasia" remains in common usage, recent evidence suggests that deficiency of any of the 10 parts of the vermis may result in a reduced vermian craniocaudal dimension. MRI demonstrates a small uplifted cerebellar vermis, often with a tegmento-vermian angle between 25 and 45 degrees, possible blunting of the fastigial recess, and an enlarged fourth ventricle with inferiorly displacement of the fourth ventricle choroid plexus. Normally, a line drawn between the fastigial point of the fourth ventricle and declive roughly bisects the cerebellum on the midline sagittal image. In inferior vermian hypoplasia, the superior portion of the vermis is relatively larger. Distinction between inferior vermian hypoplasia and Blake pouch cyst may be difficult in some cases (see also Chapter 89).

Cerebellar Dysplasia

The term cerebellar dysplasia can be defined as abnormal cerebellar cortex foliation, fissuration, or white matter arborization and can result from genetic mutations, often co-occurring with supratentorial manifestations such as polymicrogyria, cobblestone malformation, or callosal dysgenesis. Alternatively, dysplasia may result from an in utero insult (e.g., infectious, toxic, or vascular). Normally the cerebellar fissures and white matter bundles are radially oriented from the deep cerebellar nuclei on coronal images, running parallel to the calvarium on axial images. In cerebellar dysplasia, MRI may reveal focal or diffuse irregularity of the cerebellar foliar pattern or more subtle altered orientation of the cerebellar fissures. Subcortical cerebellar cysts, in addition to cerebellar dysplasia and frontoparietal polymicrogyria or cobblestone malformation, are frequently encountered in cases of *GPR56* mutation and also in disorders with muscular dystrophy (dystroglycanopathies).

Spectrum of Disease

The spectrum of disease is detailed in the preceding sections.

Differential Diagnosis

1. In utero cerebellar injury
2. PHACE syndrome
3. Rhombencephalosynapsis
4. Inferior vermian hypoplasia
5. Joubert syndrome
6. Pontocerebellar hypoplasia
7. Cerebellar dysplasia
8. Dystroglycanopathies
9. Chiari I malformation
10. Chiari II malformation

Pearls

- Congenital cerebellar malformations frequently occur in conjunction with additional anomalies of the brainstem and supratentorial brain, and thus should prompt a careful search for additional abnormalities.
- Cerebellar malformations may be the result of an in utero disruption (infection, toxin exposure, vascular insult) making acquired etiologies an important differential consideration.
- In rhombencephalosynapsis, the cerebellar hemispheres are continuous across the midline and the cerebellar vermis is either hypoplastic (partial) or absent (complete).
- In inferior vermian hypoplasia, there is less vermian tissue below than above the fastigial point-declive line on mid-sagittal images.

Signs and Complications

The signs and complications are detailed in the preceding sections.

Suggested Readings

Bahi-Buisson N, Poirier K, Boddaert N, et al: GPR56-related bilateral frontoparietal polymicrogyria: further evidence for an overlap with the cobblestone complex, *Brain* 133(11):3194–3209, 2010.

Barkovich AJ, Raybaud C. Neurocutaneous disorders. In Barkovich AJ, Raybaud C, editors, *Pediatric neuroimaging*, ed 6, 685–687, Philadelphia, 2019, Wolters Kluwer.

Kau T, Birnbacher R, Schwärzler P, et al: Delayed fenestration of Blake's pouch with or without vermian hypoplasia: fetal MRI at 3 tesla versus 1.5 tesla, *Cerebellum Ataxias* 6(1):2–7, 2019.

Paladini D, Donarini G, Parodi S, et al: Hindbrain morphometry and choroid plexus position in differential diagnosis of posterior fossa cystic malformations, *Ultrasound Obstet Gynecol* 54(2):207–214, 2019.

Pinchefsky EF, Accogli A, Shevell MI, et al: Developmental outcomes in children with congenital cerebellar malformations, *Dev Med Child Neurol* 61(3):350–358, 2019.

Poretti A, Boltshauser E, Huisman TAGM: Pre- and postnatal neuroimaging of congenital cerebellar abnormalities, *Cerebellum* 15(1):5–9, 2016.

Razek AAKA, Castillo M: Magnetic resonance imaging of malformations of midbrain-hindbrain, *J Comput Assist Tomogr* 40(1):14–25, 2016.

Robinson AJ: Inferior vermian hypoplasia - preconception, misconception, *Ultrasound Obstet Gynecol* 43(2):123–136, 2014.

Steiner JE, McCoy GN, Hess CP, et al: Structural malformations of the brain, eye, and pituitary gland in PHACE syndrome, *Am J Med Genet A* 176(1):48–55, 2018.

Whitehead MT, Choudhri AF, Grimm J, et al: Rhombencephalosynapsis as a cause of aqueductal stenosis: an under-recognized association in hydrocephalic children, *Pediatr Radiol* 44(7):849–856, 2014.

94

Holoprosencephaly

JUAN E. SMALL, MD, MSC, EMILY HAAS, MD, AND ASHA SARMA, MD

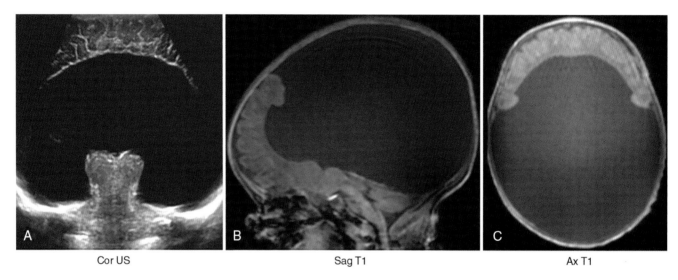

| Cor US | Sag T1 | Ax T1 |

CASE A: A 1-day-old male. Clinical concern for hydrocephalus. *Ax,* Axial; *Cor,* coronal; *Sag,* sagittal; *US,* ultrasound.

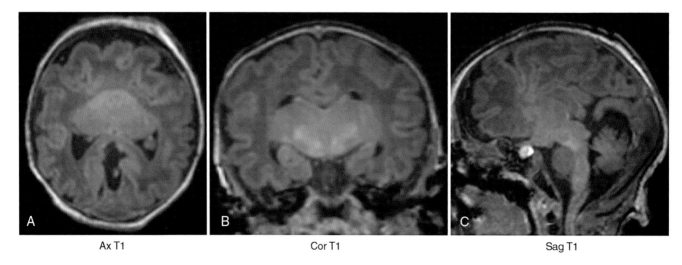

| Ax T1 | Cor T1 | Sag T1 |

CASE B: A 3-day-old female with intracranial abnormalities diagnosed on prenatal ultrasound. *Ax,* Axial; *Cor,* coronal; *Sag,* sagittal.

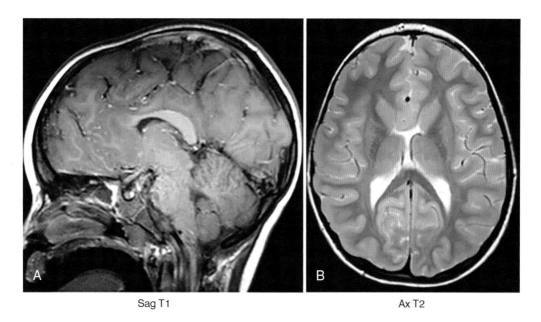

Sag T1   Ax T2

CASE C: A 4-year-old female with a seizure disorder. *Ax,* Axial; *Sag,* sagittal.

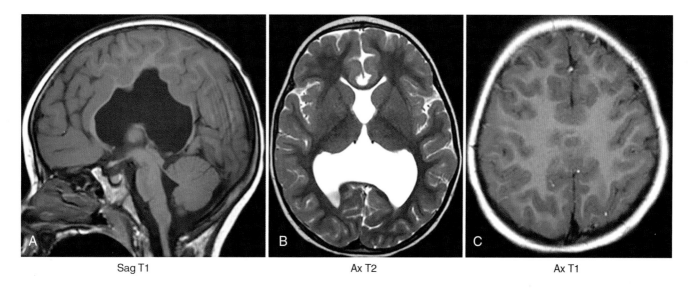

Sag T1   Ax T2   Ax T1

CASE D: A 2-year-old female with gait instability and vomiting. *Ax,* Axial; *Sag,* sagittal.

DESCRIPTION OF FINDINGS

- Case A: Crescent-shaped mantle of brain parenchyma ("pancake" brain) anteriorly with a large monoventricle/dorsal cyst. Absence of the interhemispheric fissure, septum pellucidum, and corpus callosum. Thalamic fusion, best demonstrated on the coronal US image. Significant mass effect exerted on the posterior fossa and brainstem by the large monoventricle/dorsal cyst.
- Case B: Underdevelopment and complete fusion of the frontal lobes with absence of the anterior corpus callosum and frontal horns of the lateral ventricles. At least partial thalamic fusion and some formation of the posterior interhemispheric fissure, falx, and posterior lateral ventricles.
- Case C: Absence of the genu of the corpus callosum with a truncated anterior body. Dysplastic frontal horns of the lateral ventricles with absent septum pellucidum as well as absent anterior interhemispheric falx. Azygous anterior cerebral artery. Fusion of the inferior frontal lobes, with the cortical ribbon crossing midline.
- Case D: Dysgenesis of the corpus callosum with essentially absent callosal body. Thinning of the genu and splenium. Absence of the septum pellucidum with a dysmorphic monoventricle and partial hemispheric fusion of the posterior frontal and anterior parietal lobes.

Diagnosis

Case A: Alobar holoprosencephaly
Case B: Semilobar holoprosencephaly
Case C: Lobar holoprosencephaly
Case D: Syntelencephaly (middle interhemispheric variant of holoprosencephaly)

Summary

Holoprosencephaly encompasses a range of congenital abnormalities resulting from impaired differentiation and cleavage of the forebrain (prosencephalon) during early embryogenesis. Holoprosencephaly presents with varying levels of severity, with categorization based on the degree of cerebral hemispheric separation. It is important to note the term "fusion" is frequently used in discussion; however, the true process is a lack of cleavage rather than joining of two structures. Traditionally, classification has been based on DeMyer's three degrees of severity—that is, alobar (no hemispheric separation), semilobar (some posterior hemispheric separation), and lobar (frontal and temporal lobation with a small monoventricle) (Table 94.1). Facial malformations tend to be more severe with more severe brain malformation, hence the adage, "the face predicts the brain."

Although the alobar, semilobar, and lobar categories are helpful in classifying severity of the abnormality, it is important to note that no clear distinction exists among these categories, as holoprosencephaly represents a continuum/spectrum of forebrain malformations ranging from near normal to severe abnormality. Within the spectrum of findings, certain unifying features do exist. Namely, the septum pellucidum is always absent and the olfactory bulbs and tracts are commonly absent. The corpus callosum is typically absent or incompletely formed. Notably, unlike in primary callosal hypogenesis, the posterior portion is relatively preserved in comparison to the anterior portion. In addition, the hypothalamus, neurohypophysis, and adenohypophysis are generally hypoplastic. Of note, other mild forms in the spectrum of holoprosencephaly exist, including the middle interhemispheric variant of holoprosencephaly (also referred to as syntelencephaly). Focal lack of separation has been described at many different locations in the telencephalon and may be the mildest forms of holoprosencephaly.

Alobar Holoprosencephaly

Alobar holoprosencephaly represents the most extreme and severe form, with complete lack of hemispheric cleavage. There is complete lack of separation of the cerebral hemispheres, with a single mass of brain parenchyma, typically within the anterior

---

TABLE 94.1   Holoprosencephaly Categories

Category	Septum Pellucidum	Lateral Ventricles	Third Ventricle	Thalami	Facial Anomalies	Interhemispheric Fissure and Falx	Dorsal Cyst	Vascular
Alobar	Absent	U-shaped monoventricle	Absent	Fused	Severe	Absent	92%	Dysplastic vasculature or azygos ACA
Semilobar	Absent	Posteriorly formed	Rudimentary	Variable fusion	Mild or moderately severe	Partially fused anteriorly with hypoplastic or absent anterior falx	28%	Rudimentary deep veins, azygos ACA
Lobar	Absent or dysplastic	Near normal	Near normal	May be partially fused	None or mild	Near complete formation	9%	Azygos ACA may be seen
Middle interhemispheric variant	Absent	Normal or hypoplastic frontal horns	Well formed	Fused in one-third to half of cases	None	Absent in posterior frontal and parietal region	Variable	Azygos ACA may be seen

ACA, Anterior cerebral artery.

cranial vault, ranging in shape from crescent-shaped to ball-like ("ball-in-cup" appearance). The corpus callosum is usually absent, and the thalami is fused. Absence of the septum pellucidum is seen in conjunction with a monoventricle, which often appears as a large dorsal cyst occupying a large portion of the calvarial volume. The third ventricle, falx cerebri, and interhemispheric fissure are absent. In addition, the cerebral vascular supply may consist of multiple small vessels arising from the internal carotid and basilar arteries or appear as azygous anterior circulation in less severe cases. Alobar holoprosencephaly is usually associated with severe facial anomalies such as cyclopia, proboscis, ethmocephaly, cebocephaly, cleft lip, cleft palate, and/or hypotelorism.

Semilobar Holoprosencephaly

Semilobar holoprosencephaly is the intermediate form of holoprosencephaly, characterized by partial anterior hemispheric cleavage. The septum pellucidum is absent and a monoventricle with partially formed occipital horns and rudimentary temporal horns is seen. The anterior portions of the corpus callosum are almost always absent, and partially fused thalami are characteristic. The falx and interhemispheric fissure are absent anteriorly. Patients with semilobar holoprosencephaly tend to have less severe facial anomalies, including midline cleft lip and palate and hypotelorism.

Lobar Holoprosencephaly

Lobar holoprosencephaly represents a milder form, with partial fusion (<50%) of the ventral portions of the frontal lobes. The septum pellucidum is absent, and the anterior falx and interhemispheric fissure are present, but often dysplastic. Two distinct lateral ventricles are seen with unseparated or dysplastic frontal horns, which classically demonstrate an angular shape and flattened roof, giving them a characteristic "squared" appearance. The third ventricle is generally fully formed. Dysgenesis of the anterior corpus callosum is also evident, and the basal ganglia and thalami may be partially fused. The olfactory bulbs may be normal, hypoplastic, or absent. Typically, there is no associated facial anomaly.

Middle Interhemispheric Variant Holoprosencephaly

The middle interhemispheric variant of holoprosencephaly (a.k.a., syntelencephaly) is a rare malformation characterized by lack of division across the posterior frontal and anterior parietal lobes. The sylvian fissures may be vertically oriented and cross midline in some cases. The septum pellucidum and the body of the corpus callosum are absent, with relatively normal formation of the callosal rostrum, genu, and splenium. This pattern contrasts with that of classic holoprosencephaly, as there is relative sparing of the forebrain with a well-formed anterior interhemispheric fissure. Variable formation of the falx cerebri can be seen. Gray matter heterotopia is more common than in the other types of holoprosencephaly.

Differential Diagnosis

Important considerations in the differential diagnosis include hydranencephaly, severe hydrocephalus with parenchymal volume loss, and agenesis of the corpus callosum with interhemispheric cyst. Septo-optic dysplasia shares the finding of absence of the septum pellucidum, but there is no crossing of gray matter across midline, in distinction from holoprosencephaly.

Pearls

- The *sine qua non* of holoprosencephaly is incomplete cleavage of the cerebral hemispheres. Classification is based on the degree of cleavage with a relatively wide range of findings.
- Because the septum pellucidum is absent in all cases of holoprosencephaly, identification of the septum pellucidum excludes this diagnosis.
- Fifty percent of patients with holoprosencephaly have trisomy 13 (Patau syndrome).
- Holoprosencephaly is the only brain anomaly in which the posterior corpus callosum may be formed in the absence of formation of the anterior corpus callosum.

Signs and Complications

Prognosis and complications of holoprosencephaly are dependent on disease severity and degree of hemispheric separation; however, some of the more common sequelae and complications include hydrocephalus requiring shunt placement, seizure disorders, feeding difficulties, and consequences of hypothalamic dysfunction, including homeostatic and endocrine abnormalities.

Suggested Readings

Barkovich AJ, Raybaud C. Congenital malformations of the brain and skull. In: *Pediatric neuroimaging*, ed 6,1539–2360, 2018, Lippincott Williams & Wilkins.

Calloni SF, et al: Disorders of ventral induction/spectrum of holoprosencephaly, *Neuroimaging Clin N Am* 29(3):411–421, 2019.

Hahn JS, Barnes PD: Neuroimaging advances in holoprosencephaly: refining the spectrum of the midline malformation, *Am J Med Genet C Semin Med Genet* 154C(1):120–132, 2010.

Marcorelles P, Laquerriere A: Neuropathology of holoprosencephaly, *Am J Med Genet C Semin Med Genet* 154C(1):109–119, 2010.

Simon EM, Hevner RF, Pinter JD, et al: The middle interhemispheric variant of holoprosencephaly, *AJNR Am J Neuroradiol* 23(1): 151–156, 2002.

Winter TC, Kennedy AM, Woodward PJ: Holoprosencephaly: a survey of the entity, with embryology and fetal imaging, *Radiographics* 35(1):275–290, 2015.

Yang E, Chu WCW, Lee EY: A practical approach to supratentorial brain malformation: what radiologists should know, *Radiol Clin North Am* 55(4):609–627, 2017.

95

Corpus Callosum Abnormalities

JOSEPHINE MWIKALI NDOLO, MBCHB, MMED AND ASHA SARMA, MD

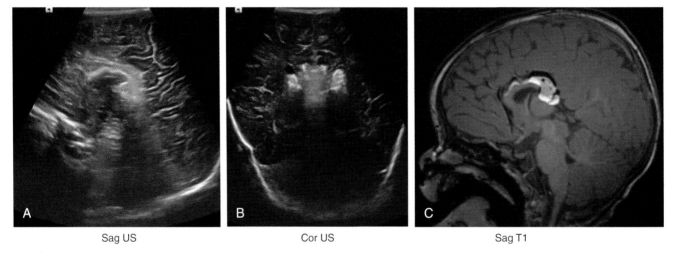

| Sag US | Cor US | Sag T1 |

CASE A: A 2-month-old male with an incidental finding on an ultrasound (A, B) performed for assessment of a scalp mass. (C) Follow-up MRI at 7 months of age. *Cor,* Coronal; *Sag,* sagittal; *US,* ultrasound.

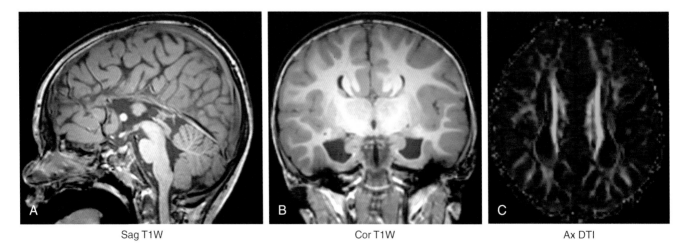

| Sag T1W | Cor T1W | Ax DTI |

CASE B: A 2-year-old male with developmental delay. *Ax,* Axial; *Cor,* coronal; *DTI,* diffusion tensor imaging; *Sag,* sagittal.

DESCRIPTION OF FINDINGS

- Case A: Ultrasound showing an echogenic midline lipoma along the course of the corpus callosum (CC), protruding into the lateral ventricles. Follow-up MRI demonstrating the midline lipoma without visualization of the splenium, consistent with callosal dysgenesis.
- Case B: Midline sagittal T1W image showing absence of the CC and cingulate gyrus and sulci with sulci "radiating" toward the third ventricle. Coronal T1W image showing widely spaced frontal horns and densely packed white matter tracts (Probst bundles) medial to the frontal horns, with characteristic "Texas longhorn" appearance. Axial DTI showing thick, uncrossed Probst bundles *(green)* medial and parallel to the lateral ventricles. Red transverse callosal fibers spanning midline are notably absent.

Diagnosis

Case A: Callosal dysgenesis with midline lipoma
Case B: Callosal agenesis

Summary

The CC is the largest of the three interhemispheric commissures (anterior commissure, hippocampal commissure, and CC). There are five named segments, from anterior to posterior, including the rostrum, genu, body, isthmus, and splenium.

Terminology surrounding commissural abnormalities is nuanced, complex, and in variable usage, which sometimes leads to confusion. These various terms are outlined in Table 95.1 and Fig. 95.4.

Anomalies of the CC are often associated with a variety of other brain malformations such as cortical malformations, midline cysts/lipomas (described in the following sections), and other posterior fossa anomalies. More than 200 named syndromes and malformations are associated with CC anomalies, for example, Chiari II malformation, Aicardi syndrome, Dandy–Walker malformation, and fetal alcohol syndrome.

Normal Immature Appearance

Although all components of the CC are formed by 20 weeks gestational age, there is substantial increase in both length and thickness of the CC until term. Rather than relying on direct visualization on the sagittal midline image, MRI evaluation of the fetal CC often relies on identification of indirect signs (see "Agenesis of the Corpus Callosum"). Following birth, the CC normally appears thin and relatively flat in neonates (Fig. 95.1). Thickening of the genu (2–3 months postnatal age) occurs prior to thickening of the splenium, which is thought to relate to early development of axonal pathways involved in basic motor and sensory function, originating from the inferior precentral and postcentral gyri. Myelination of the CC is from posterior to anterior and is normally mature around 6 to 7 months of age. The CC takes on a more adult appearance around 8 to 9 months of age (Fig. 95.2). Presence of a visible isthmus (thin segment between the body and the splenium) is variable and should not be mistaken for pathological thinning. There is wide normal variation in the appearance of the CC between individuals.

Agenesis of the Corpus Callosum

The classic appearance of agenesis of the CC includes parallel lateral ventricles located away from the midline, colpocephaly (widening of the atria and occipital horns of the lateral ventricles), "Viking helmet" or "Texas longhorn" appearance of the frontal horns on coronal images, high-riding third ventricle extending into the widened interhemispheric fissure, and sulci on the medial aspect of the hemispheres converging toward the third ventricle due to lack of formation of the cingulate gyrus and sulcus ("sunray appearance"). The "sunray" appearance is one of the hallmarks of an absent CC and (along with ventricular configuration and/or diffusion tensor imaging) can be helpful when evaluating fetuses or newborns in whom the normally thin CC may be difficult to see. "Probst bundles" are anteroposteriorly oriented white matter tracts that would normally have crossed midline to course in the contralateral hemisphere, but instead lie parallel and medial to the walls of the lateral ventricles. In callosal agenesis, these tracts thereby form intra- rather than interhemispheric connections. The parallel orientation of the lateral ventricles with colpocephaly results from abnormal white matter architecture in the posterior frontal and parietal lobes (Fig. 95.3). The white matter tracts are more densely packed anteriorly adjacent to the basal ganglia and more loosely packed posteriorly, with subsequent relative posterior ventricular prominence.

Callosal Hypogenesis/Partial Agenesis

There are various forms of hypogenesis of the CC, the most common of which is shortening, with a small or absent inferior genu or rostrum. These findings are best identified on midline sagittal MRI images.

Typically, a hypogenetic CC appears as a short, thin CC appearing as either a posterior genu and anterior body (Fig. 95.4); genu and entire body; or entire genu, body, and small splenium. The appearance of callosal anomalies in classic holoprosencephaly is atypical, as the splenium is present in the absence of a genu. In the middle interhemispheric variant of holoprosencephaly, the genu and splenium may be present without a callosal body.

Advanced imaging including diffusion tensor imaging (DTI) and tractography may allow a better understanding of

TABLE 95.1	Definition of Commissural Abnormalities
Terminology	**Definition**
Dysgenesis	Umbrella term for callosal malformations
Agenesis	Complete absence of the corpus callosum
Hypogenesis/Partial agenesis	Partial formation of the corpus callosum
Hypoplasia	Thin corpus callosum with normal anteroposterior extent

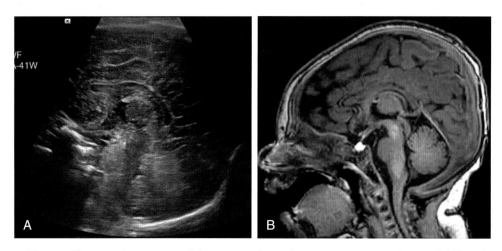

• **Fig. 95.1** The normal appearance of the corpus callosum in a term neonate on ultrasound *(US)* and sagittal *(Sag)* T1W magnetic resonance imaging.

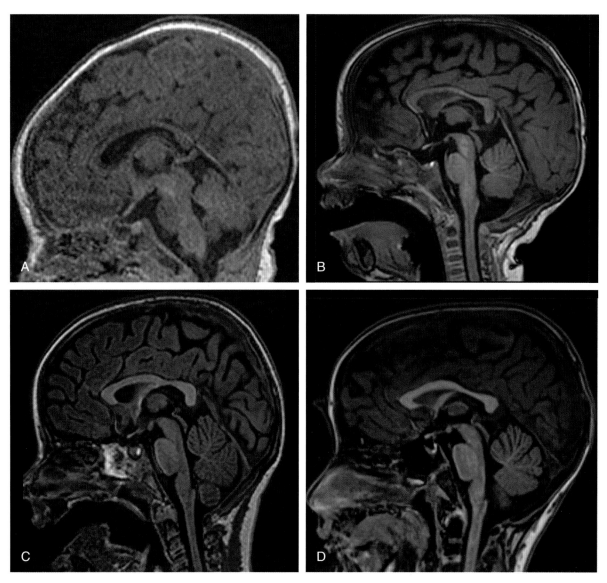

• **Fig. 95.2** Sagittal T1W images of the normal corpus callosum in (A) a neonate, (B) an 8-month-old, (C) a 2-year-old, and (D) an 8-year-old. Notice callosal thickening and development of mature morphology with advancing age.

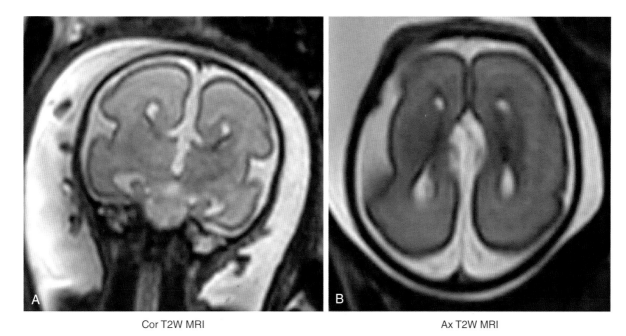

Cor T2W MRI   Ax T2W MRI

• **Fig. 95.3** Fetal magnetic resonance imaging (MRI) of a 26-week fetus undergoing evaluation for ventriculomegaly. The coronal image shows widely spaced frontal horns ("Texas longhorn" sign) and an elevated third ventricle that is contiguous with the interhemispheric fissure. The axial image demonstrates parallel lateral ventricles in this patient with callosal agenesis. The corpus callosum can sometimes be difficult to visualize on sagittal fetal MRI, and multiplanar evaluation is helpful. *Ax,* Axial; *Cor,* coronal.

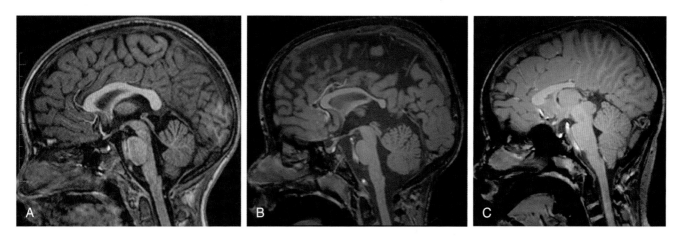

• **Fig. 95.4** Sagittal T1W MRI in three different patients. (A) Normal corpus callosum in a 10-year-old male. (B) Callosal thinning of the posterior body and splenium in a 4-year-old male with white matter injury of prematurity; note that all anatomic segments are formed. Thinning is due to Wallerian degeneration. (C) Callosal hypogenesis in a 9-year-old female with multiple brain anomalies. *Sag, Sagittal.*

intrahemispheric and interhemispheric connectivity and can help in differentiating callosal hypoplasia from hypogenesis.

Callosal Dysgenesis with Cyst or Lipoma

Callosal dysgenesis may be associated with midline cysts (agenesis of the CC with interhemispheric cyst; Fig. 95.5) or lipomas. Interhemispheric cysts associated with callosal agenesis can be communicating (type 1) or noncommunicating (type 2). The communicating cyst is a diverticulum of the ventricular system and communicates with the ventricles. A noncommunicating cyst is usually multilocular and often

associated with cortical malformations. The interhemispheric midline lipoma (tubulonodular or curvilinear) is a form of midline meningeal dysplasia that may accompany CC anomalies. However, tubulonodular lipoma can rarely be present in individuals with a normal CC.

Thin Corpus Callosum

Thinning of the CC can be focal or involve the entire CC, and can be primary or secondary. Primary thinning is due to abnormal myelination linked to hypomyelination syndromes and microcephaly (Fig. 95.6). Secondary thinning of the CC

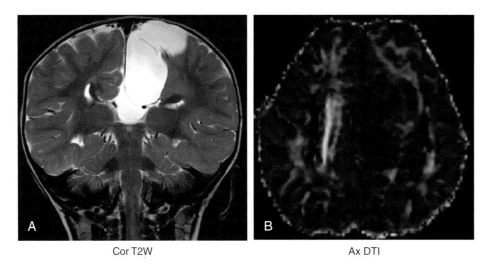

Cor T2W | Ax DTI

• **Fig. 95.5** A 12-month-old male with prenatally diagnosed ventriculomegaly and type 2 callosal agenesis with interhemispheric cyst. (A) Coronal image showing callosal agenesis, "Texas longhorn" configuration of the lateral ventricles, and a noncommunicating interhemispheric cyst. (B) Axial DTI showing uncrossed callosal fibers *(green)* medial to the corona radiata *(blue)*, with distortion of Probst bundles on the left due to the interhemispheric cyst. *Ax,* Axial; *Cor,* coronal; *DTI,* diffusion tensor imaging.

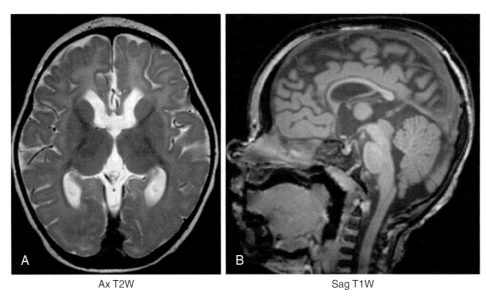

Ax T2W | Sag T1W

• **Fig. 95.6** A 15-month-old female with *FOXG1* mutation, 14q deletion, and visual impairment. Thin, foreshortened corpus callosum (especially anteriorly), small basal ganglia relative to the thalami, simplified gyral pattern, microcephaly, and dysmorphic ventricles. Callosal abnormalities are a feature of myriad genetic conditions and also may be acquired. *Ax,* Axial; *Sag,* sagittal.

can be due to injury such as white matter injury of prematurity or hypoxic ischemic encephalopathy or dysmyelinating and demyelinating conditions.

Spectrum of Disease

The spectrum of disease is detailed in the preceding section.

Differential Diagnosis

The differential diagnosis is detailed in the preceding section.

Pearls

• Classic imaging findings of callosal agenesis include parallel ventricles with colpocephaly, sulci radiating to the elevated third ventricle, and Viking helmet or Texas longhorn configuration of the lateral ventricles. These findings can be especially helpful in fetal or neonatal MRI when the CC is thin.
• Always look for additional intracranial anomalies.

Signs and Complications

Signs and complications are generally related to the associated malformations.

Suggested Readings

Andronikou S, Pillay T, Gabuza L, et al: Corpus callosum thickness in children: an MR pattern-recognition approach on the midsagittal image, *Pediatr Radiol* 45(2), 258–272, 2015.

Barkovich A: *Pediatric neuroimaging,* ed 6, Philadelphia, 2019, Lippincott Williams & Wilkins.

Edwards TJ, Sherr EH, Barkovich AJ, et al: Clinical, genetic and imaging findings identify new causes for corpus callosum development syndromes, *Brain* 137(6):1579–1613, 2014.

Glenn OA, Goldstein RB, Li KC, et al: Fetal magnetic resonance imaging in the evaluation of fetuses referred for sonographically suspected abnormalities of the corpus callosum, *J Ultrasound Med* 24(6): 791–804, 2005.

Hetts SW, Sherr EH, Chao S, et al: Anomalies of the corpus callosum: an MR analysis of the phenotypic spectrum of associated malformations, *AJR Am J Roentgenol* 187(5):1343–1348, 2006.

Manevich-Mazor M, Weissmann-Brenner A, Bar Yosef O, et al: Added value of fetal MRI in the evaluation of fetal anomalies of the corpus callosum: a retrospective analysis of 78 cases, *Ultraschall Med* 39(05): 513–525, 2018.

Neal JB, Filippi CG, Mayeux R: Morphometric variability of neuroimaging features in children with agenesis of the corpus callosum, *BMC Neurol* 15(1):116, 2015.

96

Symmetric Diffusion Abnormality in an Infant

ALEXANDRA M. FOUST, DO AND ASHA SARMA, MD

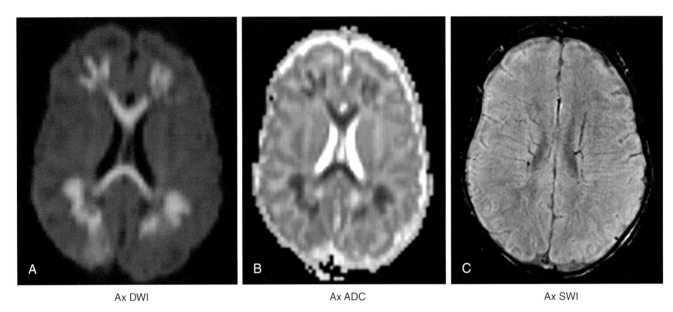

Ax DWI   Ax ADC   Ax SWI

CASE A: A 35-day-old previously healthy term male presenting with apnea. *ADC*, Apparent diffusion coefficient; *Ax*, axial; *DWI*, diffusion-weighted imaging; *SWI*, susceptibility-weighted imaging.

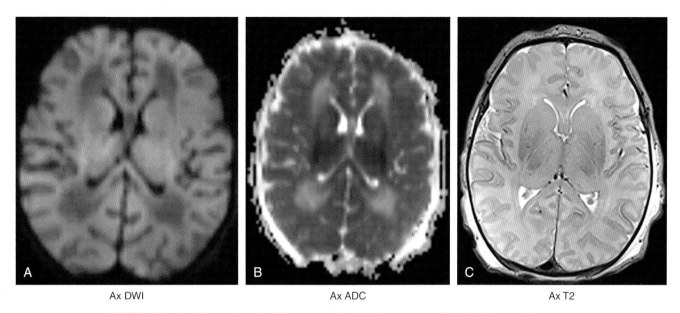

Ax DWI   Ax ADC   Ax T2

CASE B: A 3-day-old term female with nonreassuring fetal heart tones with clinical signs of distress at delivery. *ADC,* Apparent diffusion coefficient; *Ax,* axial; *DWI,* diffusion-weighted imaging.

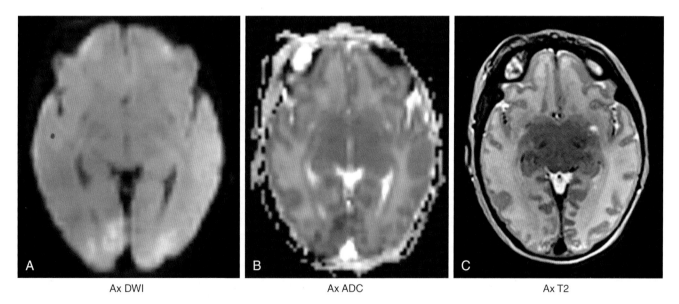

Ax DWI   Ax ADC   Ax T2

CASE C: A 3-day-old term male with hypoglycemia and new onset seizures. *ADC,* Apparent diffusion coefficient; *Ax,* axial; *DWI,* diffusion-weighted imaging.

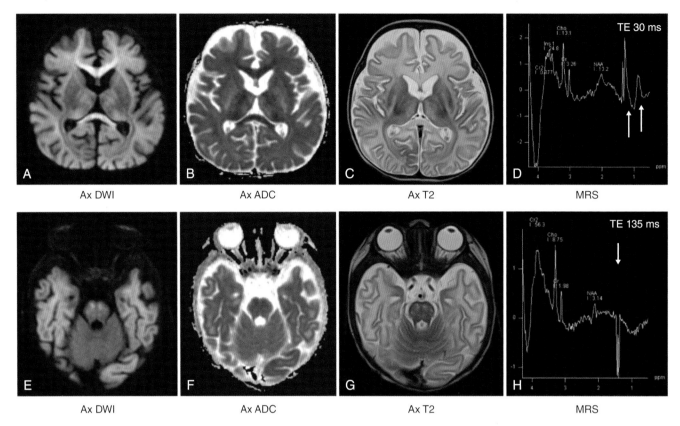

CASE D: A 3-month-old female presenting with seizures. *ADC,* Apparent diffusion coefficient; *Ax,* axial; *DWI,* diffusion-weighted imaging; *MRS,* magnetic resonance spectroscopy.

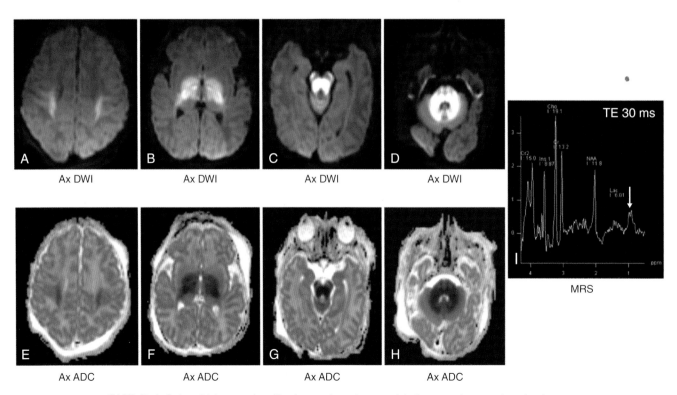

CASE E: A 9-day-old term male with abnormal newborn metabolic screening panel and seizures. *ADC,* Apparent diffusion coefficient; *Ax,* axial; *DWI,* diffusion-weighted imaging; *MRS,* magnetic resonance spectroscopy.

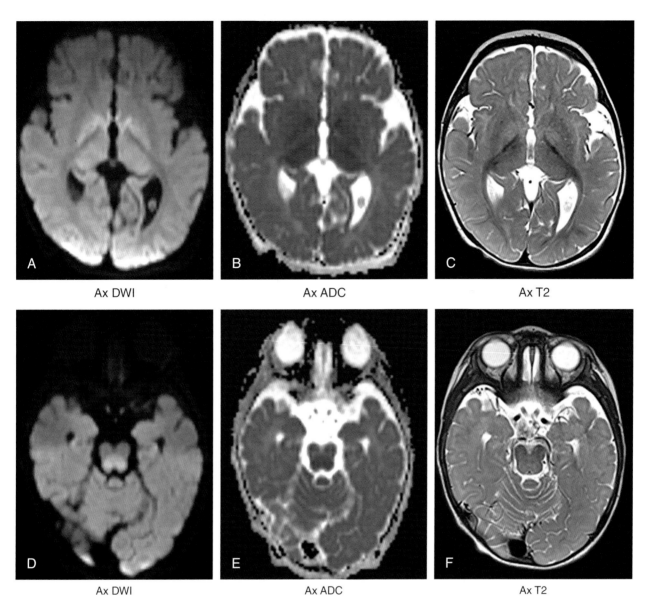

Ax DWI

Ax ADC

Ax T2

Ax DWI

Ax ADC

Ax T2

CASE F: A 9-month-old with refractory epilepsy and infantile spasms. *ADC,* Apparent diffusion coefficient; *Ax,* axial; *DWI,* diffusion-weighted imaging.

DESCRIPTION OF FINDINGS

- Case A: Axial diffusion-weighted image (A) and apparent diffusion coefficient map (B) demonstrate symmetric reduced diffusivity within the periventricular white matter of the frontal and parietal lobes in the expected distribution of the deep medullary veins. Reduced diffusivity is also observed within the genu and splenium of the corpus callosum. Axial susceptibility-weighted image (C) demonstrates symmetric prominence of the deep medullary veins in the centrum semiovale.
- Case B: Axial diffusion-weighted (A) and apparent diffusion coefficient (B) images demonstrate symmetric reduced diffusivity within the caudate heads, basal ganglia, posterior limb of the internal capsule, and thalami. Corresponding T2 prolongation is identified in the same regions (C).
- Case C: Axial diffusion-weighted (A) and apparent diffusion coefficient (B) images demonstrate relatively symmetric reduced diffusivity within the occipital lobes bilaterally. Associated T2 prolongation is also present (C), although is subtle due to the unmyelinated appearance of the white matter.
- Case D: Axial diffusion, apparent diffusion coefficient, and T2-weighted images at the level of the deep gray nuclei (A, B, C) and upper pons (E, F, G) demonstrate extensive symmetric reduced diffusivity with corresponding T2 prolongation throughout the supratentorial white matter, corpus callosum, basal ganglia, thalami, corticospinal tracts, and pontine fibers. MR spectroscopy at a short TE of 30 ms (D, *white arrow*) demonstrates a lipid-protein peak at 0.8–0.9 ppm (D, *gray arrow*) and a large lactate doublet at 1.3 ppm that inverts at the intermediate TE of 135 ms (H, *white arrow*).
- Case E: Axial diffusion-weighted (A, B, C, D) and apparent diffusion coefficient (E, F, G, H) images at the levels of the centrum semiovale (A, E), third ventricle (B, F), midbrain (C, G), and middle cerebellar peduncles (D, H) demonstrate marked symmetric reduced diffusivity involving the corticospinal tracts, globi pallidi, thalami, dorsal brainstem, and cerebellar white matter. MR spectroscopy at a short TE of 30 ms demonstrates a doublet branched chain amino acid peak at 0.9 ppm (I, *white arrow*).
- Case F: Axial diffusion, apparent diffusion coefficient, and T2-weighted images at the level of the third ventricle (A, B, C) and midbrain (D, E, F) demonstrate symmetric reduced diffusivity with subtle associated T2 prolongation within the globi pallidi, thalami, and dorsal brainstem.

Diagnosis

Case A: Neonatal parechovirus encephalitis
Case B: Profound neonatal hypoxic ischemic injury
Case C: Neonatal hypoglycemia
Case D: Mitochondrial encephalopathy (caused by a homozygous mutation of the *NARS2* gene encoding mitochondrial asparaginyl-tRNA synthetase)
Case E: Maple syrup urine disease
Case F: Vigabatrin-related brain parenchymal signal abnormality

Summary

When approaching symmetric diffusion signal abnormality in an infant, the age of the patient and clinical scenario are paramount to generating an appropriate differential diagnosis. Infectious, hypoxic, metabolic, genetic, and medication-related etiologies are important considerations.

Human Parechovirus Infection

Human parechovirus, a single-stranded ribonucleic acid (RNA) virus from the *picornavirus* family, is an important emerging cause of aseptic meningitis/meningoencephalitis during the first few months of life. Affected infants most often present with clinical findings of meningoencephalitis. MRI most frequently demonstrates reduced diffusivity involving the cerebral white matter, most commonly with a periventricular and frontoparietal predominance, with common involvement of the corpus callosum and internal capsule and signal abnormality along the course of the deep medullary veins on T1, T2, and susceptibility-weighted sequences. Similar MRI findings may be seen in enterovirus, chikungunya, and rotavirus infection. Although there is an overlap in imaging findings, absent history of perinatal depression distinguishes parechovirus infection from hypoxic ischemic injury (HII). More consistent thalamic involvement is typically seen in term HII. Diagnosis of viral encephalitis is confirmed by polymerase chain reaction–based cerebrospinal fluid (CSF) testing.

Hypoxic Ischemic Injury

HII in infants is most frequently observed in the neonatal period as a result of perinatal asphyxia, with intrauterine insults being much more common than postpartum insults. History is key to making the diagnosis in neonates, as metabolic diseases with overlapping imaging manifestations more often present after a 24- to 48-hour asymptomatic period. The imaging pattern of injury is generally bilateral and relatively symmetric, but is dependent on the degree of brain maturation (premature versus term age) as well as the severity and duration of hypoxia (Table 96.1). Regardless of the pattern of injury, diffusion-weighted imaging (DWI) is the first sequence to demonstrate abnormality, often within the first 24 hours, although optimal MRI timing is at day 3 to 5 of life when signal abnormality is at its peak (often after completion of therapeutic hypothermia). T1 and T2 hyperintensity begins to develop by the second day. MR spectroscopy performed within the first

TABLE 96.1   Patterns of Neonatal Hypoxic Ischemic Injury

Age	Severity	Pattern of Injury
Premature	Partial prolonged	*Germinal matrix and/or intraventricular hemorrhage *Periventricular white matter injury
Premature	Profound	*Deep gray matter (thalami > basal ganglia), hippocampi, dorsal brainstem, corticospinal tracts, anterior vermis **Perirolandic cortex less likely involved compared to term neonates
Term	Partial prolonged	*Parasagittal watershed cortex and subcortical white matter **Deep gray matter generally spared
Term	Profound	*Deep gray matter (basal ganglia, thalami), dorsal brainstem, hippocampi, corticospinal tracts, and possibly the perirolandic cortex

*, pertinent positive; **, pertinent negatives.

24 hours may reveal a lactate peak (doublet at 1.3 ppm), which is suggestive of a worse prognosis in term infants.

Neonatal Hypoglycemia

Transient hypoglycemia, defined as a blood glucose level of <46 mg/dL, is not uncommon even in otherwise normal term infants and frequently occurs during the first few days of postnatal life. Additionally, it may occur in the setting of HII, as affected neonates are often more susceptible to metabolic dysregulation. Although neurologic sequelae are relatively rare, the imaging pattern of bilateral posterior parietooccipital reduced diffusivity involving the subcortical white matter and possibly the adjacent cortex is suggestive, and the radiologist may be the first to raise the diagnosis. T1 shortening and T2 prolongation may also be observed. The imaging findings may be transient, as often seen in cases of rapidly recognized or mild hypoglycemia, or may progress to volume loss or cystic encephalomalacia.

Mitochondrial Encephalopathy

The term "mitochondrial encephalopathy" encompasses a heterogeneous group of disorders of intermittent or progressive brain injury caused by genetic mutations involving components of the mitochondrial respiratory chain. Various imaging appearances have been described, depending on the genetic mutation and phenotype. The subcortical/deep pattern has the most overlap with other causes of symmetric diffusion abnormality in infants with symmetric involvement of the basal ganglia, brainstem, and cerebellum. Involvement of the dentate nuclei may be helpful in distinguishing this entity from HII, hypoglycemia, and neonatal parechovirus encephalitis. Patients with mitochondrial encephalopathy often demonstrate acute episodes of deterioration during periods of stress or illness that alter the body's metabolic demands. During acute episodes, altered diffusivity is frequently observed and can present as reduced diffusivity due to cytotoxic edema, facilitated diffusivity due to interstitial edema, or a combination of both within the same region. T2 will often show increased signal in corresponding regions and arterial spin labeling may show increased perfusion. MR spectroscopy is also helpful in the acute stage to assess for the presence of lactate elevation.

Maple Syrup Urine Disease

Maple syrup urine disease (MSUD) is an autosomal recessive disorder of amino acid metabolism that results in metabolic and neurologic deterioration due to abnormal accumulation of branched chain alpha-keto acids. MSUD is currently frequently detected on routine newborn laboratory screening. Diffusion-weighted imaging demonstrates reduced diffusivity in the perirolandic white matter, basal ganglia, internal capsule, cerebral peduncles, brainstem, and cerebellar white matter (intramyelinic edema). Similar to mitochondrial encephalopathies, MSUD may also show reduced diffusivity in the dentate nuclei, which can be helpful in narrowing the differential

diagnosis. MR spectroscopy may demonstrate abnormal branched chain amino acid peaks at 0.9 ppm and/or lactate peaks at 1.3 ppm during periods of acute decompensation. Other metabolic disorders, including other organic and aminoacidopathies and urea cycle disorders, may also cause symmetric reduced diffusivity. Nonketotic hyperglycinemia is associated with callosal malformations and presents with reduced diffusivity preferentially involving structures that are myelinated at birth. An elevated glycine peak at 3.56 ppm is a characteristic finding on MR spectroscopy. Urea cycle disorders present with hyperammonemia in the neonatal period with reduced diffusivity in the basal ganglia and cortex.

Vigabatrin Toxicity

Vigabatrin, an irreversible gamma-aminobutyric acid (GABA) transaminase inhibitor clinically utilized for the treatment of infantile spasms, is associated with a characteristic asymptomatic pattern of MRI signal abnormality in nearly one-third of cases. MRI of the brain in these patients will demonstrate symmetric bilateral reduced diffusivity, often with associated T2 hyperintensity, within the globi pallidi, dorsal brainstem, thalami, and/or dentate nuclei. The signal abnormality is often reversible with cessation of the vigabatrin therapy, however, the medication does not need to be discontinued as a result of MRI signal changes.

Spectrum of Disease

The spectrum of disease is detailed in the preceding sections.

Differential Diagnosis

The differential diagnosis is detailed in the preceding sections.

Pearls

- Age and clinical presentation are important factors when evaluating an infant with symmetric diffusion signal abnormality
- Viral encephalitis, HII, and metabolic disorders have imaging overlap; however, an HII typically presents after perinatal asphyxia; metabolic disorders present with encephalopathy after a 24–48-hour asymptomatic period; and viral encephalitis presents with signs of sepsis and encephalopathy
- Symmetric posterior predominant restricted diffusivity within the first few days of life is suggestive of neonatal hypoglycemia
- Vigabatrin therapy should be considered in patients with infantile spasms and a characteristic pattern of abnormality on DWI

Signs and Complications

Symmetric restricted diffusivity often reflects a serious underlying diagnosis. Although there is some overlap in imaging appearance, certain imaging patterns are suggestive and important for radiologists to bring to clinical attention.

Suggested Readings

Amarnath C, Helen Mary T, Periakarupan A, et al: Neonatal parechovirus leucoencephalitis – radiological pattern mimicking hypoxic-ischemic encephalopathy, *Eur J Radiol* 85:428–434, 2016.

Bano S, Chaudhary V, Garga UC: Neonatal hypoxic-ischemic encephalopathy : a radiological review, *J Pediatr Neurosci* 12(1):1–6, 2017.

Bathla G, Policeni B, Agarwal A: Neuroimaging in patients with abnormal blood glucose levels, *AJNR Am J Neuroradiol* 35:833–840, 2014.

Bond KM, Brinjikji W, Eckel LJ, et al: Dentate update : imaging features of entities that affect the dentate nucleus. *AJNR Am J Neuroradiol* 38:1467–1474, 2017.

Bricout M, Grévent D, Lebre AS, et al: Brain imaging in mitochondrial respiratory chain deficiency: combination of brain MRI features as a useful tool for genotype/phenotype correlations, *J Med Genet* 51(7):429–435, 2014.

Dracopoulos A, Widjaja E, Raybaud C, et al: Vigabatrin-associated reversible MRI signal changes in patients with infantile spasms, *Epilepsia* 51(7):1297–1304, 2010.

Huang BY, Castillo M: Hypoxic-ischemic brain injury: imaging findings from birth to adulthood, *Radiographics* 28(2):417–439, 2008.

Jan W, Zimmerman RA, Wang ZJ, et al: MR diffusion imaging and MR spectroscopy of maple syrup urine disease during acute metabolic decompensation, *Neuroradiology* 45(6):393–399, 2003.

Mascalchi M, Montomoli M, Guerrini R: Neuroimaging in mitochondrial disorders, *Essays Biochem* 62:409–421, 2018.

Pearl PL, Vezina LG, Saneto RP, et al: Cerebral MRI abnormalities associated with vigabatrin therapy, *Epilepsia* 50(2):184–194, 2009.

Sarma A, Hanzlik E, Krishnasarma R, et al: Human parechovirus meningoencephalitis : neuroimaging in the era of polymerase chain reaction-based testing, *AJNR Am J Neuroradiol* 40:1418–1421, 2019.

Vannucci RC, Vannucci SJ: Hypoglycemic brain injury, *Semin Neonatol* 6:147–155, 2001.

Wong DST, Poskitt KJ, Chau V, et al: Brain injury patterns in hypoglycemia in neonatal encephalopathy, *AJNR Am J Neuroradiol* 34:1456–1461, 2013.

Yoon HJ, Kim JH, Jeon TY, et al: Devastating metabolic brain disorders of newborns and young infants, *Radiographics* 34:1257–1273, 2014.

97

Abnormal Ventricular Morphology

JENNIFER HUANG, MD, MED AND ASHA SARMA, MD

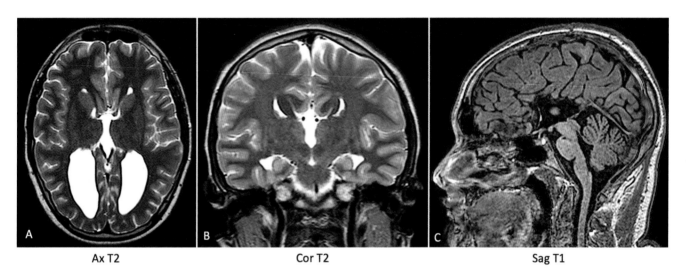

Ax T2   Cor T2   Sag T1

CASE A: A 14-year-old child presenting with headache. *Ax*, Axial; *Cor*, coronal; *Sag*, sagittal.

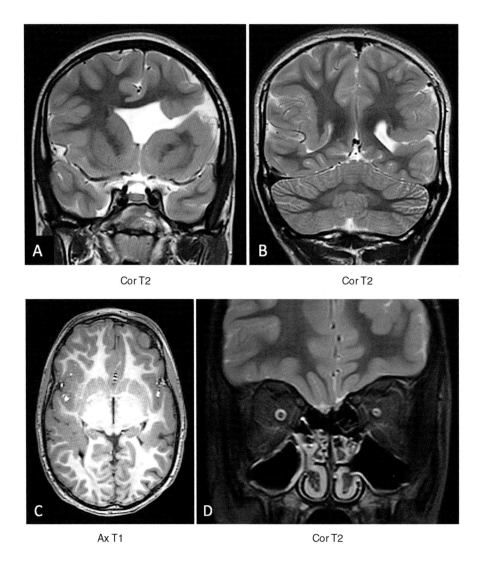

Cor T2

Cor T2

Ax T1

Cor T2

CASE B: An 8-year-old child presenting with headaches. *Ax*, Axial; *Cor*, coronal.

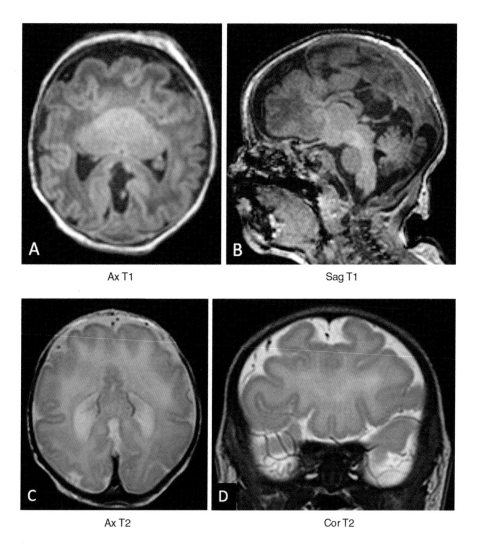

Ax T1

Sag T1

Ax T2

Cor T2

CASE C: A 3-day-old full-term infant presenting with dysmorphic features. *Ax*, Axial; *Cor*, coronal; *Sag*, sagittal.

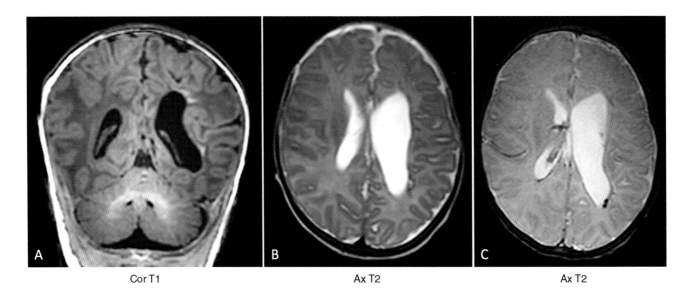

Cor T1   Ax T2   Ax T2

CASE D: A 4-week-old former term infant with possible ventriculomegaly on prenatal ultrasound. *Ax*, Axial; *Cor*, coronal.

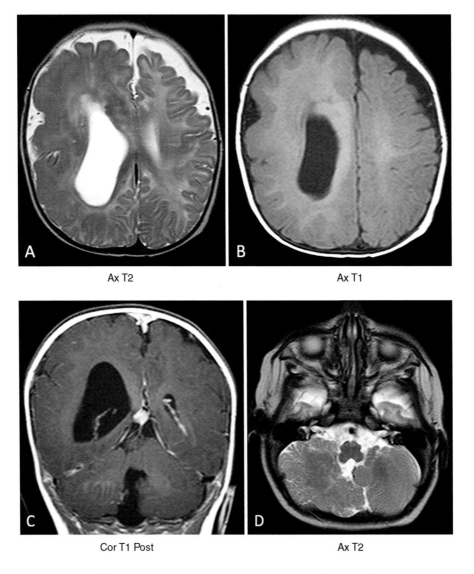

Ax T2   Ax T1

Cor T1 Post   Ax T2

CASE E: A 5-month-old child with seizures. *Ax*, Axial; *Cor*, coronal.

DESCRIPTION OF FINDINGS

- Case A: Symmetric disproportionately enlarged occipital horns (colpocephaly) of the widely spaced, parallel ("race car" sign) lateral ventricles. "Texas longhorn" appearance of the lateral ventricles on coronal imaging. Complete agenesis of the corpus callosum with absent cingulate gyrus and radial orientation of gyri toward the roof of the third ventricle ("sunray" appearance).
- Case B: Absent septum pellucidum with dysmorphic, "flat-roofed" lateral ventricles. Dipping of the inferior aspect of the frontal horns below the fornices. Bilateral closed lip schizencephaly with extensive frontoparietal and perisylvian polymicrogyria, more severe on the left. Small intraorbital and prechiasmatic optic nerves, left greater than right.
- Case C: Underdeveloped and completely fused frontal lobes as well as fused thalami. Azygos anterior cerebral artery (ACA) and absent anterior falx. Absent lateral ventricle frontal horns. Corpus callosal dysgenesis with absent anterior callosal formation.
- Case D: Moderate left periventricular white matter volume loss with punctate foci of T1 hyperintense signal in the left periventricular white matter. Foci of hemosiderin staining within the occipital horns, representing sequelae from prior intraventricular hemorrhage.
- Case E: Overgrowth of the right cerebral hemisphere with asymmetric enlargement and dysmorphic appearance of the right lateral ventricle. Areas of pachygyria in the right frontal and temporal lobes, with heterogeneous signal in the periventricular white matter consistent with heterotopias. Overgrowth and foliar disorganization of the right cerebellar hemisphere.

Diagnosis

Case A: Colpocephaly and Agenesis of the corpus callosum
Case B: Septo-optic dysplasia complex
Case C: Semilobar holoprosencephaly
Case D: Presumed in utero periventricular white matter ischemic injury
Case E: Hemimegalencephaly

Summary

Congenital ventricular abnormalities may be due to anomalies or injuries that occurred in utero. When evaluating abnormal ventricles in pediatric patients, it is important to assess ventricular size and morphology, as well as associated findings, in order to narrow the differential diagnosis.

Differential Diagnosis

Colpocephaly

Colpocephaly is a descriptive term used to describe disproportionate enlargement of the occipital horns of the lateral ventricles. It is most often associated with agenesis of the corpus callosum. Key neuroimaging findings include parallel and widely spaced lateral ventricles ("racing car" sign), best seen on axial images, as well as the characteristic "Texas longhorn" appearance of the frontal horns of the lateral ventricles on coronal images. It is important to carefully assess midline sagittal images for callosal agenesis, although in a fetus or neonate with a thin corpus callosum, identification of secondary signs may be necessary.

Septo-optic Dysplasia Complex

Septo-optic dysplasia (SOD) complex, also known as de Morsier syndrome, is a heterogeneous spectrum that is characterized by agenesis/dysgenesis of the septum pellucidum and/or the corpus callosum, optic nerve hypoplasia, and hypothalamic-pituitary dysfunction. Two out of three of these features must be present for diagnosis, and only 30% to 47% of patients meet all three criteria. The configuration of the frontal horns of the lateral ventricles is distinctive on coronal imaging when the cavum septum pellucidum is absent—the frontal horns are "boxlike" or "flat-roofed," with dipping of the inferior aspects below the level of the fornix. Ventricular "dimples" pointing toward the cleft may alert the radiologist to the presence of closed lip schizencephaly. Alternatively, there may be open lip schizencephaly, the most commonly associated malformation of cortical development. Differentiating SOD complex from lobar holoprosencephaly (HPE) may, at times, be challenging. Both entities feature absent septum pellucidum; however, the constellation of findings otherwise differs. Most importantly, no findings of midline fusion are seen in SOD complex. Optic nerve hypoplasia, seen in SOD complex, is not a typical feature of HPE (noting that this may be difficult to evaluate on imaging of infants in whom the optic nerves are normally relatively small).

Holoprosencephaly

There are several types of HPE, which exist on a spectrum and are characterized by a failure of the developing brain to cleave into two distinct hemispheres. Clinically, HPE is often associated with facial malformations such as hypotelorism, pyriform aperture stenosis, and solitary central mega incisor. All types of HPE feature an absent septum pellucidum, which may occasionally lead to difficulty in distinguishing it from the SOD complex, as described previously. Ventricular abnormalities in HPE vary by form. The most severe form, alobar HPE, features a single midline forebrain mass ("disc" or "pancake" brain) with a monoventricle posteriorly ("ball-in-cup" appearance), and sometimes a large dorsal cyst. In the intermediate form, semilobar HPE, there may be relatively well-formed posterior structures, including the posterior portions of the lateral ventricles, without normal formation of the anterior lateral or third ventricles. In lobar HPE, there is <50% frontal midline fusion (roughly), and there is some formation of the third ventricle and frontal horns of the lateral ventricles (although with dysmorphic appearance). Identification of an azygos anterior cerebral artery can be another helpful clue to diagnosis in subtle cases.

Presumed In Utero Venous Infarct

In Utero Periventricular White Matter Ischemic Injury with associated ex vacuo ventricular dilatation may occur due to arterial or venous infarction. An arterial infarct tends to correspond to an arterial vascular territory, while a venous infarct is confined to a medullary venous territory, with sparing of the cortex and basal ganglia. In some cases, evidence of remote germinal matrix hemorrhage can be identified. The mechanism of venous infarction is similar to that seen in preterm infants with grade IV germinal matrix hemorrhage (periventricular medullary venous infarction due to venous hypertension caused by intraventricular hemorrhage). The resultant ventricular configuration is also similar, with an outward convex contour of the body of the enlarged lateral ventricle, squaring of the posterior body, and sometimes, adjacent T2 hyperintense gliosis. Clinical presentations are variable and may include spastic hemiplegia. In contradistinction to hemimegalencephaly, ipsilateral white matter volume will be decreased rather than increased, the frontal horn will have a relatively normal contour, and signs of prior hemorrhage may be evident on T2-weighted or hemosiderin sensitive MRI.

Hemimegalencephaly

Hemimegalencephaly represents hamartomatous overgrowth of part or all of a cerebral hemisphere due to a defect in neuronal proliferation, migration, and organization. The most common clinical presentations are intractable seizures and developmental delay, with approximately 50% associated with skin lesions or truncal/extremity overgrowth (including syndromes with mutations involving genes in the PI3K/AKT/mTOR pathway, such as tuberous sclerosis). Imaging shows an enlarged cerebral hemisphere. There is a wide spectrum of clinical and imaging manifestations. The lateral ventricle tends to be enlarged to a similar degree as the affected hemisphere and the frontal horn demonstrate a bizarre configuration, with straightening, superolateral angulation, which is best demonstrated on coronal images. Although usually enlarged, the dysmorphic ventricle may also be small or normal in caliber. As opposed to in utero infarction, the affected white matter has increased (rather than decreased) volume. The gray matter may be normal or affected by variable cortical malformations, such as pachygyria, polymicrogyria, or heterotopia. Abnormal white matter signal intensity in the affected hemisphere is also common.

Spectrum of Disease

The spectrum of disease is detailed in the preceding section.

Pearls

- The various entities that cause congenitally abnormal ventricular morphology may appear similar on imaging; therefore, careful evaluation of additional imaging findings in each case is necessary to arrive at an accurate diagnosis.

- Absent septum pellucidum can be seen in both SOD complex and HPE. Optic nerve hypoplasia is more commonly seen in SOD complex and there are no signs of midline fusion.
- When unilateral lateral ventriculomegaly is encountered, look carefully at the adjacent white matter. Hemimegalencephaly will feature increased white matter volume, while white matter injury of prematurity demonstrates gliosis and white matter volume loss.

Signs and Complications

- Colpocephaly: Enlarged occipital horns in association with callosal dysgenesis
- SOD complex: Absent septum pellucidum +/− corpus callosum, optic nerve hypoplasia, hypothalamic-pituitary abnormalities; associated with malformations of cortical development such as schizencephaly and PMG.
- HPE: Spectrum of incomplete separation of two cerebral hemispheres; associated with facial malformations and azygos ACA.
- White matter injury of prematurity: Enlarged lateral ventricle with ipsilateral white matter volume loss; evidence of prior intraventricular hemorrhage (IVH.)
- Hemimegalencephaly: Enlarged, dysmorphic lateral ventricle with straightened, superolaterally angulated frontal horn. Variable anatomic distribution of abnormalities and cortical malformations.

Suggested Readings

Alam A, Sahu S: Magnetic resonance imaging in evaluation of periventricular leukomalacia, *Med J Armed Forces India* 66(4):374–380, 2010.

Benson JC, Nascene D, Truwit C, et al: Septo-optic dysplasia: assessment of associated findings with special attention to the olfactory sulci and tracts, *Clin Neuroradiol* 29(3):505–513, 2019.

Esenwa CC, Leaf DE: Colpocephaly in adults, *BMJ Case Rep.* 2013: bcr2013009505, 2013.

Flores-Sarnat L: Hemimegalencephaly: part 1. Genetic, clinical, and imaging aspects, *J Child Neurol* 17(5):373–384, discussion 384, 2002.

Kirton A, Shroff M, Pontigon A-M: Risk factors and presentations of periventricular venous infarction vs arterial presumed perinatal ischemic stroke, *Arch Neurol* 67(7):842–848, 2010.

Winter TC, Kennedy AM, Woodward PJ: Holoprosencephaly: a survey of the entity, with embryology and fetal imaging, *RadioGraphics* 35(1):275–290, 2015.

98
Periventricular Nodularity

JOSEPHINE MWIKALI NDOLO, MBCHB, MMED AND ASHA SARMA, MD

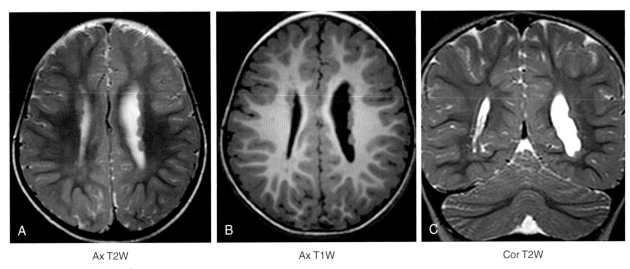

| Ax T2W | Ax T1W | Cor T2W |

CASE A: A 1-year-old male with a history of seizures. *Ax*, Axial.

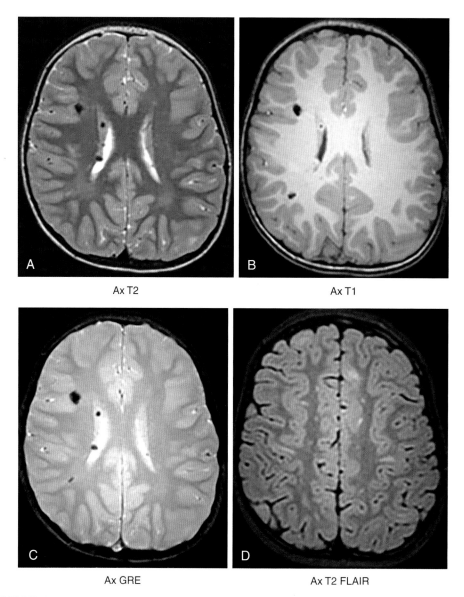

CASE B: A 5-year-old with seizures and intellectual disability. *Ax,* Axial; *FLAIR,* fluid attenuated inversion recovery; *GRE,* gradient recalled echo.

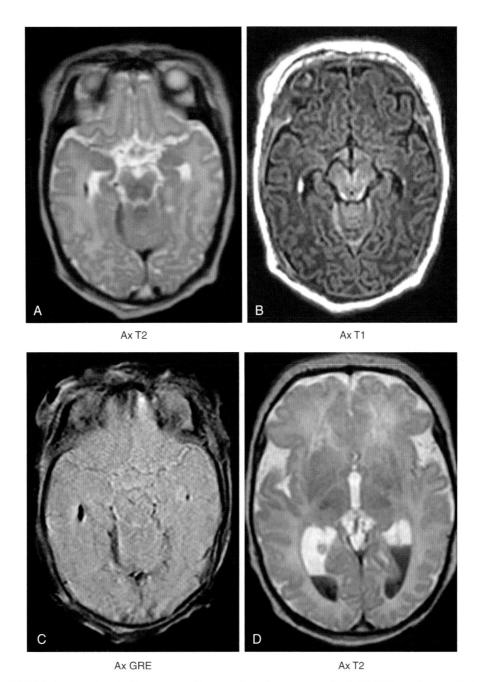

Ax T2   Ax T1

Ax GRE   Ax T2

CASE C: A 4-month-old with a history of intraventricular hemorrhage. *Ax,* Axial; *GRE,* gradient recalled echo.

DESCRIPTION OF FINDINGS

- Case A: MRI of the brain demonstrates nodularity along the ventricular margins bilaterally that is isointense to gray matter on all sequences, most prominent along the left ventricular wall. Additionally, gray matter heterotopia is also seen in the right frontal white matter extending to the subcortical white matter, best seen on the axial T1 image.
- Case B: MRI of the brain demonstrates subependymal nodules that are hypointense on T2, hyperintense on T1, and demonstrating blooming artifact on the gradient refocused echo (GRE) sequence reflecting calcification. Multiple white matter hyperintensities are seen on the axial fluid attenuated inversion recovery (FLAIR) sequence corresponding to cortical tubers. The cortical/subcortical tubers are helpful in distinguishing subependymal nodules of tuberous sclerosis from adherent clot.
- Case C: Two foci of T2 hypointensity, T1 hyperintensity, and corresponding susceptibility artifact along the ventricular walls, right larger than left. The layering blood products in the occipital horns of the lateral ventricles aid in confidently making the diagnosis.

Diagnosis

Case A: Subependymal heterotopia
Case B: Subependymal nodules in tuberous sclerosis
Case C: Intraventricular hemorrhage

Summary

The main differential considerations for periventricular nodularity in the pediatric population are subependymal heterotopia (SEH), subependymal nodules (SEN), and subependymal giant cell astrocytoma (SEGA); in tuberous sclerosis complex (TSC), intraventricular hemorrhage, and ependymal spread of tumor.

Subependymal Heterotopia

Gray matter heterotopia is due to abnormal neuronal migration. It is commonly associated with other brain anomalies such as Chiari II malformation, cephaloceles, cerebellar hypoplasia, fragile X syndrome, and agenesis of the corpus callosum (Fig. 98.1), just to name a few. Gray matter heterotopia has been classified into subependymal (periventricular), subcortical, and band types. SEH is the most common type. It is characterized by nodularity along the margins of the lateral ventricles. SEH is most commonly located at the trigone and occipital horns of lateral ventricles. On imaging, foci of SEH appear as smooth, round, often clustered masses that are

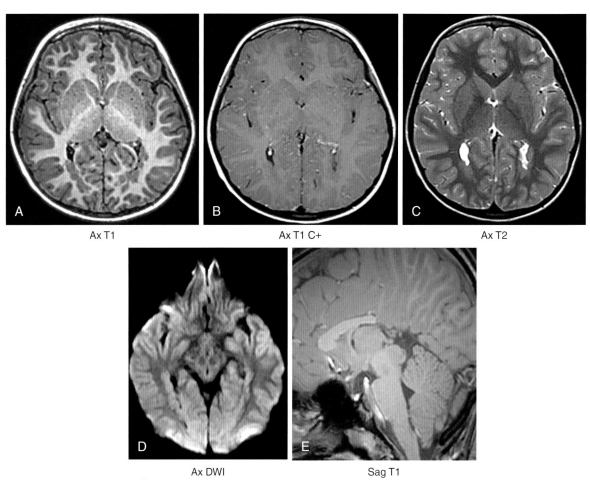

Ax T1   Ax T1 C+   Ax T2

Ax DWI   Sag T1

• **Fig. 98.1** A 5-year-old with subependymal heterotopia. The posterior periventricular nodularity is isointense to gray matter on all sequences without postcontrast enhancement (B). On the DWI sequence (D), the heterotopic gray matter is relatively bright compared to the adjacent white matter. Also seen is the associated partial agenesis of the corpus callosum (E) with absence of the posterior body and splenium. *Ax,* Axial; *DWI,* Diffusion-weighted imaging; *Sag,* Sagittal.

isointense to gray matter on all sequences. They may be single or extensive and multiple. They may protrude into the ventricular lumen or extend into the adjacent white matter. Diffusion-weighted imaging (DWI) may be helpful in detecting small foci of SEH, which are relatively bright compared to adjacent white matter and similar to cortex (Fig. 98.1D). SEH does not enhance after administration of intravenous contrast (Fig. 98.1B) and does not calcify, allowing differentiation from SEN of TSC, which are variably calcified and enhancing. SEN of TSC are concentrated along the caudates and more irregular in shape, with their long axes perpendicular to the ventricular wall.

Subependymal Nodules (Tuberous Sclerosis Complex)

TSC is an autosomal dominant genetic disorder characterized by variable benign hamartoma development in several organs, including the brain, heart, skin, eyes, kidney, lung, and liver. Intracranially, the main findings are cortical tubers, SENs, and SEGAs. SENs are collections of swollen glial cells and giant cells, usually located in the former location of the germinal matrix, concentrated along the caudates. SENs often calcify, usually after the first year of life. Their appearance on MRI changes as the adjacent brain myelinates. In infants, the SENs are hyperintense on T1-weighted imaging and hypointense on T2-weighted imaging relative to the unmyelinated white matter and can at times be confused for subependymal hemorrhage. As brain myelination progresses, the SENs become isointense to white matter and are most apparent on T1-weighted imaging where they stand out against low-intensity CSF. Enhancement after administration of intravenous contrast is variable, ranging from none to intense, but has no clinical significance. Recognition of additional findings of tuberous sclerosis (TS) in the brain or other organs can be helpful in differentiating SENs from other causes of periventricular nodularity. Calcified SENs may mimic periventricular calcifications that occur in congenital cytomegalovirus (CMV) infection; however, additional typical features of congenital CMV can help distinguish the two entities.

SENs can progress to SEGAs, from which they are histologically indistinguishable. A SEGA is defined as an enlarging SEN located near the foramen of Monro. On imaging, one can differentiate SEGA from SEN on the basis of the progressive growth, location, larger size, and potential for mass effect. Growth is the most reliable distinguishing feature. Neither the degree of enhancement nor signal intensity is helpful in making the distinction. Given the location near the foramen of Monro (Fig. 98.2), SEGAs can lead to obstructive hydrocephalus. Serial imaging is recommended to monitor growth of SENs and potential transformation into SEGA.

Intraventricular Hemorrhage

Hemorrhage in the preterm infant typically begins in the germinal matrix, classically at the caudothalamic groove. The germinal matrix is the source of future neuronal and glial cells in the

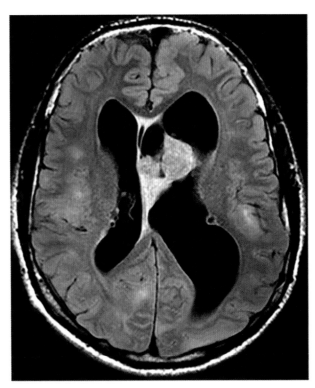

Ax FLAIR

• **Fig. 98.2** A large, lobulated FLAIR hyperintense lesion in the region of the left foramen of Monro consistent with a subependymal giant cell astrocytoma in a 16-year-old male with tuberous sclerosis. Smaller subependymal nodules are also seen bilaterally, including cortical and subcortical tubers. *Ax,* Axial; *FLAIR,* fluid attenuated inversion recovery.

immature brain, and this embryonic structure usually involutes by 34-weeks gestation. The propensity to bleed is due to fragile vessels in the germinal matrix and lack of cerebral arterial autoregulation. As mentioned earlier, intraventricular hemorrhage with clot adhering to the walls of the ventricles can appear similar to SENs in fetuses or newborns, particularly if other features of TS are not evident. Hemorrhage in the germinal matrix can extend to the lateral ventricle and, at times, results in nodularity along the lateral ventricular wall. Intraventricular hemorrhage can also occur for other reasons, including choroid plexus hemorrhage due to parturitional stress. Intraventricular clot can be distinguished from the aforementioned causes based on the following features:

• Location (often dependent without tendency for appearance in the caudothalamic grooves)
• Lack of signs of TS
• Typically more amorphous shape
• Characteristic blood signal intensity (including blooming artifact, recalling that SENs typically do not calcify in the first year of life)
• Resolution over serial examinations.

Ependymal Tumor Metastasis

Ependymal spread of tumor can appear as nodular foci along the walls of the ventricles (Fig. 98.3). Ependymal tumor

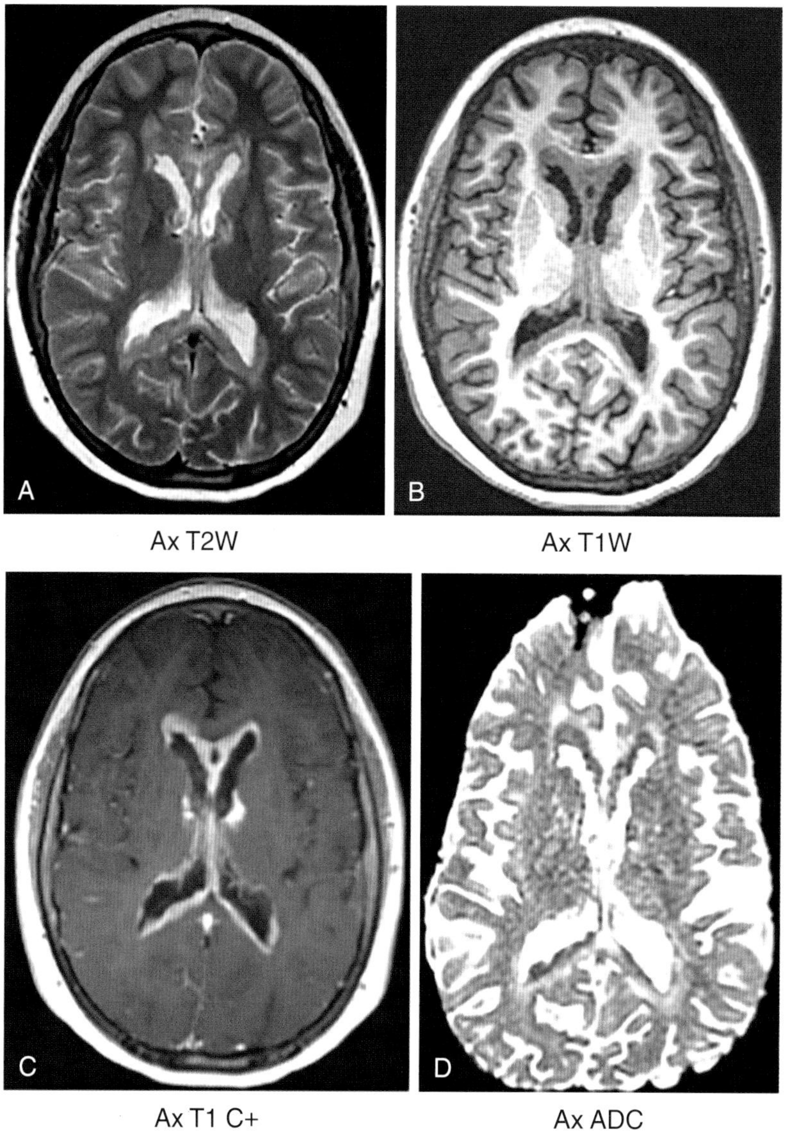

• **Fig. 98.3** A 16-year-old with disseminated germ cell tumor presenting with thick, enhancing diffuse periventricular nodularity with decreased diffusivity as seen on the ADC map (D). *ADC,* Apparent diffusion coefficient; *Ax,* Axial.

deposits typically stand out against suppressed CSF on FLAIR, with otherwise variable signal characteristics and enhancement dependent on characteristics of the primary tumor. Postcontrast FLAIR may increase the conspicuity of lesions in some cases. The presence of additional lesions or history of a primary malignancy may be key in making the diagnosis.

Spectrum of Disease

The spectrum of disease is detailed in the preceding section.

Differential Diagnosis

The differential diagnosis is detailed in the preceding section. See Table 98.1 for a brief summary.

Pearls

- SEH is gray matter-isointense on all sequences and does not enhance. Lack of enhancement, lack of calcification, location, and identification of associated brain findings are key when distinguishing between SEH and TS-related SENs.
- Progressive growth on serial imaging is the most reliable feature for distinguishing SEGAs from SENs. The degree of enhancement and signal characteristics are not helpful features for distinguishing SEGAs from SENs.

Signs and Complications

Signs and complications are generally related to the associated malformations.

TABLE 98.1 Differentiating Between the Various Causes of Periventricular Nodularity

	Gray Matter Heterotopia	Subependymal Nodules	Intraventricular Hemorrhage
Signal characteristics	Matches gray matter on all sequences	Depends on brain myelination and/or calcification	Depend on the age of the blood
Enhancement	None	Variable but common	None
Calcification	Never	Common	None
Location	Anywhere; Commonly at the trigone and occipital horns of lateral ventricles	Usually concentrates around caudates	Often dependent in the lateral ventricles; resolves over serial exams

Suggested Readings

Donkol R, Moghazy KM, Abolenin A: Assessment of gray matter heterotopia by magnetic resonance imaging, *World J Radiol* 4(3):90–96, 2012.

Stein JR, Reidman DA: Imaging manifestations of a subependymal giant cell astrocytoma in tuberous sclerosis, *Case Rep Radiol* 1–5, 2016, 3750450.

Barkovich A: *Pediatric neuroimaging*, ed 6, Philadelphia, 2019, Lippincott Williams & Wilkins.

99
Congenital Fluid-Filled Cranial Vault

KAI WANG, MD AND ASHA SARMA, MD

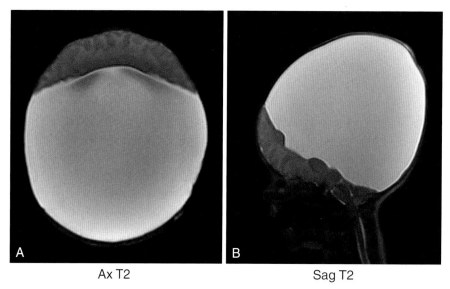

Ax T2   Sag T2

CASE A: A 1-month-old male with macrocephaly and abnormal prenatal ultrasound. *Ax*, Axial; *Sag*, sagittal.

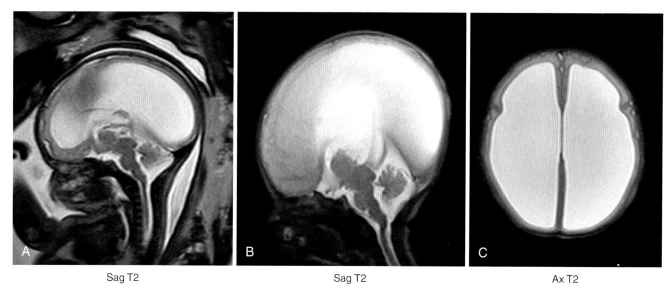

Sag T2   Sag T2   Ax T2

CASE B: A 31-week gestational age male fetus (left); neonate (two right images) with prenatally diagnosed hydrocephalus. *Ax*, Axial; *Sag*, sagittal.

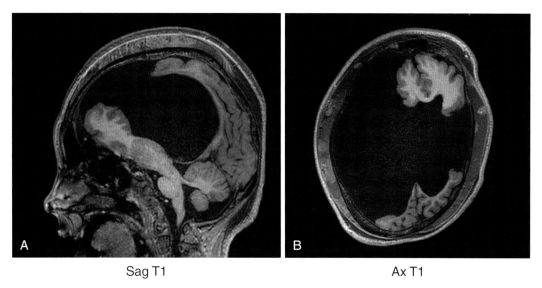

Sag T1

Ax T1

CASE C: A 10-year-old female with history of seizure and developmental delay. *Ax*, Axial; *Sag*, sagittal.

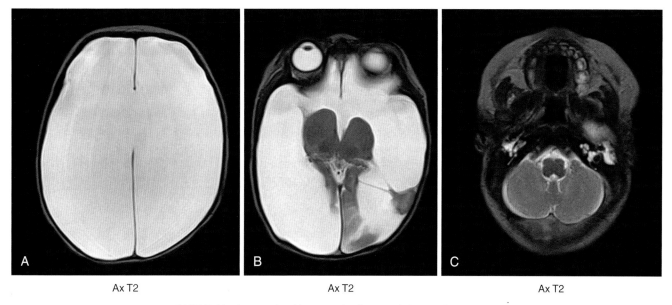

Ax T2

Ax T2

Ax T2

CASE D: Newborn male with prenatally diagnosed abnormality. *Ax*, Axial.

DESCRIPTION OF FINDINGS

- Case A: Continuous cerebral tissue extending across the midline, without normal cleavage of the hemispheres. Absent midline structures, including the corpus callosum, falx, and interhemispheric fissure. Large dorsal cyst in communication with a large monoventricle.
- Case B: Marked supratentorial ventricular enlargement with thinning of the cerebral mantle. Thickened tectum. Absent cerebrospinal fluid (CSF) signal in the cerebral aqueduct.
- Case C: Bilateral transmantle clefts extending from the lateral ventricles to the convexity subarachnoid spaces. The clefts are lined by gray matter with polymicrogyria rather than dysplastic white matter. Absent septum pellucidum. No findings of midline fusion.
- Case D: Absent parenchyma supplied by anterior circulation, with preservation of the brain parenchyma supplied by the vertebrobasilar system (central gray nuclei and cerebellum).

Diagnosis

Case A: Alobar holoprosencephaly
Case B: Congenital X-linked hydrocephalus due to *L1CAM* mutation
Case C: Open-lip schizencephaly
Case D: Hydranencephaly

Summary

Multiple entities may present with fluid-filled appearance of the cranial vault in the neonatal period, including alobar holoprosencephaly (HPE), congenital hydrocephalus, bilateral open-lip schizencephaly, and hydranencephaly. In all of these conditions, much of the normal brain architecture, such as the ventricular system, cavum septum pellucidum, and corpus callosum, may be malformed or destroyed. Although these processes may bear resemblance to one another, knowledge of specific distinguishing neuroimaging features may increase diagnostic accuracy. These disorders may be due to underlying genetic abnormalities or acquired in utero insult. In all of these conditions, affected pediatric patients may need CSF diversion procedures.

Alobar Holoprosencephaly

HPE is caused by the total or partial failure of separation of the prosencephalon into two separate cerebral hemispheres. HPE is a spectrum of disease: from most to least severe, the most common subtypes include alobar, semilobar, and lobar types. Currently, more severe variants of HPE tend to be diagnosed by fetal ultrasound. Alobar HPE is characterized by absence of cleavage of the cerebral hemispheres, resulting in a "pancake," "ball," or "cup" appearance of the parenchyma within the anterior cranial vault. A single large monoventricle is commonly associated with a large dorsal cyst that may exert mass effect and cause macrocrania. Alobar HPE may be distinguished from other entities in the differential diagnosis by complete continuity of gray and white matter across the midline and absence of the falx cerebri. Facial anomalies such as hypotelorism or cyclopia, nasal malformation such as proboscis, and single central maxillary mega incisor may also be seen.

Congenital Hydrocephalus

Severe congenital hydrocephalus is caused by various combinations of abnormal CSF circulation (e.g., congenital aqueductal obstruction from various causes, including X-linked aqueductal stenosis due to *L1CAM* mutation) and failure of CSF resorption (e.g., from infection or intracranial hemorrhage), among other factors. It can present with massive ventriculomegaly with little recognizable normal cerebral tissue. Severe hydrocephalus can sometimes be differentiated from hydranencephaly by recognition of a thin cerebral mantle pressed against the inner table of the calvarium; however, confident distinction is not always possible. Unlike in HPE, the falx is intact.

Bilateral Open-Lip Schizencephaly

Schizencephaly is a neuronal migration disorder that may be due to genetic causes or various insults occurring before neuronal migration is complete. Schizencephaly is characterized by a cleft connecting the ventricles to the subarachnoid space. In distinction to porencephaly (encephalomalacia and gliosis occurring after completion of neuronal migration, on a spectrum with hydranencephaly), the cleft in schizencephaly is lined by abnormal gray matter (usually polymicrogyria) rather than gliotic white matter. However, differentiation may not always be possible by neuroimaging. Subtypes include closed-lip and open-lip schizencephaly. In open-lip schizencephaly, the CSF-filled cleft may be very large and lead to difficulty in distinction from other causes of fluid-filled cranial vault. However, identification of abnormal gray matter lining the cleft margins leads to accurate diagnosis. Presence of the interhemispheric fissure and falx distinguishes severe bilateral open-lip schizencephaly from alobar HPE.

Hydranencephaly

Hydranencephaly is the most severe form of bilateral cerebral destruction and is thought to result from severe in utero anterior cerebral circulation infarction leading to liquefactive necrosis of affected brain structures during the second trimester of gestation. Brain structures supplied by the posterior cerebral arteries are relatively preserved. Therefore, hydranencephaly is characterized by absence of the cerebral hemispheres with intact falx cerebri, brainstem, and cerebellum. In contradistinction to alobar HPE, the thalami tend to be preserved and completely cleaved, and temporo-occipital parenchymal remnants are common. Importantly, the falx is present. Unlike in congenital hydrocephalus, no thinned cerebral mantle is appreciable.

Spectrum of Disease

The spectrum of disease is detailed in the preceding sections.

Differential Diagnosis

1. Encephaloclastic porencephaly
2. Syntelencephaly

3. Septooptic dysplasia
4. Cystic encephalomalacia

Pearls

- Midline fusion differentiates alobar HPE from other causes of fluid-filled cranial vault.
- Presence of thin cerebral mantle tissue distinguishes severe hydrocephalus from hydranencephaly.
- Bilateral open-lip schizencephaly is identified based on abnormal gray matter lined CSF-filled clefts connecting the ventricles and subarachnoid spaces.
- In severe cases, it may be difficult to differentiate among congenital hydrocephalus, bilateral open-lip schizencephaly, and hydranencephaly, and findings may occur in combination.

Signs and Complications

They are detailed in the preceding section.

Suggested Readings

Cecchetto G, Milanese L, Giordano R, et al: Looking at the missing brain: hydranencephaly case series and literature review, *Pediatr Neurol* 48(2):152–158, 2013.

Griffiths PD, Jarvis D: In utero MR imaging of fetal holoprosencephaly: a structured approach to diagnosis and classification, *AJNR Am J Neuroradiol* 37(3):536–543, 2016.

Patel SK, Yuan W, Mangano FT: Advanced neuroimaging techniques in pediatric hydrocephalus, *Pediatr Neurosurg* 52(6):436–445, 2017.

Richieri-Costa A, Ribeiro LA: Single maxillary central incisor, holoprosencephaly, and holoprosencephaly-like phenotype, *Am J Med Genet A* 140(23):2594–2597, 2006.

Stopa J, Kucharska-Miąsik I, Dziurzyńska-Białek E, et al: Diagnostic imaging and problems of schizencephaly, *Pol J Radiol* 79:444–449, 2014.

Yang E, Chu WCW, Lee EY: A practical approach to supratentorial brain malformations: what radiologists should know, *Radiol Clin North Am* 55(4):609–627, 2017.

100
Asymmetric Cerebral Hemispheres

JOSEPHINE MWIKALI NDOLO, MBCHB, MMED AND ASHA SARMA, MD

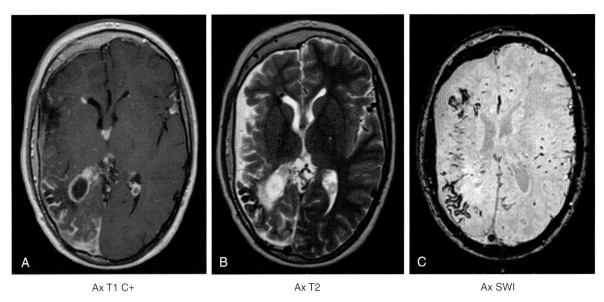

Ax T1 C+   Ax T2   Ax SWI

CASE A: A 17-year-old male with a history of seizures. *Ax*, Axial, *SWI*, susceptibility weighted imaging.

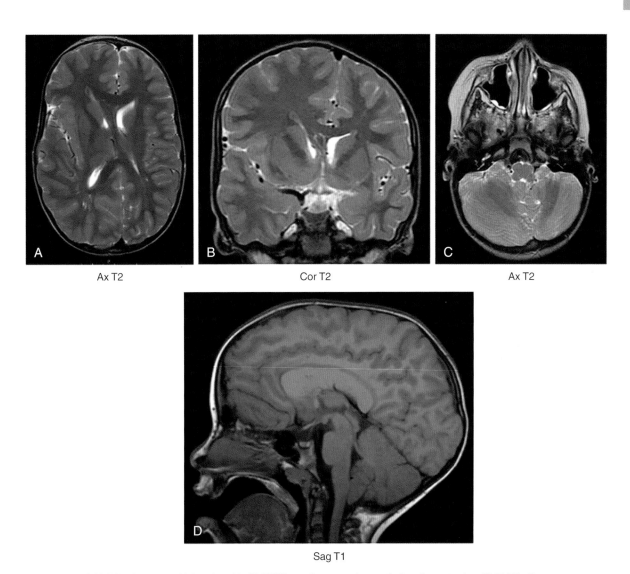

Ax T2   Cor T2   Ax T2

Sag T1

CASE B: A 4-year-old female with CLOVES syndrome and somatic hemihypertrophy. *CLOVES,* Congenital lipomatous asymmetric overgrowth of the trunk with lymphatic, capillary, venous, and combined-type vascular malformations, epidermal naevi, scoliosis/skeletal and spinal anomalies. *Ax,* Axial; *Cor,* coronal; *Sag,* sagittal.

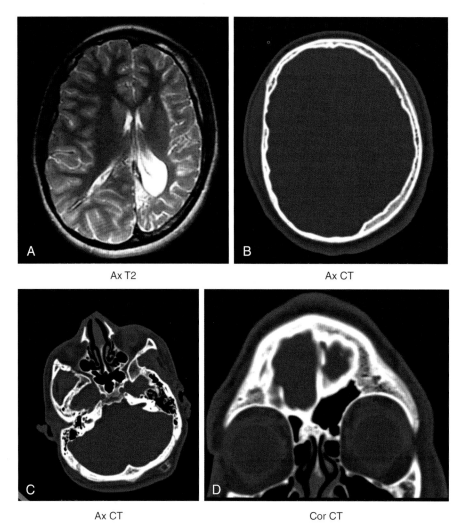

Ax T2

Ax CT

Ax CT

Cor CT

CASE C: A 14-year-old male with cerebral palsy. *Ax,* Axial; *Cor,* coronal; *CT,* Computed tomography.

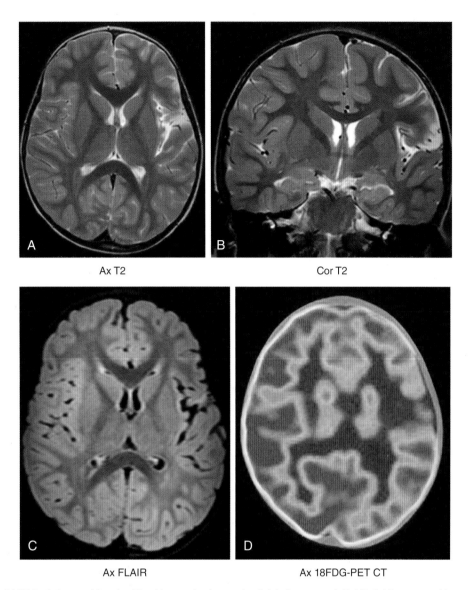

Ax T2	Cor T2
Ax FLAIR	Ax 18FDG-PET CT

CASE D: A 5-year-old male with a history of seizures. *Ax,* Axial, *Cor,* coronal; *FLAIR,* fluid attenuated inversion recovery.

DESCRIPTION OF FINDINGS

- Case A: Right cerebral volume loss and leptomeningeal hyperenhancement, with avid enhancement of the ipsilateral choroid plexus. Calcifications in the ipsilateral cerebral cortex on susceptibility weighted imaging (SWI).
- Case B: Enlargement of the right cerebral and cerebellar cortex with broad gyri. Enlarged, dysmorphic ipsilateral lateral ventricle with characteristically "pointed" frontal horn. Enlarged ipsilateral cerebellar hemisphere. Abnormally thickened corpus callosum.
- Case C: Left cerebral volume loss with enlargement of the left lateral ventricle. Ipsilateral calvarial thickening, ipsilateral paranasal sinus and mastoid sinus hyperpneumatization, and elevated left orbital roof.
- Case D: Left periinsular region volume loss and T2 hyperintensity with corresponding decreased *fluorodeoxyglucose* (FDG) uptake on positron emission tomography (PET).

Diagnosis

Case A: Sturge–Weber syndrome (SWS)
Case B: Hemimegalencephaly
Case C: Dyke–Davidoff–Masson syndrome (DDMS) due to remote unihemispheric ischemic injury
Case D: Rasmussen encephalitis

Summary

Asymmetry of the cerebral hemispheres can be caused by hemiatrophy or hemihypertrophy (as in hemimegalencephaly). The etiologies of childhood cerebral hemiatrophy are diverse but can generally be grouped into congenital and acquired types. In congenital conditions, cerebral damage is usually due to intrauterine vascular injury. Acquired causes include trauma, intracranial hemorrhage, Rasmussen encephalitis, phakomatosis (such as SWS), neoplasms (such as basal ganglia germinoma), and infection (such as TORCH [toxoplasmosis, other infections, cytomegalovirus, and herpes simplex virus] syndrome, HIV). Evaluation of the ventricles (e.g., is the larger ventricle ipsilateral or contralateral to the larger hemisphere?), identification of associated features (e.g., encephalomalacia, gliosis, enhancement, cortical malformations), and assessment of the skull, paranasal sinuses, and mastoid air cells, may be helpful in determining which hemisphere is abnormal and narrowing the differential diagnosis.

Hemimegalencephaly

Hemimegalencephaly is hamartomatous overgrowth of all or part of a cerebral hemisphere, with focal or diffuse neuronal migration or organizational defects within the affected hemisphere. There are three types: isolated, syndromic, and total hemimegalencephaly. The isolated group is a sporadic disorder without cutaneous or systemic involvement. The syndromic type is associated with other clinical features in conditions such as PIK3CA-*R*elated *O*vergrowth *S*pectrum disorders (PROS), neurofibromatosis type 1, and tuberous sclerosis. Of note, syndromic hemimegalencephaly confers a worse prognosis than the isolated type. The third and least common type is total hemimegalencephaly, in which there is also enlargement of the ipsilateral half of the brainstem and cerebellum.

Affected children present with macrocephaly at birth or infancy, which is occasionally erroneously clinically suspected to represent hydrocephalus. Intractable seizures also begin at an early age.

On imaging, there is characteristic enlargement of all or part of a cerebral hemisphere, usually with associated cortical malformation. The most typical appearance of the cortical malformation is thickened cortex with broad gyri, shallow sulci, and indistinct cortical–white matter junction. The gyral pattern may also appear normal, or with polymicrogyria or agyria. On magnetic resonance imaging (MRI), the white matter is often heterogeneous, with variable degrees of T2 hyperintensity due to heterotopia or gliosis. The white matter of the affected hemisphere may also show signs of advanced myelination for age. Patients with agyria tend to have mild-to-moderate hemispheric enlargement, while those with polymicrogyria have more severe hemispheric enlargement. Rarely, both hemispheres may be affected, although almost always asymmetrically.

Importantly, in hemimegalencephaly, the ipsilateral ventricle is characteristically enlarged and the frontal horn appears straight and pointed superiorly and anteriorly. This finding distinguishes hemimegalencephaly from atrophy of the contralateral hemisphere, in which the ventricle in the *smaller* hemisphere is larger due to ex vacuo dilatation.

Rasmussen Encephalitis

Rasmussen encephalitis (RE) is a rare but severe immune-mediated, chronic inflammatory, progressive brain disorder. The etiology is unknown, but autoimmunity associated with persistent viral infection (e.g., upper respiratory infection) has been implicated. Clinically, RE is characterized by drug-resistant focal/partial motor epilepsy (epilepsia partialis continua), followed by hemiparesis and progressive cognitive decline. Patients are typically normal until the onset of seizures, usually between 14 months and 14 years.

Initial imaging is typically normal. Over time, cortical edema, cortical/subcortical T2W hyperintensity, and eventual unilateral progressive cerebral atrophy develop (See Fig. 100.1). There is usually periinsular predominant distribution of abnormalities, with frontal and temporal lobes being the most commonly affected. Most patients will also develop hyperintensity and atrophy of the ipsilateral caudate and putamen. It is important to remember that increasing simple partial seizures in a previously healthy child with normal initial neuroimaging should raise suspicion for RE.

Sturge-Weber Syndrome

SWS is a neurocutaneous syndrome. Although various theories exist as to the underlying cause, this disorder is widely thought to arise from abnormal cortical venous development with resultant pial vascular malformation ("angiomatosis"), cortical anoxia, and development of collateral venous drainage pathways. Angiomatosis involves the face, the choroid of the eye, and leptomeninges (Fig. 100.2). The typically associated facial

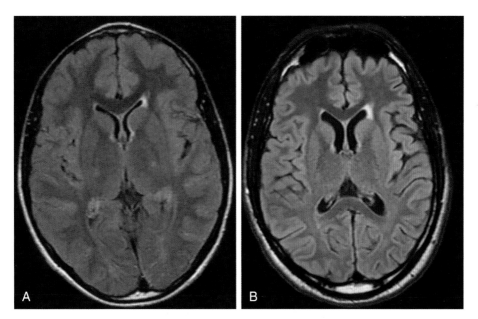

• **Fig. 100.1** A child with Rasmussen Encephalitis. (A) Normal FLAIR MRI brain on the left. (B) Follow-up imaging 5 years later shows subtle left periinsular predominant volume loss. *FLAIR MRI,* Fluid attenuated inversion recovery magnetic resonance imaging.

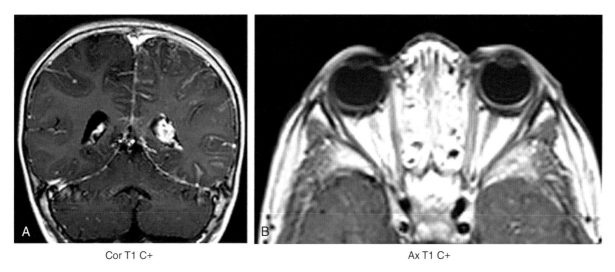

Cor T1 C+   Ax T1 C+

• **Fig. 100.2** (A) Left leptomeningeal angiomatosis with an enlarged and hyperenhancing ipsilateral choroid plexus in Sturge–Weber syndrome. (B) Subtle enhancement of the left posterior globe due to choroidal angioma. *Ax,* Axial; *Cor,* Coronal.

port-wine stain is a capillary malformation that can involve any part of the face but is most characteristically found in the distribution of the ophthalmic division of the trigeminal nerve (the eye and forehead region).

Leptomeningeal angiomatosis is unilateral in 80% to 90% of patients, and bilateral in 10% to 20%. On postcontrast images, the angioma appears as an area of enhancement filling in the subarachnoid space, covering the gyri and sulci. Enlarged deep medullary veins, the collaterals through which venous blood travels from the superficial to deep venous system in the absence of normally developed cortical veins, are seen deep to pial angioma. The ipsilateral choroid plexus is also commonly enlarged, with hyperplasia also resulting from

diversion of venous flow. Calcifications that occur in the cerebral cortex underlying the pial angioma, with a posterior predominance (characteristically, "tram-track" cortical calcifications), are the most common finding on computed tomography (CT). Eventually, the ipsilateral cerebral hemisphere becomes atrophic in most patients. Enhancement of the pial angioma may be inconspicuous if the affected hemisphere is markedly atrophic and heavily calcified.

It is important to remember that imaging findings in infants may differ compared to those in older children. In infancy, MR imaging may be normal, and follow-up imaging is recommended if SWS is suspected clinically. MRI may be optimized by including contrast-enhanced T2-weighted fluid-attenuated inversion recovery (FLAIR) images, which improve detection of subtle leptomeningeal enhancement and differentiation from normal vascular enhancement when compared to T1-weighted post-contrast images. Accelerated white matter myelination may also be seen as one of the early imaging findings in infancy, best seen as accentuated T2 shortening and decreased diffusivity in the white matter on diffusion tensor imaging. The hypermyelination may result from abnormal venous congestion or recurring seizures. Ipsilateral T2-hyperintense marrow signal and marrow enhancement are observed in most patients. In younger patients, this may be the only finding and can provide an early diagnostic clue. Secondary compensatory skull changes to cerebral atrophy, including calvarial thickening and hyperpneumatization of sinuses (as seen in DDMS) have also been described.

Dyke-Davidoff-Masson Syndrome

The term "Dyke–Davidoff–Masson syndrome" refers to a set of conditions with different etiologies, all of which lead to unilateral cerebral atrophy, ipsilateral calvarial hypertrophy, and hyperpneumatization of the paranasal sinuses and mastoid air cells. DDMS is caused by cerebral insult that occurs in utero or during early life, in early stages of calvarial maturation. The brain parenchyma demonstrates signs of remote encephaloclastic injury (e.g., encephalomalacia, gliosis), enlargement of the lateral ventricle and ipsilateral sulci, atrophy of the ipsilateral cerebral peduncle (Wallerian degeneration), and atrophy of the contralateral cerebellum. Calvarial findings include ipsilateral calvarial thickening, ipsilateral paranasal sinus and mastoid hyperpneumatization, and elevated ipsilateral greater sphenoid wing, petrous ridge, and orbital roof. Finding the enlarged ventricle in the smaller hemisphere is another feature that helps to differentiate unilateral volume loss from hemimegalencephaly.

Spectrum of Disease

The spectrum of disease is detailed in the preceding section.

Differential Diagnosis

The differential diagnosis is detailed in the preceding section.

Pearls

- In hemimegalencephaly, a helpful classic imaging finding is a dysmorphic enlarged ventricle in the larger hemisphere. Identification of somatic overgrowth, ipsilateral cortical malformation, and ipsilateral cerebellar and brainstem enlargement are potentially useful clinical and imaging features.
- Initial imaging in RE is typically normal. Subsequent imaging shows unilateral progressive cerebral volume loss, predominantly in the periinsular region. Serial imaging and close correlation with clinical and electroencephalographic findings are often needed to make the diagnosis.
- SWS is most often characterized by unilateral cerebral volume loss. Additional distinctive features include "tram-track" calcification, enhancing pial and choroidal angiomas, enlarged deep venous collaterals, and ipsilateral enlarged choroid plexus.
- DDMS is characterized by unilateral cerebral atrophy due to an encephaloclastic insult in early life. Ipsilaterally enlarged ventricle due to hemispheric volume loss, calvarial hypertrophy, and hyperpneumatization of the paranasal sinuses and mastoid air cells are helpful clues to the diagnosis.

Signs and Complications

Signs and complications are generally related to the associated malformations or injuries.

Suggested Readings

Broumandi, DD, Hayward UM, Benzian JM, et al: Best cases from the AFIP: hemimegalencephaly, *Radiographics* 24(3):843–848, 2004.

Varghese B, Aneesh M, Singh N, et al: A case of Rasmussen encephalitis: the differential diagnoses and role of diagnostic imaging, *Oman Med J* 29(1):67–70, 2014.

Barkovich A: *Pediatric neuroimaging*, ed 6, 2019, Lippincott Williams & Wilkins.

101
Cortical Malformations

JENNIFER HUANG, MD, MED AND ASHA SARMA, MD

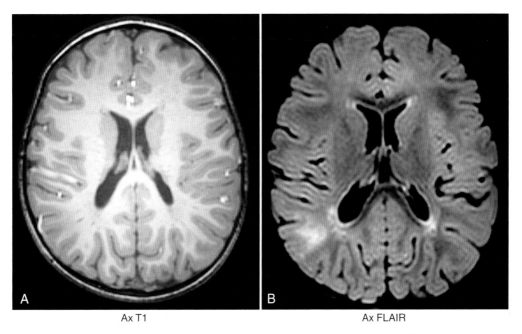

Ax T1   Ax FLAIR

CASE A: A 2-year-old otherwise healthy child with seizure and fever. *Ax,* Axial; *FLAIR,* fluid attenuated inversion recovery.

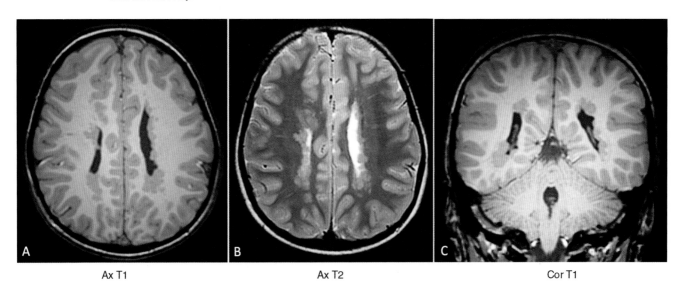

Ax T1   Ax T2   Cor T1

CASE B: A 6-year-old child with headache and developmental delay. *Ax,* Axial; *Cor,* coronal.

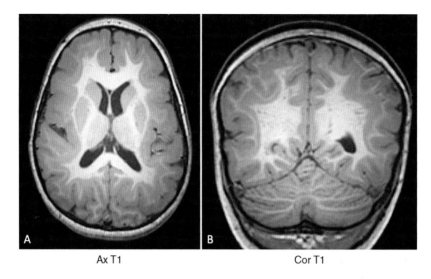

Ax T1   Cor T1

CASE C: A 3-year-old child presenting with epilepsy and developmental delay. *Ax*, Axial; *Cor*, coronal.

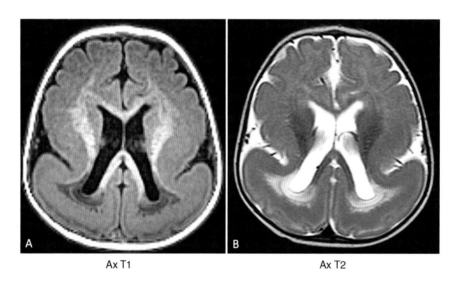

Ax T1   Ax T2

CASE D: A 7-month-old infant presenting with developmental delay. *Ax*, Axial.

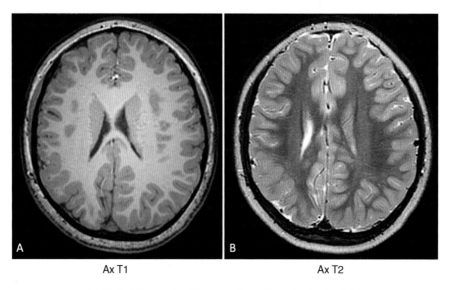

Ax T1   Ax T2

CASE E: A 7-year-old child presenting with epilepsy. *Ax*, Axial.

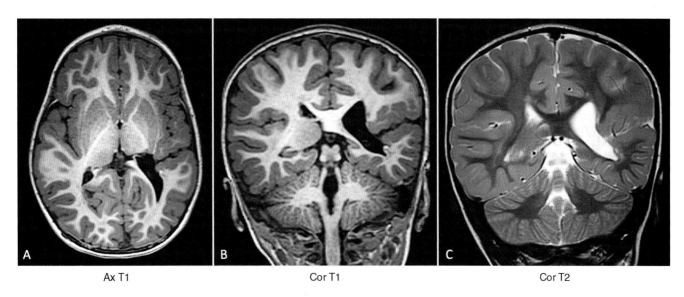

Ax T1   Cor T1   Cor T2

CASE F: A 3-year-old child presenting with intermittent/transient left eye esotropia and nystagmus. *Ax*, Axial; *Cor*, coronal.

DESCRIPTION OF FINDINGS

- Case A: Focal cortical/subcortical T2 prolongation in right parietal lobe with blurring of the gray-white matter junction and transmantle sign (wedge-shaped T2/fluid attenuated inversion recovery [FLAIR] hyperintense signal radially oriented toward the ipsilateral ventricle).
- Case B: Numerous nodular foci of gray matter in the bilateral subependymal regions in a patient with callosal dysgenesis (not pictured).
- Case C: Band of heterotopic gray matter deep to the cortex.
- Case D: Posterior agyria and less pronounced anterior gyral simplification. From outer to innermost, characteristic pattern of thin cortex, subjacent T2 hyperintense "cell sparse zone," thick band of heterotopic gray matter, and dysplastic white matter.
- Case E: Thickened, nodular cortex with shallow sulci and increased gyral frequency, with associated abnormal sulcation in the right parietooccipital region.
- Case F: Thin, CSF-containing cleft lined with abnormal gray matter with polymicrogyria (PMG), connecting the convexity subarachnoid space with the lateral ventricle. "Dimpled" appearance of the ventricular margin pointing into the cleft.

Diagnosis

Case A: Focal cortical dysplasia (type IIb)
Case B: Periventricular ventricular nodular heterotopia
Case C: Band heterotopia
Case D: Lissencephaly (*L1S1/PAFAH1B1*-associated)
Case E: Polymicrogyria
Case F: Schizencephaly

Summary

Malformations of cortical development (MCD) are a heterogeneous and large group of disorders of disrupted cerebral cortical formation. These malformations result from aberrations in three major stages of cortical development: (1) cell proliferation and apoptosis; (2) cell migration; and (3) postmigrational development. Classification is based on the stage that is first affected, as the initial disruption may have effects on subsequent stages of development.

There are numerous underlying causes, including genetic, infectious, vascular, and metabolic entities. Manifestations may include abnormal cortical structure or gray matter heterotopia, and sometimes abnormal brain size (micro- or megalencephaly). Although clinical presentations vary, affected pediatric patients may present with epilepsy, developmental delay or intellectual disability, or cerebral palsy. Up to half of drug-resistant epilepsies requiring surgical treatment are caused by MCD. Accurate radiological diagnosis is key in guiding genetic testing and treatment planning, especially in the context of epilepsy surgery. Active research into the genetic and mechanistic underpinnings of MCDs is ongoing, leading to rapidly changing systems of classification. This chapter covers a sample of more commonly encountered entities. A comprehensive discussion of etiopathogenesis and current classification of MCDs is beyond the scope of this clinically focused text, but may be found in the excellent article by Severino and colleagues that is cited below.

Importantly, the imaging appearance of cortical malformations may change rapidly across fetal and early postnatal life due to developmental changes including sulcation and progression of myelination. Postnatally, magnetic resonance imaging (MRI) assessment is generally the most accurate in early infancy or after completion of myelination (which occurs around 2 years of age), when gray-white differentiation is maximal. In the intermediate time frame, the gray-white boundary may be difficult to visualize, necessitating MRI follow-up.

A few key features of assessment include (1) relative head size (normocephaly, microcephaly, macrocephaly); (2) gyral pattern (normal, simplified, or abnormal gyral pattern); (3) presence of heterotopia (discussed further later); (4) identification of associated malformations (e.g., posterior fossa or callosal malformations); and (5) correlation with clinical data (e.g., side of hemiplegia, seizure semiology, electroencephalographic findings).

Differential Diagnosis

Focal Cortical Dysplasia

Focal cortical dysplasia (FCD) refers to a heterogeneous group of focal cortical malformations, which are characterized by cortical architectural abnormalities and/or cytological abnormalities. There are three subgroups of FCD, categorized at the pathology level. Type I refers to alterations in cortical layering, either columnar/radial or laminar/tangential. Type II, the most common, describes disruption of cortical lamination with abnormal cell types, while type III refers to type I FCD with an additional brain lesion (i.e., neoplasm) in the same lobe. The cortical tubers of tuberous sclerosis are considered a subtype of FCD IIb due to the histological and imaging similarities. Imaging features of FCD include cortical thickening, blurring of the gray-white matter junction, abnormal sulcal or gyral pattern, cortical or subcortical signal abnormality, and transmantle sign (radially oriented T2/FLAIR hyperintense signal in subcortical white matter pointing toward the ipsilateral ventricle). Of note, these imaging findings may appear different in unmyelinated brains, often showing hypointense T2 and hyperintense T1 signal intensity in involved areas. As many of these imaging features can be very subtle and therefore overlooked, further evaluation with surgical EEG, hybrid imaging such as MRI/positron emission tomography (PET), and/or multidisciplinary discussions is often necessary.

Gray Matter Heterotopia

Gray matter heterotopia, mainly due to impaired cell migration, manifests as clusters of normal neurons in abnormal locations and is classically categorized based on morphology and location. Regardless of the location, the key distinguishing imaging feature is isointensity with the cerebral cortex on all magnetic resonance pulse sequences. Periventricular nodular heterotopia (PVNH) is the most common type, representing nodular areas of ectopic gray matter lining the ventricular wall.

Subcortical heterotopia is a broad term referring to conglomerates of gray matter within the white matter of bilateral cerebral hemispheres, which include transmantle and ribbon-like heterotopia, as well as cerebral hamartomas.

Lissencephaly-Pachygyria Spectrum

Lissencephaly is a disorder of neuronal migration that includes a spectrum of agyria (absent gyration) to pachygyria (reduced gyration). Although both lissencephaly and PMG feature thickened cortices, lissencephaly demonstrates absent or decreased number of sulci (agyria and pachygyria, respectively) resulting in a smooth and thickened appearance of the cortex. The key to differentiating lissencephaly from PMG is to look for the simplified smooth gyral pattern in lissencephaly compared to the nodular disorganized gyral folds of PMG. Another potentially useful distinguishing feature is to look at the sylvian fissures, which will be shallow and vertically oriented in lissencephaly. The gray-white matter junction is smooth and there may be decreased white matter volume. Lissencephaly was historically categorized into two groups; however, it is now recognized that cobblestone malformation (previously lissencephaly type II) represents a different pathophysiology than other forms of lissencephaly, and therefore this categorization has been discarded. Subcortical band heterotopia (SBH) is a malformation that is considered part of the lissencephaly-pachygyria spectrum due to common underlying genetic etiologies. It is characterized by a "double cortex," with a thick symmetric subcortical gray matter band and thin cortex. At first glance, this thickened appearance may appear similar to PMG, but the differentiating feature is the white matter layer between the gray matter band heterotopia and the overlying cortex.

Polymicrogyria

PMG is a cortical malformation with variable appearance. The term refers to excessively small and numerous gyri, and this is traditionally thought of as a disorder of late neuronal migration and cortical organization, although this has been disputed in some literature. There are many genetic and nongenetic causes, e.g., chromosomal abnormalities, in utero infections, and exposure to teratogens. PMG can be unilateral, bilateral, or multifocal, and when bilateral, it is often seen symmetrically. The most common location is in the perisylvian regions, particularly along the posterior aspect. Thin-section T1- and T2-weighted imagings are complementary in establishing the diagnosis. On thin-section imaging, PMG is seen as irregular gyri, while on thick-section imaging, it appears as a thickened nodular cortex due to its innumerable and disorganized gyral folds. PMG is more often focal and/or asymmetric, while pachygyria, which can also appear as a thickened cortex, is more frequently bilateral and symmetric.

Schizencephaly

Schizencephaly is a disorder of neuronal migration, resulting in a full-thickness parenchymal cleft that extends from the cortical surface to the ventricle, and which is lined by dysplastic gray matter, often PMG. Schizencephaly likely results from an early prenatal focal injury to the germinal matrix or infarct in an immature cerebrum, with replacement of involved tissue by malformed cortex. Patients often present with seizures and developmental delay. There are two types: closed lip and open lip, with closed lip referring to the cleft walls being closely apposed, while open lip implying wider separation of the walls by a larger CSF-filled cleft. A clue in identifying subtle closed-lip schizencephaly is to look for a dimple in the normally smooth contours of the walls of the lateral ventricles. Multiplanar imaging is obligatory as subtle abnormalities may be overlooked if the plane of imaging is the same as the plane of the cleft. Most common in the frontoparietal lobes near the central sulcus, schizencephaly is seen bilaterally in up to 50% of patients, and when seen unilaterally, there is often contralateral PMG, suggesting the two disorders are on a spectrum. Important associations include septo-optic dysplasia (in 70% of cases—absent septum pellucidum and/or corpus callosum, optic nerve hypoplasia, hypothalamic-pituitary axis abnormalities).

Dysgyria

Dysgyria is a recently introduced term that encompasses a nonspecific malformation with dysmorphic cortex but with an imaging appearance not typical for PMG, pachygyria, or simplified gyral pattern. Imaging may demonstrate normal cortical thickness but with a disordered gyral pattern, including abnormalities of sulcal depth and orientation, smooth cortical surface, or narrow gyri separated by deep or shallow sulci. These can be diffuse or localized. The full range of disorders in which dysgyria is seen is not yet known, but was first described in association with mutations of the tubulin genes and dystroglycanopathies.

Differential Diagnosis

1. Tuberous sclerosis: Includes FCD IIb with the syndrome, differentiated from sporadic cases of FCD IIb by additional associated imaging findings, including subependymal nodules and subependymal giant cell astrocytoma.
2. Glioneuronal tumor: May be difficult to differentiate from FCD and may also be seen in association; possible clues include older age at onset of seizures, higher uptake on (11) C-methionine PET.
3. Stenogyria/polygyria: Differs from PMG as the cortex is histologically normal in organization. Imaging demonstrates multiple narrow gyri separated by shallow sulci. Associated with Chiari II malformation.
4. Porencephaly: Differs from schizencephaly as the cleft is not lined by gray matter, but instead, gliotic white matter. May result from a later developmental insult.

Pearls

Malformation	Etiopathological Considerations	Key Imaging Findings
Microcephaly	Reduced proliferation or increased apoptosis Genetic and acquired causes (including congenital cytomegalovirus infection)	• Small head circumference • May have normal or abnormal cortex
Macrocephaly and brain overgrowth spectrum	Increased proliferation or decreased apoptosis Associations including *PTEN*, *PI3K* mutation	• Increased head circumference • May have normal cortex or be associated with cortical malformations or white matter signal abnormalities • Posterior fossa structures less commonly involved
Focal cortical dysplasia	Disordered cortical lamination +/− abnormal cell types Associated with tuberous sclerosis, neurofibromatosis type II	• Focal cortical thickness abnormality • Abnormal gyral and sulcal pattern • Gray-white matter junction blurring • "Transmantle" sign
Gray matter heterotopia	Impaired neuronal migration Extensive PVNH associated with *FLNA* mutation	• Conglomerates of gray matter in heterotopic locations, which follow cortex on all MR sequences
Lissencephaly-pachygyria	Impaired neuronal migration Mutations including *LIS1*, *DCX*	• Thickened cortex with absent or reduced gyration • Subcortical band heterotopia on same spectrum
Cobblestone malformation	Neuronal overmigration Associated with dystroglycanopathies, Zika virus infection	• Undersulcated cerebral surface with mild to moderate cortical thickening • Micronodular cortical surface on thin-section MRI due to overmigration of neurons beyond pial limiting membrane • Posterior fossa abnormalities: brainstem cleft, cerebellar microcysts
Polymicrogyria	Impaired neuronal migration and organization Numerous associations	• "Thickened" overfolded cortex with excessive small gyri • Most commonly along sylvian fissures
Schizencephaly	Impaired neuronal migration Associated with septo-optic dysplasia	• Parenchymal cleft extending from cortex to ventricles, lined by dysplastic gray matter, often PMG
Dysgyria	Impaired neuronal migration and organization	• Abnormal gyral pattern with abnormal sulcal depth or orientation, not meeting criteria for other MCD types

Signs and Complications

The signs and complications are detailed in the preceding section.

Suggested Readings

De Ciantis A, Barkovich AJ, Cosottini C, et al: Ultra-high-field MR imaging in polymicrogyria and epilepsy, *AJNR Am J Neuroradiol* 36(2):309–316, 2015.

Di Donato N, Chiari S, Mirzaa GM, et al: Lissencephaly: expanded imaging and clinical classification, *Am J Med Genet A* 173(6):1473–1488, 2017.

Donkol RH, Moghazy KM, Abolenin A: Assessment of gray matter heterotopia by magnetic resonance imaging, *World J Radiol* 4(3):90–96, 2012.

Severino M, Geraldo AF, Utz N, et al: Definitions and classification of malformations of cortical development: practical guidelines, *Brain* 143(10):2874–2894, 2020.

Stopa J, Kucharska-Miąsik I, Dziurzyńska-Białek E, et al: Diagnostic imaging and problems of schizencephaly, *Pol J Radiol* 79:444–449, 2014.

102

Hippocampal and Perihippocampal Lesions

JENNIFER HUANG, MD, MED AND ASHA SARMA, MD

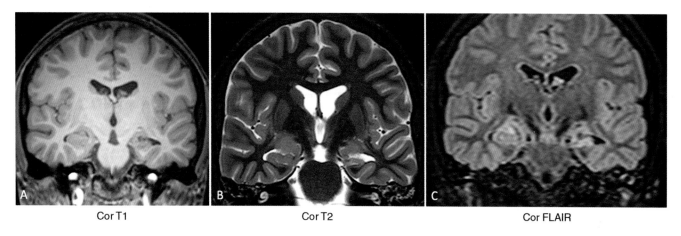

Cor T1   Cor T2   Cor FLAIR

CASE A: A 15-year-old child with seizures. *Cor,* Coronal; *FLAIR,* fluid attenuated inversion recovery.

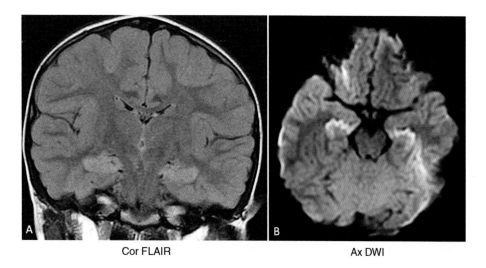

Cor FLAIR   Ax DWI

CASE B: A 29-month-old child with status epilepticus. *Ax,* Axial; *Cor,* coronal; *DWI,* diffusion-weighted imaging; *FLAIR,* fluid attenuated inversion recovery.

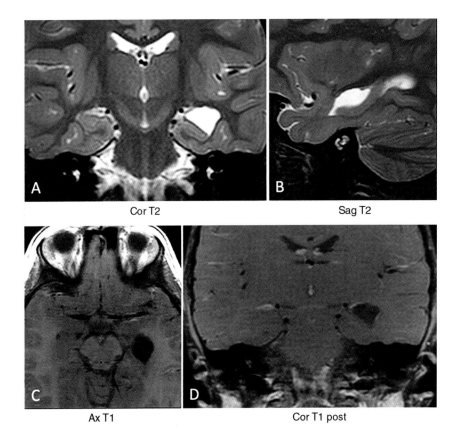

Cor T2

Sag T2

Ax T1

Cor T1 post

CASE C: A 16-year-old child with headaches. *Ax,* Axial; *Cor,* coronal; *Sag,* sagittal.

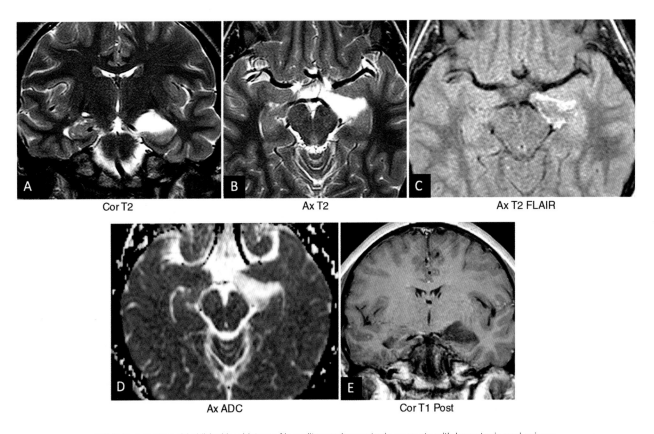

Cor T2

Ax T2

Ax T2 FLAIR

Ax ADC

Cor T1 Post

CASE D: A 3-year-old child with a history of hereditary spherocytosis presents with hypertonia and seizure. *ADC,* Apparent diffusion coefficient; *Ax,* axial; *Cor,* coronal; *FLAIR,* fluid attenuated inversion recovery.

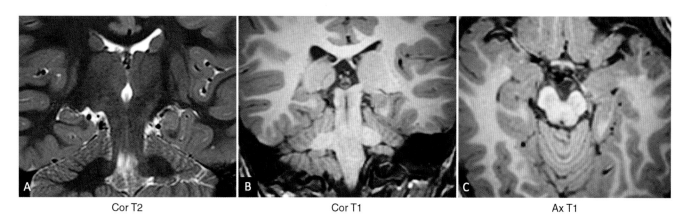

Cor T2   Cor T1   Ax T1

CASE E: A 6-year-old child with seizures. *Ax*, Axial; *Cor*, coronal.

DESCRIPTION OF FINDINGS

- Case A: Asymmetrically small size and hyperintensity of the left hippocampus on T2-weighted imaging and fluid-attenuated inversion recovery (FLAIR) with loss of normal hippocampal architectural features. Normal right hippocampus. Relative prominence of the temporal horn of the left lateral ventricle due to volume loss.
- Case B: Symmetric, cortically based reduced diffusivity in both hippocampi with swollen, hyperintense appearance of the hippocampi and parahippocampal gyri on FLAIR.
- Case C: cerebrospinal fluid (CSF)-isointense, nonenhancing, spindle-shaped lesion with complete suppression on FLAIR imaging in right medial temporal lobe causing minimal mass effect on the left hippocampus.
- Case D: Well-defined, T2-hyperintense, T1-hypointense, nonenhancing mass with incomplete suppression on FLAIR imaging and without restricted diffusion in the left mesial temporal lobe. Minimal mass effect without surrounding edema.
- Case E: Globular-appearing left hippocampus with vertical orientation of the collateral sulcus. Preserved hippocampal architecture and signal without dilatation of the temporal horn.

Diagnosis

Case A: Mesial temporal sclerosis
Case B: Status epilepticus
Case C: Choroid fissure cyst
Case D: Dysembryoplastic neuroepithelial tumor (DNT)
Case E: Incomplete hippocampal inversion

Summary

Temporal lobe epilepsy is the most common focal epilepsy in pediatric patients, often prompting imaging evaluation of the brain in order to identify a causal structural abnormality. The hippocampus of the temporal lobe consists of two interlocking gray matter folds. It lies immediately below the temporal horn of the lateral ventricle and arches around the mesencephalon (hence the term "mesiotemporal"). Evaluation of hippocampal lesions relies on accurate identification of the three anatomic components of the hippocampus (head, body, and tail) and nearby landmarks. Abnormalities in this region most commonly present clinically as partial complex seizures that can be localized via surface electroencephalography.

Temporal lobe epilepsy has a fairly broad variety of causes, including mesial temporal sclerosis, tumors, malformations of cortical development, vascular malformations, trauma, and infection. MRI is the imaging modality of choice in evaluating the temporal lobe, specifically including thin-section, oblique coronal sequences oriented perpendicular to the long axis of the hippocampus.

Differential Diagnosis

Mesial Temporal Sclerosis

Mesial temporal sclerosis (MTS) describes the finding associated with hippocampal neuronal loss and gliosis related to seizures. Patients often present with a history of childhood seizures. Coronal T2-weighted and FLAIR images are the most sensitive in detecting MTS. Imaging findings may be extremely subtle in the early stages, and patients may initially present with seizure-related hippocampal swelling and signal abnormality on T2-weighted imaging, FLAIR, and diffusion-weighted imaging (DWI). While comparison with the contralateral side may be useful, MTS is bilateral in 10% to 20% of cases, which may occasionally lead to misinterpretation as normal. MTS is characterized by abnormal T2 prolongation, decreased hippocampal volume, and loss of the normal hippocampal architecture. Secondary signs include ipsilateral atrophy of the fornix and mammillary body and enlargement of the temporal horn of the ipsilateral lateral ventricle. Dual pathology with a second epileptogenic lesion (such as focal cortical dysplasia) may be seen in up to 15% of cases, and these lesions should be actively sought on MRI evaluation for accurate treatment planning.

Status Epilepticus

The imaging findings in status epilepticus may mimic MTS, with T2 hyperintense appearance of the hippocampi. However, unlike in MTS, patients with status epilepticus will not have atrophy or architectural distortion of the hippocampus. Additionally, cortically based low diffusivity may be present due to cytotoxic edema in the acute stage of status epilepticus. These seizure-related changes will typically resolve on follow-up imaging within days to weeks after treatment of the seizures. However, in some cases, hippocampus involvement of status epilepticus can lead to MTS. In the acute setting, in a patient who is actively seizing, MRI is often ordered to look for an underlying causative lesion. Hippocampal low diffusivity can also be seen in global hypoxic injury (involving both gray and white matter) or transient global amnesia. Patients with hippocampal injury due to hypoxia will often have coexistent findings in other ischemia-sensitive structures such as the globi pallidi. Transient global amnesia is a disorder of older adults who present with self-limited memory loss, in which characteristic dot-like foci of low diffusivity are transiently present.

Choroid Fissure Cyst

Choroid fissure cysts (CFCs) are benign extraaxial neuroepithelial cysts within or near the choroidal fissure, the CSF-containing groove that runs immediately above the hippocampal fimbriae. Most cases are asymptomatic and found incidentally. On imaging, CFCs typically appear as small (1 to 2 cm in diameter), well-circumscribed, cystic lesions that are located medial to the lateral ventricle temporal horn, between the hippocampus and diencephalon. In addition to being found in this characteristic location, CFC follows CSF on all sequences (including FLAIR), is nonenhancing, and demonstrates a classic spindle shape on sagittal images. These features are key in differentiating CFC from other cystic-appearing structures in this region, including neoplasms (usually without suppression on FLAIR and sometimes enhancement) and hippocampal sulcus remnant cysts (smaller and often more numerous). Typically, no treatment is needed, although some authors propose surgical resection in rare cases of CFC causing significant mass effect in patients with intractable epilepsy.

Dysembryoplastic Neuroepithelial Tumor

The majority of patients with dysembryoplastic neuroepithelial tumors (DNTs) present in childhood (mean age of 10 years) with partial complex seizures. DNT most commonly occurs in the cortex of the medial temporal lobe (50% to 80%), with the second most common location being in the frontal lobe (33%). Classically, this cortically based mass "points" toward the ventricle with a wedge-shaped morphology, which is thought to relate to its origin from dysplastic cells in the germinal matrix that migrate toward the cortex. As a frequent trigger of intractable epilepsy, DNT is often small at presentation. DNT should be considered in a child or adolescent with partial complex epilepsy who is found to have a multilobular, cystic-appearing, or "bubbly" T2/FLAIR-hyperintense cortically based mass within the temporal lobe with minimal surrounding edema. Unlike nonneoplastic lesions such as CFC and arachnoid cyst, DNT does not suppress on FLAIR, and facilitated diffusion can distinguish DNT from epidermoid. Characteristic morphology and infrequent enhancement frequently differentiate DNT from other low-grade epilepsy-associated temporal lobe neoplasms, such as ganglioglioma and pleomorphic xanthoastrocytoma (PXA) although imaging is imperfect in distinguishing among low-grade epilepsy associated tumors due to overlapping findings.

Incomplete Hippocampal Inversion

Incomplete hippocampal inversion (IHI), or "hippocampal malrotation," results from failure of complete inversion of the hippocampus during fetal development. This results in a medially displaced, rounded, and globular-appearing hippocampus with associated vertically oriented collateral sulcus, more commonly seen on the left. The fornix may be inferiorly displaced. The hippocampus itself demonstrates normal signal intensity, however, there is blurring of the normal hippocampal internal architecture. Comparison with the contralateral side, if normal, can be helpful. The role of IHI in the pathogenesis of epilepsy is controversial. A recent systematic review by Mutti, et al. reported that IHI is commonly observed in patients with malformations of cortical development, especially periventricular nodular heterotopia or polymicrogyria. However, weak increased odds of epilepsy in individuals with IHI suggest that isolated IHI is not a strong independent predictor for epilepsy development.

Spectrum of Disease

The spectrum of disease is detailed in the preceding section.

Pearls

- In pediatric patients who present with seizures localized to the temporal lobes, low-grade neoplasms and cortical dysplasias are more common causes of temporal lobe epilepsy compared to MTS. It is important to remember that lesions may co-occur.
- Careful evaluation of hippocampal anatomy and comparison to the contralateral side is imperative in the diagnosis of MTS, which can exhibit subtle findings early in the course of disease.
- Choroid fissure cyst is typically an asymptomatic, incidental finding that can be distinguished based on its characteristic location above the hippocampal fimbriae, as well as spindle-shaped morphology and isointensity to CSF.
- DNT, ganglioglioma, and PXA commonly manifest as cortically based temporal masses that may be difficult to distinguish on imaging, however, some differentiating features may include "bubbly" appearance with wedge-shaped morphology in DNT and enhancement and/or calcification in ganglioglioma and PXA.
- IHI has a questionable association with temporal lobe epilepsy.
- Status epilepticus is a mimic of MTS and can be differentiated by lack of hippocampal architectural distortion and atrophy, as well as cortically based restricted diffusion.

Signs and Complications

The signs and complications are detailed in the preceding sections.

Suggested Readings

Achour A, Mnari W, Miladi A, et al: Temporal choroidal fissure cyst: a rare cause of temporal lobe epilepsy, *Pan Afr Med J* 36:120, 2020.

Cury C, Toro R, Cohen F, et al: Incomplete hippocampal inversion: a comprehensive MRI study of over 2000 subjects, *Front Neuroanat* 9:160, 2015.

Dekeyzer S, De Kock I, Nikoubashman O, et al: "Unforgettable" – a pictorial essay on anatomy and pathology of the hippocampus, *Insights Imaging* 8(2):199–212, 2017.

Granados Sánchez AM, Orejuela Zapata JF: Diagnosis of mesial temporal sclerosis: sensitivity, specificity and predictive values of the quantitative analysis of magnetic resonance imaging, *Neuroradiol J* 31(1):50–59, 2018.

Kim J-A, Chung JI, Yoon PH, et al: Transient MR signal changes in patients with generalized tonicoclonic seizure or status epilepticus: periictal diffusion-weighted imaging, *AJNR Am J Neuroradiol* 22(6):1149–1160, 2001.

Mutti C, Ricco M, Bartolini Y, et al: Incomplete hippocampal inversion and epilepsy: a systematic review and meta-analysis, *Epilepsia* 62(2):383–396, 2021.

Raz E, Kapilamoorthy TR, Gupta AK, et al: Case 186: dyscmbrioplastic neuroepithelial tumor, *Radiology* 265(1):317–320, 2012.

103

Leukodystrophies

AHMAD AMER, MD, HALYNA POKHYLEVYCH, MD, SWAPNIL KHOSE, MD, MPH, AND JASON M. JOHNSON, MD, MBA

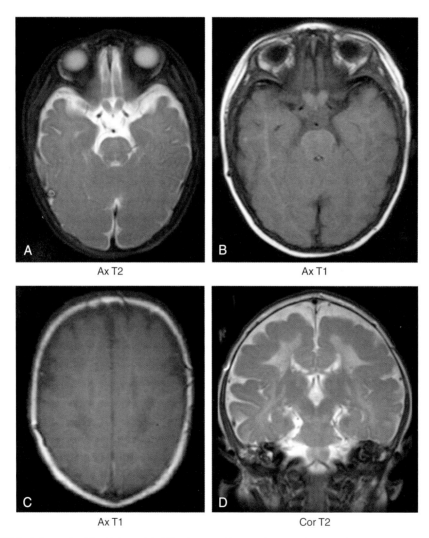

Ax T2

Ax T1

Ax T1

Cor T2

CASE A: A 6-month-old with hyperirritability, increased muscular tone, fever, and developmental arrest. *Ax,* Axial; *Cor,* coronal. (Courtesy Christopher Filippi, MD).

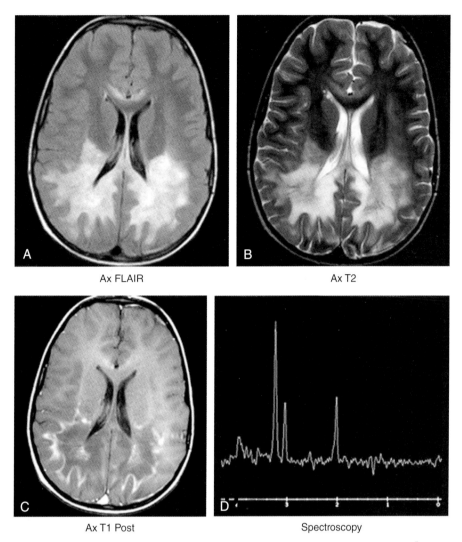

Ax FLAIR

Ax T2

Ax T1 Post

Spectroscopy

CASE B: Normal development until 6 years of age, and then rapid onset of dementia, progressive neurologic decline, and adrenal insufficiency. *Ax,* Axial; *FLAIR,* fluid level attenuation inversion recovery.

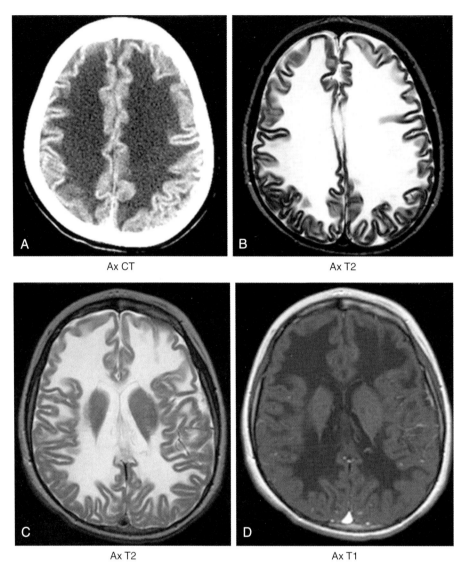

A — Ax CT

B — Ax T2

C — Ax T2

D — Ax T1

CASE C: A 4-year-old with ataxia, spasticity, deterioration following minor head trauma and febrile illness. *Ax*, Axial; *CT*, Computed tomography.

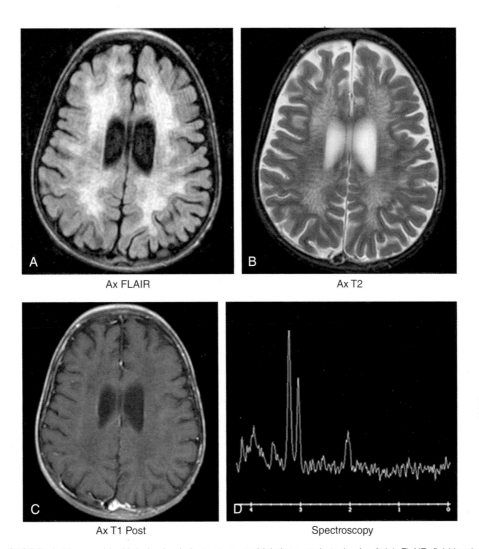

Ax FLAIR

Ax T2

Ax T1 Post

Spectroscopy

CASE D: A 12-year-old with behavioral changes, pyramidal signs, and ataxia. *Ax,* Axial; *FLAIR,* fluid level attenuation inversion recovery.

DESCRIPTION OF FINDINGS

- Case A: Magnetic resonance (MR) imaging reveals symmetric bilateral enlargement of the optic nerves with diffuse, symmetric periventricular white matter T1 hypointensity. Coronal T2-weighted imaging (T2WI) displays confluent, symmetric deep periventricular hyperintensity that spares the subcortical U-fibers. The coronal T2WI also demonstrates T2 hypointense signal and decreased size of the bilateral thalami.
- Case B: T2-fluid-attenuated inversion recovery (T2/FLAIR) and T2W MR images show symmetric, confluent, abnormal, high signal intensity in the parietooccipital white matter with involvement of the splenium of the corpus callosum. On the postcontrast images, a "leading edge" of enhancement is identified. Proton magnetic resonance spectroscopy (MRS) shows marked reduction of the N-acetylaspartate (NAA) (2.0 ppm) and elevation of choline (3.2 ppm) within the affected region of the brain.
- Case C: Unenhanced axial CT image shows diffuse white matter hypoattenuation. This white matter abnormality is better appreciated as hyperintense white matter signal on T2W MRI. T2W and T1W postcontrast images at the level of the diencephalon show preservation of the ependyma with relatively normal size and morphology of the ventricles. No leading edge of enhancement is seen on postcontrast imaging.
- Case D: FLAIR and T2WI show confluent hyperintense signals in a striated or "tigroid" pattern in the periventricular and deep white matter of the cerebral hemispheres, with sparing of the subcortical U-fibers. Postcontrast imaging reveals no abnormal white matter enhancement. Proton MRS shows marked reduction of the NAA (2.0 pp) and elevation of choline (3.2 ppm) within the affected region of the brain. There were no cerebellar or basal ganglia changes (not shown).

Diagnosis

Case A: Krabbe disease
Case B: Classic childhood cerebral X-linked adrenoleukodystrophy
Case C: Vanishing white matter disease
Case D: Metachromatic leukodystrophy

Summary

Leukodystrophies are a variably defined group of rare, progressive, metabolic, genetic diseases that variably affect the brain, spinal cord, and peripheral nerves. Depending on the disease, gray matter may be involved in addition to white matter. This challenging topic is broad and yet also nuanced and is covered in greater detail in the neuroradiology literature. Although we do not aim to cover this topic comprehensively, we would like to discuss a few helpful points relating to more common disorders that may help to establish an accurate initial diagnosis and complement confirmatory clinical and genetic testing. A stepwise approach is essential to interpreting imaging studies of patients with leukodystrophies.

Key steps include determining:

1. patient age and clinical presentation
2. whether there is white matter and/or gray matter involvement (including involvement of specific tracts and nuclei and sparing of others)
3. whether there is peripheral nervous system involvement
4. if brain involvement is patchy or confluent
5. the overall pattern of disease

Patients may present with many different patterns of white matter involvement, and thus evaluation for other characteristics is necessary. Those characteristics include enhancement, presence of lesions with signal intensity similar to that of cerebrospinal fluid, susceptibility-weighted MRI signal intensity abnormalities, abnormal MR spectroscopy, and spinal cord involvement.

Aside from considering that the most common imaging presentation of leukodystrophy is nonspecific, it is often quite useful to specifically look for either the subtle or uncommon features that lead to specific diagnosis. This approach is best applied early in the course of disease. Many metabolic brain disorders are indistinguishable later in the course of disease when nonspecific findings such as volume loss and gliosis predominate. Serial or evaluation of remote prior imaging may be helpful.

Clinical features such as presence or absence of macrocephaly can help, particularly in entities such as Canavan and Alexander diseases in which the head size is typically large. It is important that some leukodystrophies have variable forms that may present with different clinical and imaging patterns and in patients of different ages (e.g., X-linked adrenoleukodystrophy [ALD] and Alexander disease).

Perhaps the most commonly identified highly specific imaging appearance is that of X-linked ALD (Case 2), most commonly exhibiting in its early stages a preference for the callosal splenium and posterior white matter with enhancement representing demyelination along the leading edge.

Metachromatic leukodystrophy (MLD), one of the more common of the dysmyelinating disorders, is known for its "butterfly-shaped," confluent, central cerebral white matter T2 hyperintensities, and also the "tigroid" pattern of radial stripes caused by white matter sparing in the perivenular regions. Although these two characteristics are typical for MLD, they are not specific. Both of these have been described in various, albeit less common, other entities (see the Spectrum of Disease section). In distinction from classical Alexander disease and X-linked ALD, there is no anterior (Alexander) or posterior (X-linked ALD) predominance. Alexander disease may also present with irregularities along the margins of the lateral ventricles ("ventricular garland" sign) and signal abnormalities or volume loss in the medulla and spinal cord.

In the context of leukodystrophy, optic nerve enlargement is a pathognomonic finding for globoid cell leukodystrophy (Krabbe disease) (Case 1). This disorder most commonly presents with fever and hyperirritability in an infant. Thalamic hyperattenuation and low signal on T2WI are also common findings, and there may also be enlargement and abnormal enhancement of the spinal nerve roots.

Although the disorder is exceedingly rare, the imaging appearance of vanishing white matter disease (Case 3) is quite striking. The white matter appears to have "vanished," as the signal intensity of white matter tracts is virtually isointense to that of CSF. Although most intracranial processes with parenchymal volume loss eventually lead to ex vacuo dilatation of the ventricular system, it is remarkable that the ependymal lining of the ventricles remains in place.

Spectrum of Disease

Many of the leukoencephalopathies have different appearances when imaged at different time points over the course of the illness. Imaging early may be more useful than imaging at end stages when many diseases appear similar. There can also be substantial overlap in the appearance of chronic leukodystrophies. For example, these cases of primary central nervous system vasculitis with secondary white matter disease (Fig. 103.1) and chronic ALD (Fig. 103.2) show diffuse periventricular signal abnormality with global volume loss with a "tigroid" appearance of the white matter. This appearance is also associated with MLD.

Selected Differential Diagnoses

Adrenomyeloneuropathy
Childhood cerebral X-linked ALD
Adult cerebral X-linked ALD
Female heterozygote form of ALD
Vanishing white matter disease/ovarioleukodystrophy
Megalencephalic leukoencephalopathy with subcortical cysts (Van der Knaap disease)
MLD
Alexander disease
Leukodystrophy with neuroaxonal spheroids
Vanishing white matter disease
Hypomyelinating disorders (e.g., Pelizaeus–Merzbacher disease)
Globoid cell leukodystrophy (Krabbe disease)
Canavan disease
Glutaric aciduria type 1
Mitochondrial disorders

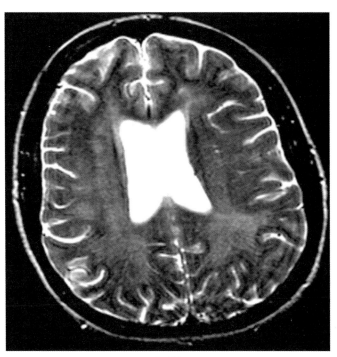

Ax T2

• **Fig. 103.2** Chronic adrenoleukodystrophy. *Ax*, Axial.

Pearls

- A stepwise approach to the leukodystrophies is important, as described previously.
- More specific features may be evident earlier in the disease process; end-stage features tend to show more overlap.
- Contrast enhancement also may help narrow the differential diagnosis; thus, all patients with an unknown leukoencephalopathy should have contrast-enhanced imaging at least once during their evaluation.
- MR spectroscopy may also be helpful.

Some Highly Diagnostic Imaging Findings

Globoid cell leukodystrophy (Krabbe disease)—optic nerve enlargement, abnormal thalami and symmetric basal ganglia and deep white matter involvement, spinal nerve root enlargement and hyperenhancement.

ALD—parietooccipital symmetric white matter disease with enhancing leading edge and involvement of the callosal splenium.

Vanishing white matter disease—symmetric, bilateral diffuse white matter abnormality within the white matter appearing isointense to CSF on MR and isodense to CSF on CT. T2/FLAIR imaging is key in differentiating from hydrocephalus.

MLD—diffuse symmetric white matter abnormality involving the frontal and posterior white matter with radial stripes in the perivenular region, which is specific for this disorder. However, these findings also overlap with findings in the late stages of several other disorders.

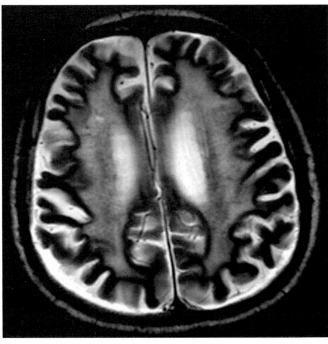

Ax T2

• **Fig. 103.1** Primary central nervous system vasculitis with secondary white matter disease. *Ax*, Axial.

Megalencephalic leukoencephalopathy with subcortical cysts—anterior temporal white matter cysts.

Signs and Complications

A patient's initial presentation is often nonspecific. Initial neuroimaging should exclude a central nervous system mass, infarction, or hydrocephalus, which are much more common.

Sudden changes in patient neurological status should raise suspicion for an acute neurological process as in other patients with metabolic disease. When treated with bone marrow transplantation, patients with leukodystrophies are at increased risk of central nervous system vasculitis and complications of immunosuppression, including bacterial, fungal, and viral infections.

Suggested Readings

Barkovich A: *Pediatric Neuroimaging*, ed 6, Philadelphia, 2018, Lippincott Williams & Wilkins.

Costello DJ, Eichler AF, Eichler FS: Leukodystrophies: classification, diagnosis, and treatment, *Neurologist* 15(6):319–328, 2009.

Resende LL, de Paiva ARB, Kok F, et al: Adult leukodystrophies: a step-by-step diagnostic approach, *Radiographics* 39(1):153–168, 2019.

van der Knaap MS, Bugiani M: Leukodystrophies: a proposed classification system based on pathological changes and pathogenetic mechanisms, *Acta Neuropathol* 134(3):351–382, 2017.

Yang E, Prabhu SP: Imaging manifestations of the leukodystrophies, inherited disorders of white matter, *Radiol Clin North Am* 52(2):279–319, 2014.

104

Congenital Infections

JOSEPHINE MWIKALI NDOLO, MBCHB, MMED AND ASHA SARMA, MD

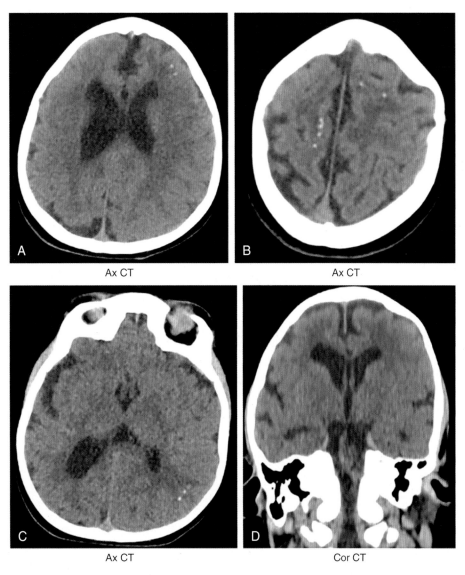

Ax CT

Ax CT

Ax CT

Cor CT

CASE A: Neonate with microcephaly. History travel to Brazil in the second trimester of pregnancy. *Ax,* Axial, *Cor,* coronal; *CT,* Computed tomography. (Case courtesy of Daniel Noujaim, MD and Dr. Pablo Coimbra.)

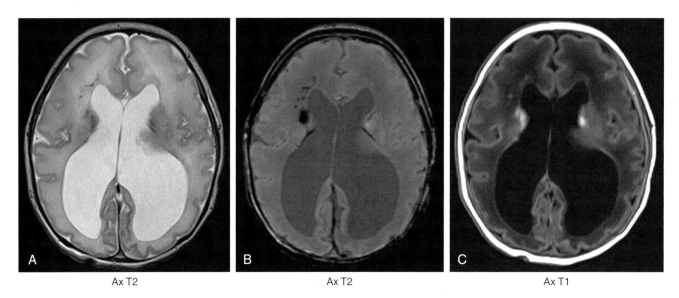

Ax T2   Ax T2   Ax T1

CASE B: A 2-day-old child with chorioretinitis. *Ax,* Axial. (Case courtesy of Alexandra Foust, DO and Dr Pablo Coimbra, Boston Children's Hospital.)

DESCRIPTION OF FINDINGS

- Case A: Computed tomography (CT) head images demonstrate micro-cephaly, gyral broadening, and gray-white calcifications. These features are most in keeping with Zika virus infection.
- Case B: Imaging demonstrates parenchymal calcifications and marked ventriculomegaly. Note the absence of cortical malformations. These, to-gether with the provided history of chorioretinitis, are imaging hallmarks of congenital toxoplasmosis.

Diagnosis

Case A: Zika
Case B: Toxoplasmosis

Summary

The acronym "TORCH" is a mnemonic used to refer to congenital infections such as <u>T</u>oxoplasmosis, <u>O</u>ther infections (such as syphilis, varicella-zoster, and parvovirus B19), <u>C</u>ytomegalovirus (CMV), and <u>H</u>erpes simplex virus.

Importantly, clinical and neuroradiological manifestations of these infections may vary depending coincident timing of infection with key developmental processes during gestation. For example, infections that occur early in the first trimester may result in spontaneous abortion, those that occur during the early second trimester during cortical development may result in cortical malformations (gliosis and encephalomalacia are less likely to occur due to immature immune status), and those that occur during the third trimester may result in disruption of myelination and more familiar encephaloclastic manifestations.

The classic clinical findings in patients with TORCH infections include rash and neonatal ocular findings. Zika has emerged as an important "other" congenital infection that fits well into the category of TORCH infection.

Congenital toxoplasmosis, CMV, and Zika, can bear superficial resemblance to one another due to the presence of intracranial calcification. Assessing the following three factors can be helpful for differentiating among them: (1) head size; (2) presence or absence of cortical malformations; (3) location of parenchymal calcifications.

In addition, we shall review findings in congenital and neonatal herpes encephalitis, as it is a common and potentially devastating infection. This summary is not meant to be comprehensive, but focuses on some more commonly encountered and distinctive entities.

Spectrum of Disease

Congenital Cytomegalovirus Infection

CMV is the most common congenital infection worldwide. Microcephaly is a key clinical manifestation. Intracranial findings include ventriculomegaly, periventricular calcifications, basal ganglia calcifications, migrational anomalies, and white matter disease. Periventricular calcifications are typically chunky (see Fig. 104.1), while basal ganglia calcifications are punctate. The latter point can help to distinguish CMV from other entities with more florid basal ganglia calcification.

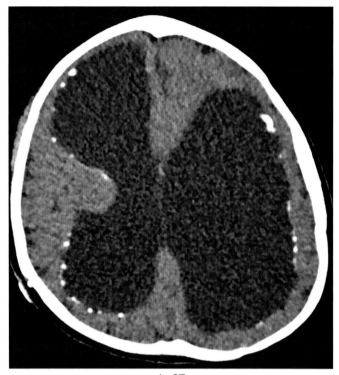

Ax CT

• **Fig. 104.1** Computed tomography image of the head demonstrates ventriculomegaly and periventricular calcifications in this patient with congenital cytomegalovirus infection. *Ax,* Axial; *CT,* Computed tomography. (Case courtesy Aashim Bhatia, MD, MS)

White matter abnormalities, seen as hyperechogenicity on ultrasound and increased signal intensity on T2-weighted images, occur in approximately 22% of patients. There is predominant posterior white matter involvement with reported sparing of the immediate periventricular and subcortical white matter. Anterior temporal white matter disease with cyst formation is almost pathognomonic for CMV infection. Anterior temporal cysts may be more conspicuous in utero due to progressive ventriculomegaly.

Infections in the early second trimester (<18 weeks) present with more severe findings, including microcephaly, lissencephaly, pachygyria, cerebellar hypoplasia, and ventriculomegaly, delayed myelination, and periventricular calcification. Late second trimester infections will present with polymicrogyria, schizencephaly, cerebellar hypoplasia, and ventriculomegaly. Third trimester infections are characterized by delayed myelination, dysmyelination, and white matter disease. Migrational anomalies are rare in the third trimester, as neuronal growth and migration are essentially complete at the time of infection.

Systemic symptoms include sensorineural hearing loss (SNHL), hepatosplenomegaly, hepatitis, thrombocytopenic purpura, and other hematologic abnormalities. SNHL, common in children with congenital CMV, can be progressive or fluctuate. On imaging, the inner ear structures are usually normal, likely indicating cellular level damage that is beyond the resolution of available imaging modalities.

In summary, imaging hallmarks of congenital CMV infection include microcephaly, periventricular and fine basal ganglia calcifications, cortical malformations, and white matter signal abnormality with anterior temporal cysts.

Congenital Toxoplasmosis

Toxoplasmosis, the second most common congenital infection worldwide, is the result of in utero infection with the parasite *Toxoplasma gondii*. The classic triad of chorioretinitis, hydrocephalus, and cerebral calcifications is rare (see Case B). The intracranial parenchymal calcifications are due to focal brain necrosis, resulting in nodular rather than punctate calcifications. These calcifications tend to be randomly distributed rather than periventricular (as in CMV) or predominantly at the gray and white matter junction (as in Zika). Hydrocephalus, due to ependymal inflammation, results in obstruction at the level of the foramen of Monro and/or the cerebral aqueduct. Hydrocephalus may result in macrocephaly (in contrast to microcephaly in CMV and Zika). Unlike in CMV and Zika, cortical malformation is not typically associated with congenital toxoplasmosis.

Infection before 20 weeks gestational age typically results in severe manifestations, such as extensive "tram-track" calcifications, ventriculomegaly, and porencephaly. Imaging findings of infections occurring between 20- and 30-weeks gestational age include sparse periventricular calcifications and hydrocephalus. In the third trimester, infections lead to parenchymal calcifications without ventricular dilatation.

Extracranial manifestations such as hepatomegaly, ascites, and increased placental thickness are suggestive of the disease.

In summary, imaging hallmarks of congenital toxoplasmosis include randomly distributed, chunky parenchymal calcifications, macrocephaly due to hydrocephalus, and absence of cortical malformations.

Congenital Zikavirus Infection

Zika infection is exceptionally neurotoxic and characteristically results in severe microencephaly, an abnormal head shape with overriding sutures, a cupped appearance of the occipital bone extending higher than the adjacent parietal bones, and redundant skin folds.

Manifestations of Zika infection later in gestation include ventriculomegaly, coarse calcifications predominantly at the gray, white matter junction, and cortical malformations such as cobblestone malformation. Abnormalities of the corpus callosum, ranging from dysgenesis to agenesis, have also been reported in the majority of affected neonates.

Two characteristics that can help differentiate Zika from the rest of the TORCH infections are severe microcephaly with a partially collapsed skull and a cupped appearance to the sutures and calcifications predominantly at the gray and white matter junction (Table 104.1).

Congenital and Neonatal HSV Infection

Congenital and neonatal herpes simplex virus (HSV) infections are commonly caused by HSV 2. Clinicians have to maintain a high index of suspicion as only two-thirds of infants have the herpetic skin rash. In contrast to HSV 1

TABLE 104.1 Differentiating Between CMV, Toxoplasmosis and Zika on Imaging

	Microcephaly	Calcifications	Migrational Anomalies
CMV	Present; especially in first trimester infections	Periventricular	+++
Toxoplasmosis	Macrocephaly due to hydrocephalus	random	−
Zika	Severe; deformed skull with overlapping sutures	Gray/white junction	+++

CMV, Cytomegalovirus.

encephalitis in adolescents and adults, the insula, temporal lobe, and limbic system may be spared and other regions of the brain are more likely to be involved. Though the imaging characteristics of congenital and neonatal HSV are variable, the most common imaging findings are cerebral edema and leptomeningeal enhancement, early restricted diffusion, and areas of hemorrhage. Though the cerebral edema can be diffused, there has been a reported preponderance for the periventricular white matter. Several months later, gyriform calcification of the cortex, cortical thinning, white matter atrophy, and multicystic encephalomalacia occur.

Differential Diagnosis

The differential diagnosis is detailed in the preceding section.

Pearls

Head size, type and location of calcifications, and presence or absence of cortical malformations are helpful for differentiating among congenital infections. The timing of infection influences the ultimate clinicoradiological manifestations.

Signs and Complications

Signs and complications are generally related to the associated malformations.

Suggested Readings

Levine D, Jani J, Castro-Aragon I, et al: How does imaging of congenital Zika compare with imaging of other TORCH infections?, *Radiology* 285(3):744–761, 2017.

Fink K, Thapa MM, Ishak GE, et al: Neuroimaging of pediatric central nervous system cytomegalovirus infection, *Radiographics* 30(7): 1779–1796, 2010.

Barkovich A: *Pediatric neuroimaging*, ed 6, Philadelphia, 2019, Lippincott Williams & Wilkins.

105

Congenital Arterial Anastomosis

ROBERT CHEN, MD AND DAVID WEI WEN, MBBS, FRCR

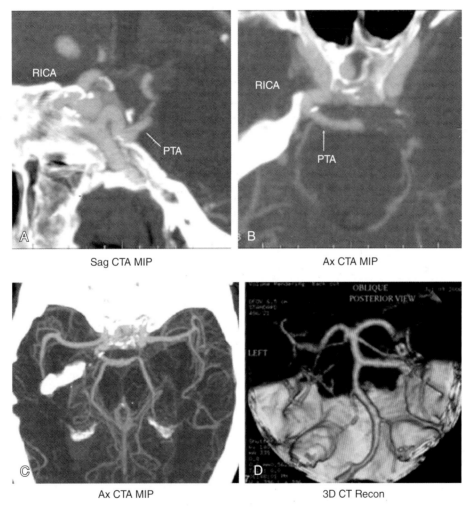

Sag CTA MIP

Ax CTA MIP

Ax CTA MIP

3D CT Recon

CASE A: Incidentally noted imaging finding. *Ax*, Axial; *CT*, Computed tomography; *CTA*, CT angiography; *MIP*, maximum intensity projection; *PTA*, persistent trigeminal artery; *Recon*, reconstruction; *RICA*, right internal carotid artery.

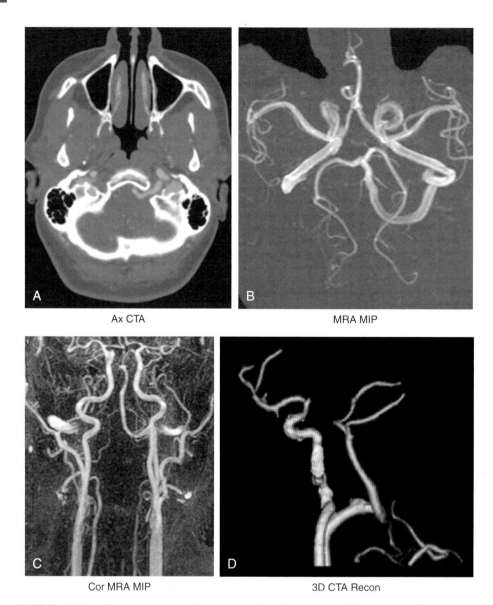

Ax CTA

MRA MIP

Cor MRA MIP

3D CTA Recon

CASE B: Incidentally noted imaging finding. *Ax*, Axial; *Cor*, coronal; *CTA*, Computed tomography angiography; *MIP*, Maximum intensity projection; *MRA*, magnetic resonance angiography; *Recon*, reconstruction.

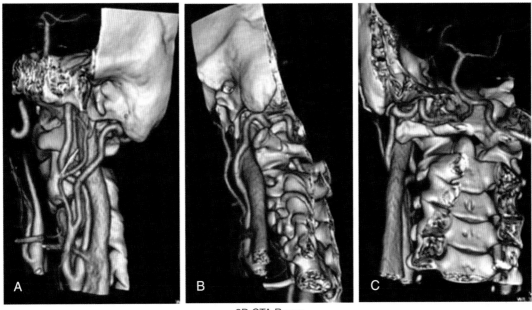

3D CTA Recon

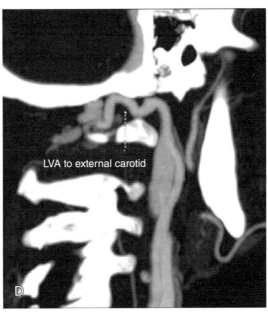

CTA MIP

CASE C: Incidentally noted imaging finding. *CTA,* Computed tomographic angiography; *LVA,* left vertebral artery; *MIP,* maximum intensity projection; *Recon,* reconstruction.

DESCRIPTION OF FINDINGS

- Case A: Multiplanar thick maximum intensity projections and a three-dimensional (3D) volume–rendered image demonstrate a large anomalous vessel arising from the petrocavernous junction of the right ICA, near the posterior genu. It takes a parasellar course around the dorsum sellae to join the mid basilar artery and is consistent with a persistent trigeminal artery.
- Case B: Axial source computed tomography angiography, magnetic resonance angiography, and 3D volume–rendered images demonstrate an anomalous vessel from the left ICA coursing through an enlarged hypoglossal canal and connecting with the proximal basilar artery. Its path through the hypoglossal canal is a clue that this vessel is a persistent hypoglossal artery.
- Case C: 3D volume–rendered images and sagittal maximum intensity projection demonstrate a robust vessel arising from the left external carotid artery, coursing horizontally across the atlantooccipital space, and giving rise to the left intradural vertebral artery, diagnostic of a type 2 proatlantal artery.

Diagnosis

Case A: Persistent trigeminal artery
Case B: Persistent hypoglossal artery
Case C: Proatlantal artery

Summary

Carotid-basilar connections typically are transient anastomoses between the anterior and posterior cerebral circulations that exist for only 7 to 10 days during the formation of the embryo in the first trimester. During this short window, the embryo grows from 3 to 4 mm to approximately 12 to 15 mm in size. Four transient fetal carotid-basilar connections exist, which include (from superior to inferior) the trigeminal, otic, hypoglossal, and proatlantal intersegmental arteries. Aside from the proatlantal intersegmental artery, they are named for the cranial nerves they follow. The purpose of these transient connections is to supply blood to the hindbrain by diverting blood from the carotids to the posterior circulation while the developing vertebrobasilar systems begin to form. The posterior communicating arteries begin to develop when the embryo is 5 mm in size, which is approximately the same time as the carotid-basilar connections begin to disappear and the vertebrobasilar system begins to develop (with fusion of the paired dorsal longitudinal arteries, forming the basilar artery, and the longitudinal connections between the cervical intersegmental arteries, forming the vertebral arteries). The otic artery regresses first, followed by the hypoglossal, trigeminal, and proatlantal intersegmental arteries. In a small percentage of people, the carotid-basilar connections fail to regress and persist into adulthood. These anastomoses are usually clinically insignificant; however, they have been associated with other neurovascular abnormalities, such as aneurysms, and sometimes can alter the management of neurointerventional and neurosurgical procedures.

The trigeminal artery, which is the most common of these fetal connections to persist into adulthood, represents 85% of all persistent fetal anastomoses. It has been reported in 0.1% to 1.0% of the adult population. The trigeminal artery arises from the petrocavernous junction of the internal carotid artery (ICA) near the posterior genu and connects with the mid basilar artery between the superior cerebellar and anterior inferior cerebellar arteries. When present, this vessel may have a parasellar course around the posterior clinoid process or may run through a canal through the bony dorsum sellae (as described in the Spectrum of Disease section). The importance of the trigeminal artery lies in its association with other vascular anomalies. Aneurysms may arise from the trigeminal artery itself (in 2% of cases), typically at the junction of the ICA and trigeminal artery but may also occur along the trunk of the trigeminal artery and at the junction of basilar and trigeminal arteries. Aneurysms may also arise elsewhere within the cerebral circulation (reported in 14% to 32% of cases). This large percentage, however, is probably exaggerated because it was derived from a number of biased case studies that favored the inclusion of cerebral aneurysms in association with a trigeminal artery. Case reports also link trigeminal arteries with arteriovenous malformations, brain tumors, moyamoya disease, facial hemangiomas, Dandy-Walker syndrome, Sturge-Weber syndrome, carotid-cavernous fistulas, cranial nerve symptoms such as tic douloureux, and vascular anomalies such as hypoplastic/aplastic posterior communicating and vertebral arteries. Identification of an intrasellar trigeminal artery is crucial for presurgical planning of any transsphenoidal pituitary surgery.

The remaining persistent fetal connections are less common than the persistent trigeminal artery. Persistent hypoglossal artery, which is the next most prevalent, is seen in approximately 0.027% to 0.26% of adults. It arises from the cervical ICA around the C1–C2 level and courses superiorly to pass through an enlarged hypoglossal canal, joining with the proximal basilar artery. On very rare occasions, the hypoglossal artery can arise from the external carotid artery.

The proatlantal intersegmental artery arises more inferiorly than the hypoglossal artery, roughly around the C2–C3 level. The proatlantal intersegmental artery is classically differentiated from the hypoglossal artery by its more posteriorly and horizontally oriented course. It enters the skull base via the foramen magnum and typically anastomoses more proximally than the hypoglossal artery, around the horizontal portion of the vertebral artery.

Although the proatlantal intersegmental artery is rare, with only about 40 cases reported in the literature since 1999, it is important to take note of this particular fetal connection for preinterventional and presurgical planning purposes and because of its reported association with aneurysms. Two types of proatlantal intersegmental arteries have been described, with type 1 arising from the ICA and type 2 arising from the external carotid artery (as described in the Spectrum of Disease section).

The otic artery is the rarest fetal connection to persist into adulthood, with only a handful of cases reported in the literature. Some experts do not believe it actually exists. It is reported to arise from the petrous ICA and parallel the eighth nerve complex, passing through the internal auditory canal before joining the proximal basilar artery.

Spectrum of Disease

The trigeminal artery may take two main directions with respect to the dorsum sellae, with the posterior communicating artery either coursing posterolaterally around it or passing directly through it to anastomose with the mid basilar artery. A Saltzman classification for trigeminal arteries also exists: Saltzman type 1 is associated with hypoplastic/aplastic proximal basilar and posterior communicating arteries, with the trigeminal artery being the sole supply to the posterior cerebral arteries, and Saltzman type 2 consists of patent posterior communicating arteries that supply the posterior cerebral arteries, with the trigeminal artery supplying the superior cerebellar arteries.

Two types of proatlantal intersegmental arteries exist, arising from either the ICA (type 1) or external carotid artery (type 2). They are fairly similar in prevalence. The type 1 proatlantal intersegmental artery arises from the caudal portion of the ICA around C2–C3, courses anterior to the vertebral bodies, and makes a characteristic horizontal suboccipital sweep over the atlas before entering the foramen magnum. The type 2 proatlantal artery arises from the external carotid artery around C2–C3 and takes a more lateral course than its type 1 counterpart. It courses obliquely across C1–C2 and also enters through the foramen magnum, anastomosing with the horizontal portion of the vertebral artery.

Differential Diagnosis

1. **Trigeminal artery**
2. **Otic artery**
3. **Hypoglossal artery**
4. **Proatlantal intersegmental artery**

Pearls

- Four transient vascular connections that link the anterior and posterior cerebral circulations in the developing first-trimester embryo occasionally may persist into adulthood.
- Aside from the proatlantal intersegmental artery, the carotid-basilar connections are named according to the cranial nerves they parallel (trigeminal, otic, and hypoglossal arteries).
- Although these vascular anomalies are usually incidental and clinically insignificant, they may be associated with other neurovascular abnormalities such as aneurysms, and their presence may impact treatment planning.
- Persistent trigeminal artery accounts for 85% of persistent carotid-basilar connections and is seen in 0.1% to 1.0% of the adult population. An increased incidence of cerebral aneurysms may exist. The remaining three persistent carotid-basilar connections are much less common.

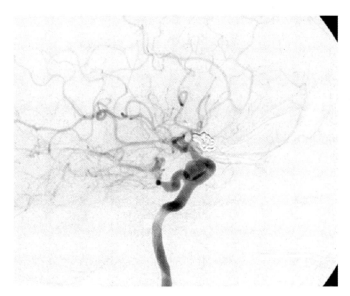

• **Fig. 105.1** A lateral angiogram demonstrates an ectatic vessel coursing posteriorly from the petrocavernous junction, characteristic of a persistent trigeminal artery. Note the large fusiform paraclinoid aneurysm, as well as prior surgical clipping of a middle cerebral artery aneurysm. Persistent trigeminal arteries have been associated with cerebral aneurysms.

Signs and Complications

The persistent trigeminal artery is associated with the characteristic "Neptune's trident" sign on the lateral projection (Fig. 105.1). It may be associated with a higher incidence of cerebral aneurysms and also has been linked with brain tumors, moyamoya disease, carotid-cavernous fistulas, facial hemangiomas, Dandy-Walker malformation, Sturge-Weber syndrome, and tic douloureux. When the trigeminal artery takes an intrasellar course, knowledge of this carotid-basilar connection is crucial.

The type 1 proatlantal intersegmental artery has a classic suboccipital sweep as it crosses horizontally between the occiput and atlas, differentiating it from the hypoglossal artery, which also arises from the cervical ICA. As with persistent trigeminal artery, some case reports suggest a possible association of this particular anomaly with cerebral aneurysms. Ligating the external carotid artery or performing a carotid endarterectomy without prior knowledge of a proatlantal intersegmental artery could possibly have devastating consequences. In addition, posterior fossa ischemia can result from a steno-occlusive lesion along the carotid artery, proximal to the origin of a persistent carotid-basilar connection. This may have implications for endovascular revascularization therapy.

Suggested Readings

Ali S, Walker MT: Bilateral persistent trigeminal arteries associated with bilateral carotid aneurysms, *J Vasc Interv Radiol* 18:692–694, 2007.

Cloft HJ, Razack N, Kallmes DF: Prevalence of cerebral aneurysms in patients with persistent primitive trigeminal artery, *J Neurosurg* 90:865–867, 1999.

Diana F, Mangiafico S, Valente V, et al: Persistent trigeminal artery aneurysms: case report and review of the literature, *J Neurointerv Surg* 11:1261–1265, 2019

Gumus T, Onal B, Ilgit ET: Bilateral persistence of type 1 proatlantal arteries: report of a case and review of the literature, *AJNR Am J Neuroradiol* 25:1622–1624, 2004.

Luh GV, Dean BL, Tomsick TA, et al: The persistent fetal carotid-vertebrobasilar anastomoses, *AJR Am J Roentgenol* 172:1427–1432, 1999.

Namba K: Carotid-vertebrobasilar anastomoses with reference to their segmental property, *Neurol Med Chir (Tokyo)* 57, 267–277, 2017.

Purkayastha S, Gupta AK, Varma R, et al: Proatlantal intersegmental arteries of external carotid artery origin associated with Galen's vein malformation, *AJNR Am J Neuroradiol* 26:2378–2383, 2005.

Uchino A: Carotid-vertebrobasilar anastomosis: Magnetic resonance and computed tomographic angiographic demonstration, *Jpn J Radiol*, 37(8):565–578, 2019.

106
Spinal Dysraphism

JENNIFER HUANG, MD, MED AND ASHA SARMA, MD

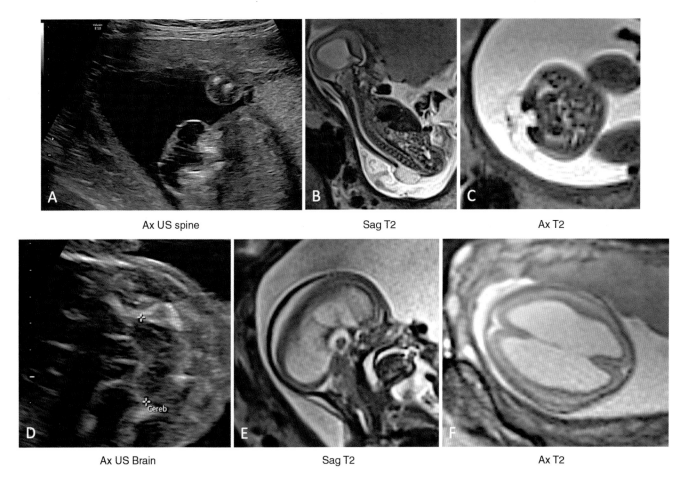

Ax US spine	Sag T2	Ax T2

| Ax US Brain | Sag T2 | Ax T2 |

CASE A: A 22-week gestational age fetus with elevated maternal alpha fetoprotein. *Ax*, Axial; *Sag*, sagittal; *US*, ultrasound.

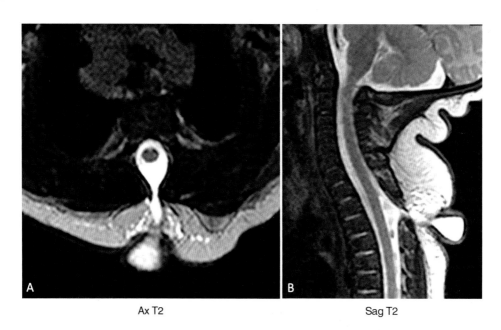

Ax T2   Sag T2

CASE B: A 1-month-old infant with thoracic skin appendage on exam. *Ax*, Axial; *Sag*, sagittal.

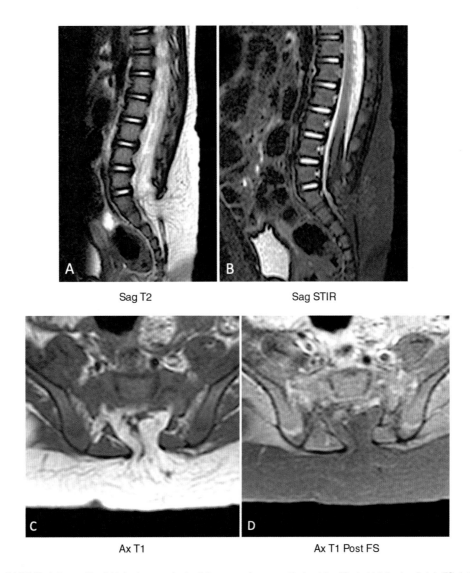

Sag T2   Sag STIR

Ax T1   Ax T1 Post FS

CASE C: A 5-month-old infant presents for follow-up of a sacral bulge identified at birth. *Ax*, Axial; *FS*, fat saturated; *Sag*, sagittal; *STIR*, short-tau inversion recovery.

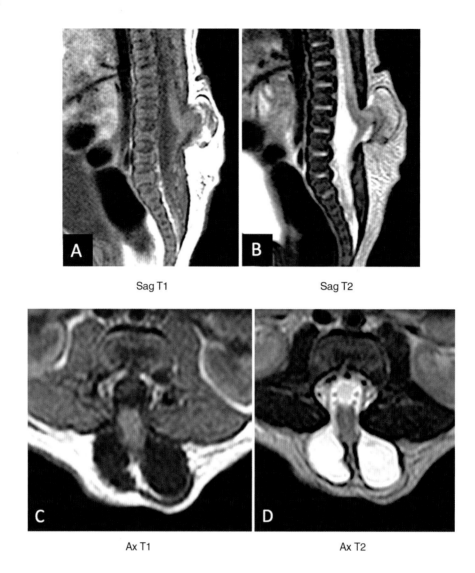

Sag T1   Sag T2

Ax T1   Ax T2

CASE D: A 1-day-old infant born with skin covered lumbar swelling. *Ax*, Axial; *Sag*, sagittal.

DESCRIPTION OF FINDINGS

- Case A: Open spinal dysraphic defect of the lumbosacral spine with posteriorly protruding sac containing cerebrospinal fluid (CSF) and neural placode. No overlying subcutaneous fat or skin. Associated "banana" configuration of the cerebellum, downward displacement of the cerebellum and brainstem, small posterior fossa, and obstructive hydrocephalus.
- Case B: Closed dysraphism posteriorly at the level of T2–T3 with extension of the subarachnoid space through the interspinous space into the subcutaneous fat. Skin covered 1 cm outpouching of CSF. No neural elements contained within the sac. Normal spinal cord morphology and conus position (not pictured).
- Case C: Closed dysraphism with fat directly abutting the spinal cord. No protrusion of neural elements or the subarachnoid space. Cord-lipoma interface located within the spinal canal. Overlying subcutaneous fat covering the dysraphic defect.
- Case D: Closed dysraphism at the L3–L4 level. CSF-containing sac protrudes through open posterior elements of L3 and L4. Linear lipomatous component within the posterior aspect of the sac, with the cord-lipoma interface outside of the vertebral canal. Skin and subcutaneous soft tissues cover the defect.

Diagnosis

Case A: Myelomeningocele (with associated Chiari II malformation)

Case B: Meningocele
Case C: Lipomyelocele
Case D: Lipomyelomeningocele

Summary

After congenital heart disease, neural tube defects are the second most common type of congenital anomaly. Spinal dysraphisms (SDs), or neural tube defects, are congenital malformations involving the spine.

There are three main stages of spinal cord development—gastrulation, primary neurulation, and secondary neurulation. Primary and secondary neurulation are key embryological processes involved in the development of SDs. Primary neurulation involves formation of the neural plate, which bends and closes (neurulation) and subsequently separates from the cutaneous ectoderm (dysjunction) to form the neural tube. Finally, in secondary neurulation, a caudal cell mass is formed, which differentiates to form the conus medullaris and filum terminale (Fig. 106.1). The caudal cell mass also gives rise to anorectal and urogenital structures, as well as caudal musculoskeletal spinal structures. Because secondary neurulation is considered

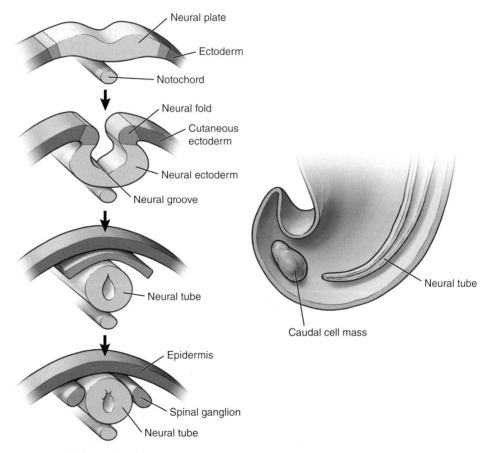

• **Fig. 106.1** A. Formation of the neural tube:
1. In the first step of primary neurulation, neuroectodermal tissue separates from the ectoderm and thickens into the neural plate.
2. The neural plate invaginates inwards to create a neural groove.
3. The neural crest closes (neurulation) to form the neural tube.
4. In the final step, the neural tube separates from the cutaneous ectoderm (dysjunction).
B. In secondary neurulation, the caudal cell mass differentiates to form the conus medullaris and filum terminale, as well as the anorectal and urogenital structures and caudal musculoskeletal spinal structures.

a more disorganized embryological process, lumbosacral spinal anomalies are more frequently encountered than cervicothoracic anomalies. Anorectal and urogenital anomalies are commonly associated with SDs due to common embryological origin of these structures and the caudal intraspinal structures.

SD can be broadly categorized into two types: open and closed. Open SD refers to nonskin–covered interface of the thecal sac and neural placode with the external environment (Fig. 106.2), whereas closed SD occurs when the sac is covered by skin and/or subcutaneous fat (Fig. 106.3). *Open SDs include myelomeningocele, myelocele, and hemimyelomeningocele, while closed SDs can be further subcategorized into defects with or without a subcutaneous mass.* Closed SDs often have an associated cutaneous marker (e.g., sacral dimple, hairy tuft) in 43% to 95% of cases. SD is usually diagnosed via antenatal US or MR, and postnatal imaging of open SD is rarely performed prior to surgery, primarily due to infection risk. At some centers, fetal myelomeningocele repair may be performed. Postnatally, presurgical imaging is often performed in cases of closed SD.

Exposure of the neural tissues to the environment can lead to physical injury as well as chemical injury from amniotic fluid. Therefore, open SDs confer a worse prognosis than closed SDs. The clinical severity depends on the segment of spinal cord involved, placode size, and degree of damage. Because the lumbosacral segment is most commonly involved, the typical clinical picture includes motor and sensory deficits of the lower extremities and bowel and bladder incontinence.

Because SD encompasses a broad and variable spectrum of abnormalities, the terminology can sometimes be confusing. To avoid confusion, first characterize whether the spinal dysraphism is open or closed, then carefully evaluate whether there is protrusion of the subarachnoid space in order to arrive at an accurate diagnosis. The etymological roots for fat (lipo-), spinal cord (myelo-), and the subarachnoid space (-meningo) are added to "-cele" (swelling) in order to name the anomaly. So-called simple and complex dysraphic states (closed defects without a subcutaneous mass) are addressed in Chapter 107.

Differential Diagnosis

The differential diagnosis is detailed in the preceding section.

Spectrum of Disease

Myelomeningocele

The most common open SD is myelomeningocele, occurring in approximately 0.6 to 1.0 in 1000 live births and accounting for more than 98% of cases. These anomalies are due to failure of neurulation and dysjunction of the neural tube. The two main defining features are: (1) exposure of the neural placode to the external environment and (2) expansion of the subarachnoid space. Both the spinal cord (myelo-) and CSF-containing sac (meningo-) are herniated posteriorly,

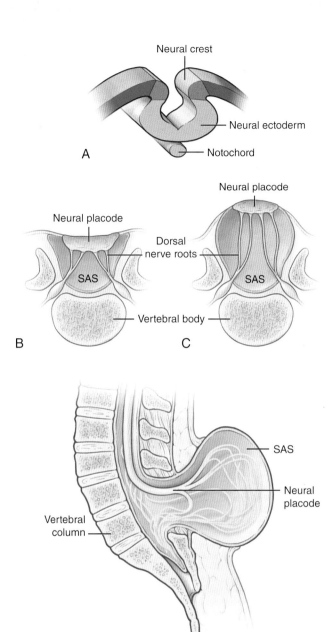

• **Fig. 106.2** A. Open spinal dysraphism occurs when the neural tube fails to close completely (failure of neurulation), with the neural folds remaining in continuity with the cutaneous ectoderm (non-dysjunction). The terminology pertaining to open spinal dysraphism depends on the position of the neural placode relative to the skin surface. The term "myelocele" (B, axial schematic) refers to a malformation with location of the neural placode flush with the skin surface, while "myelomeningocele" (C, axial schematic, D, sagittal schematic) refers to a neural placode protruding above the skin surface, with accompanying protrusion of the subarachnoid space.

creating a nonskin–covered mass. The lumbosacral region is the most common location (45%), followed by the thoracolumbar (30%) and lumbar (20%) regions. Patients with myelomeningocele have Chiari II malformation, with associated hindbrain herniation and other abnormalities such as hydrocephalus, and it has been suggested that the underlying etiology is abnormal CSF dynamics from an in utero CSF leak resulting from the open spinal dysraphism. Developments in

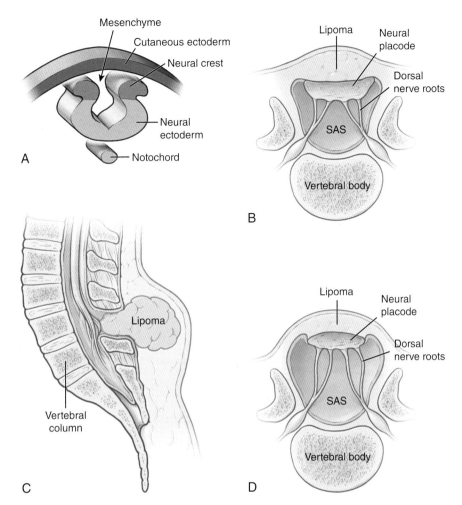

• **Fig. 106.3** A. Closed spinal dysraphism results from premature separation of the neural crest from the cutaneous ectoderm (premature dysjunction), which allows mesenchyme to enter the potential space, adhere to the potential space, and subsequently to differentiate into fat. The terminology depends on the location of the cord-lipoma interface relative to the vertebral canal. Lipomyelocele (B, axial schematic, C, sagittal schematic) is a malformation with the cord-lipoma interface at the level of the neural arches. This is sometimes referred to as a "transitional lipoma". A lipomyelomeningocele (D, axial schematic) is a malformation with position of the cord-lipoma interface outside of the vertebral canal, with accompanying posterior herniation of the subarachnoid space.

fetal surgery have made in utero repair of the neural tube defect possible. Improved neurological outcomes and decreased need for CSF diversion have been reported.

Myelocele

Another open spinal dysraphism, myelocele, is closely related to myelomeningocele, although much rarer. The differentiating feature is that, in myelomeningocele, the neural placode protrudes above the skin surface, while in myelocele, it is flush with the skin surface. This is due to a lack of posterior expansion of the subarachnoid space in myelocele compared to myelomeningocele.

Meningocele

"Meningocele" refers to herniation of a CSF-filled sac without involvement of the spinal cord.

Lipoma With Dural Defect

Lipoma with dural defect falls into the category of closed SDs with subcutaneous mass and comprises a spectrum of abnormalities that differ from each other by position of the spinal cord-lipoma interface. These anomalies occur due to premature dysjunction: mesenchyme enters the potential space, adheres to the neural placode, and subsequently differentiates into fat. This includes lipomyelomeningocele and lipomyelocele. On imaging, an intradural fatty mass attached to the spinal cord is referred to as the cord-lipoma complex.

In lipomyelomeningocele, the cord-lipoma (lipo- myelo-) interface is located outside of the vertebral canal due to posterior herniation of the subarachnoid space (-meningocele). This differs from lipomyelocele, in which the cord-lipoma interface lies at the level of the neural arches and the closely related lipomyeloschisis, where the cord-lipoma interface is within the spinal canal.

Pearls

- Open SD features exposure of the neural sac to the external environment, whereas closed SD is characterized by overlying skin and/or subcutaneous tissue. Open SDs are commonly associated with Chiari II malformation and generally confer a worse prognosis than closed SDs.
- When an exposed neural placode is encountered, consider where the neural placode is located. In myelomeningocele, the placode protrudes above the skin surface due to posterior expansion of the subarachnoid space, while in myelocele, the placode is flush with the skin surface.
- An intradural fatty mass attached to the spinal cord is considered lipomyelomeningocele if the cord-lipoma interface is outside of the vertebral canal and lipomyelocele if the cord-lipoma interface is at the level of the neural arches/within the spinal canal.

Signs and Complications

- There is frequent association of SD with other anomalies, including genitourinary and anorectal malformations.

- Closed SD is often associated with a cutaneous lesion that is identified on clinical examination. Initial evaluation with ultrasound can be helpful in neonates before ossification of the posterior elements.

Suggested Readings

Kumar J, Afsal M, Garg A: Imaging spectrum of spinal dysraphism on magnetic resonance: A pictorial review, *World J Radiol* 9(4):178190, 2017.

Rufener SL, Ibrahim M, Raybaud CA, et al: Congenital spine and spinal cord malformations—pictorial review, *AJR Am J Roentgenol* 194 (3_supplement): S26–S37, 2010.

Trapp B, de Andrade Lourenção Freddi T, et al: A practical approach to diagnosis of spinal dysraphism, *Radiographics* 41(2):559–575, 2021.

107

Complex Spinal Dysraphism

JENNIFER HUANG, MD, MED AND ASHA SARMA, MD

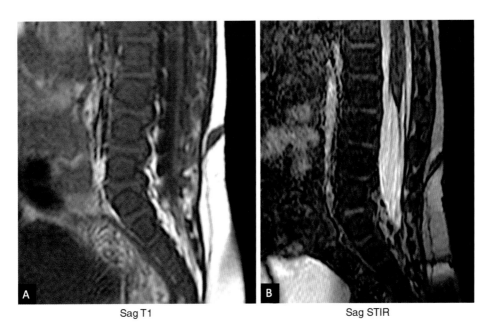

Sag T1   Sag STIR

CASE A: A 3-day-old full-term infant with midline lumbar skin dimple. *Sag*, Sagittal; *STIR*, short tau inversion recovery.

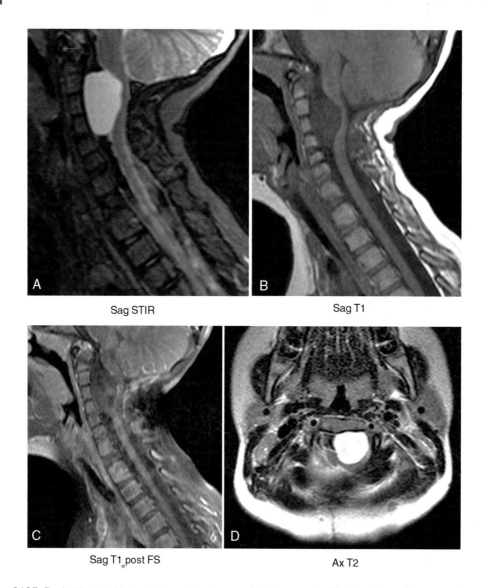

CASE B: A 17-year-old presenting with decreased balance and difficulty with motor processing. *Ax*, Axial; *FS*, fat saturated; *Sag*, sagittal; *STIR*, short tau inversion recovery.

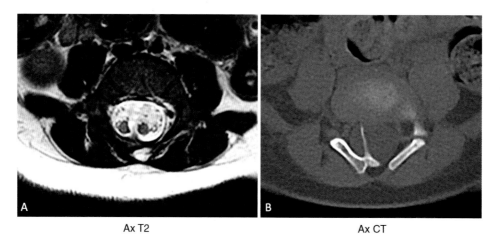

CASE C: A 14-month-old child with congenital scoliosis and rib anomalies. *Ax*, Axial; *CT*, Computed tomography.

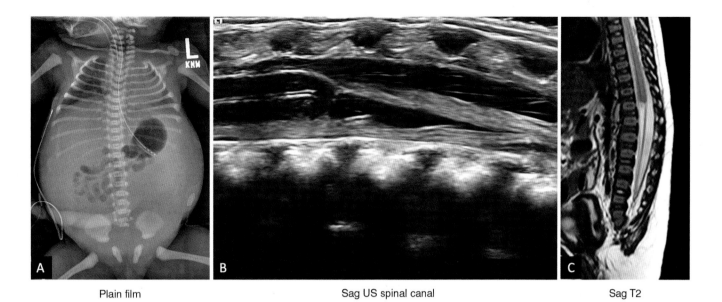

Plain film   Sag US spinal canal   Sag T2

CASE D: A premature neonate with multiple anomalies. *Sag*, Sagittal; *US*, ultrasound.

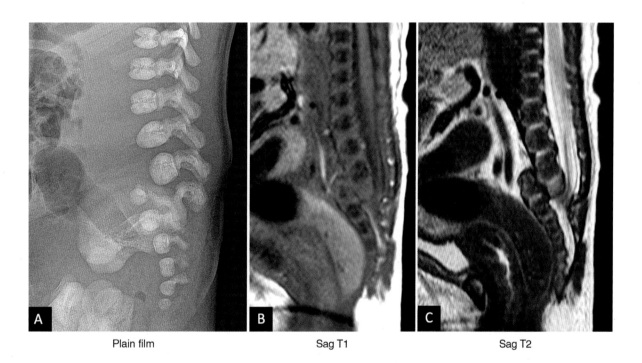

Plain film   Sag T1   Sag T2

CASE E: A full-term neonate with multiple congenital anomalies. *Sag*, Sagittal.

DESCRIPTION OF FINDINGS

- Case A: Hyperintense tract in the dorsal subcutaneous fat at the level of L4 to L5, extending toward the spinal canal. Within the thecal sac, a hypointense linear structure extends toward the dorsal aspect of the conus, joining at approximately L1 to L2. Conus termination at L2 to L3.
- Case B: Ovoid, CSF-isointense intradural extramedullary cystic mass compressing the ventral aspect of the cervical spinal cord. Multiple hypoplastic, incompletely segmented cervical vertebrae, which are smoothly remodeled.
- Case C: Split lumbar spinal cord with two distinct hemicords. Thin bony septum crossing the spinal canal and dividing the cord.
- Case D: Sacrum below the S1 level is absent. Blunted or "cigar-shaped" appearance of the conus medullaris, which ends at the T12 level.
- Case E: Hypoplastic L5 vertebral body with posterior subluxation of the upper lumbar spine relative to the segment below the dysgenetic level. Dysmorphic, rounded, and expanded appearance of L3 and L4 vertebral bodies. Narrowing of the central canal at the dysmorphic L4/L5 joint. Conus ends at the L2 level.

Diagnosis

Case A: Dermal sinus tract
Case B: Neurenteric cyst
Case C: Split cord malformation
Case D: Caudal regression syndrome
Case E: Segmental spinal dysgenesis

Summary

Spinal dysraphisms (SDs) can be broadly categorized into open- and-closed SDs. Closed SD can be further grouped into those with and without a subcutaneous mass. The latter group includes simple and complex dysraphic states. The simple category includes filar/intradural lipomas, tight filum terminale, and persistence of the terminal ventricle (which is considered a normal variant). The complex group includes dorsal dermal sinus, anomalies caused by abnormal notochordal splitting (neurenteric cyst, split cord malformation), and anomalies caused by abnormal segmental notochordal formation (caudal regression syndrome [CRS], segmental spinal dysgenesis [SSD]). Most of these diagnoses have a fairly characteristic and distinct appearance and therefore can usually be easily differentiated; however, in some cases, they may overlap or coincide with additional abnormalities, making evaluation more challenging.

Dermal Sinus Tract

The term "dermal sinus tract" refers to an epithelial-lined fistulous connection between the neural tissue and the skin surface. Most commonly in the lumbosacral region, they are frequently associated with spinal dermoid or epidermoid cysts. Due to the risk of infection related to a direct communication between the neural tissue and cutaneous surface, surgical repair is necessary. These lesions may also cause tethered cord syndrome. It is important to determine the extent of the dermal sinus tract for preoperative planning, as intradural extension of the tract warrants surgical exploration and excision. Thin-section, heavily

T2-weighted steady state sequences (e.g., constructive interference in steady state [CISS], balanced fast field echo [BFFE]) may be especially helpful.

Neurenteric Cyst

Neurenteric cysts are rare foregut duplication cysts that are composed of heterotopic endodermal tissue and within the spectrum of malformations related to abnormal splitting of the notochord early in embryogenesis. The majority of neurenteric cysts are solitary intradural and extramedullary lesions (90%), although there are rare cases of multiple lesions along the spinal axis. Most patients present with waxing and waning myelopathic symptoms. Most commonly, these cysts present as a cerebrospinal fluid (CSF)-isointense lesion predominantly located ventral to the cord. There may be ventral communication with the thorax or abdomen through an anomalous vertebral body or associated thoracic or abdominal foregut duplication cysts. When large, they may cause mass effect on the surrounding structures. Common associations include SD, scoliosis, and Klippel–Feil syndrome (as seen in case A). Other spinal malformations, including split cord malformation, lipoma, and dermal sinus tract, are also associated.

Split Cord Malformation

Split cord malformation is another complex SD that is associated with abnormal notochordal splitting. It is characterized by separation of the spinal cord into two hemicords. It is rarely a diagnostic dilemma, as the appearance on imaging is very characteristic. There are two types. The term "type 1" refers to two hemicords, each contained in a distinct dural tube and separated from the other by an osseous or cartilaginous septum. In type 2, the single dural tube contains both hemicords, which may be separated by a fibrous septum. Patients with split cord malformation may be asymptomatic or may present with a variety of clinical symptoms, including pain, motor or sensory deficits, and autonomic dysfunction. There is a high association with other spinal malformations, characteristically including segmentation anomalies with intersegmental laminar fusion. CT or T2*-weighted MRI may be useful for imaging the associated septum. Surgical excision of the intervening septum is the treatment of choice.

Caudal Regression Syndrome

CRS is a spectrum of structural defects, ranging from partial to total agenesis of the caudal spine. Motor deficits correspond to the level of vertebral agenesis. There are many associated anomalies, which include pulmonary, anorectal, genitourinary, and musculoskeletal abnormalities. CRS may also coexist with other spinal anomalies, such as myelomeningocele, diastematomyelia, and tethered cord. CRS may be isolated or part of a syndrome, such as VACTERL and Currarino triad (partial sacral agenesis, anorectal malformation, and presacral mass). Severe cases are often identified in utero or at birth, although mild cases may not be diagnosed until adulthood. Approximately

20% of CRS cases are associated with maternal diabetes (either type 1 or type 2). Imaging appearance may vary depending on the severity of regression. Group 1 CRS manifests on imaging with major sacral deformities and high-lying, blunt cord terminus (cigar-shaped conus medullaris), whereas group 2 CRS demonstrates less severe sacral anomalies and a tapered, low-lying and elongated appearance of the distal cord with tethering. Management of genitourinary and gastrointestinal associations is often the primary goal, with surgical treatment utilized to improve neurological function if needed.

Segmental Spinal Dysgenesis

A rare congenital spinal anomaly, SSD, is characterized by localized spinal agenesis or dysgenesis and congenital kyphoscoliosis. CRS and SSD may represent different phenotypes of a single spectrum of segmental spine/cord anomalies, with the location of abnormal development along longitudinal axis determining the malformation type (intermediate segment derangement leads to SSD; caudal segment leads to CRS). Unless there is concurrent CRS, the distal spinal bony architecture in SSD is usually normal. SSD may be associated with abnormal development of the spinal cord and nerve roots, such as low-lying cord segment or hypoplastic or absent spinal cord. The cord may be relatively normal in appearance, inferior to the level of dysgenesis. The severity of clinical deficits, which can include clinical kyphosis, spastic paraplegia, and neurogenic bladder, correlates with the degree of morphologic derangement. Plain radiographs or CT may be useful to characterize the bone abnormalities, but MR is preferred for detection of spinal cord abnormalities and should always be performed at presentation. Treatment is aimed at maintaining spinal stability and preventing progressive kyphosis, with early spinal fusion with or without cord decompression.

Spectrum of Disease

The spectrum of disease is detailed in the preceding section.

Pearls

- Most of the complex SDs have characteristic imaging appearances that rarely present a diagnostic dilemma.

- Many of these entities may coincide or present with associated anomalies, therefore careful imaging evaluation of the whole spine is necessary to determine the full extent of disease for comprehensive diagnosis and treatment planning.

Signs and Complications

- Dermal sinus tract: Frequently associated with dermoid/epidermoid; intradural extension needs surgery to decrease risk of infection. Thin-section heavily T2-weighted steady state MRI sequences are recommended.
- Neurenteric cyst: Usually intradural/extramedullary, ventrally located nonenhancing cyst that is typically associated with vertebral anomalies; may communicate with posterior mediastinum or abdomen.
- Split cord malformation: May be associated with a fibrous or osseous septum.
- CRS: Associated with VACTERL and Currarino triad.
- SSD: May be in the same spectrum as CRS; segmental spine/cord anomaly with normal distal spine osseous architecture.

Suggested Readings

Barkovich AJ, Edwards M, Cogen PH: MR evaluation of spinal dermal sinus tracts in children, *AJNR Am J Neuroradiol* 12(1):123–129, 1991.

Borkar SA, Mahapatra AK: Split cord malformations: a two years experience at AIIMS, *Asian J Neurosurg* 7(2):56–60, 2012.

Boruah DK, Dhingani DD, Achar S, et al. Magnetic resonance imaging analysis of caudal regression syndrome and concomitant anomalies in pediatric patients, *J Clin Imaging Sci* 6:36, 2016.

Rufener SL, Ibrahim M, Raybaud CA, et al: Congenital spine and spinal cord malformations—pictorial review, *Am J Roentgenol* 194(Suppl 3):S26–S37, 2010.

Savage JJ, Casey JN, McNeill IT, et al: Neurenteric cysts of the spine, *J Craniovertebr Junction Spine* 1(1):58–63, 2010.

Tortori-Donati P, Fondelli MP, Rossi A, et al: Segmental spinal dysgenesis: neuroradiologic findings with clinical and embryologic correlation, *Am J Neuroradiol* 20(3):445–456, 1999.

108

Pediatric T2 Hyperintense Spinal Cord Lesion

KAI WANG, MD AND ASHA SARMA, MD

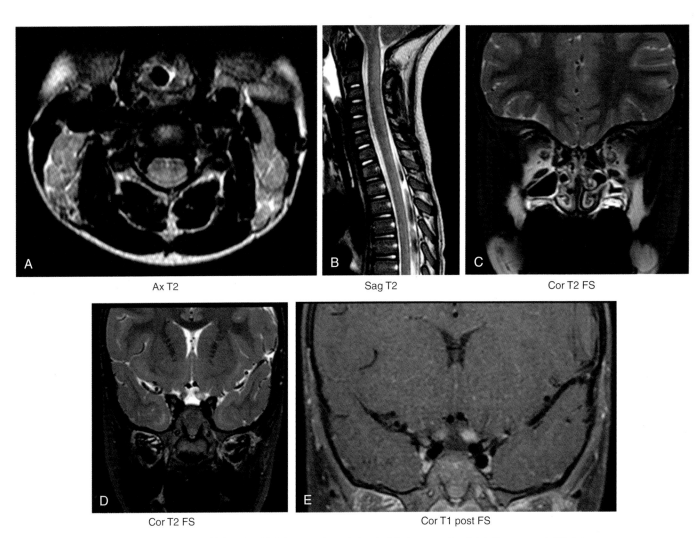

Ax T2

Sag T2

Cor T2 FS

Cor T2 FS

Cor T1 post FS

CASE A: A 4-year-old female with left eye pain and visual disturbances. *Ax,* Axial; *Cor,* coronal; *FS,* fat saturated; *Sag,* sagittal.

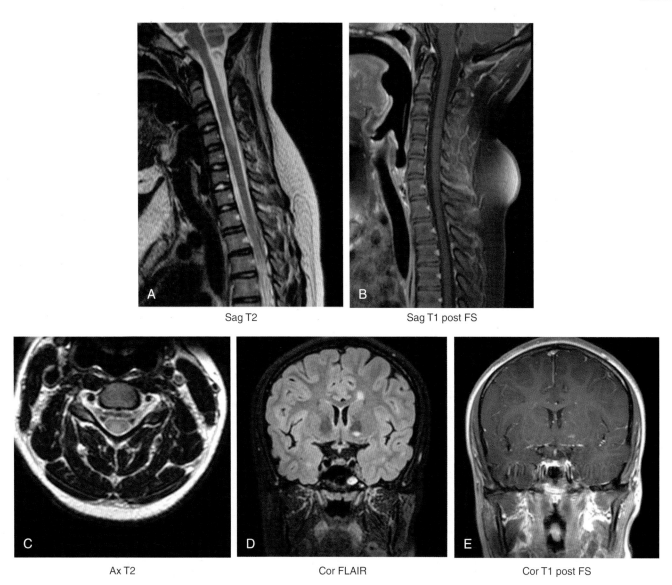

Sag T2   Sag T1 post FS

Ax T2   Cor FLAIR   Cor T1 post FS

CASE B: A 15-year-old male with gradually worsening ataxia and fatigue. *Ax,* Axial; *Cor,* coronal; *FLAIR,* fluid attenuated inversion recovery; *FS,* fat saturated; *Sag,* sagittal.

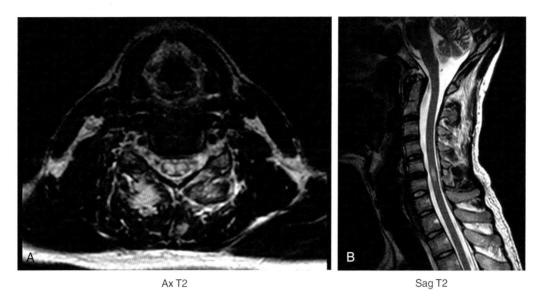

Ax T2   Sag T2

CASE C: A 28-year-old male with history of IV drug use with sudden onset paralysis and urinary retention. *Ax,* Axial; *Sag,* sagittal.

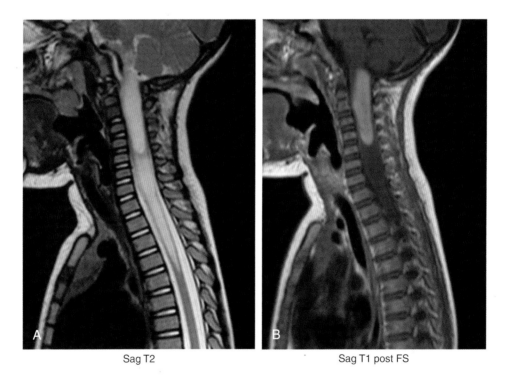

Sag T2   Sag T1 post FS

CASE D: A 3-year-old male with gait disturbances. *FS,* fat saturated; *Sag,* sagittal.

DESCRIPTION OF FINDINGS

- Case A: Ill-defined, mildly expansile T2 hyperintense lesion in the cervical spinal cord. Expansile longitudinally extensive T2 prolongation and enhancement in the left greater than right optic nerves that involves the prechiasmatic segments and chiasm.
- Case B: Multiple T2 hyperintense lesions involving the periventricular and juxtacortical white matter. Short segment (less than two vertebral body levels) T2 hyperintense lesion involving the dorsal cord.
- Case C: Central cord T2 hyperintense lesion with characteristic "owl's eye" appearance, predominantly involving the central gray matter with mild circumferential cord expansion.
- Case D: Expansile, homogeneously enhancing, T2 hyperintense intramedullary cervical cord lesion with associated adjacent cord edema or "presyrinx."

Diagnosis

Case A: Longitudinally extensive transverse myelitis: neuromyelitis optica spectrum disorder (NMOSD)
Case B: Short segment cord lesion: multiple sclerosis (MS)
Case C: Spinal cord infarct
Case D: Spinal cord astrocytoma (pilocytic astrocytoma)

Summary

T2 hyperintense lesions of the spinal cord result from a variety of underlying conditions, including mechanical (compressive edema or altered cerebrospinal fluid (CSF) dynamics, i.e., syrinx or presyrinx), ischemic, infectious, inflammatory (e.g., demyelinating), and neoplastic conditions. If there is volume loss with chronic symptoms, myelomalacia from a chronic or remote insult may be considered. With an acute presentation, there is frequently a nonspecific appearance that can make the diagnosis challenging. Brain and orbital imaging may show more distinctive lesions and, thus, provide increased specificity in many cases. IV gadolinium is often needed for complete characterization, and diffusion-weighted imaging (DWI) may be added in cases where acute spinal cord infarct is suspected. In addition, identification of clinical syndromes and laboratory testing of CSF or serum for antibody-based biomarkers in suspected demyelinating syndromes is generally needed to narrow diagnostic differential possibilities. Differentiation is important due to differing treatment considerations. An additional differential consideration is spinal dural arteriovenous fistula with cord edema (look for prominent flow voids).

Long-Segment Cord Demyelinating Lesions

Long-segment cord lesions can be found in multiple pediatric demyelinating disorders, including acute demyelinating encephalomyelitis (ADEM), neuromyelitis optica spectrum disorder (NMOSD), anti-myelin oligodendrocyte (MOG) antibody disorder (MOG-AD), and idiopathic transverse myelitis. Longitudinally extensive transverse myelitis (LETM) is defined as confluent T2 prolongation involving more than three vertebral segments.
ADEM: ADEM is an immune-mediated demyelinating disorder that is associated with antigenic challenge from a febrile illness or vaccination. It is classically monophasic (although recurrent and multiphasic forms have also been described) and is most common in children under 10 years of age. The typical presentation is with a febrile illness and acute neurologic deficits, importantly, including encephalopathy. Spinal cord involvement is seen in 10% to 30% of cases. Brain lesions are classically multifocal indistinct ovoid lesions >2 cm, asymmetrically involving the cerebral white matter, with additional lesions in a central, juxtacortical, periventricular, brainstem, and cerebellar distribution.
NMOSD: Common manifestations of NMOSD include transverse myelitis and optic neuritis. A distinctive biomarker associated with NMOSD is anti-AQP4 (aquaporin 4 water channel) antibody, although the syndrome is also associated with anti-MOG antibody in a subset of cases. A distinctive pattern of cerebral lesions with high expression of AQP4 water channels, including along the margins of the third ventricle, hypothalamus, periaqueductal gray matter, and area postrema, has been described. Distinctive clinical features include intracranial optic neuritis (most often bilateral, long-segment posterior optic neuritis that may extend to the chiasm), spinal cord syndrome, and area postrema syndrome. LETM lesions involve more than half of the cord cross-sectional area with central gray matter predominance, with cord swelling and variable enhancement.
MOG-AD: MOG-AD is a more recently described demyelinating syndrome, characterized by the presence of positive serum anti-MOG antibody. Due to the broad variety of associated clinical and imaging manifestations, and antibody testing is currently performed in cases of suspected pediatric demyelinating disease with features not suggestive of multiple sclerosis. Affected patients older than 10 years of age are more likely to present with optic neuritis (especially with a bilateral, anterior, longitudinally extensive pattern) and LETM than those under 9 who tend to present with ADEM-like syndrome. In MOG-AD LETM, there is a predilection for lesions involving the lower cord and conus.
Idiopathic Transverse Myelitis: Idiopathic ATM is a monophasic demyelinating disease of the spinal cord that is usually seen in pediatric patients. As manifestations overlap with other diseases, it is currently considered a diagnosis of exclusion. Patients most often present with a prodromal viral-like illness with a sensory deficit including loss of pain and temperature sensation. Expansile LETM involving nearly the whole cross-sectional area of the cord, sometimes with a central dot sign of preserved gray matter on axial images. There is variable enhancement. The imaging appearance overlaps with viral myelitis.

Multiple Sclerosis

Multiple sclerosis (MS) is the most common demyelinating disease of the spinal cord and may occur in any portion of the cord. Although mostly a disease of early adulthood, approximately 5% of patients have symptoms beginning in childhood.

Children are more likely to have atypical presentations, for example, with altered mental status, lethargy, or seizure.

MS lesions are characteristically disseminated in space and time. MS spinal cord lesions are usually more focal and involve only 1 to 2 vertebral body segments. They are most usually found in a cervical or cervicothoracic distribution. Other demyelinating diseases of the spinal cord tend to have more expansile lesions and involve greater than 2 vertebral body levels. MS predominantly affects the peripheral aspect of the spinal cord and with involvement of less than half of the cord cross-sectional area. MS is more likely to have asymptomatic cord lesions than other pediatric demyelinating syndromes.

On postcontrast magnetic resonance imaging (MRI) images, MS lesions may demonstrate homogeneous, nodular, or ring-like (characteristically "incomplete ring") enhancement during the acute or subacute phases. In chronic MS, cord atrophy can be seen. Although isolated spinal cord involvement is possible, it makes up less than one-third of all MS cases. Most commonly spinal cord MS lesions are associated with intracranial and/or optic nerve demyelinating lesions.

Spinal Cord Infarct

Spinal cord infarcts are rare in pediatric patients. They are more common in adults with aortic pathologies. The typical presentation is of abrupt-onset weakness and loss of sensation, with pain and rapid progression. The classic MRI appearance is T2 hyperintensity of the anterior horn cells within the central cord, in a central "owl's eye" pattern. Typically, lesions involve less than one vertebral body segment of cord length, and the most common location is in the distal thoracic cord which represents a watershed territory. Low diffusivity may be seen on MRI. Vascular anomalies and fibrocartilaginous embolism are among the causes that have been described in pediatric patients.

Spinal cord Astrocytoma

Spinal cord astrocytoma typically presents as homogeneous expansion of the spinal cord, most commonly affecting the cervical spinal cord. Enhancement is variable based on tumor type, with pilocytic tumors in pediatric patients often exhibiting homogeneous enhancement and diffuse astrocytoma typically showing no or minimal enhancement. Syrinx or tumoral cysts are common. Although usually less than four vertebral levels are involved, there can be more extensive, even holocord involvement. Contrast-enhanced MRI is important to identify a tumor located within a syrinx. It can be difficult to differentiate between transverse myelitis and astrocytoma on initial study, although transverse myelitis typically has a faster clinical progression and responds to immunosuppressive therapies such as steroids. Spinal cord ganglioglioma can also appear similar.

Spectrum of Disease

Detailed in the preceding sections.

Differential Diagnosis

Detailed in the preceding sections.

Pearls

- Demyelinating diseases may affect patients of any age; however, the relative incidences of different disorders, clinicoradiologic spectrum, treatment, and prognostic considerations differ between children and adults.
- Short segment spinal cord lesions <1 vertebral body level in length are typical of MS.
- There is a broad differential diagnosis for longitudinally extensive spinal cord lesions, including multiple demyelinating disorders and tumors. Clinical correlation including antibody biomarker testing is frequently needed for evaluation, and serial imaging is also often needed to determine the course of the findings.
- "Owl's eye" pattern of central cord signal abnormality is typical of spinal cord infarct.
- Contrast-enhanced spinal cord imaging should be performed to evaluate for tumors in case with syrinx of unknown etiology.

Signs and Complications

Detailed in the preceding section.

Suggested Readings

Baumann M, Grams A, Djurdjevic T, et al: MRI of the first event in pediatric acquired demyelinating syndromes with antibodies to myelin oligodendrocyte glycoprotein, *J Neurol* 265(4):845–855, 2018.

Borisow N, Mori M, Kuwabara S, et al: Diagnosis and treatment of NMO spectrum disorder and MOG-encephalomyelitis, *Front Neurol* 9:888, 2018.

Faguy K: Multiple sclerosis: an update, *Radiol Technol* 87(5):529–550, 2016.

Gaitán MI, Yañez P, Paday Formenti ME, et al: An optimized MRI technique to detect the central vein sign in MS plaques, *AJNR Am J Neuroradiol* 41(3):456–460, 2020.

Khoueiry M, Moussa H, Sawaya R: Spinal cord infarction in a young adult: What is the culprit? *J Spinal Cord Med* 44(6):1015–1018, 2021.

Koelman DL, Mateen FJ: Acute disseminated encephalomyelitis: current controversies in diagnosis and outcome, *J Neurol* 262(9):2013–2024, 2015.

Wang C, Greenberg B: Clinical approach to pediatric transverse myelitis, neuromyelitis optica spectrum disorder and acute flaccid myelitis, *Children (Basel)* 6(5):70, 2019.

Wingerchuk DM, Lennon VA, Pittock SJ, et al: Revised diagnostic criteria for neuromyelitis optica, *Neurology* 66(10):1485–1489.

Zalewski NL, Rabinstein AA, Krecke KN, et al: Characteristics of spontaneous spinal cord infarction and proposed diagnostic criteria, *JAMA Neurol* 76(1):56–63, 2019.

109

Odontoid: Acute Versus Chronic Fragmentation

JUAN E. SMALL, MD, MSC, EMILY HAAS, MD, AND ASHA SARMA, MD

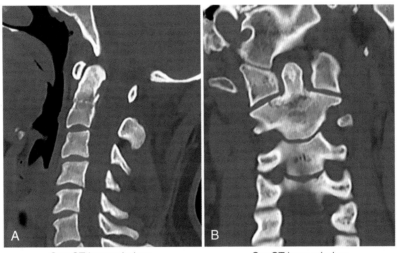

Sag CT bone window

Cor CT bone window

CASE A: A 19-year-old female presenting after trauma. *Cor,* Coronal; *CT,* Computed tomography; *Sag,* sagittal.

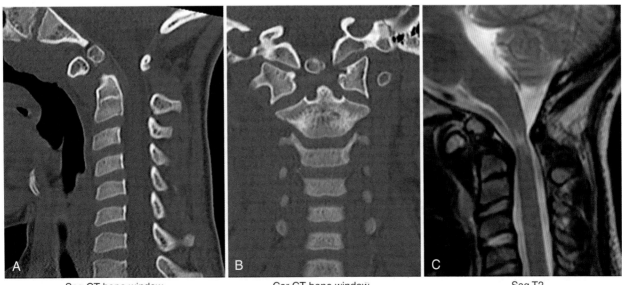

Sag CT bone window

Cor CT bone window

Sag T2

CASE B: A 10-year-old male with spondyloepiphyseal dysplasia presenting with bilateral upper extremity pain. *Cor,* Coronal; *CT,* Computed tomography; *Sag,* sagittal.

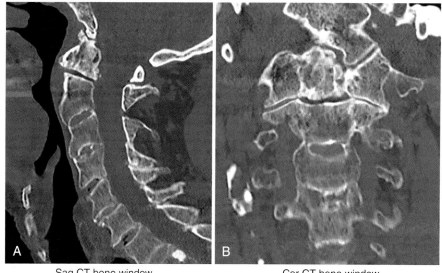

Sag CT bone window   Cor CT bone window

CASE C: A 90-year-old male presenting after a ground-level fall. *Cor,* Coronal; *CT,* Computed tomography; *Sag,* sagittal.

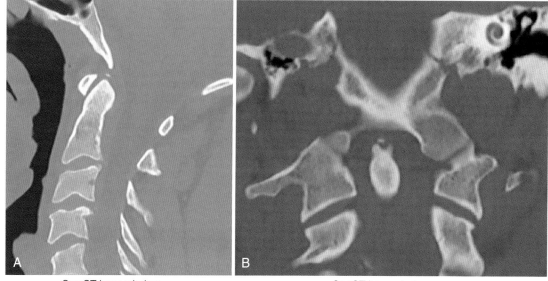

Sag CT bone window   Cor CT bone window

CASE D: A 26-year-old male presents after being struck by a vehicle. *Cor,* Coronal; *CT,* Computed tomography; *Sag,* sagittal.

DESCRIPTION OF FINDINGS

- Case A: Sharp, lucent fracture line extending through the dens/superior C2 vertebral body with extension into the right lateral mass. There is a relatively narrow fracture gap, and the fractured dens has a "matching" vertebral body donor site.
- Case B: Smooth, well-corticated, round os odontoideum (dystopic) is seen superior to a hypoplastic den. The os is not fused to the clivus or C1 ring in this particular case. The anterior arch of C1 is hypertrophic, and there is anterior subluxation of C1 with moderate narrowing of the spinal canal at this level. The degree of cord compression is best demonstrated on the sagittal MR image, with increased signal noted in the cervical cord.
- Case C: Transversely oriented, narrow, well-corticated fracture plane extends through the base of the dens. The non-united dens appear fused to the C1 anterior arch, and there is minimal posterior displacement of this complex with respect to the C2 vertebral body.
- Case D: Small, corticated ossific fragment is seen at the tip of the dens and is much smaller than the os noted in Case B.

Diagnosis

Case A: Acute type III dens fracture
Case B: Os odontoideum (dystopic)
Case C: Chronic type II dens fracture
Case D: Persistent ossiculum terminale

Summary

Acute and Chronic Odontoid Fractures

The odontoid process of the C2 vertebral body represents a key structure contributing to rotational motion at the craniocervical junction. It is sometimes difficult but nevertheless important to be able to differentiate among acute and chronic and/or developmental odontoid pathologies. Acute fractures generally exhibit sharp margins without cortication, and the fracture fragments typically "match" in morphology to their respective donor sites. Surrounding soft tissue edema (best seen on MRI) further supports the diagnosis of acute traumatic injury. Odontoid fractures can be separated into three types. In brief, a type I odontoid fracture represents an avulsion fracture at the tip of the dens, a type II fracture represents a transverse fracture at the base of the dens, and a type III fracture extends into the superior body of C2. Difficulty often arises when differentiating chronic, undiagnosed fractures from developmental variants because of the bone remodeling over time, with development of sclerosis or cortication along the fracture fragments. Matching morphology of the fracture fragment to the donor site and a (generally) narrow gap between the two are helpful features favoring fracture.

Os Odontoideum

Chronic or congenital/developmental anomalies, including os odontoideum and persistent ossiculum terminale, tend to demonstrate smooth, well-corticated margins. Os odontoideum presents as a round or oval, well-corticated ossicle with borders that do not directly match up with the remainder of the C2 vertebral body. It is separated from adjacent bone by a wider gap than that typically seen in chronic fracture. As such, it is identified as a separate piece of well-corticated bone that is usually posteriorly located with respect to the (often hypertrophic) C1 anterior arch, reflecting the long-standing nature of this process. The etiology of os odontoideum is controversial, although most investigators favor trauma that has occurred before the age of 5 to 6 years over congenital malformation as the underlying etiology. In either case, failure of fusion of the odontoid process with the axis has occurred, leading to the appearance of an ossicle adjacent to the C2 vertebral body. Typically, odontoid hypoplasia ultimately results in atlantoaxial instability due to lack of normal anchoring of the transverse atlantal ligament. Therefore, when it is encountered, flexion-extension radiographs for assessment of craniocervical junction stability may be indicated. Although the os odontoideum may vary in size, it is usually smaller than the expected size of a normal dens. Os odontoideum has been reported with increased frequency in conditions such as Morquio syndrome, multiple epiphyseal dysplasia, trisomy 21, and Klippel–Feil syndrome.

It is important to note that the os odontoideum may be located at the expected anatomic position of the dens (orthotopic) or at a position other than the expected anatomic position (dystopic), most commonly near the foramen magnum, where it may fuse with the clivus. The orthotopic os has the potential to fuse with the anterior arch of C1, in which case the two move as a single unit. Although often exhibiting a smooth margin, os odontoideum can also have an irregular shape, with narrow separation from and interdigitation with the anterior C1 arch. This relatively characteristic finding is termed the "jigsaw" sign.

Persistent Ossiculum Terminale

Not all separate, well-corticated ossific structures in the region of the dens represent os odontoideum. Persistent ossiculum terminale results from failure of fusion of the secondary ossification center at the tip of the dens with the odontoid by 12 years of age. This secondary ossification center usually appears by age 3 and gradually fuses with the body of the odontoid. Persistent ossiculum terminale tends to be smaller than os odontoideum and generally lies above the level of the transverse ligament. Therefore, it is typically not associated with atlantoaxial instability. The dens itself also appears significantly less truncated than in cases of os odontoideum. In addition, well-corticated margins suggest an ossicle rather than a type I avulsion fracture of the dens.

Spectrum of Disease

The spectrum of disease is detailed in the preceding section.

Differential Diagnosis

The differential diagnosis is detailed in the preceding section.

Pearls

- Acute dens fracture
  - Sharp, radiolucent margins without cortication
  - Fracture fragments match in morphology to their donor site with a relatively narrow fracture plane/gap
  - Surrounding soft tissue edema further supports an acute traumatic injury
- Chronic dens fracture
  - Sclerosis along the fracture fragments
  - Matching morphology of the fracture fragment to the donor site, again with a narrow fracture plane/gap
- Os odontoideum
  - Round or oval, smooth, well-corticated margins
  - Borders do not directly match up with the remainder of the C2 vertebral body
  - C1 anterior arch often hypertrophic
  - Os may be orthotopic or dystopic
  - May be associated with atlantoaxial instability
  - "Jigsaw" sign is characteristic: os may have irregular shape and interdigitating joint line with the anterior arch of C1
- Persistent ossiculum terminale
  - Smaller than os odontoideum and generally not associated with atlantoaxial instability
  - Dens markedly less truncated than in the case of an os odontoideum
- Well-corticated margins suggest ossiculum terminale rather than type I dens fracture

Signs and Complications

Signs and complications are generally related to atlantoaxial instability and mass effect on the cord.

Suggested Readings

Arvin B, Fournier-Gosselin MP, Fehlings MG: Os odontoideum: etiology and surgical management, *Neurosurgery* 66(Suppl 3):22–31, 2010.

Buyukkaya A, Yazgan O, Yazgan S, et al: Characteristic imaging findings of os odontoideum, *Spine J* 14(12):3052–3053, 2014.

Hedequist DJ, Mo AZ: Os odontoideum in children, *J Am Acad Orthop Surg* 28(3):e100–e107, 2020.

Jain N, Verma R, Garga UC, et al: CT and MR imaging of odontoid abnormalities: a pictorial review, *Indian J Radiol Imaging* 26(1):108–119, 2016.

Offiah CE, Day E: The craniocervical junction: embryology, anatomy, biomechanics and imaging in blunt trauma, *Insights Imaging* 8(1): 29–47, 2017.

O'Brien WT Sr, Shen P, Lee P: The dens: normal development, developmental variants and anomalies, and traumatic injuries, *J Clin Imaging Sci* 5:38, 2015.

Perdikakis E, Skoulikaris N: The odontoid process: various configuration types in MR examinations, *Eur Spine J* 23(5):1077–1083, 2014.

Pryputniewicz DM, Hadley MN: Axis fractures, *Neurosurgery* 66(Suppl 3):68–82, 2010.

110

Pediatric Nasofrontal Mass

JUAN E. SMALL, MD, MSC, EMILY HAAS, MD, AND ASHA SARMA, MD

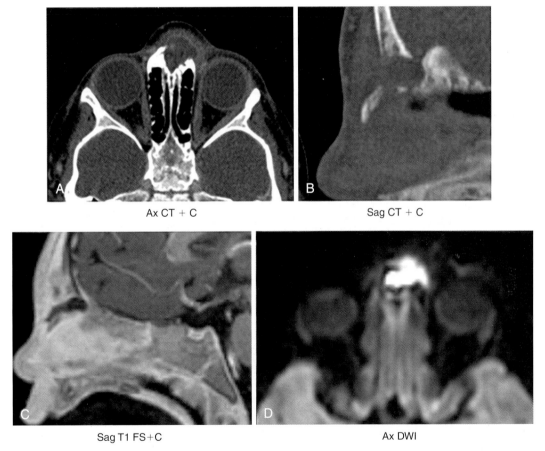

Ax CT + C

Sag CT + C

Sag T1 FS+C

Ax DWI

CASE A: A toddler presents with several days of swelling and purulent discharge from a hair-containing cutaneous pit at the nasion. *Ax,* Axial; *C+,* post-contrast; *CT,* Computed tomography; *DWI,* diffusion-weighted imaging; *FS,* fat saturated; *Sag,* sagittal.

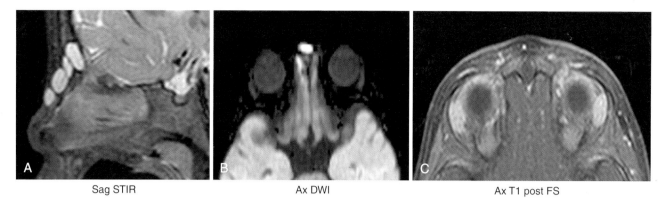

Sag STIR   Ax DWI   Ax T1 post FS

CASE B: A 12-month-old male with a nasal mass. *Ax,* Axial; *+ C,* post-contrast; *DWI,* diffusion-weighted imaging; *FS,* fat saturated; *MRI,* magnetic resonance imaging; *Sag,* sagittal; *STIR,* short tau inversion recovery.

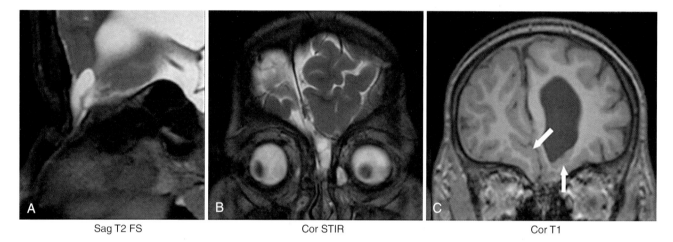

Sag T2 FS   Cor STIR   Cor T1

CASE C: A School-age child with no prior access to medical care presenting with vision loss and headaches. *Cor,* Coronal; *FS,* fat saturated; *Sag,* sagittal; *STIR,* short tau inversion recovery.

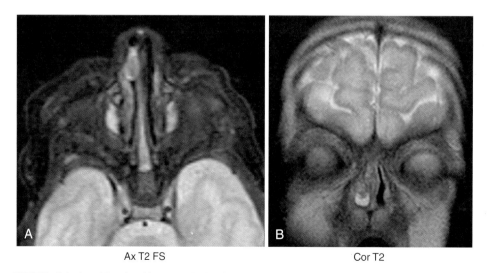

Ax T2 FS   Cor T2

CASE D: A 1-day-old male with a mass in the right nasal cavity that was discovered on newborn exam. *Ax,* Axial; *Cor,* coronal; *FS,* fat saturated.

DESCRIPTION OF FINDINGS

- Case A: Erosive mass-like lesion located at the nasal bridge with surrounding inflammatory changes and a contiguous tract extending to a widened foramen cecum. MR images also demonstrate inflammatory changes along the tract extending to the frontal dura. Low diffusivity within the lesion.
- Case B: Lobulated midline cystic, nonenhancing mass with associated reduced diffusion, traversing the glabella. The lesion is closely associated with frontal dura but without parenchymal involvement.
- Case C: Small frontal cerebrospinal fluid (CSF)-containing congenital cephalocele with associated right inferior frontal polymicrogyria, gray matter heterotopia along the inferior aspect of the left lateral ventricle, and ventriculomegaly.
- Case D: Small mass in the right nasal cavity, which is near-isointense to brain parenchyma, with a small amount of surrounding fluid. The mass was resected with pathology, confirming neuroglial tissue.

Diagnosis

Case A: Nasal dermal sinus tract (infected)
Case B: Nasal epidermoid/dermoid
Case C: Frontal cephalocele
Case D: Nasal glial heterotopia (formerly known as nasal glioma)

Summary

Congenital midline nasofrontal masses are relatively uncommon lesions that usually present in infancy or early childhood. There are three major differential diagnostic considerations: nasal dermal sinus or dermoid/epidermoid, nasofrontal or nasoethmoidal cephalocele, and nasal glial heterotopia (formerly known as nasal glioma). Familiarity with the embryogenesis of the nasofrontal region is essential to understanding these entities. Early in development, a nasofrontal fontanelle (termed the fonticulus nasofrontalis) transiently separates the developing inferior frontal bone from the nasal bone. As this transient fontanelle forms, a funnel-like dural projection/diverticulum extends toward the nasal region through the foramen cecum, which is a midline opening anterior to the ethmoidal crista galli. The apex of this projection briefly extends through the prenasal space to the skin in the region of the nasal bridge. Subsequently, it involutes as the nasal process grows. The nasofrontal fontanelle subsequently fuses to form the frontonasal suture.

Failure of the dural diverticulum to regress can result in midline abnormalities, such as a nasal cephalocele, nasal dermoid, or nasal glial heterotopia (nasal glioma). In general, a persistent dural diverticulum that contains meninges and/or brain parenchyma represents a frontal cephalocele (Fig. 110.1A), whereas regression of the diverticulum with a detached brain parenchymal remnant at the developmental apex of the diverticulum represents nasal glial heterotopia (nasal glioma) (Fig. 110.1C). Additionally, focal adherence of the ectoderm along the course of the diverticulum may result in a dermoid/epidermoid cyst and/or dermal sinus tract (Fig. 110.1B).

Across this spectrum of pathologies, the most important imaging feature to ascertain is the presence or absence of intracranial extension. Connection between the mass and the anterior cranial fossa must be detected, as it may be a portal for intracranial infection. Moreover, a different surgical approach is needed for complete resection.

Dermal Sinus and Dermoid/Epidermoid

The presence of a dermal sinus with or without a congenital inclusion cyst, such as dermoid or epidermoid cyst, can result from retention of dermal elements as the embryogenic dural diverticulum regresses. Associated dermoid or epidermoid cysts can occur anywhere along the dural tract, from the nasal soft tissues to the intracranial compartment. Approximately half of affected patients have a dimple or pit at the nasal bridge. Lesions may also manifest themselves with sebaceous discharge or presence of hair. Some cases come to clinical

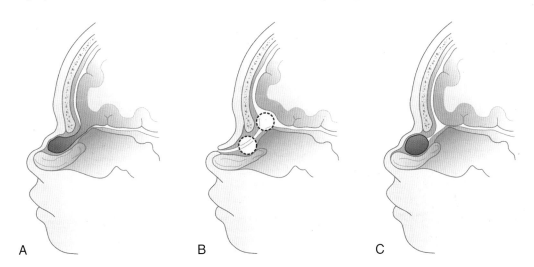

• **Fig. 110.1** Failure of regression of the embryonic frontonasal dural diverticulum can lead to: (A) a nasal encephalocele, in which a persistent dural diverticulum contains meninges and brain parenchyma; (B) a nasal dermoid/epidermoid, which may occur anywhere along the course of the regressing dural diverticulum; or (C) a nasal glial heterotopia, in which a brain parenchymal remnant is left behind near the developmental apex of the embryologic diverticulum.

attention due to complications, which can include meningitis, cavernous sinus thrombosis, and periorbital cellulitis. Important CT findings that raise sensitivity for intracranial extension include bifid crista galli and widened foramen cecum (Fig. 110.2; noting that the radiologist should be aware that the cribriform plate is not fully ossified in infants—thin-section T2-weighted imaging or contrast-enhanced CT may be helpful to troubleshoot). Although epidermoid is more likely to exhibit similar attenuation to water on CT and low diffusivity on MRI, and dermoid is more likely to contain fat, in practice, imaging assessment is considered unreliable for differentiating between the two. Histopathologic assessment can more accurately identify the dermal appendages that distinguish a dermoid cyst. Additionally, treatment does not differ between dermoid and epidermoid. Therefore, many radiologists use the terminology "dermoid or epidermoid" in reporting.

Congenital Cephalocele

Congenital cephalocele represents a defect in the skull with extension of meninges and/or brain parenchyma. Specific to the discussion of nasofrontal masses and anterior cephaloceles, frontoethmoidal cephaloceles can be further subdivided into frontonasal, nasoethmoidal, and naso-orbital cephaloceles. Frontonasal cephaloceles represent protrusion of intracranial contents through the nasofrontal fontanelle (persistent fonticulus frontonasalis) into the region of the glabella (Fig. 110.3). Nasoethmoidal cephaloceles represent protrusion of contents through the foramen cecum and prenasal space, with extension toward the nasal bridge. The description "naso-orbital" refers to protrusion into the orbit via the lacrimal bone. Crucial to the imaging diagnosis of anterior cephaloceles is the identification of continuity with the intracranial subarachnoid space (meningocele) and/or brain parenchyma (encephalocele).

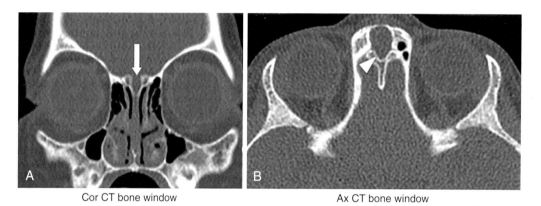

Cor CT bone window   Ax CT bone window

• **Fig. 110.2** Identifying intracranial extension of a nasofrontal mass is a key component of imaging evaluation. Bifid appearance of the crista galli *(arrow)* and a widened foramen cecum *(arrowhead)* are helpful features that may raise your level of suspicion. *Ax,* Axial; *Cor,* coronal; *CT,* Computed tomography.

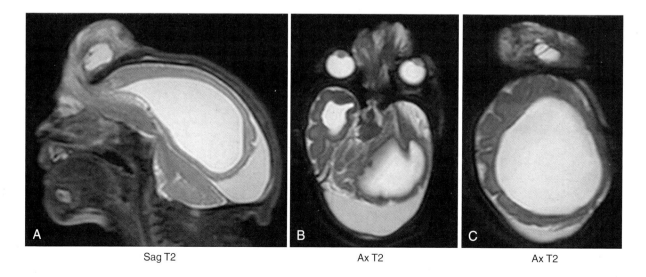

Sag T2   Ax T2   Ax T2

• **Fig. 110.3** Large frontonasal encephalocele containing a large portion of dysplastic brain parenchyma and ventricle. Associated hydrocephalus and markedly distorted cerebral anatomy. *Ax,* Axial; *Sag,* sagittal.

Additionally, it is important to be aware of other anomalies that are frequently seen in conjunction with cephaloceles, including facial abnormalities such as cleft lip and palate, optic nerve hypoplasia, dysgenesis of the corpus callosum, malformations of cortical development, and dysfunction of the hypothalamic-pituitary axis.

Nasal Glial Heterotopia

Nasal glial heterotopia can be thought of simply as a cephalocele that has been "pinched off" during development, losing its connection with the intracranial contents. Because this entity is nonneoplastic, the term nasal "glial heterotopia" is preferred over the historically used term "nasal glioma." Nasal glial heterotopia generally appears on imaging as well-circumscribed, round or polypoid, nonenhancing neurogenic dysplastic tissue that demonstrates variable signal intensity. Lesions are more likely to be located off-midline than dermoid/epidermoid, and may be intra-nasal, extra-nasal, or combined in location. A fibrous stalk is occasionally seen. Occasional enhancement within these lesions may reflect sequestered choroid plexus.

Spectrum of Disease

The spectrum of disease is described in the preceding section, with additional examples depicted in Figs. 110.2 and 110.3.

Differential Diagnosis

Additional nasofrontal region lesions in infants may include nasolacrimal duct cysts (mediocanthal region and inferior nasal cavity), vascular malformations, and neoplasms such as hemangioma and myofibroma.

Pearls

- Identification of a bifid or dystrophic crista galli and enlarged foramen cecum strongly suggests the presence of a congenital midline nasofrontal lesion.
- Dermoid and epidermoid are difficult to reliably distinguish on imaging and have similar treatment considerations, and therefore, many practitioners prefer not to differentiate between the two in reporting. The presence of low diffusivity on MRI favors epidermoid and fat contents favor dermoid.
- A nonenhancing lesion that is iso- to hyperintense to brain parenchyma on T2-weighted MRI in an off-midline location suggests nasal glial heterotopia.
- Herniating brain parenchyma and/or CSF through an anterior skull defect is diagnostic of a cephalocele.
- Pitfall: Incomplete ossification of the cribriform plate within the first year of life should not be mistaken for bony defect on CT.

Suggested Readings

Ginat DT, Robson CD: Diagnostic imaging features of congenital nose and nasal cavity lesions, *Clin Neuroradiol* 25(1):3–11, 2015.

Gnagi SH, Schraff SA: Nasal obstruction in newborns, *Pediatr Clin North Am* 60(4):903–922, 2013.

Hedlund G: Congenital frontonasal masses: developmental anatomy, malformations, and MR imaging, *Pediatr Radiol* 36:647–662, 2006.

Kadom N, Sze RW: Radiological reasoning: pediatric midline nasofrontal mass, *AJR Am J Roentgenol* 194(Suppl 3):WS10–WS13, 2010.

Rodriguez DP, Orscheln ES, Koch BL: Masses of the nose, nasal cavity, and nasopharynx in children, *Radiographics* 37: 1704–1730, 2017.

Saettele M, Alexander A, Markovich B, et al: Congenital midline nasofrontal masses, *Pediatr Radiol* 42(9):1119–1125, 2012.

Sefidbakht S, Iranpour P, Keshavarz P, et al: Fetal MRI in prenatal diagnosis of encephalocele, *J Obstet Gynaecol Can* 42(3):304–307, 2019.

111

Pediatric Globe Lesions

SCOTT EDWARD HUNTER, MD, MBA

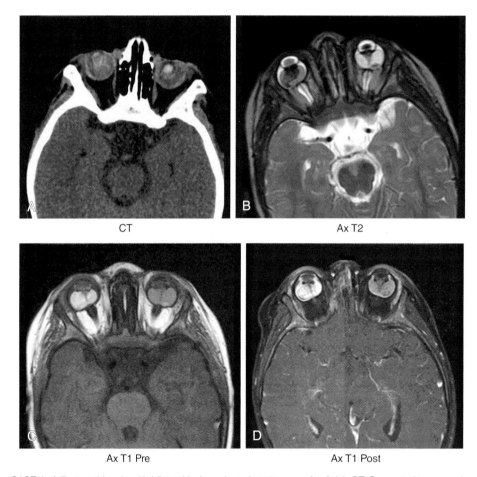

CT

Ax T2

Ax T1 Pre

Ax T1 Post

CASE A: A 7-year-old male with bilateral leukocoria and nystagmus. *Ax,* Axial; *CT,* Computed tomography.

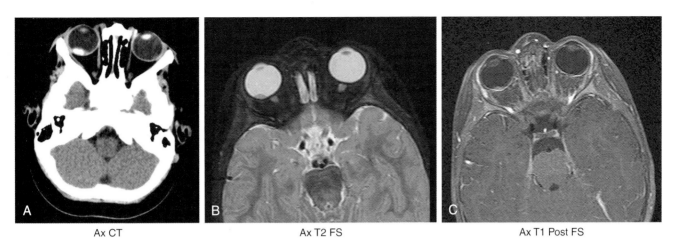

Ax CT   Ax T2 FS   Ax T1 Post FS

CASE B: A 2-year-old male with right-sided leukocoria. *Ax,* Axial; *CT,* computed tomography; *FS,* fat saturated.

DESCRIPTION OF FINDINGS

- Case A: An axial CT image through the orbits shows small globes bilaterally with abnormal retrolental soft tissue density. Axial T2-weighted MRI more clearly reveals a triangular configuration of this T2-hypointense intraocular soft tissue. T1-weighted precontrast and postcontrast images show abnormally hyperintense vitreous with mild enhancement within the left retrolental soft tissue.
- Case B: Axial CT image demonstrates a calcified lentiform mass in the normal-sized right globe. Axial T2-weighted MRI shows corresponding T2 hypointensity of the lesion relative to the surrounding vitreous. An axial T1-weighted postcontrast image demonstrates mild enhancement.

Diagnosis

Case A: Persistent fetal vasculature
Case B: Retinoblastoma

Summary

Lesions of the pediatric globe encompass a broad range of pathologies. However, characteristic imaging findings often permit conclusive diagnosis in conjunction with the clinical examination.

Retinoblastoma

Retinoblastoma is the most common intraocular malignancy of childhood, constituting 3% of cancers in children younger than 15 years. Caused by mutations in both copies of the *RB1* tumor suppressor gene, the tumor occurs in both heritable and nonheritable forms. About 40% of children with retinoblastoma have the heritable form of the condition. Bilateral or multifocal cases occur far more commonly in the heritable form. So-called "trilateral" retinoblastoma occurs when bilateral ocular disease coexists with a suprasellar or pineal small round blue cell tumor. The vast majority of cases are diagnosed before the age of 5 years, with heritable forms typically diagnosed earlier than nonheritable forms.

On CT, retinoblastoma typically appears as a nodular, calcified lesion of the posterior globe. Indeed, calcification is a hallmark finding that is present in 95% of cases and usually distinguishes retinoblastoma from other common tumor-like lesions of the posterior globe. CT is more sensitive for calcification than MRI, but CT has the disadvantage of ionizing radiation. In current practice, ocular ultrasound performed by ophthalmologists is most commonly utilized in initial imaging evaluation and is useful for detecting calcification. On MRI, retinoblastoma is hyperintense to vitreous on T1-weighted sequences and hypointense to vitreous on T2-weighted sequences. Enhancement is a characteristic finding. Importantly, MRI is far more sensitive than CT for detecting extraocular and subarachnoid spread. Therefore, even cases diagnosed on CT typically require MRI of the orbits and brain for more definitive delineation of tumor extent.

Persistent Fetal Vasculature

Persistent Fetal Vasculature (PFV), which has also been called persistent hyperplastic primary vitreous or PHPV, constitutes the second most common cause of pediatric leukocoria behind retinoblastoma. This congenital ocular lesion is caused by incomplete regression of the embryonic ocular blood supply. Unilateral in more than 90% of cases, PFV is a nonhereditary condition that typically is detected at birth or within the first few weeks of life. Two clinically important forms of PFV exist: an anterior form and a posterior form. In the anterior form, the persistent vitreous lies in the retrolental space, is supplied by the ciliary artery, and has no posterior globe abnormalities. The posterior form, by contrast, represents persistent hyaloid vasculature on the optic disk. The posterior form carries a worse prognosis because of the higher incidence of tractional retinal detachment and abnormalities of the optic disk. Most patients have a combination of the two forms. CT demonstrates microphthalmia in the majority of cases, usually with abnormal retrolental soft tissue corresponding to the primary vitreous. This soft tissue often exhibits a cone-shaped configuration with a linear band extending to the posterior pole of the globe. This morphology, sometimes referred to as the "martini glass" sign, is characteristic and is more sensitively detected by MRI. MRI also has the advantage of more clearly displaying subtle associated abnormalities of the lens and retrolental space. The persistent vitreous often exhibits enhancement on MRI after administration of gadolinium.

Spectrum of Disease

Intraocular lesions of the pediatric population constitute a broad spectrum of diseases, encompassing vascular, infectious, and neoplastic abnormalities. Ophthalmologic examination often yields the common finding of leukocoria, and because biopsy carries a high risk, imaging often is pivotal to the diagnosis.

Vascular lesions of the pediatric globe include Coats disease, an idiopathic primary retinal vascular anomaly with retinal telangiectasias often resulting in retinal detachment (Fig. 111.1). Coats disease is unilateral in 90% of cases. CT typically reveals mildly and diffusely hyperattenuating vitreous without calcification. Rarely, very advanced cases with osseous metaplasia of the retinal pigment epithelium may show calcification. However, this pattern of calcification is thin and linear and conforms to the contour of the globe in a pattern distinct from that seen in persons with retinoblastoma. MRI may more sensitively reveal retinal detachment with T1- and T2-hyperintense subretinal fluid. Thin linear enhancement of the thickened retina often may be observed. Ultrasound may depict partial or total retinal detachment.

Infectious lesions include *Toxocara* endophthalmitis, a granulomatous reaction caused by exposure to the larval form of the parasite *T. canis or T. cati*, as well as toxoplasmosis infection resulting from in utero or acquired exposure to *T. gondii*. Patients with *Toxocara* infections may have a history

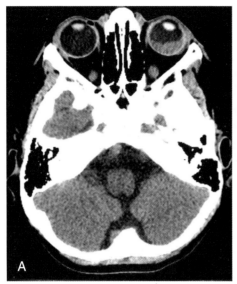 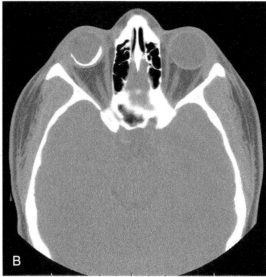

• **Fig. 111.1** Coats disease. (A) A 3-year-old male with decreased vision in the left eye. An axial computed tomography image through the globes reveals asymmetric hyperattenuation of an otherwise unremarkable left globe. (B) Computed tomography of a different patient with right-eye blindness reveals the thin, linear pattern of calcification seen in an advanced case of Coats disease with osseous metaplasia of the retinal pigment epithelium. (A, Courtesy Dr. Tina Young-Poussaint.)

of exposure to a dog or a sandbox, because infection occurs via fecal-oral transmission, often from a canine host. These lesions often are nonspecific in appearance; CT may reveal a hyperattenuating globe with or without a discrete mass. The absence of calcification is important in differentiating this process from retinoblastoma. MRI is far more sensitive in demonstrating a centrally located enhancing mass in the vitreous, often with T1 isointensity and mild T2 hyperintensity. Moderate uveoscleral enhancement may be seen, as may enhancement of a granuloma. Ocular toxoplasmosis, by contrast, manifests as a chorioretinitis resulting from in utero or acquired infection by *T. gondii*. Imaging manifestations typically are those of chronic inflammation and scarring, including microphthalmia, as well as retinal traction and detachment (Fig. 111.2).

Neoplastic lesions of the pediatric globe may include medulloepithelioma. These rare tumors, which may be benign or malignant, originate from nonpigmented epithelium of the ciliary body. There is an increased incidence in patients with *DICER1* mutation-associated tumor predisposition syndrome. On CT, they may appear as irregular dense masses about the ciliary body. MRI reveals the masses to be T1 hyperintense and T2 hypointense. Cystic components also may be visualized more sensitively by MRI. Avid enhancement is characteristic.

Differential Diagnosis

1. Retinoblastoma
2. Persistent fetal vasculature
3. Coats disease
4. *Toxocara* endophthalmitis
5. Congenital ocular toxoplasmosis

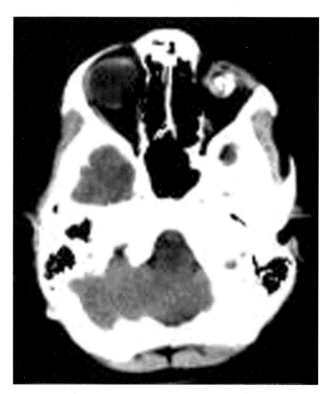

• **Fig. 111.2** Ocular toxoplasmosis. An axial computed tomography image through the globes demonstrates left-sided microphthalmia and calcification in this patient with in utero toxoplasmosis infection and ocular manifestations.

6. Medulloepithelioma
7. Astrocytic hamartoma (associated with tuberous sclerosis)
8. Incontinentia pigmenti
9. Retinopathy of prematurity
10. Morning glory disc anomaly

Pearls

- Morphology: Retinoblastomas often are nodular in contour and lie along the posterior pole of the globe. PFV typically is conical in shape, with a fibrous band extending to the posterior pole of the globe (martini glass sign). Coats disease usually presents without a definable mass, instead of appearing as a diffuse change in attenuation or signal of the vitreous. *Toxocara* endophthalmitis may appear on MRI as a centrally located, noncalcified mass with moderate enhancement. Congenital toxoplasmosis with ocular manifestations may reveal microphthalmia from chronic scarring, as well as evidence of retinal traction and detachment. Medulloepitheliomas generally are unilateral tumors arising from the ciliary body or iris, although they rarely may arise from the retina or optic nerve head, making the distinction from retinoblastoma difficult.
- Enhancement: Retinoblastoma usually is characterized by moderate or avid enhancement. The retrolental soft tissue of persistent fetal vasculature often enhances, with avidity dependent on its degree of vascularity. In Coats disease, linear enhancement may be seen along the border between the subretinal exudates and the remaining vitreous. *Toxocara* endophthalmitis may be associated with moderate uveoscleral enhancement or enhancement of a granuloma. Medulloepitheliomas exhibit moderate homogeneous enhancement.
- Calcification: Retinoblastoma exhibits punctuate or speckled calcification in more than 90% of cases. Advanced cases of Coats disease may exhibit curvilinear peripheral calcification in rare cases when osseous metaplasia of the retinal pigment epithelium is present. Medulloepithelioma may be associated with dystrophic calcifications about the ciliary body. Patients with toxoplasmosis who have repeated episodes of chorioretinitis may have dystrophic calcification from chronic scarring. End-stage ocular disease with phthisis bulbi (often a sequela of retinopathy of prematurity) is usually calcified and associated with markedly small globe size. Calcification is rare in the remaining entities described in this chapter.
- Demographics: Retinoblastoma is diagnosed before 5 years of age in more than 90% of cases, with an average age at diagnosis of approximately 18 months. PFV is congenital and usually is noted at birth or within the first few weeks of life. Coats disease peaks in incidence between the ages of 6 and 8 years and affects boys eight times as frequently as girls. *Toxocara* endophthalmitis occurs most often in children aged 5 to 10 years. Congenital ocular toxoplasmosis usually is detected at birth or shortly thereafter. Medulloepithelioma peaks in incidence between the ages of 4 and 12 years.

Signs and Complications

Retinoblastoma presents with leukocoria in more than half of cases, and strabismus is the second most common presentation, occurring in approximately 20% of cases. The disease carries an excellent prognosis when only a noninvasive intraocular tumor is identified. However, extraocular disease carries a poor prognosis. Intraarterial chemotherapy (IAC) delivered directly into the ophthalmic artery is often the preferred first-line treatment for locally advanced unilateral tumors without evidence of cancer beyond one eye. Systemic intravenous chemotherapy (IVC) remains a key treatment for less advanced cases of bilateral and germline retinoblastoma. Plaque radiation therapy often plays a role as secondary treatment for small- or medium-sized tumors that are chemoresistant. Cryotherapy and photocoagulation may be used as alternative treatments for small tumor deposits, depending on the distribution. Enucleation may be pursued when preservation of vision is not possible.

PFV generally presents with leukocoria and microphthalmia. Complications are far more frequently encountered in the posterior form of the disease. When untreated, the disease often is complicated by recurrent hemorrhage and secondary glaucoma, often resulting in phthisis bulbi or requiring enucleation. Surgery often preserves vision in patients with the anterior form of the disease.

Coats disease is generally a progressive process and often leads to complications such as retinal detachment and visual loss. Therapy depends heavily on the progression of disease. In the absence of retinal detachment, conservative therapy such as photocoagulation or cryoablation of aberrant retinal telangiectasias is used, often in conjunction with intraocular injections of antivascular endothelial growth factor (anti-VEGF) agents. After retinal detachment, surgery is of diminished utility. Some patients may require enucleation for painful glaucoma.

Toxocara endophthalmitis may occur in the absence of systemic infection and usually presents with unilateral visual loss. Pain and redness also are common presenting symptoms. The inflammatory response often is complicated by vitreous membranes or tractional retinal detachment, which generally leads to blindness when untreated. Acute infection may be treated with albendazole and local or systemic corticosteroids, whereas lesions associated with vitreous membranes may require a vitrectomy to repair tractional retinal detachments.

Congenital toxoplasmosis often manifests with bilateral chorioretinitis, causing symptoms in more than 90% of those affected. Common symptoms include visual loss, eye pain, and photophobia. Retinal detachment may occur after acute episodes of inflammation. Infants with inactive chorioretinal scarring from congenital infection may experience reactivation later in life. Antiparasitic therapy is unable to restore vision that is lost as a result of prior episodes of scarring. If untreated, up to 60% of these patients may progress to severe vision loss.

Medulloepitheliomas often present with pain and vision loss, along with leukocoria. Management includes observation, enucleation, radiation, and resection. Enucleation is common because these tumors often are detected late. However, treatment strategies are based on tumor size and the potential for preservation of vision.

Suggested Readings

Apushkin MA, Apushkin MA, Shapiro MJ, et al: Retinoblastoma and simulating lesions: role of imaging, *Neuroimaging Clin N Am* 15(1): 49–67, 2005.

Barkovich J: *Pediatric neuroimaging*, ed 4, Philadelphia, 2005, Lippincott Williams & Wilkins.

Castillo M, Wallace DK, Mukherji SK: Persistent hyperplastic primary vitreous involving the anterior eye, *AJNR Am J Neuroradiol* 18(8): 1526–1528, 1997.

Chung EM, Specht CS, Schroeder JW: Pediatric orbit tumors and tumorlike lesions: neuroepithelial lesions of the ocular globe and optic nerve, *Radiographics* 27:1159–1186, 2007.

de Graaf P, van der Valk P, Moll AC et al: Contrast-enhancement of the anterior eye segment in patients with retinoblastoma: correlation between clinical, MR imaging, and histopathologic findings, *AJNR Am J Neuroradiol* 31(2):237–245, 2010.

Hosten N, Liebig T: *CT of the head and spine*, New York, 2002, Thieme.

Mafee MF, Valvassori GE, Becker M: *Imaging of the head and neck*, New York, 2005, Thieme.

Müller-Forell WS, editor: *Imaging of orbital and visual pathway pathology, medical radiology series*, Berlin, 2002, Springer-Verlag.

Razek AA, Elkhamary S: MRI of retinoblastoma, *Br J Radiol* 84(1005): 775–784, 2011.

Sansgiri RK, Wilson M, McCarville MB, et al: Imaging features of medulloepithelioma: report of four cases and review of the literature. *Pediatr Radiol* 43, 1344–1356, 2013.

Schueler AO, Hosten N, Bechrakis NE, et al: High resolution magnetic resonance imaging of retinoblastoma, *Br J Ophthalmol* 87(3):330–335, 2003.

Silvera VM, Guerin JB, Brinjiki W, Dalvin LA: Retinoblastoma: What the neuroradiologist needs to know, *AJNR Am J Neuroradiol* 42 (4): 618–626, 2021.

Steidl S, Hartnett ME: *Clinical pathways in vitreoretinal disease*, New York, 2003, Thieme.

Tortori-Donati P, Rossi A, Biancheri R: *Pediatric neuroradiology*, Berlin, 2005, Springer-Verlag.

Wilson ME, Saunders RA, Trivedi RH: *Pediatric ophthalmology: current thought and a practical guide*, Heidelberg, 2009, Springer-Verlag.

Yang X, Wang C, Su G: Recent advances in the diagnosis and treatment of Coats' disease, *Int Ophthalmol* 39:957–970, 2019.

Abbreviations

ADC	Apparent diffusion coefficient		**FS**	Fat suppressed
CISS	Constructive interference in steady state		**GRE**	Gradient refocused echo
CNS	Central nervous system		**HU**	Hounsfield units
CPA	Cerebellopontine angle		**ICA**	Internal carotid artery
CSF	Cerebrospinal fluid		**MRI**	Magnetic resonance imaging
CT	Computed tomography		**PET**	Positron emission tomography
DWI	Diffusion-weighted imaging		**ROI**	Region of interest
FDG	Fluorodeoxyglucose		**SCC**	Squamous cell carcinoma
FIESTA	Fast imaging employing steady-state acquisition		**STIR**	Short T1 inversion recovery
FLAIR	Fluid attenuated inversion recovery			

Index

Page numbers followed by *b* indicate boxes; *f,* figures; and *t,* tables.